FIMS
SPORTS MEDICINE
MANUAL:
EVENT PLANNING
AND EMERGENCY CARE

FIMS
SPORTS MEDICINE
MANUAL:
EVENT PLANNING
AND EMERGENCY CARE

Senior Editor

David O'Sullivan McDonagh, MD

Editors

Professor Lyle J.Micheli, MD
Professor Walter R. Frontera, MD, PhD
Professor Fabio Pigozzi, MD
Katharina Grimm, MD
Charles F. Butler, MD
Professor Angela D.Smith, MD
Richard Budgett, MD
Costas Parisis, MD
Professor Inggard Lereim, MD

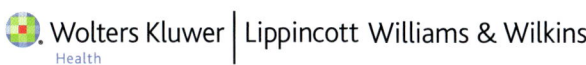
. Wolters Kluwer | Lippincott Williams & Wilkins
Health

Philadelphia · Baltimore · New York · London
Buenos Aires · Hong Kong · Sydney · Tokyo

Acquisitions Editor: Robert A. Hurley
Project Manager: David Murphy
Marketing Manager: Lisa Lawrence
Design Manager: Holly McLaughlin
Manufacturing Manager: Benjamin Rivera
Production Services: SPi Global

Printed in China

Library of Congress Cataloging-in-Publication Data
FIMS sports medicine manual : event planning and emergency care / senior editor, David O'Sullivan McDonagh.
      p. ; cm.
   Sports medicine event manual
   ISBN 978-1-58255-873-8 (alk. paper)
   1. Sports medicine—International cooerpation. 2. Sports injuries. I. McDonagh, David O'Sullivan.
II. International Federation of Sports Medicine. III. Title: Sports medicine event manual.
   [DNLM: 1. Sports Medicine—methods. 2. Athletic Injuries. 3. International Cooperation.
4. Physician's Role. 5. Practice Management, Medical—organization & administration. QT 261]
   RC1210.F56 2011
   617.1'027—dc23
                                                                                    2011015850

To purchase additional copies of this book, call our customer service department at (800) 638-3030 or fax orders to (301) 223-2320. International customers should call (301) 223-2300.

Visit Lippincott Williams & Wilkins on the Internet: at LWW.com. Lippincott Williams & Wilkins customer service representatives are available from 8:30 am to 6 pm, EST.

10 9 8 7 6 5 4 3 2 1

RRS1109

To Eileen

Go n-éiri an bóther leat.

Senior Editor, Editors, Contributing Authors, Reviewers

Senior Editor

David O'Sullivan McDonagh, MD

Consultant, Accident and Emergency Department, University Hospital, Trondheim, Norway
Assistant Professor, NTNU (the University of Science and Technology) Trondheim, Norway
Chair, FIBT (Bobsleigh and Skeleton) Medical Committee
Secretary, AIBA (International Boxing Association) Medical Commission
Winter Olympic International Federations representative to FIMS
Physician for the Top Athlete Program in central Norway
Head of the Scientific and Education Committee, EFSMA (European Federation of Sports Medical Associations)
Member, Norwegian Antidoping Tribunal
Member ICC (International Cricket Council) Antidoping Tribunal
Past Team Physician, Norwegian Boxing team, Nordic Combined team, Bobsled and Luge team
Member, Norwegian Rugby Union medical committee
Physician for the Olympic Athlete Program in central Norway
Deputy CMO at the Lillehammer 1994 Olympic Winter Games
CMO/Deputy CMO for World Ice Hockey Championships, 2 World Nordic Skiing Championships and over one hundred other World Cup, World Championships events in various sports
Advisor to 5 Olympic Games organization committees

Editors

Professor Lyle J. Micheli, MD

Director, Boston Children's Hospital
Associate Clinical Professor of Orthopaedic Surgery, Harvard Medical School, Boston, Massachusetts
Vice President of FIMS
Past President, American College of Sports Medicine (ACSM)

Professor Fabio Pigozzi, MD

Professor IUPM, Rome, Italy
Chair, (UIPM) Modern Pentathlon Medical Committee
President FIMS

Professor Walter R. Frontera, MD

Dean, University of Puerto Rico School of Medicine, San Juan, Puerto Rico
Past President of FIMS
Past President, ACSM

Katharina Grimm, MD

Head Medical Office, FIFA

Charles F. Butler, MD

Chairman AIBA (International Boxing Association) Medical Commission
Member AIBA Executive Committee

Professor Angela D. Smith, MD
University of Pennsylvania, School of Medicine
Children's Hospital, Philadelphia, Pennsylvania
Chair Education Commission FIMS 2002–2009
Past President, ACSM

Richard Budgett, MD
Chief Medical Officer, British Olympic Association
Chief Medical Officer, London 2012 Summer, Olympics
Member FIBT Medical Committee
Gold Medal Olympian

Professor Inggard Lereim, MD
Orthopaedic Department, NTNU, Trondheim, Norway
Vice Chair, FIS (Skiing) Medical Committee
Chief Medical Officer Lillehammer 1994 Olympic Winter Games

Costas Parisis, MD
Chair, FIBA (International Basketball Association) Medical Committee
Chief Medical Officer, Athens 2004 Olympic Summer Games

Contributing Authors

Abdelhamid Khadri, Vice-President AIBA (Boxing) Medical Commission, Rafat, Morocco

Abel Wakai, St. James's Hospital, Dublin, Ireland

Alain Lacoste, Chair FISA (Rowing) MC, France

Andreas Niess, German Athletics Team, University of Tübingen, Germany

Ann Quinn, ITF (Tennis) Medical Commission, Australia

Anthony F. Clough, Dental Lead London 2012, University College London, England

Babette Pluim, ITF, Royal Netherlands Lawn Tennis Association, Netherlands

Bernard Montalvan, ITF (Tennis) Medical Commission, France

Bredo Knudtzen, Former Team Physician Norwegian National Ice Hockey Team, Norway

Brian Hainline, ITF (Tennis) Medical Commission, USA

Charles Butler, Chair AIBA (Boxing) Medical Commission, Michigan, USA

Clint Readhead, SA Rugby Medical Association Committee Member, South Africa

Colin Fuller, FIFA/IRB, University of Nottingham, England.

Constantine Au, Sports Medicine Subcommittee, College of Emergency Medicine, Hong Kong

Costas Parisis, Chair FIBA (Basketball) MC, Greece

Craig Ferrel, Chair FEI (Equestrian Sports) Medical Committee, USA

Dave Miley, ITF (Tennis) Medical Commission, Ireland

David Townend, Associate Professor Maastricht University, Netherlands

Demetrios G. Pyrros, President World Association of Disaster Medicine, Greece

Demitri Constantinou, FIFA Medical Centre, University of Witwatersrand, Johannesburg, SA

Derek McCormack, Glasgow Celtic FC, Scotland

Didier Rousseau, Chair JIF (Judo) MC, France

Dominique Sprumont, University of Neuchatel, Switzerland

Don McKenzie, Chair ICF (Canoeing) MC, Canada

Dory Boyer, Deputy CMO, VANOC, Canada

Doug Hiller, Chief Medical Officer ITU (Triathlon), Waimea, Hawaii

Eanna Falvey, IRB, University College Cork, Ireland

Emin Ergen, Chair FITA (Archery) MC, Turkey

Eugene Byrne, USA Bobsleigh, Member FIBT and FIL MC, USA

Evan L. Lloyd, Chair WCF (Curling) MC, Scotland

Fabio Pigozzi, IOC, EOC, FIMS, UIPM, Italy.

Fook Wong, Chair FIH (Field Hockey) MC, USA

Francois Gnamian, Chair IHF (Handball) MC, Ivory Coast

Gary Mak, Consultant Cardiologist for the Hong Kong Sports Institute, Hong Kong

George Ruijsch van Dugteren, Chair FIE (Fencing) MC, South Africa

Geraint Fuller, Consultant Neurologist, Gloucester, UK

Gianfranco Beltrami, Chair IBAF (Baseball) MC, Italy

Gordon Bosworth, physiotherapist to the Canadian Skating Team, UK

Gurchuran Singh, Chair BWF (Badminton) MC, Malaysia

Heinz Günter, Chair FIBA (Basketball) MC, Austria

Herbert Hoerterer, Chair FIS (Skiing) MC, Germany

Hiu-fai Ho, Sports Medicine Subcommittee, Hong Kong College of Emergency Medicine

Iain Higgins, In-house sports lawyer, ICC (International Cricket Council), Dubai, UAE

Inggard Lereim, Vice Chair FIS (Skiing) MC, Norway

Jack Taunton, Chief Medical Officer, VANOC—2010 Olympic Games, Vancouver, Canada

James R. Andrews, Medical Director, LPGA (Golf), Alabama, USA

James M. Lally, Chair ISSF (Shooting) MC, USA

James Macdonald, Team Physician University of California, Santa Cruz , USA

James Sekajugo, Uganda Health Ministry, Kampala, Uganda

James A. Whiteside, American College of Sports Medicine, Alabama, USA

Jan Hoff, University of Science and Technology, NTNU, Trondheim, Norway

Jane Moran, Chair ISU (Skating) MC, Canada

Jean Francois Kahn, Chair ITTF (Table Tennis) MC, France

Jean-Luc Dion, Team Dentist, Quebec Nordiques (NHL), Quebec City, Canada

Jim Carrabre, Chair IBU (Biathlon) MC, USA

Jim Thorne, Ice Hockey Canada Men's Olympic Team, Calgary Flames Hockey Club (NHL)

Jiri Dvorak, FIFA Medical Committee, Switzerland

Joseph Cummiskey, IOC MC, FIMS Executive Committee, President EFSMA, Ireland

Jon Patricios, Sports Concussion South Africa, Johannesburg, South Africa

Johan-Arnt Hegvik, Anesthetics Dept, Trondheim University Hospital, Norway

John M. Ryan, MO Leinster Rugby Football Team, Irish Hockey Union, Ireland

Jörg Ellermeyer, Chair FIL (Luge) MC, Germany

Juan Manuel Alonso, Chair IAAF (Athletics) MC, Spain

Julia Alleyne, Canadian Skating Team, University of Toronto, Canada

Justin Durandt, SA Rugby Medical Association Committee Member, South Africa

Karl Weber, ITF (Tennis) Medical Commission, Germany

Kathryn E. Ackerman, Harvard University, Boston, USA

Kathleen A. Stroia, ITF (Tennis) Medical Commission, USA

Kenneth Wu, Sports Medicine Subcommitttee, College of Emergency Medicine, Hong Kong

Kjell Løfors, Norwegian Boxing Union MC, Norway

Lars Engebretsen, Ullevål University Hospital, Oslo, IOC, Norway

Lars Kolsrud, Olympic Athlete Program, Norway.

Lars Toft, Chief Physician, SOS International, Denmark

Marc Demars, Chair FILA (Wrestling) MC, France

Margo Mountjoy, FINA (Swimming) MC, IOC, Canada

Mark Aubry, IOC, Chair IIHF (Ice Hockey) MC, Canada

Maria Rizzo, Department of Health Sciences, University of Rome, Italy

Mario Zorzoli, Chair UCI (Cycling) MC, Switzerland

Martin Schwellnus, IOC, Stellenbosch University, South Africa

MG Molloy, Medical Officer International Rugby Board (IRB), Ireland

Michael McNamee, Centre for Philosophy, Humanities and Law, University of Wales, UK

Michel Binder, Member FIG (Gymnastics) Medical Committee, France

Michel Leglise, IOC Medical Committee, Chair FIG MC, France

Miguel Crespo, ITF (Tennis) Medical Commission, Spain

Nicky Dunn, ITF (Tennis) Medical Commission, United Kingdom

Nils Ericsson, Head of Emergency Department, Trondheim, Norway

Nils Kaehler, VP, Norwegian Motorcross Federation, Norway

Paul Piccininni, IOC Medical Committee, Toronto, Canada

Peter Giannoudis, President British Trauma Society, UK

Peter Harcourt, Chair ICC's Medical Committee (Cricket), Victoria, Australia

Peter Jenoure, University of Basel, WADA List Committee, EFSMA, Switzerland

Peter van de Vliet, International Paralympic Committee, Belgium

Pierre d'Hemecourt, Medical Director Boston Marathon., USA

Pierre Viviers, SA Rugby Medical Association Committee Member, South Africa

J. Preston Wiley, IRB, University of Calgary, Canada

Ray Padilla, Dentist, LA Galaxy, USA Men's and Women's Soccer, Los Angeles, USA

Rene Fasel, President, IIHF, Member IOC, President – AOWS), Switzerland

Roald Bahr, Chair FIVB (Volleyball) MC, IOC Medical Committee, Norway

Roger Hackney, Surgeon, British Olympic Association, Leeds, England

Scott Kincade, University of Texas South Western, Dallas, Texas,USA

Sergio Migliorini, Chair ITU (Triathlon) MC, Italy

Shane Brun, Team Physician Australian National Soccer Team, Australia.

Stefano Dragoni, Chair ITU (Triathlon) MC, Italy

Stuart Miller, ITF (Tennis) Medical Commission, United Kingdom

Suzanne Shepherd, Department Emergency Medicine, University of Pennsylvania, USA

Tai-wai Wong, HK Association of Sports Medicine, Hong Kong

Tim Wood, ITF (Tennis) Medical Commission, Australia

Terence Babwah, FIFA (Football) MC, Trinidad

Trygve Moe, Consultant Psychiatrist, Friskvern, Oslo, Norway

Victor Lun, University of Calgary, Canadian Bobsleigh, Speed Skating Teams, Calgary, Canada

Vlad Haralambie, FIBT MC, Romanian Motorsports Federation, Romania

Wayne Viljoen, South African Rugby Medical Association Committee Member, South Africa

Wayne Derman, University of Cape Town, SA Olympic Team 2000, 2004, South Africa

Willy Pieter, University of Asia and the Pacific, Pasig City, MM, Philippines

Thank you to:

Paul McCrory, Winne Meeuwisse, Karen Johnston, Jiri Dvorak, Mark Aubry, Michael G Molloy and Robert Cantu for allowing us to print the contents of the 3rd International Conference on Concussion in Sport, Zurich, November 2008

Reviewers

Are Holen, Vice Dean, Faculty of Medicine, NTNU, Trondheim, Norway

Arild Aamodt, Head of Orthopedic Department, St. Olavs University Hospital, Trondheim, Norway

Bredo Knudtzen, Former Team Physician Norwegian National Ice Hockey Team, Norway

Christian Schneider, German Bobsleigh Federation, Schōn Klinik, Munich, Germany

David Mulder, McGill University, Montreal, Canada

Ian Cohen, University of Toronto, Toronto, Canada

Irene Skaget, Vinje Ambulance Service, Trondheim, Norway.

Lars Jacob Stovner, Professor of Neurology, NTNU, Trondheim, Norway

Jan Mjønes, Head of Urology Department, NTNU, Trondheim, Norway

Jan Kristian Damås, Dept of Infectious Medicine, NTNU, Trondheim, Norway

Jørn-Terje Iversen, Vinje Ambulance Service, Trondheim, Norway

Julia Alleyne, Canadian Skating Team, Women's College, University of Toronto, Canada

Ketil Holen, Rosenborg Football Team, Trondheim, Norway

Kjell Løfors, Ophthalmology Department, NTNU, Norwegian Boxing Union, Norway

Kristian Bjerva, Clinical Chemistry Department, St. Olavs University Hospital, Trondheim, Norway

Kristin Ryggen, Dermatology Department, St. Olavs University Hospital, Trondheim, Norway

Mike Wilkinson, Deputy CMO, VANOC, Vancouver, Canada

Mohamed Mydin Musa, President SSEMM, Prof, Help University, Kuala Lumpur, Malaysia

Sven Erik Gisvold, Professor of Anesthetics, NTNU, Trondheim, Norway

Svein A. Nordbø, Microbiology Department, St. Olavs University Hospital, Trondheim, Norway

Talia Alenabi, Secretary General, Asian Federation of Sports Medicine, Tehran, Iran

Tomm Müller, Department of Neurosurgery, St. Olavs Hospital Trondheim, Norway

Vegard Bugten, ENT Department, NTNU, Trondheim, Norway

Foreword

I would like to congratulate Dr. McDonagh on the production of this important work. Sport at all levels relies on medical experts to plan and execute efficient and effective services to ensure the health of our athletes. As President of an International Federation that conducts sporting events in many countries, I am keenly aware of the importance of ensuring that athletes receive consistent care of the highest quality, wherever they may be training or competing.

Dr. McDonagh addresses an array of essential issues including planning the medical aspects of sporting events and on-field treatment of injured or ill athlete. These topics and skills are crucial ones that all event physicians need to master. This seminal work demonstrates Dr. McDonagh's continued leadership in developing the field of sports medicine for the benefit of sport and athletes. This manual will be an invaluable tool for medical professionals to provide the highest quality care at sporting events of all kinds.

The FIBT is delighted to play its part in promoting excellence and best practices in the conduct of sporting events and in supporting projects that will advance the care of athletes within the Olympic Movement.

Robert H. Storey
Honorary President FIBT

The sport of boxing has significant focus on safety and fair play. To ensure the highest level of athlete safety in the competition environment, we need experienced and professional medical members on site so that when an injury or other health incidence occurs, the medical staff can handle and resolve the issue effectively. Antidoping work plays a prominent role in assuring that all boxers are competing in a setting of fair play. The medical aspect of doping therefore is crucial to any competition and sport.

I am pleased to have Dr. McDonagh on the AIBA Medical Commission as his main area of expertise has been event management and the emergency treatment of athletes. I believe that the boxers will be greatly benefited by his contribution in AIBA.

It is delightful to see that this book will be published to train and educate more good sports medical doctors. I hope this manual will be widely used by the medical jury for the benefit of our beloved sport and athletes.

Dr. Ching Kuo Wu
AIBA President
IOC Member

As President of the International Federation of Sports Medicine and also on behalf of all the FIMS Executive Committee and Standing Commissions, I am very happy to congratulate Dr. McDonagh for having promoted this important editorial initiative, the *FIMS Sports Medicine Manual: Event Planning and Emergency Care*.

In the last few years, the International Federation of Sports Medicine has intensified its efforts in disseminating the principles of motivation, performance, and health aspects for all people engaged in sport and physical activity. In this context, the sport physicians' work has to be dedicated to the protection of the athletes' health, including planning the medical aspects of sport events and on-field medical treatment, in order to allow athletes to safely compete in all national and international sports events.

Therefore, FIMS has focused its energies on supporting educational initiatives with the goal of promoting continuous professional development and on supporting editorial initiatives as well as Team Physician Courses.

In conclusion, I am sure that this book will be very much acclaimed by all the members of FIMS and I would recommend it to the broader fraternity of sports medicine throughout the world.

Prof. Fabio Pigozzi
Professor of Internal Medicine, University of Rome "Foro Italico"
Chairman, Union International de Pentathlon Moderne (UIPM) Medical Committee
President, FIMS

Preface

While the concept and tasks of the team physician are well defined, few books address the specific tasks of the event physician (EP). Many sports physicians may be supercompetent in their own specialty, back in the hospital environment, but being the sole physician at a smaller sports event, without any laboratory or radiological facilities and no support from colleagues or even ambulance staff, may pose demanding challenges on an EP. Due to the difficulty of enticing qualified personnel to attend relatively unattractive sporting events, it is not unusual to have an EP with little knowledge or experience of sports medicine managing an event.

At larger sports events, the opposite may be the case, with athletes having access to a multiplicity of specialists at a luxurious new clinic.

There are specific problems and challenges encountered before and during a sports event, both managerial and therapeutic, situations that the EP may not have encountered previously.

The aim of this manual is to describe some of the roles of an EP and to offer a practical approach to event organization as well as giving an update on effective on-site diagnosis and treatment.

In these days of superspecialists, the need for "generalists" with knowledge of how to diagnose and treat a broad range of acute conditions is still necessary, remembering the old adage "Common conditions are common."

In all the years I have worked with athletes, I have been presented with a panorama of different complaints and conditions, some major but most minor, by nervous and apprehensive athletes—before, during, or after an event. On many occasions, support and encouragement have been as effective as any pill. On other occasions, I have been involved with life-threatening unstable cervical fractures and major pneumothoraces, as dramatic a situation as one can possibly experience.

One has to be prepared for the worst at any moment, and yet, these dramatic events are rare and often few and far between. As a good anesthetist colleague once said to me, "being an anesthetist is 90% routine and 10% chaos." I think this adage could well be transferred to the EP.

The doctor–athlete relationship is at times different from other doctor–patient relationships. Usually, when an athlete contacts a physician before an event, the athlete has one goal: to be able to participate in the competition. Whereas most illnesses are treated with some form of rest, the athlete usually wants symptomatic relief in order to continue in the sports event, preferably optimally, and is quite happy to let injury repair or illness improvement take place after the event. The EP's task is to accommodate this wish within the bounds of ethically accepted norms, but it is also the EP's task to advise against further participation (or even remove the athlete from the event if rules allow) when further participation would have deleterious effects on the athlete's health. This can be a fine balance particularly on the eve of an Olympic final or World Championships.

In this manual, we will address the following subjects:

Section 1: Planning the Medical Aspects of a Sports Event

Section 2: Evaluating and Treating Athlete Injuries and Illnesses at a Sporting Event

Section 3: The "Return-to-Play" Conundrum

Section 4: Sport Medical Equipments and Diagnostic Tests

Invariably, when covering a wide and varied number of topics, certain issues will be addressed in detail, others less so, and some totally ignored. I have included the topics that I consider to be relevant based on my experience. Obviously, if you live in Norway, the chance of being bitten by a poisonous snake is not very likely, yet if you live in parts of northern India or Bangladesh, this is a real danger. If you live in Oman, you will surely yawn, or smile, through the section on working in extreme cold. This is the nature of the beast when writing for an international audience.

No manual on emergency sports medicine would be complete without a decent section on fractures and orthopedic problems, but I have also included many other relevant areas that are not often covered in sports medical textbooks. Emergency Sports Medicine is not all about the treatment of injuries; in fact, in my experience, medical conditions are just as common, particularly if an event is spread over several days. Ideally, the perfect EP would be a specialist in anesthesiology, cardiology, respiratory medicine, family medicine, neurosurgery, ENT, physical medicine, dentistry, psychology, and orthopedics. The only way forward is that we all become a little bit better at more things.

Regarding references, my editors have advised me to avoid long reference lists to ease the flow of the text and also in the name of brevity. Hopefully this does not compromise the quality of contents. A list of recommended reading is given at the end of each chapter.

I would like to thank all of the 110 contributing authors and the 33 reviewers for their contributions.

I would like to thank my editors Walter, Fabio, Lyle, Angela, Richard, Charles, Inggard, and Costas for their excellent reviewing work and advice during this long process and in particular Katharina Grimm from FIFA for dedicated work above and beyond the call of duty.

I would like to thank Costas Christodoulakis for helping to get the whole project started.

I would like to thank Kevin, Birgitte, Kirsten, Magnus, Grete, John, Trish, Anne, Henry, Niall, Mary Jo, Brian, Deirdre, Nils Ericsson, and Knut Johannessen for all the help they have given, in their own different ways. I would like to thank the staff of both the A+E and Orthopedic Depts for their help and assistance down through the years.

Well, enough of this weary tome.

Nobody reads these introductions anyway. To those of you who do, I hope you find something of interest in this manual. I would greatly appreciate any comments from readers, in particular those from far off lands with issues that I have not adequately addressed.

There will be a second edition in 3 or 4 years.

I can be reached at the following e-mail: mcdonagh@ntnu.no

All profits from the sales of this manual will go to FIMS for the promotion of education and research in sports medicine.

Best Regards
David McDonagh, MD

Contents

CHAPTER 1

The Planning of Mass Participation Events

Contributed by David McDonagh, Deputy CMO, Lillehammer 1994 Olympic Winter Games; Costas Parisis, CMO, Athens 2004 Olympic Summer Games; Demetrios G. Pyrros, Deputy CMO, Athens 2004 Olympic Summer Games

Reviewers: Richard Budgett, CMO, London 2012 Olympic Summer Games, and Mike Wilkinson, Deputy CMO, Vancouver 2010 Olympic Winter Games

Larger sporting events such as World and Continental Championships, Olympic Games, etc., require many years of preparation and planning. For the Olympic Games, work often starts 5 or 6 years before. It is important that medical personnel are involved early on in the process so that medical facilities can be incorporated into structural, staffing, budgets plans, etc.

Based on our own experiences with the organization of Olympic Games and World Championships, here is a model for a medical services plan with suggested tasks, milestones, and completion dates. Now, while this program may appear excessively advanced and overdimensioned when considering minor sporting events, the issues addressed are often present at smaller sports events, though on a much reduced scale. What needs to be kept in mind at all times, and what will always affect the "legislated" medical coverage required, are the International Sports Federation (IF) rules. It is incumbent on any event planner to be fully versed in these requirements and rules and to convey their contents onto the event medical teams.

1.1 MILESTONES

5–6 Years Before Olympic Games

a) Choose the chief medical officer (CMO).

b) Choose secretary or medical services coordinator—preferably with hospital experience and bookkeeping skills

c) Appoint medical services manager—full-time

d) Select head of doping control program—due to increasing antidoping complexity, this is by necessity becoming a full-time position—to fall under Medical Services

e) Enter into negotiations with regional and national government health authorities to clearly identify each other's role in the delivery of medical services.

f) Establish fora whereby all topics relating to Games medical services can be discussed, plans can be made, and individual responsibilities clearly defined (financially and organizationally).

g) Initiate appropriate contract work between the different authorities.

h) Make arrangements for medical services for the organizing committee employees, as many may have migrated from other parts of the country or from other major games. The CMO and the subsequent medical staff must not become the organization's private physician.

3–4 Years Pregames

a) Participate at arena meetings.

b) Prepare guidelines for medical/antidoping staff.

c) Prepare emergency/disaster management plans.

d) Prepare volunteer accommodation, accreditation, and transport plans.

e) Final contract work with governmental and local health authorities

f) Final contract work with paramedic suppliers

g) Final contract work with ambulance suppliers

h) Final contract work with helicopter suppliers

i) Final contract work with military, if necessary

j) Final contract with antidoping authority

k) Final contract work with antidoping lab

l) New staff: Emergency nurse with 113 or emergency ward experiences

m) Polyclinic nurse or manager—to have responsibility for equipping the polyclinic 3 months before the start of the Games and working at the clinic during the Games: volunteer initially?; full time 6 to 8 months before Games.

3–2 Years Pregames

a) Recruitment of medical staff for the arenas

b) Recruitment of antidoping staff for the arenas

c) Quantify volume of medical equipment.

d) Initiate radio-telecommunication plans.

e) Budget/cost control

f) Establish contact with national medical governing bodies and insurance companies so that all issues regarding the delivery of medical services (including services to nonnationals) are discussed and ensure that all areas of potential conflict are addressed.

g) Establish contact with national and local medical and public health authorities to develop plans for the prevention and treatment of infectious diseases in the athlete and volunteer population.

h) Develop plans for a volunteer health program for the period of the Games.

i) Conclude contracts.

2–1 Year Before Games

a) Completion of medical staffing/antidoping staffing (names and addresses)

b) Completion of equipment ordering

c) Prepare work rotas for all medical staff

d) Prepare work rotas for all antidoping staff

e) Prepare work rotas for all polyclinic staff

f) Budget/cost control

g) Liaise with visiting IFs and national team physicians

Final 18 Months Before the Games

a) Testing of arenas, staff training—including antidoping personnel through smaller test events

b) Equipment delivered partially to arena—final delivery 1 month before

c) Completion of medical manuals

d) Completion of polyclinic

e) Establish warehouse or logistics plan for supplementing depleted stocks

f) Ongoing work with public health and safety authorities

g) Budget/cost control

1.2 AMBULANCES

Number of Ambulances: The ambulance service will serve two separate groups: (a) the athletes (team staff is usually included) and (b) everybody else. It is essential that an agreement on the roles, responsibilities, required numbers, and qualifications of all the ambulances and associated staff be established early.

Many IFs require two ambulances to be present at televised sporting events—either due to the fact that many athletes are participating in high-velocity sports (most winter sports) and thus the risk of multiple injuries (e.g., bobsleigh, soccer, downhill skiing) or due to the fact that the departure of an ambulance from the track may oblige the event organizer to stop the event due to Federation regulations.

At larger events or where local bylaws stipulate, separate ambulance services are required for the spectators; crowd size can vary up to 100,000 people and more. Not all ambulances have the same equipment standards and this topic is discussed in more detail in Chapter 7.

1.3 MEDICAL STAFF

The number of volunteers required varies from event to event. At the Olympic Games, there can be as many as 3,000 medical volunteers, whilst a local football game may require only two or three medical personnel.

Physicians and Nurses

Physicians will be primarily responsible for medical emergencies as well as other medical issues. Nurses will play a vital role in terms of triage, medical documentation, and in delivering medical care in conjunction with physicians.

Number of Physicians: The more competent the paramedics are, the less is the need for a large array of physicians, though physicians should always be present when there are large crowds or physical sports. The requirements for physicians and their qualifications will vary by sport and sporting federation. In most countries the medical director is always a physician.

Role and Duties: Physicians are often divided into two groups: those responsible for treating spectators and volunteers and those responsible for treating the athletes (team staff). The physician responsible for athlete care has an important role and must offer expert medical care when requested to athletes and if necessary lifesaving medical services to those in need. Athletes may request assistance before, during, or after an event. Some federations require that athletes be controlled by a physician before an event (e.g., boxing). On other occasions, an athlete may need an examination to ensure that he or she is fit to participate, particularly if he or she has recently been injured or ill. In my opinion, the physician should not demand to examine an athlete unless stipulated by Federation rules. A situation can arise whereby an event physician (EP) can suddenly see a nearby spectator in need of emergency medical intervention. He may have to vacate his athlete physician role to offer lifesaving medical treatment. This is obviously

the correct thing to do; however, in these extreme circumstances, he should inform his superiors by radio/phone that he is leaving his post, that assistance is required at a particular location, and that a substitute may be required at his post.

Number of Nurses: The requirement for nurses will vary both by sport and event size. It is our experience that an experienced nurse is able to provide care on a wide range of medical issues and can be invaluable for both the planning of event coverage and for the delivery of comprehensive care at the events to both athletes and spectators.

EMTs/Paramedics

Assistants will be helpful in transporting individuals to medical tents and assisting medical professionals in obtaining equipment and performing emergency medical procedures.

Number of Paramedics: As a rule, you allow for two paramedics per ambulance. Preferably, one of the paramedics will have advanced skills but should at least be able to give oxygen via a mask from a tank and be competent in fracture immobilization and laceration bandaging.

In a large stadium, one or two teams can be placed on the field/track in case of injury to athletes.

Different countries have different practices, but generally it is a good idea to have some paramedic teams in the spectator areas, particularly if there are large crowds, icy steps, abundant alcohol, etc. At larger events, there may be up to five to six teams spread around the arena.

The EMT's/paramedic's role has to be agreed upon beforehand. As a rule, the EMT will be a part of the team that has first contact with the athlete and offers medical assistance if necessary. In many countries EMTs/paramedics are well versed in athlete rescue, life support procedures, the care of spinal injuries, and even the administration of medications. Many are more experienced than physicians at intubation and CPR. Standards must be evaluated before an event and precise roles, field of play (FOP) access rules, and treatment procedures and protocols must be completed, distributed, and rehearsed before the event.

EMT/Paramedic Titles: It can be very confusing when working with different ambulance services and paramedics due to the array of titles. Try to define the level of care a paramedic can provide: Here is an example of the variety of titles within the London Ambulance Services: ambulance attendant (PTS), emergency care assistant/A&E support, emergency medical dispatcher (EMD1, EMD2, EMD3, EMD4), clinical support advisor (working as the CSD/clinical support desk in EOC), clinical telephone advisor (CTA), emergency medical technician (EMT1, EMT2, EMT3, EMT4), student paramedic, paramedic, emergency care practitioner (ECP), HEMS paramedic, hazardous area response team (HART) operative, tactical support officer (TSO), team leader, training officer, duty station officer (DSO), area operations manager (AOM).

Don't nod and agree; ask!

Sports Trainers

Certified athletic trainers, massage therapists, and chiropractors can be invaluable in terms of massaging, stretching, and providing medical modalities (such as ice) at larger events. Podiatrists, too, can be invaluable to care for the large volume of foot and ankle complaints, ranging from blisters to sprains, that present at large running events.

Physiotherapists

Contributed by Gordon Bosworth, former physiotherapist to the British Olympic Team, and now physiotherapist for the Canadian Speed Skating Team

The physiotherapist has several functions at a major sporting event, notwithstanding the treatment of his or her athletes. The Winter Sports Arena is very different to most sporting arenas; the venues alone pose several challenges to athletes and support teams. You should be thinking of the following:

■ Services and expertise available at the location

■ Nearest hospital

■ Ambulance or alternative transport for injured athletes

■ EMS

■ Understand the psychological and physical pressure on the athletes.

■ Ensure you have relevant first aid skills and equipment available.

■ Warm-up areas should be sourced and the athletes monitored throughout the warm-up for safety and the early signs of injury.

■ Be capable of working in the cold and on uneven terrain from time to time.

■ Be conscious of the equipment used by the athletes and the potential for this to cause injury during setup and practice.

■ Consider voltage and ampere differences when travelling; in some countries you may need a transformer.

■ Ensure that the team bag has sufficient medications given the number of countries travelled in a season.

■ Clothe yourself appropriately; you need to be comfortable and able to sustain your body temperature during long events and sometimes difficult conditions. You must be able to function at any time and in any conditions where the event is held.

If you are working as part of a larger medical team, certain emergency situations will be covered; however, when alone, be clear on the emergency procedures at each venue. Familiarize yourself with the venue to ensure you can position yourself to gain greatest and quickest access to your athletes during practice and competition. Check your emergency bag daily and ensure you are properly equipped to deal with any and all potential problems.

Athletes carrying minor injuries will require on-site work and encouragement in order to both train and compete. The management of the athlete is paramount. Often it is a case of reassuring them it is OK. You spend much of your time giving motivational support when athletes are carrying minor injuries.

Know your sport and your athletes. You will seldom be in a venue alone; other physiotherapists and physicians will likely be around. Get to know who they are as they will have invaluable local knowledge, and remember that working together, especially in emergency situations, facilitates proper care.

Treating athletes on location can be arduous. There are seldom areas to place your treatment table and you may need to improvise. You should do a thorough reconnoiter of the venue, if possible, prior to the team starting training. Know your access points when track side; know the rules regarding going onto/into the track. Remember that at winter venues the areas of competition typically cover several kilometers (e.g., bobsleigh, skiing, etc.), hence the importance of knowing your venue, access, and vantage points. Ideally you should be in radio contact with your team members and, if possible, with the start/finish area. Communication systems should be in place to enable contact, but make sure you are radio competent. Ensure that you can make yourself understood; language can be a problem, and although most countries speak English, you should make sure you can be understood by key emergency aid personnel in the local language.

Make sure that you are up-to-date with CPR and life support. You need to be confident and competent to cope. Be prepared to improvise and lend support elsewhere if required, as you may have to perform several roles in a team.

I have alluded to the treatment of the athlete in venue—what is and is not available/possible. Decision-making processes may change somewhat in different situations. There is much you can do to prevent injury but the constraints of this chapter do not allow me to go into detail. Given the difficulties outlined, preventative measures must be prioritized.

Regular, simple biomechanical checks can be easily and quickly performed to determine if an athlete is likely to be injured during training. The following may be useful in this regard:

- Sacroiliac joint loading function tests.

- Muscle timing/firing, especially gluteal/VMO

- Foot function/compression/position tests

- Shoulder girdle function/position

Sports in which there is a danger of crashing are also fraught with problems. Brush up on basic trauma management and attend a course. At major events there will be specialists available; know who they are and where they are located.

Factors that influence medical staffing numbers are

- High-velocity/low-velocity sport (e.g., speed skating contra table tennis)

- On land or on water

- Sports with frequent/dangerous injuries

- Size of arena/track distance (e.g., marathon, cross-country skiing)

- Federation rules/International Olympic Committee (IOC) rules

- Tradition

- National regulations

- Number of spectators

For example, staffing of a major stadium with 70,000 people during the Olympic Games, the following staffing levels are not unusual, and are often higher:

Spectator Medical Services:

- Six to eight teams of 2 first aid responders (e.g., Red Cross), 2 teams per tier

- Doctors: 1 for each tier, total 3 to 4, accompanied by a nurse

- Medical tent/cabin/room: 2 doctors, 4 nurses, 4 paramedics—to treat spectators and also as a backup in case of emergency. The "room" staff can rotate with the stadium staff so they can experience some of the Games.

- Due to fallout (sickness, etc.), it is a good idea to have medical and paramedical staff in reserve.

- Ambulances: minimum 2, often 4, staffed by 2 ambulance personnel each

- Ambulance standard, Europe: CEN 1 to 2; ambulance standard, United States: BLS and ALS

- Subtotal: doctors: 5; nurses: 9; first aid responders: 24; ambulance paramedics: 8; ambulances: 4

Athlete Medical Services:

- Athletics arena: 2 teams, 1 team at each end of stadium by the track, composed of 1 doctor, 1 anesthetic nurse, 2 paramedics (*Note: Different sports have different requirements, for example, boxing, judo, wrestling, etc., have staff ringside*)

- Athletes' medical room: 2 doctors, 2 nurses, 1 physiotherapist/sports masseur

- Ambulances: 2, staffed by 2 ambulance paramedics each

- Subtotal: doctors: 4; nurses: 4; physiotherapist/masseur 1; ambulance paramedics: 4; ambulances: 2; ambulance standard: CEN 1 to 2

Total: doctors: 9; Nurses: 13; first aid responders: 28; ambulance paramedics: 12; ambulances: 6, physiotherapist/masseur: 1; ambulances: 6 × 1.5 (sickness, unavailability, etc.) – 56 volunteers × 1.5 = 84

1.4 EMERGENCY SPORTS MEDICINE TRAINING COURSES

Many courses are available to train medical personnel in various forms of patient treatment. These synonyms can be confusing. Here are some of the terms:

- BLS: Basic Life Support

- ALS: Advanced Life Support

- ACLS: Advanced Cardiac Life Support—manage a patient's airway, initiate IV access, read and interpret electrocardiograms, understanding of emergency pharmacology
- ATLS: Advanced Trauma Life Support—a program based on trauma therapy whereby one treats the greatest threat to life first

1.5 FIMS EMERGENCY SPORTS MEDICINE COURSES

FIMS have recently created the Emergency Sports Medicine Course. The course focuses totally on emergency medical procedures and is an invaluable tool for EPs. At the time of printing, FIMS is cooperating with several IFs in producing specific courses for specific sports and several federations are now looking at making this course mandatory for physicians wishing to participate in major championships.

Day 1

8:30–8:45	Opening	
8:45–9:00	Basics of emergency care	15 minutes
9:00–10:15	Dislocations in sport: Workshop: Diagnosis and management Shoulder, AC joint, elbow, hand, hip, patella, toe injuries	75 minutes
10:30–12:00	**Group 1**	
	Neck, spinal, extremity injuries: Workshop	
	Practical treatment: Cervical collars, immobilization, vacuum splints, backboards, lifting techniques: Workshop	90 minutes
	Group 2	
	Sudden cardiac arrest, airway management: Workshop	90 minutes
13:00–14:00	Injuries and illnesses: Face, nose and eye, throat	60 minutes
14:00–14:45	Acute muscle, tendon injuries: Diagnosis and treatment	45 minutes
15:00–15:45	Ankle, knee, and shoulder injuries: Treatment, including taping	45 minutes
16:00–17:00	Thorax, abdominal, pelvic injuries: Diagnosis and treatment	60 minutes

Day 2

08:30–08:50	Control of bleeding, IV fluid treatment	20 minutes
09:00–10:30	**Group 2**	
	Neck, spinal, extremity injuries: Workshop	
	Practical treatment: Cervical collars, immobilization, vacuum splints, backboards, lifting techniques.	90 minutes
	Group 1	
	Sudden cardiac arrest, airway management: Workshop	90 minutes
10:45–11:15	Wound care, suturing, taping, antibiotics, vaccines	30 minutes
11:15–12:00	Disaster medicine, stadium disasters, planning, management	45 minutes
13:30–14:30	Head injuries, concussion, treatment, RTP guidelines	60 minutes
14:50–15:50	The collapsed athlete	60 minutes
16:00–16:15	Emergency medications in sport	15 minutes
16:15–16:45	WADA: The doping control procedure, the list	30 minutes
16:45–17:30	Treating patients from abroad: Ethical issues in emergency care	45 minutes

1.6 BUILDING THE TEAM: TEAMWORK AND POSITIVE FEEDBACK

The medical director has a major task in recruiting the right number of staff, the right number of specialists, and not least, the right people. At the Olympic Games it is vital to choose the best people to be the venue medical managers (VMM). These physicians will be responsible for the medical services at their own venue. They should have a sports medicine background, have respect in the sports medical community, be hard workers, and have good management skills. It is important that these VMMs participate in the planning of the medical services at an early stage, to gain knowledge of the complexity of the sport and to help design the venue facilities to have optimal treatment facilities. Fortunately, plans from previous Olympics and World Championships are usually available, and the IOC in particular is most helpful in supplying detailed information. The chairpersons of the various IF medical committees also have detailed information about the individual sports and should be contacted for their advice and approval.

Staffing requirements at a venue may vary from Games to Games, depending on a number of factors, such as the distance to the nearest hospital, the distance to the nearest neurologic unit, the availability of helicopters, etc.

The VMM needs to have good personnel management skills and needs to be able to create an ethos of enthusiasm, loyalty, quality, and flexibility. In "selling" the Games to volunteers, it is not unusual to sell the concept of the "Great Olympic Experience." Staff may become extremely disheartened if they are stuck in a parking lot outside a stadium for 14 days, or at an event they have absolutely no interest in. Do not underestimate our colleagues' needs for praise, motivation, variation, and not least, the social experience—the feeling of being part of a team. If the medical volunteers feel that the job they do is not appreciated, or if they consider themselves to be unfairly treated ("Why do I always get the 6:00 AM shift?" or "Why do I always have to stand out here and freeze at −30 degrees?" or "Why do those guys sit in the tent all day drinking coffee?"), then they become disgruntled and may decide to go home.

The VMM has an important leadership task. It can be a good idea to have a highly qualified and respected professor as a VMM (commanding loyalty by status), but equally it can be useful to have a physician with long experience and knowledge of the actual venue sport. It depends on the individual as much as on his or her background.

Once chosen, the VMM has to develop a staffing plan. Staffing guidelines should be delivered by the medical director, the IOC, the relevant IF, etc. The VMM needs to estimate how many and what kind of medical staff is needed (sports medicine physicians, primary care physicians/GPs, orthopedists, anesthesiologists, etc.). Similarly, plans must be made for support medical staff—nurses, paramedics, physiotherapists, athletic trainers, etc.

The VMM needs to plan where staff are to be located, and this is usually done in conjunction with the venue management team, the IOC, and IF experts.

The whole question of equipment type, equipment volume and placement must be also be addressed.

Once the venue medical plan has been completed, the task of choosing appropriate individuals begins. The team will then need to get together

on several occasions and should have a minimum of one, but preferably several, training/bonding sessions at the venue. The best form of training is a live event and the IFs often plan events in the season before the Games to allow for this type of training. Medical staff need to gain venue geographical location knowledge (how to get from A to B) as well as sport-specific treatment guidelines. This is also a vital part of the teambuilding process.

Motivational and inclusive leadership will make the event a once-in-a-lifetime experience for all who participate. Poor leadership and lack of consideration will certainly lead to burnout, absenteeism, and service of inferior quality. Remember, at the Olympic Games, most of the staff are volunteers and are offering their own time and money to be there.

Finally, I would like to emphasize how important it is for the VMM to have good relationships with the rest of the venue management team, as the medical team is only a part of the whole process. We are a small, but important, cog in the wheel. Sporting events are about sports and not primarily about sports medicine, but it is important for the medical team to be comfortably integrated into the rest of the venue team.

1.7 LIAISE WITH VISITING IFS AND NATIONAL TEAM PHYSICIANS

This is an area of potential conflict; however, as with all aspects of planning, it is important to enter into early dialogue with the IFs and national teams' medical staff. While an Olympic Games may be organized by the IOC, during the Games each sport is actually run by the IF in cooperation with the local organizing committee.

Each sport has its own IF, and these bodies run the sport. They organize World Cups and World Championships. When the Olympic Games come along, it is important for the VMM to enter into *early* dialogue with the chairpersons of the IFs' medical committees, as these physicians have an in-depth knowledge of their sports and the needs of their IF's athletes.

They can give excellent advice and practical tips to the organizers, advice that can be incorporated into one's medical plans.

However, I can also remember several occasions where IFs were asked to participate in the medical event planning and did not, but then turned up at a major event and caused all sorts of problems for the event organizers.

These situations can be avoided by early communication and dedicated cooperation with the IF medical chairpersons. These auspicious gentlemen and ladies have enormous experience and knowledge of their sports and can be of great help to EP newcomers.

Early in the organization process, the EP and the IF representatives must agree upon the levels of treatment that will be offered. Thereafter, a medical plan should be developed and approved.

Guidelines made by organizers must not be "over the top."

There is, more often than not, an element of overreaction by the organizing medical staff, particularly at the start of a major event. Athletes can be sent to unnecessary hospital and laboratory investigations due to overenthusiastic staff.

Not all athletes who fall need helicopter transfer to the nearest neurologic unit. MRI scans and ultrasound tests are not necessary for all injuries.

Remember, in the lead-up to a major event, athletes have strict training and rest regimes; the last thing they need is to spend 5 or 6 hours unnecessarily in a hospital. This has happened to some of my athletes. Good intentions by the organizers may inadvertently create unnecessary negativity, and you start the Games on a bad note. So, avoid exaggeration.

On occasions, difficulties can arise with visiting team physicians. This situation usually arises if the visiting physician has not received, or has not read, the pregames information package regarding visiting physicians' rights and responsibilities. I have seen visiting team physicians completely override the host medical staff, demanding various forms of treatment, sometimes excellent, sometimes unheard of by the rest of the medical world. These situations can be extremely difficult for the friendly, well-drilled host rescue teams. I have even done it myself (shame on me). These are difficult situations. My only advice here is to iron out potential conflict areas before the event at the team physicians meeting. It is important to have defined the following issues:

a) Who will perform emergency intervention procedures? This is usually the task of the host staff.

b) Who will offer nonemergency medical care? This is usually the task of the team physician.

c) Who will decide return-to-play issues? This is usually the task of the team physician; however many team physicians prefer that the EP takes this responsibility. If this is the case, it is important that any liability issues be well defined prior to the request and event. In some cases, the IF's physician has the last word.

At the Olympic Games in Lillehammer, all the visiting physicians were obliged to come to one of the Olympic Village polyclinics to receive their temporary medical licenses. This allowed a colleague and myself to converse with each visiting physician, to establish a rapport, and to discuss potential areas of conflict. We had no conflicts during the Games. It is more difficult to do this at a Summer Games due to the number of venues, but my advice is still the same: establish contact when issuing the temporary licenses.

1.8 STAFF ROTATION

Try to avoid moving staff from one venue to another. Familiarity breeds content, and venue knowledge is vital for optimal response. However, if boredom and tedium (overworked or underemployed) are becoming an issue, and there is a danger of losing volunteer medical staff, then venue rotation may be a valuable option. Wait as long as you can; for example, wait until the second week of the Olympic Games before starting rotation, if at all.

1.9 FOR HOW LONG SHOULD MEDICAL SERVICES BE AVAILABLE?

The EP and paramedics should be present at least 60 minutes before the event starts. At major events, particularly outdoor events, it can be a good idea to have staff arrive 90 minutes before the event starts. This allows for a short briefing, equipment and staff transfer, and on-site preparation. It is also a great opportunity to review any changes for the day's plan and to practice any emergency procedures or FOP access issues. In some sports, athletes arrive an hour or more before the event start. Medical staff should be present at least 30 minutes before the athletes and/or spectators arrive.

After the event is over, keep athlete services available for at least 30 minutes after the award ceremony and until all athletes have left the venue. Spectator services should be available until all spectators have left the venue. Conclude the service by having a 5- to 10-minute meeting with all medical staff to give reports; collect logs, statistics, and equipment lists; and confirm that all staff will be returning the next day.

1.10 TRAFFIC CONTROL

Traffic control is an important topic to have thought through before an event. The major concern is that ambulance access and exit routes will be blocked by either spectators or traffic. The usual congestion sites are

- Getting from the location on the track back to the venue exit road, sometimes via the medical station. At larger events there should be a dedicated road for venue vehicles.

- Getting onto the main road outside the venue can be difficult. A policeman/woman at such a junction can be amazingly helpful. Speak to the police or traffic experts in your organizing committee. Make sure that ambulances have access to traffic control via the radio system.

1.11 TIMING OF EVENTS AND COOPERATION WITH LOCAL WEATHER AUTHORITIES

Usually the timing of major events is controlled by the local organizing committee in conjunction with a representative from the IF and media. While many factors may influence the start time (finance, ticket sales, TV, etc.) the EP should make it clear that certain climatic conditions will effect athletes' performance and health (e.g., do not start a marathon at 1 PM in Texas in August due to the heat, or avoid start times in the tropics where athletes can slip on at wet road surfaces if there are afternoon rains.) It is better to have discussed these issues in the initial planning phase when planners are open to creative thoughts than nearer the event when times and schedules have been cemented.

1.12 MEDICAL LOG

During a large sports event it is important to keep a medical log. The reasons are obvious: not only as an operational tool during an event or as a statistical tool after the event, but also to keep track of individual incidents. It is important to know where the athlete is in the treatment chain; a log allows one to give information to coaches, family, etc. One has also documented the chain of response in case of later review.

Keeping a careful log allows one to have an overview of staff reserves and of how many staff members are available to be relocated in case of a major incident. By analyzing the medical log at the end of the day, one can evaluate the need for extra (or less) staff, equipment, materials, medications, etc. I would strongly advise that an experienced person is placed in charge of this important task.

1.13 ATHLETE INJURY FORMS

Basically, athletes and EPs come in contact with each other at three different sites: on the track or FOP, at the venue medical room, or at the athlete polyclinic.

For venue medical room and polyclinic consultations, all medical entries should be made electronically on a computer-based medical records system. The medical director should have prepared a minimum standard for what is acceptable patient documentation. Staff need to be trained in the use of this medical software. This may take time, so be prepared.

For field-side consultations, which are usually fewer than at the stations listed above, it is sufficient to complete a standardized paper journal after the athlete has been treated or transferred to the next level of care. If it is a busy station, then it is often easier to have a checklist so you can simply check off boxes, but written text is always necessary. The more severe the injury, the greater the likelihood that the medical journal will be reviewed, so spend some time documenting your findings, diagnosis, treatment, and further treatment suggestions. Note the time of consultation start and finish. It is also an advantage to have some form of injury severity scale. Always complete the journal by describing how the consultation ended: the athlete returned to play; the athlete retired and did not seek or need further consultation; the athlete was transferred by ambulance to hospital, radiology, lab, etc.; athlete care was transferred to the team physician. Get the athlete to sign the treatment document before leaving the medical room.

On returning to the venue medical center, always transfer the contents of the paper journal to the computer-based system.

Keep the paper journals in the paper archive.

1.14 INJURY SEVERITY SCALES

There are several injury severity scales by which one can evaluate injuries. None of these different scales are perfect, as they are all open to individual interpretation. These scales may be useful in emergency scenarios, particularly when there are multiple injuries, or when reviewing statistics. The medical director must decide before the competition which scale is to be used.

Some of the different scales are listed below.

Abbreviated Injury Scale

The Abbreviated Injury Scale (AIS) is an anatomical scoring system first introduced in 1969.

Injuries are ranked on a scale of 1 to 6: 1 is minor, 2 is moderate, 3 is serious, 4 is severe, 5 is critical, and 6 is an unsurvivable injury.

Injury Severity Score

The Injury Severity Score (ISS) is a useful anatomical scoring system that can provide an overall score for patients with multiple injuries. Each injury is given an AIS score for the major body regions (head, face, chest, abdomen, pelvis + extremities, external). The three most severely injured body region scores are then squared to give the ISS score.

New Injury Severity Score

The New Injury Severity Score (NISS) was developed in 1997 and is a modification of the ISS. It was developed to improve upon the ISS (see Appendix).

Glasgow Coma Scale

The Glasgow Coma Scale (GCS) has been a useful tool for many years; it is still considered to be an important weapon in the EP's arsenal. The problem with the GCS is that it has been designed to evaluate trauma 6 hours after the injury, and not immediately after an event. The GCS is composed of three parameters: eye response, verbal response, and motor response. Scores are between 3 and 15, the higher the better. A score of 13 or 14 may indicate a mild brain injury; 9 to 12, a moderate brain injury; and 8 or less, a severe brain injury.

Eye Response (4)
1. No eye opening
2. Eye opening to pain
3. Eye opening to verbal command
4. Eyes open spontaneously

Verbal Response (5)
1. No verbal response
2. Incomprehensible sounds
3. Inappropriate words
4. Confused
5. Orientated

Motor Response (6)
1. No motor response
2. Extension to pain
3. Flexion to pain
4. Withdrawal from pain
5. Localizing pain
6. Obeys commands

Organ Injury Scales

The Organ Injury Scales measure organ injury with a grade from 1 to 6. Injuries may also be divided by mechanism or by anatomic description. (See Appendix.)

1.15 DAILY VENUE REPORTS

The day's event should be concluded with a staff meeting. Each team should deliver a report on the number and severity of injuries, hospital admissions or referrals, and other special situations. There should be a short review of staffing and staff location plans. Is everything working OK or not? A list of used equipment should be delivered; supplies should be replenished before the next day's event. Staff rotas for the next day should be confirmed and a start time agreed upon. Radios must be delivered so that batteries can be charged.

At the end of the staff meeting, the VMM must then send his report to the medical director, who in turn makes his daily report to the organizing committee and/or the IF/IOC.

1.16 COMPUTER-BASED MEDICAL RECORDS

It can take some time for medical staff to learn and to become proficient in new medical software, so allow time for training in the pregames period.

Journal security and safety issues must be addressed.

Remember, all medical personnel must sign confidentiality agreements.

1.17 LIAISE WITH VISITING SCIENTIFIC RESEARCH GROUPS

At major events there are often visiting scientific groups conducting research programs. These studies maybe include injury statistical analysis and biomechanical studies. Try to assist these groups, as they are usually conducting important medical studies. (See Chapter 14 by Prof. Colin Fuller.)

1.18 MEDICAL STAFF CLOTHING AND VISIBILITY

You can have the best equipment and staff in the world, but if you have inadequate footwear and poor quality gloves (working in water, freezing cold), your ability to perform in cold wet climates is extremely reduced. Particularly, if patients have to be lifted and carried out of ditches or up steep hills, rescue can become exhausting for medical staff.

Staff working in extreme heat and sun should be supplied with loose-fitting, appropriate clothing. Sun block, sunglasses and caps are vital. Correct clothing is essential.

Remember also that staff may have to work both indoors and outdoors so correct clothing has to be available. It is not unusual to have a 20°C to 30°C temperature difference between in- and outdoors. Laundry facilities must be provided for staff volunteers. After 10 days of wearing the same shirt, staff can begin to look a bit scruffy, so facilities must be provided and must be used.

Visibility

Medical staff are often clothed similarly to other volunteers. There are advantages (volunteers get highly desired clothing) and disadvantages (clothing design can often be a bit "loud" and not always something you would wear after the event). If medical staff are required to wear the standard volunteers clothing, then they should at least have an outer vest with the "Star of Life" or similar recognizable markings, so that they can be instantly recognizable and easily seen in throngs of spectators.

Event clothing is not always practical for medical personnel: we need plenty of pockets and clothing that is appropriate for indoor and outdoor temperatures. Sometimes, the EP must argue that medical personnel wear clothing that is practical for their work even if this contrasts with standard uniforms.

Medical rooms, tents, etc., should be marked by large signs or flags that are visible from a distance and can stand out in a dense crowd. Signs should not be similar to other event signs; they should be easily distinguishable as being medical.

1.19 ACCREDITATION

Access to various zones of a sports arena during a major event is extremely restricted, with good reason. While it is important to allow medical personnel access to all parts of an arena, it is not necessary (in fact totally undesirable) to have medics wandering around in the technical rooms and dressing rooms, VIP dining areas, and other restricted areas. As medical personnel, we do not want TV cameras near the athletes' medical room filming injured sports stars. At the same time, you do not want medical staff wandering into a camera shot with "Hello Mom" placards.

Medical staff should stay at their stations and not pose behind Usain Bolt receiving his medals.

Different zones are given different number and letter codes. Before the Games all medical staff will have to receive an accreditation card. They will have to go through a registration process weeks or months before the Games, then turn up at an accreditation center before the Games, be photographed, and receive their accreditation cards. All staff must wear these cards around their necks at all times. At some events, pregames accreditation is possible (Fig. 1.1).

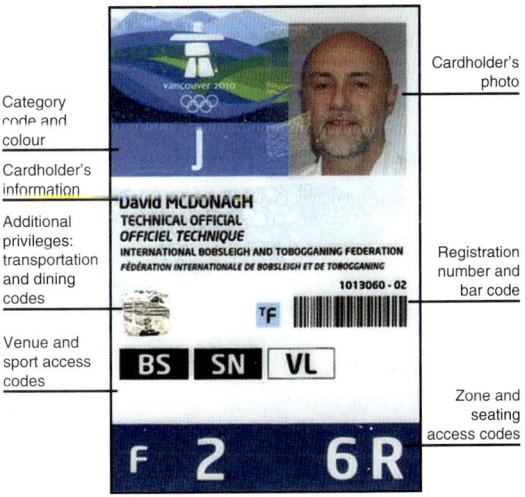

Olympic Identity and Accreditaion Card for the Vancouver 2010 Olympic Winter Games

FIGURE 1.1.

Each accreditation card will have written on it which arenas one has access to and to which zones (usually a number or symbol) within the arena one is allowed to enter.

Only very few are allowed access to all zones of an arena; only very few need access to all zones. Obviously police and medics should have this access—the so-labeled O accreditation. In emergency situations medics will usually be allowed access to any zone. As a rule, staff should wait to be called onto the track/field, etc., by a responsible official.

The VMM must keep stringent control and ensure that staff do not abuse their accreditation—after all, emergency interventions at most events are rare.

The VMM must also explain to the medical staff before the Games that the number of zones you have been given access to has nothing to do with the individual physician's academic qualifications or external appearance. Zone accreditation is based on function and has nothing to do with an order of merit. I have been approached by an eminent professor who was deeply offended at having a "lesser" accreditation than one of the paramedics. Oh, the joys of management.

If you have two teams at track side, then no other medics should be allowed into this area except in case of an emergency. Even the most hardnosed security officer will almost always allow medical personnel access. Special access armbands are often issued by security staff to allow entry into in the inner sanctuaries and these are often issued on a daily basis to the track-side medical teams.

Finally, do not lose your accreditation card. My advice is to have the accreditation card around your neck at all times—well, maybe not in the shower. You will not believe how stressed you are every morning going to work: late to bed; Where is my phone? Where is my money? Where are my food coupons? Where is my radio? Are my batteries charged? Which jacket did I leave my keys in? What pocket? Where is my extra hat, T-shirt, gloves, sunglasses, sun screen, camera, whatever?

Believe me, it's a real hassle. Remember: no card, no access, no matter who you are.

You will not be allowed on special volunteer buses, trains, etc.: *nada*.

Remember also to check the lanyard or neck strap that holds your card. Some of these have a little black notch in the middle, and these are designed to loosen. Sports tape—can be used to strengthen this notch.

1.20 TEMPORARY MEDICAL LICENSES AND INSURANCE FOR VISITING PHYSICIANS

During large sporting events, it is usual to issue medical licenses for visiting nonnational physicians to allow them to practice medicine legally on their own nationals before and during the event. Visiting physicians must apply for these licenses from the host nation's national health authorities many months in advance. Insurance matters must be addressed and the visiting physicians must receive information well in advance of the Games about what rights and facilities they will have on entering the host nation. As a rule, foreign physicians are only allowed to treat athletes from their own country; they may issue prescriptions that can be delivered at a specific pharmacy. Usually they have to approach a host physician if medical tests are to be conducted outside of the polyclinic/event hospital. A meeting between the host medical staff and visiting physicians is usually arranged, just before commencement of the Games.

1.21 MEDIA/PRESS RELEASES

It can be quite tempting for those not used to media exposure to make statements to TV and newspapers reporters. Who does not want to show off to friends and family ("Look, I finally made it!")? However, off-the-cuff comments can often end up with exaggerated responses in the media and one may end up suffering a correcting statement from one's superiors—this can be quite an embarrassing experience.

Before the 1994 Winter Olympics, in an attempt to prevent the spread of communicable diseases, we installed condom machines at the Olympic Village and at official residencies. When asked by the press if we would place a machine at the Olympic Family Hotel, I replied that we would of course place a machine there if one did not exist from before. Big deal! Within 2 days, my name appeared around the world in various unflattering forms (e.g., "Condoms for Samaranch," "IOC to be given free condoms," "Irish doctor recommends condoms to IOC boss," etc.). I received telephone calls from around the world. It lasted for a week. My moment of fame! Not quite.

Another example was during another major sports event. An athlete was transferred to hospital due to an ankle injury. The EP (who had not seen the athlete) was told by another source that the athlete probably had a femur fracture. The EP then held a 10-minute ad hoc press conference informing about the possible life-threatening and career-ending consequences of a femoral shaft fracture (arterial bleeding etc.). Headlines went national and international: "Athlete X's career ends after fatal broken leg injury," "Athlete X out of Championships due to broken leg," etc. The day after, athlete X returned to competition with a minor ankle sprain and won a medal.

Conclusion: Say nothing unless you have to; check your facts before you do so (check the medical log, speak to the treating physician), and always speak in moderation ("The athlete has been sent hospital for further checks"). Fortunately, most organizations recommend that one spokesperson be responsible for conversing with the media. My advice is to leave press statements to the appointed press officers or the medical director.

1.22 LANGUAGE AND CULTURAL DIFFICULTIES

Language differences do not usually create great difficulties, as a rule. If you have seen the injury, then the path to diagnosis is usually clear. If not, then one can usually get some kind of history by physical demonstration.

The problem gets worse when nonacute conditions have to be diagnosed, and almost impossible if there are psychiatric problems present. Translators are necessary in certain instances, and if you are running a mass participation event, then a corps of translators should be available. At smaller events these services are not usually available. Ask other volunteers, ground staff, etc., if someone speaks the language. In today's multinational world, it is not unusual to find someone who speaks the athlete's language. If nobody can, then look for some of the athlete's team members or staff. If all fails, then a translator can be contacted, but this often costs money and it can take time to get hold of the right person. One can always give up and send the patient to the local hospital where translator services might be available.

The idea that cultural differences are a source of potential conflict is, in my opinion, exaggerated, and I have never found these to be a hindrance.

1.23 INCIDENT MANAGEMENT—MEDICAL DISPATCH

The whole of the medical team should have radio access. Some doctors have appalling radio skills and may need to be allocated to experienced radio operators who can manage the radios for them.

There should be a dedicated medical channel. Only the medical staff is allowed to use this channel.

At an event, it is important to create a medical dispatch unit. This unit should be composed of three persons: an experienced medical dispatch nurse, an experienced dispatch ambulance paramedic, and an experienced doctor. At very large events, a fourth person may be present to manage the medical log.

The unit should be physically placed in a room near the main venue organization team in case of a major disaster or in case of radio failure. This room must have good sound insulation and should be suitably equipped with maps of the arena, local region, hospital locations, etc., as well as with telephones, Internet access, and internal event TV.

The medical dispatch is the central address for all medical requests and contacts.

Any medical team requiring assistance must contact medical dispatch, which then decides if a patient will be treated locally, transferred to the arena medical rooms, or directly transferred to hospital. The dispatch has control over all human resources, motorized resources and equipment.

Emergency messages from other event volunteers or staff should be channeled to the event medical dispatch unit.

The dispatch unit must also have contact with the local communal or municipal emergency medical dispatch unit in order to coordinate ambulance, helicopter and hospital services in the best possible way.

1.24 MEDICAL TREATMENT ROOMS AND MEDICAL EQUIPMENT

Room Requirements/Dimensions

- 36 m² for athletes' medical room (standard for all arenas)

- 36 m² for spectators' medical room (standard for all arenas)

- 62 m² for doping control room (in main arena, smaller elsewhere)

Room Equipment—Olympic Standard, Minimum Standard

(See attached list in Appendix.)

Personnel Equipment

Aspects to be considered:

Number of doctors, nurses, paramedics, first aid responders

Equipment standard

Kit out backpacks to doctors, nurses, paramedics, first aid responders containing portable and lightweight equipment. The contents of the backpacks will vary according to the individual's qualifications.

Belt packs and fanny packs are usually standard and can contain items for personal use, for example, water bottles, snacks, sunglasses, and gloves.

(See list, as approved by FIS and developed by I. Lereim and D. McDonagh, in Appendix.)

1.25 EQUIPMENT DELIVERY

Ordered equipment should be delivered in crates that include shelves and should be packed in such a way that the crates, when opened, are actually stand-alone units ready for use, thus negating the need for extensive packing and unpacking of medical equipment. Obviously, product numbering makes reordering and stocktaking much easier.

1.26 STANDARDIZATION OF EQUIPMENT

The contents of crates and their placement in medical rooms should be standardized and identical, thus allowing medical staff, in the event of them being moved to another arena, the familiarity with equipment that is necessary if one is to function optimally in an emergency situation.

1.27 USE OF EQUIPMENT

Do not open sealed equipment and medications unless absolutely necessary.

Equipment that is not used can be resold after an event.

Daily preevent equipment test: always test vital equipment before the start of an event. In particular check

- Oxygen tanks
- Otoscope and ophthalmoscope batteries
- Laryngoscope bulbs
- Splints and pumps
- Medications and infusion fluids

(Note on infusion liquids and cold climates: liquids can and do freeze. The last thing a hypothermic, shocked, hypovolemic patient needs is a bolus of cold infusion fluid.)

1.28 DISPOSABLES

Medical litter is unsightly and potentially dangerous. Demand that all staff pick up their own medical litter. Sharps must be disposed of and destroyed in a correct and safe fashion.

1.29 CHECKLISTS

All disposable materials and medications used should be compiled on a list. This list can be sent daily (or less frequently) by fax or email to the central warehouse and refills can be ordered.

1.30 EQUIPMENT REFILL/WAREHOUSE

At large events it is important to have a store of disposable materials and medications. Refill orders should be sent in by a particular time each day, allowing new products to be delivered to the stadium during the nighttime. Refilling then takes place before the start of competition the next day.

1.31 DERIGGING AND RESALE

After an event has been completed, a major derigging operation is initiated. This process can begin already 1 hour after the final event, and rooms, etc., are literally stripped bare of all equipment, including telephones and other electronic equipment. The urgency and speed at which these derigging exercises occur is often quite staggering, and one often wonders why it takes months to kit out rooms but takes only hours to empty them. In all honesty, this haste is present to prevent theft.

1.32 BUDGET

Athlete medical room cost per room × total no. of rooms ....
Spectator medical room cost per room × total no. of rooms ....

Portable medical equipment rule of thumb
One rucksack + resuscitation bag
per doctor ....
One rucksack per paramedic ....
Polyclinic ....
Doping control officer costs ....
Lab costs for doping controls—urine/blood ....
Expenses for training medical staff (events/
meetings, with travel/food/accommodation) ....
Equipment for medical staff (e.g., bag/belt pack,
reflex jacket, water bottle) ....
Helicopter rental ....
Ambulance hire ....
First aid responder costs ....
Travel/representation ....

First Subtotal:
Forgotten: + 10%

Second Subtotal:
Safety margin: + 10%

Final Total:

1.33 LOST CHILDREN SERVICE

Children and the elderly can get lost in large crowds, so a system should be put into place that allows wayward spectators to be registered and found. Many volunteer organizations have experience with this type of work, and they should be encouraged to have stations available outside major events venues. These organizations should have visible and recognizable flags above their stations as well as complete telephone lists to the organization ground staff.

1.34 POTENTIAL AREAS OF CONFLICT

If the standard of health care at an event is not sufficient, then the EP should raise the matter with the event organizer. Items that can be the source of conflict often include the

- Number of medical staff
- Qualifications of medical staff
- Level of ambulance sophistication
- Equipment standard
- Safety aspects

If the event organizer chooses to listen to the EP and adopt his or her suggestions, then well and good. If not, the EP may remind the organizer that he or she may be held legally responsible for negligence in the event of a serious incident. This has often a sobering effect on organizers, but it is a tactic that should not be overplayed.

There is a fundamental difference between debating the inherent danger of certain sports and a perceived lack of safety standards at an individual event, compared with safety norms at similar events in the region. Some gentle-souled physicians may consider boxing or rugby to be potentially life threatening (I don't want to get into that discussion), while some grizzled veterans on the organizing committee may consider modern sport to be too gentle and safety orientated. If the EP has ethical problems regarding certain sports, then there are other fora at which these topics should be debated. The EP has the right to withdraw his or her services if the level of medical preparation is perceived to be inadequate.

Physician qualifications and experience: Certain federations and nations have specific qualification requirements for the EP (see Chapters 76 and 77). There is a growing trend for IFs and event organizers to demand that EPs are competent in rescue skills.

Conflict with team personnel: There are many potential areas of conflict within teams, and sometimes the EP becomes involved. Team trainers will, as a rule, have their athletes' back in training and competition as soon as possible. This is not always in an athlete's best interest and conflict between a team leader and a team physician may occur— the EP may be asked for a second opinion. On other occasions a team will not have a physician at all, and again the EP must prioritize the patient's health ahead of team aspirations.

Conflicts can occur between the EP and visiting team physicians, but a preevent discussion about the delegation of responsibilities usually has a clarifying effect. On other occasions, there may be "command" issues between physicians and paramedics or other groups. The overall medical responsibility for the treatment of athletes at a sports event should rest with a physician. However, physicians do not necessarily have to be involved in all aspects of rescue and treatment. Experienced and qualified paramedics can have an important role to play and can be more experienced than some physicians in certain procedures. Clarify these issues before the event.

Appendix

Team Physician Consensus Statement

Mass Participation Event Management for the Team Physician: A Consensus Statement

DEFINITION

Mass participation event management is medical administration and participant care at these sporting events. Medical management provides safety advice and care at the event that accounts for large numbers of participants, anticipated injury and illness, variable environment, repeated games or matches, and mixed age groups of varying athletic ability. This document does not pertain to the care of the spectator.

GOAL

The goal is to assist the team/event physician in providing medical care during mass participation events. The physician's role is to organize a medical team that facilitates event safety, provides medical care, makes return-to-participation decisions, and acts as the event medical spokesperson. To accomplish this goal, the team physician should have knowledge of and be involved with

- Administrative matters concerning the event
- Medical care and protocols
- Hydration and fluid replacement

SUMMARY

This document provides an overview of select medical issues that are important to team physicians who are responsible for mass participation event management. It is not intended as a standard of care, and should not be interpreted as such. This document is only a guide, and as such, is of a general nature, consistent with the reasonable, objective practice of the healthcare professional. Individual treatment will turn on the specific facts and circumstances presented to the physician. Adequate insurance should be in place to help protect the physician, the athlete, and the sponsoring organization.

This statement was developed by a collaboration of six major professional associations concerned about clinical sports medicine issues; they have committed to forming an ongoing project-based alliance to bring together sports medicine organizations to best serve active people and athletes. The organizations are American Academy of Family Physicians, American Academy of Orthopaedic Surgeons, American College of Sports Medicine, American Medical Society for Sports Medicine, American Or-

thopaedic Society for Sports Medicine, and the American Osteopathic Academy of Sports Medicine.

EXPERT PANEL

Stanley A. Herring, M.D., Chair, Seattle, Washington
John A. Bergfeld, M.D., Cleveland, Ohio
Lori A. Boyajian-O'Neill, D.O., Kansas City, Missouri
Peter Indelicato, M.D., Gainesville, Florida
Rebecca Jaffe, M.D., Wilmington, Delaware
W. Ben Kibler, M.D., Lexington, Kentucky
Francis G. O'Connor, M.D., Fairfax, Virginia
Robert Pallay, M.D., Hillsborough, New Jersey
William O. Roberts, M.D., St. Paul, Minnesota
Alan Stockard, D.O., San Marcos, Texas
Timothy N. Taft, M.D., Chapel Hill, North Carolina
James Williams, M.D., Cleveland, Ohio
Craig C. Young, M.D., Milwaukee, Wisconsin

ADMINISTRATION

A well developed and properly executed medical plan will provide on-site care for participants with the additional goals of reducing patient load on area emergency facilities and providing rapid access to these facilities for participants in need of more advanced care. The unique aspects of mass participation event planning include access to and communication with the "field of play" (e.g., 42 km of city streets, several acres of soccer pitches, multiple tennis courts, open water sports, or back-country trails), a wide variation in the number and ability of competitors, and differences in the type and volume of injury and illness.

General Administration.

It is *essential* to:

- Develop an agreement concerning medical care and administrative responsibilities between the medical team and the organizing body
- Assess potential environmental conditions and site and event risk factors
- Organize the medical team before the event

- Notify police, fire and rescue departments and emergency medical facilities of time, location and access to the event and the expected number of casualties
- Develop and communicate medical protocols to include directing acute on-site care, determining who needs to be transported, as well as limits to participation or return-to-play
- Plan for operations, transportation, communication, and command and control
- Develop an adverse event protocol for deaths or catastrophic illness or injuries that addresses confidentiality, medical reporting, and public disclosure
- Adhere to the principles of the Health Insurance Portability and Accountability Act (HIPAA)
- Develop and maintain medical and event records
- Follow modified universal precautions protocol for the handling and disposal of body fluids and contaminated medical waste and all other principles of Occupational Safety and Health Administration (OSHA) standards
- Confirm and adhere to medical policies of applicable governing bodies
- Provide all-area access credentials to the medical team

It is *desirable* to:

- Organize the medical team at least six months before the event
- Schedule the event when historical environmental conditions are most favorable
- Schedule the start time to accommodate the safest start and finish times for elite through novice competitors
- Develop a tracking system so family members can find injured or ill participants
- Conduct a postevent review of the medical care, administrative plan and budget
- Review and analyze event injury, illness, and environmental data
- Prepare a summary report

Hazardous Condition Plan.
Hazardous conditions pose a risk to event participants beyond the inherent risk of the activity and to support staff involved in the event.

It is *essential* to:

- Develop a modification or cancellation policy for the event when hazardous conditions exist
- Hot conditions: determine an ambient temperature and relative humidity cut-off appropriate for the sport, age, and abilities of the participants
- Cold conditions: determine an ambient temperature and windchill cut-off that is appropriate for the sport, age, abilities of the participants, and location (latitude, altitude)
- Suspend activities when lightning and thunder are present ("if you can hear it, clear it"), and resume activity after 30 min without lightning and thunder

- Consider other sport-specific conditions, such as air quality, traction, water conditions, wind speed, and visibility
- Announce the risks of current and anticipated competitive environment at the start

It is *desirable* to:

- Publish hazardous condition protocol in advance
- Monitor conditions on-site with a wet-bulb globe thermometer or ambient temperature–relative humidity device, and lightning warning system
- Develop an on-site communications system for changing conditions

Competitor Education.
Preevent and on-site participant education may reduce injury risk and improve safety.

It is *essential* to develop a method to inform participants of:

- Inherent event risks
- Safety measures to reduce individual risk
- Anticipated environmental conditions and site risks
- Risks of over and under hydration where applicable
- Fitness recommendations for the event
- Location and identification of medical facilities and personnel

It is *desirable* to provide in advance:

- Health and safety material to all participants and coaches
- Equipment and clothing recommendations
- A method for participants to convey significant medical information

Competition Site Preparation.
Site preparation positions medical resources and personnel and facilitates safety for competitors and support staff.

It is *essential* the competition site:

- Be inspected to reduce injury risks
- Be accessible to medical team and support staff
- Include designated access and egress points for emergency medical services
- Include major and minor medical aid stations that are clearly identified, strategically placed with controlled entry, and easily accessible to injured or ill participants, medical team, and support staff
- Include a transportation plan for well and injured/ill competitors both on-site and between the event site and the emergency facility
- Include a communications plan to direct emergency care and link medical sites and personnel
- Include hydration fluids that are available for participants, medical team, and support staff

It is *desirable* the competition site:

- Include food, shelter, and sanitation facilities for competitors, medical team, and support staff

- Include parking/venue passes, locations and maps for medical team and support staff

Staffing for Medical Areas.

Staffing for mass participation events should be based on anticipated medical event requirements, anticipated injury and illness, and planned level of medical care delivery. These decisions are made in advance by the event medical director and are frequently based upon historical event data.

It is *essential* the medical team:

- Include a medical director
- Provide basic first aid and cardiopulmonary resuscitation (CPR)
- Provide event-specific medical and musculoskeletal care
- Include support staff who possess specific skills to access all areas of the course

It is *desirable* the medical team:

- Provide early defibrillation
- Provide advanced cardiac life support and advanced trauma life support
- Provide intravenous fluid administration for non life-threatening illness
- Include non-medical staff to assist medical providers

Equipment and Medical Supplies.

The medical team requires equipment and supplies in the major and minor medical aid stations. The requirements may differ based on the mass participation event, the number of competitors, and the type and volume of injury and illness.

It is *highly desirable*, depending upon the mass participation event, that the major medical aid station:

- Be contained and offer privacy and protection from environment
- Have the following supplies:
  - Medical supplies, including automatic or manual external defibrillator, airway kit, intubation equipment, pocket venti-mask, rectal thermometers, blood pressure cuff, stethoscope, pen light, oxygen and oxygen delivery system, intravenous fluids and administration kits, medications (advanced cardiac life support drugs, aspirin, dextrose 50% in water, albuterol inhaler, epinephrine 1:1000 SQ, antihistamine, diazepam, glucagon, and magnesium sulfate), glucose monitor, sodium monitor, and oxygen saturation monitor, and as indicated, cricothyrotomy kit and immersion tubs
  - Musculoskeletal supplies, including ice, plastic bags, splints, slings, braces, crutches, athletic tape, blister care products, elastic bandages, and suture materials
  - Other supplies, including shelter, stretchers, cots, blankets, towels, chairs, tables, security fencing, heating and cooling equipment, generator or electricity source, lights, sharps box, gloves, contaminated waste disposal, waterless soap, portable sink, toilet, and as indicated, back boards and semi-rigid neck collars.

It is *desirable*:

- Other supplies included for game-day preparation be available for the major medical aid station [See "Sideline Preparedness for the Team Physician"]
- The minor medical aid stations provide basic first aid supplies for medical and musculoskeletal conditions.

MEDICAL CARE

Medical care at mass participation events is best delivered by predetermined protocols. These protocols direct acute on-site care, determine who needs to be transported, and determine limits to participation or return-to-play. While some events may require preparticipation screening, in general, it is neither practical nor cost effective.

Medical Care Delivery.

It is *essential* to provide on-site:

- Basic first aid and CPR
- Event-specific medical and musculoskeletal care

It is *desirable* to provide on-site:

- Early defibrillation
- Advanced cardiac life support and advanced trauma life support
- Intravenous fluid administration for non life–threatening illness
- Hyper- and hypothermia evaluation and initial care
- Hyponatremia evaluation and initial care

Limits to Event Participation and Return-To-Play.

It is *essential* the medical team:

- Be authorized to evaluate the injured or ill participant and limit participation or determine return-to-play

It is *desirable* the medical team:

- Has facilities and equipment for evaluation on-site.
- Publish criteria for limits to participation or return-to-play

HYDRATION AND ENERGY REPLACEMENT

Events should have fluids (and food if indicated) available for safe participation. Fluids should be easily accessible and strategically placed. Six to 12 oz. (180–360 mL) of fluid should be available for every 15–20 min of continuous activity. Excessive fluid intake may result in hyponatremia.

It is *essential* to:

- Provide fluids for competitors, medical team, and support staff
- Provide additional fluid choices containing carbohydrate and sodium for events involving continuous activity lasting more than 1 h
- Encourage participants to replace sweat losses during activity and replace weight loss postevent

It is *desirable* to:

- Cool fluids to 59–72°F (15–22°C) for optimal palatability and absorption

- Publish the fluid types and location before the event
- Utilize carbohydrate and salt solutions for optimal palatability and absorption containing:
- 25–50 mmol·L^{-1} sodium, 2–8% carbohydrate for pre-event and event
- 50–100 mmol·L^{-1} sodium postevent (with normal diet)

AVAILABLE RESOURCES

Ongoing education pertinent to the team physician is essential. Information regarding team physician–specific educational opportunities can be obtained from the six participating organizations:

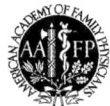

- American Academy of Family Physicians (AAFP)
  11400 Tomahawk Creek Pkwy
  Leawood, KS 66211
  800-274-2237
  www.aafp.org

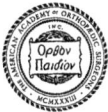

- American Academy of Orthopaedic Surgeons (AAOS)
  6300 N River Rd
  Rosemont, IL 60018
  800-346-AAOS
  www.aaos.org

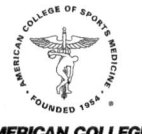

- American College of Sports Medicine (ACSM)
  401 W Michigan St
  Indianapolis, IN 46202
  317-637-9200
  www.acsm.org

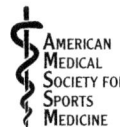

- American Medical Society for Sports Medicine (AMSSM)
  11639 Earnshaw
  Overland Park, KS 66210
  913-327-1415
  www.amssm.org

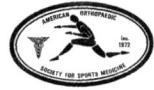

- American Orthopaedic Society for Sports Medicine (AOSSM)
  6300 N River Rd, Suite 500
  Rosemont, IL 60018
  847-292-4900
  www.sportsmed.org

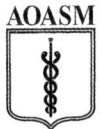

- American Osteopathic Academy of Sports Medicine (AOASM)
  7600 Terrance Ave., Suite 203
  Middleton, WI 53562
  608-831-4400
  www.aoasm.org

SELECTED READINGS

AMERICAN ACADEMY OF PEDIATRICS COMMITTEE ON SPORTS MEDICINE FITNESS. Human immunodeficiency virus in the athletic setting. *Pediatrics* 1991;88:640–641.

AMERICAN COLLEGE OF SPORTS MEDICINE. Sideline preparedness for the team physician: a consensus statement. *Med. Sci. Sports Exerc.* 33:846–849, 2001.

AMERICAN MEDICAL SOCIETY FOR SPORTS MEDICINE, AMERICAN ACADEMY OF SPORTS MEDICINE. Human immunodeficiency virus and other blood-borne pathogens in sports. *Clin. J. Sports Med.* 5:199–204, 1995.

ARMSTRONG, L. E., Y. EPSTEIN, J. E. GREENLEAF, et al. American College of Sports Medicine position statement on heat and cold illnesses during distance running. *Med. Sci. Sports Exer.* 28:i–x, 1996.

BECKER, K. M., C. L. MOE, K. L. SOUTHWICK, and J. N. MACCORMACK. Transmission of Norwalk virus during a football game. *NEJM* 343:1223–1227, 2000.

CASA, D. J., J. ALMQUIST, S ANDERSON, et al. Inter-Association task force on exertional heat illnesses consensus statement. *NATA NEWS* June 2003;24–29.

CIANCA, J. C., W. O. ROBERTS, and D. HORN. Distance running: organization of the medical team. In: *Textbook of Running Medicine*, F. G. O'Connor and R. P. Wilder (Eds.). New York: McGraw-Hill, 2001, p. 489.

COVERTINO, V. A., L. E. ARMSTRONG, and E. F. COYLE. Exercise and fluid replacement. *Med. Sci. Sports. Exerc.* 28:i–vii, 1996. ELIAS, S., W. O. ROBERTS, and D.C. THORSON. Team sports in hot weather: guidelines for modifying youth soccer. *Phys. Sportsmed.* 19:67–80, 1991.

GRANGE, J. T. Planning for large events. *Curr. Sports. Med. Rep.* 1:156–161, 2002.

JASLOW, D., A. YANCY, and A. MILSTEN. *Mass Gathering Medical Care: The Medical Director's Checklist for the NAEMSP Standards and Clinical Practice Committee*. Lenaxa, Kansas: National Association of Emergency Medical Services Physicians, 2000.

JASLOW, D., M. DRAKE, and J. LEWIS. Characteristics of state legislation governing medical care. *Prehosp. Emerg. Care.* 3:316–320, 1999.

KIBLER, W. B., B. P. LIVINGSTON, and J. MCMULLEN. Tournament coverage. In: *The U.S. Soccer Sports Medicine Book*, W. E. Garrett, D. T. Kirkendall, and S. R. Contigulia (Eds.). Baltimore: Williams and Wilkins, 1996, pp. 165–174.

MAKDISSI, M., and P. BRUKNER. Recommendations for lightning protection in sport. *Med. J. Aust.* 177:35–37, 2002.

MELLION, M. B., W. M. WALSH, C. MADDEN, M. PUTUKIAN, and G. L. SHELTON (Eds.). *Team Physician's Handbook*. Philadelphia: Hanley & Belfus, Inc., 2002.

MONTAIN, S. J., M. N. SAWKA, and C.B. WEGNER. Hyponatremia associated with exercise: risk factors and pathogenesis. *Exer. Sports Sci. Rev.* 29:113–117, 2001.

O'CONNOR, F. G., S. PYNE, F. H. BRENNAN, T. A. ADIRIM. Exercise-associated collapse: an algorithmic approach to race day management. *The American Journal of Medicine and Sports.* V:212–217, 2003.

O'CONNOR, F. G., J. P. KUGLER, and R. G. ORISCELLO. Sudden death in young athletes: screening for the needle in a haystack. *Am. Fam. Phys.* 57:2763–2770, 1998.

ROBERTS, W. O. A twelve year profile of medical injury and illness for the Twin Cities Marathon. *Med. Sci. Sports Exerc.* 32:1549–1555, 2000.

ROBERTS, W. O. Administration and medical management of mass participation endurance events. In: *Team Physician's Handbook*, M. B. Mellion, W. M. Walsh, C. Madden, M. Putukian, and G. L. Shelton (Eds.). Philadelphia: Hanley & Belfus, Inc., 2002.

ROBERTS, W. O. Exercise associated collapse in endurance events: a classification system. *Phys. Sportsmed.* 17:49–55, 1989.

ROBERTS, W. O. Mass-Participation Events. In: *Handbook of Sports Medicine, 2nd Edition*, W. A. Lillegard, J. D. Butcher, and K. S. Rucker (Eds.). Boston: Butterworth-Heinemann Publications, 1998, pp. 27–45.

ROBERTS, W. O. Medical management and administration for long distance road racing. In: *IAAF Medical Manuel for Athletics and Road Racing Competitions: A Practical Guide*, C. H. Brown and B. Gudjonsson (Eds.). Monaco: International Amateur Athletic Federation, 1998.

SPEEDY, D. B., T. D. NOAKES, N. E. KIMBER, et al. Fluid balance during and after an ironman triathlon. *Clin. J. Sports Med.* 11:44–50, 2001.

SPEEDY, D. B., T. D. NOAKES, and C. SCHNEIDER. Exercise-associated hyponatremia: a review. *Emerg. Med.* 13:17–27, 2001.

U.S. TENNIS ASSOCIATION. *Emergency Care Guidelines*. Key Biscayne, FL: USTA, 2004.

YOUNG, CC. Extreme sports: injuries and medical coverage. *Curr. Sports Med. Rep.* 1:306–311, 2002.

Sideline Preparedness for the Team Physician: A Consensus Statement

DEFINITION

Sideline preparedness is the identification of and planning for medical services to promote the safety of the athlete, to limit injury, and to provide medical care at the site of practice or competition.

GOAL

The safety and on-site medical care of the athlete is the goal of sideline preparedness.

To accomplish this goal, the team physician should be actively involved in developing an integrated medical system that includes the following:

- Preseason planning
- Game-day planning
- Postseason evaluation

SUMMARY

The objective of the Sideline Preparedness Statement is to provide physicians who are responsible for making decisions regarding the medical care of athletes with guidelines for identifying and planning for medical care and services at the site of practice or competition. It is not intended as a standard of care and should not be interpreted as such. The Sideline Preparedness Statement is only a guide, and as such, is of a general nature, consistent with the reasonable, objective practice of the health care professional. Individual treatment will turn on the specific facts and circumstances presented to the physician at the event. Adequate insurance should be in place to help protect the physician, the athlete, and the sponsoring organization.

The Sideline Preparedness Statement was developed by a collaboration of six major professional associations concerned about clinical sports medicine issues; they have committed to forming an ongoing project-based alliance to bring together sports medicine organizations to best serve active people and athletes. The organizations are: American Academy of Family Physicians, American Academy of Orthopaedic Surgeons, American College of Sports Medicine, American Medical Society for Sports Medicine, American Orthopaedic Society for Sports Medicine, and American Osteopathic Academy of Sports Medicine.

EXPERT PANEL

Stanley A. Herring, M.D., Chair, Seattle, Washington
John Bergfeld, M.D., Cleveland, Ohio
Joel Boyd, M.D., Edina, Minnesota
Per Gunnar Brolinson, D.O., Toledo, Ohio
Timothy Duffey, D.O., Columbus, Ohio
David Glover, M.D., Warrensburg, Missouri
William A. Grana, M.D., Oklahoma City, Oklahoma
Brian C. Halpern, M.D., Marlboro, New Jersey
Peter Indelicato, M.D., Gainesville, Florida
W. Ben Kibler, M.D., Lexington, Kentucky
E. Lee Rice, D.O., San Diego, California
William O. Roberts, M.D., White Bear Lake, Minnesota

PRESEASON PLANNING

Preseason planning promotes safety and minimizes problems associated with athletic participation at the site of practice or competition.

The team physician should coordinate:

- Development of policy to address preseason planning and the preparticipation evaluation of athletes
- Participation of the administration and other key personnel in medical issues
- Implementation strategies

Medical Protocol Development

It is essential that:

- Prospective athletes complete a preparticipation evaluation

In addition, it is desirable that:

- The preparticipation evaluation be performed by an M.D. or D.O. in good standing with an unrestricted license to practice medicine
- A comprehensive preparticipation evaluation form be used (*e.g.*, the form may be found in *Preparticipation Physical Evaluation, 2nd edition*. New York: McGraw Hill Publishing, 1997.)
- The team physician has access to all preparticipation evaluation forms
- The team physician review all preparticipation evaluation forms and determine eligibility of the athlete to participate
- Timely preparticipation evaluations be performed to permit the identification and treatment of injuries and medical conditions

Administrative Protocol Development

It is essential for the team physician to coordinate:

- Development of a chain of command that establishes and defines the responsibilities of all parties involved
- Establishment of an emergency response plan for practice and competition
- Compliance with Occupational Safety and Health Administration (OSHA) standards relevant to the medical care of the athlete
- Establishment of a policy to assess environmental concerns and playing conditions for modification or suspension of practice or competition

- Compliance with all local, state and federal regulations regarding storing and dispensing pharmaceuticals
- Establishment of a plan to provide for proper documentation and medical record keeping

In addition, it is desirable for the team physician to coordinate:

- Regular rehearsal of the emergency response plan
- Establishment of a network with other health care providers, including medical specialists, athletic trainers and allied health professionals
- Establishment of a policy that includes the team physician in the dissemination of any information regarding the athlete's health
- Preparation of a letter of understanding between the team physician and the administration that defines the obligations and responsibilities of the team physician

GAME-DAY PLANNING

Game-day planning optimizes medical care for injured or ill athletes.

The team physician should coordinate:

- Game-day medical operations
- Game-day administrative medical policies
- Preparation of the sideline medical bag and sideline medical supplies

Medical Protocol

It is essential for the team physician to coordinate:

- Determination of final clearance status of injured or ill athletes on game day before competition
- Assessment and management of game-day injuries and medical problems
- Determination of athletes' same-game return to participation after injury or illness
- Follow-up care and instructions for athletes who require treatment during or after competition
- Notifying the appropriate parties about an athlete's injury or illness
- Close observation of the game by the medical team from an appropriate location
- Provision for proper documentation and medical record keeping

In addition, is it desirable for the team physician to coordinate:

- Monitoring of equipment safety and fit
- Monitoring of postgame referral care of injured or ill athletes

Administrative Protocol

It is essential for the team physician to coordinate:

- Assessment of environmental concerns and playing conditions
- Presence of medical personnel at the competition site with sufficient time for all pregame preparations

- Plan with the medical staff of the opposing team for medical care of the athletes
- Introductions of the medical team to game officials
- Review of the emergency medical response plan
- Checking and confirmation of communication equipment
- Identification of examination and treatment sites

In addition, it is desirable for the team physician to coordinate:

- Arrangements for the medical staff to have convenient access to the competition site
- A postgame review and make necessary modifications in medical and administrative protocols

On-Site Medical Supplies

The team physician should have a game-day sideline medical bag and sideline medical supplies. Following are lists of medical bag items and medical supplies for contact/collision and high-risk sports.

It is highly desirable for the medical bag to include:

General

- Alcohol swabs and povidone iodine swabs
- Bandage scissors
- Bandages, sterile/nonsterile, Band-Aids
- D-50%-W
- Disinfectant
- Gloves, sterile/nonsterile
- Large bore angiocath for tension pneumothorax (14 to 16 gauge)
- Local anesthetic/syringes/needles
- Paper
- Pen
- Sharps box and red bag
- Suture set/steri-strips
- Wound irrigation materials (*e.g.*, sterile normal saline, 10- to 50-cc syringe)

Cardiopulmonary

- Airway
- Blood pressure cuff
- Cricothyrotomy kit
- Epinephrine 1:1000 in a prepackaged unit
- Mouth-to-mouth mask
- Short-acting beta agonist inhaler
- Stethoscope

Head and Neck/Neurologic

- Dental kit (*e.g.*, cyanoacrylate, Hank's solution)
- Eye kit (*e.g.*, blue light, fluorescein stain strips, eye patch pads, cotton tip applicators, ocular anesthetic and antibiotics, contact remover, mirror)
- Flashlight
- Pin or other sharp object for sensory testing
- Reflex hammer

It is highly desirable for sideline medical supplies to include:

General

- Access to a telephone
- Extremity splints
- Ice
- Oral fluid replacement
- Plastic bags
- Sling

Head and Neck/Neurologic

- Face mask removal tool (for sports with helmets)
- Semirigid cervical collar
- Spine board and attachments

In addition, it is desirable for the medical bag to include:

General

- Benzoin
- Blister care materials
- Contact lens case and solution
- % Ferric subsulfate solution (*e.g.*, Monsel's for cauterizing abrasions and cuts)
- Injury and illness care instruction sheets for the patient
- List of emergency phone numbers
- Nail clippers
- Nasal packing material
- Oto-ophthalmoscope
- Paper bags for treatment of hyperventilation
- Prescription pad
- Razor and shaving cream
- Rectal thermometer
- Scalpel
- Skin lubricant
- Skin staple applicator
- Small mirror
- Supplemental oral and parenteral medications
- Tongue depressors
- Topical antibiotics

Cardiopulmonary

- Advanced Cardiac Life Support (ACLS) drugs and equipment
- I.V. fluids and administration set
- Tourniquet

In addition, it is desirable for sideline medical supplies to include the following:

General

- Blanket
- Crutches
- Mouth guards
- Sling psychrometer and temperature/humidity activity risk chart
- Tape cutter

Cardiopulmonary

- Automated external defibrillator

Head and Neck/Neurologic

- A sideline concussion assessment protocol

There are many different sports, levels of competition, and available medical resources that must all be considered when determining the on-site medical bag and sideline medical supplies.

POSTSEASON EVALUATION

Postseason evaluation of sideline coverage optimizes the medical care of injured or ill athletes and promotes continued improvement of medical services for future seasons.

The team physician should coordinate:

- Summarization of injuries and illnesses that occurred during the season
- Improvement of the medical and administrative protocols
- Implementation strategies to improve sideline preparedness

Medical Protocol

It is essential for the team physician to coordinate:

- Postseason meeting with appropriate team personnel and administration to review the previous season
- Identification of athletes who require postseason care of injury or illness and encourage followup

In addition, it is desirable for the team physician to coordinate the following:

- Monitoring of the health status of the injured or ill athlete
- Postseason physicals
- Off-season conditioning program

Administrative Protocol

It is essential for the team physician to coordinate:

- Review and modification of current medical and administrative protocols

In addition, it is desirable for the team physician to coordinate:

- Compilation of injury and illness data

CONCLUSION

This Consensus Statement outlines the essential and desirable components of sideline preparedness for the team physician to promote the safety of the athlete, to limit injury, and to provide medical care at the site of practice or competition. This statement was developed by the collaboration of six major professional associations concerned about clinical sports medicine issues: American Academy of Family

Physicians, American Academy of Orthopaedic Surgeons, American College of Sports Medicine, American Medical Society for Sports Medicine, American Orthopaedic Society for Sports Medicine, and American Osteopathic Academy of Sports Medicine.

Ongoing education pertinent to the team physician is essential. Information regarding team physician specific educational opportunities can be obtained from the six participating organizations:

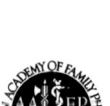

- American Academy of Family Physicians
  11400 Tomahawk Creek Pkwy.
  Leawood, KS 66211-2672
  1-800-274-2237
  www.aafp.org

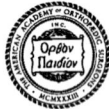

- American Academy of Orthopaedic Surgeons
  6300 N. River Rd.
  Rosemont, IL 60018
  1-800-346-AAOS
  www.aaos.org

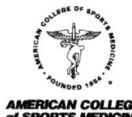

- American College of Sports Medicine
  401 W. Michigan St.
  Indianapolis, IN 46202
  (317) 637-9200
  www.acsm.org

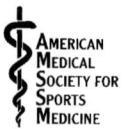

- American Medical Society for Sports Medicine
  11639 Earnshaw
  Overland Park, KS 66210
  (913) 327-1415
  www.amssm.org

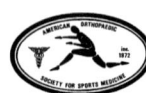

- American Orthopaedic Society for Sports Medicine
  6300 N. River Rd., Ste. 200
  Rosemont, IL 60018
  (847) 292-4900
  www.sportsmed.org

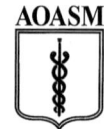

- American Osteopathic Academy of Sports Medicine
  7611 Elmwood Ave., Ste. 201
  Middleton, WI 53562
  (608) 831-4400
  www.aoasm.org

Medical Services Planning at Smaller Sports Events

Contributed by David McDonagh, Deputy CMO, Lillehammer 1994 Olympic Winter Games

Reviewer: Mike Wilkinson, Deputy CMO, Vancouver 2010 Winter Olympic Games, Canada

2.1 TIMING

For smaller events, it is preferable to book medical/ambulance staff at least 3 months before the event. It is not always easy to find an EP, and most physicians are busy people, so preemptive planning is always wise. Similarly, ambulance services should be planned well in advance to ensure availability and to prepare budget costs.

2.2 MEDICAL STAFF

The amount of staff required can vary from event to event. Sometimes the EP is alone, sometimes accompanied by some first aid responders, and sometimes with one or two ambulances and paramedics. There are many factors that affect the numbers of personnel to be employed: tradition, economy, availability, and not least local, national, and international regulations.

Smaller events require less planning and organization but are often more demanding on the EP if a medical situation arises.

2.3 NUMBER OF AMBULANCES/ PARAMEDICS/PHYSICIANS

Many sports today require two ambulances to be present at televised sporting events—either due to the fact that many athletes are participating in high-velocity sports and that there is a risk of multiple injuries or due to the fact that the departure of an ambulance from the track may compromise national or international regulations and thus oblige the event organizer to stop the event.

A motorized buggy for athlete transport from the field can be useful, particularly when treating spinal or cardiac patients.

Also, services are often required by law and services must be sufficient to treat spectators needs.

Number of Paramedics

As a rule, two paramedics per ambulance are preferable: One to drive and one to assist the EP or monitor the patient under transport. One of the paramedics should at least be able to administer oxygen via a mask from a tank and be competent in fracture immobilization and wound care.

Number of Physicians

At most smaller events, one physician and one staffed ambulance will usually suffice. When crowds are larger than 2,000–3,000 spectators, then one may have to consider the need for providing spectator medical services. International Federations seldom make specific demands regarding the need for spectator medical services but usually expect these services to be available at international events. For more local events, local traditions and practices should be followed. Again, the more competent the paramedics, the less the need for physicians, though physicians should always be present when there are large crowds or physically demanding contact sports.

Factors that influence medical staffing numbers:

- High-velocity/low-velocity sport
- On land or on water

- Sports with frequent/dangerous injuries
- Size of arena
- Track distance: Marathon, cross-country skiing, etc.
- Federation rules
- IOC rules
- Tradition
- National regulations
- Number of spectators

2.4 FOR HOW LONG SHOULD MEDICAL SERVICES BE AVAILABLE?

For smaller events, it is usually sufficient for the EP and paramedics to be present 30 minutes to 60 minutes before the start of the event.

2.5 CHECKLIST: ONE WEEK (OR MORE) BEFORE EVENT START

- Check your doctor's bag for medications (outdated?), bandages, bulbs. Order new materials.
- Telephone numbers: Event organizer, ambulance service, local hospital, helicopter
- Inform organizers of need for radios and telephones.
- Medical room inspection to discover what equipment is available.
- Site inspection: Where to place ambulance, evacuation routes, etc.

2.6 CHECKLIST: ON THE EVENT DAY

- Check your doctor's bag before leaving home for medications (cold medications in the fridge?). It is always a good idea to check ophthalmoscope/otoscope/laryngoscope batteries/bulbs the day before. Charge up your cell phone.
- Remember telephone lists.
- Collect and check radios, if available at venue.
- With the radio functioning, inform the event manager of your arrival and confirm the presence of the ambulance/paramedics.

- Final inspection of medical room, ambulance, oxygen tanks.
- Site inspection: Confirm ambulance placement, evacuation routes, etc.

As you can see, there is quite a checklist to be completed here, so 30 minutes offers too little time for the perfectionist. An hour is more appropriate. If one spends a little time in preparation before the event, one can avoid a lot of stress and unnecessary delays during an emergency treatment.

2.7 ROOM EQUIPMENT

See Chapter 74.

2.8 PERSONNEL EQUIPMENT

See Chapter 74.

2.9 ACSM—SIDELINE PREPAREDNESS FOR THE TEAM PHYSICIAN: A CONSENSUS STATEMENT

The ACSM consensus statement addresses "game-day" planning tasks for the team physician and gives a full list of necessary tasks that need to be completed. However, without being a semantic pedant, the ACSM uses the term *team physician* as an all-encompassing title, and it is obvious that a physician who works with a team cannot take responsibility for other athletes, spectators, etc. So, there is a need for clarification of medical responsibilities and titles that reflect these responsibilities.

In the "ACSM:Sideline Preparedness for the Team Physician: A Consensus Statement," the following tasks are listed.

The team physician should coordinate:

- Game-day medical operations
- Game-day administrative medical policies
- Preparation of the sideline medical bag and sideline medical supplies

Medical Protocol

It is essential for the team physician to coordinate:

- Determination of final clearance status of injured or ill athletes on game day before competition

- Assessment and management of game-day injuries and medical problems
- Determination of athletes' same-game return to participation after injury or illness
- Follow-up care and instructions for athletes who require treatment during or after competition
- Notifying the appropriate parties about an athlete's injury or illness
- Close observation of the game by the medical team from an appropriate location
- Provision for proper documentation and medical record keeping

In addition, is it desirable for the team physician to coordinate:

- Monitoring of equipment safety and fit
- Monitoring of postgame referral care of injured or ill athletes

Administrative Protocol

It is essential for the team physician to coordinate:

- Assessment of environmental concerns and playing conditions

- Presence of medical personnel at the competition site with sufficient time for all pregame preparations
- Plan with the medical staff of the opposing team for medical care of the athletes
- Introductions of the medical team to game officials
- Review of the emergency medical response plan
- Checking and confirmation of communication equipment
- Identification of examination and treatment sites

In addition, it is desirable for the team physician to coordinate:

- Arrangements for the medical staff to have convenient access to the competition site
- A postgame review and make necessary modifications in medical and administrative protocols

On-site Medical Supplies

- The team physician should have a game-day sideline medical bag and sideline medical supplies.

CHAPTER **3**

Contributed by Demetrios G. Pyrros, President, World Association for Disaster and Emergency Medicine (WADEM); Deputy CMO, Athens 2004 Summer Olympic Games, Greece

Reviewers: David McDonagh, Deputy CMO, Lillehammer 1994 Olympic Winter Games; and Mike Wilkinson, Deputy CMO, Vancouver 2010 Winter Olympic Games, Canada

Disaster/Major Incident Planning

There are more than 45 definitions of the term *disaster*, and even the term itself is not generally accepted since some authors in the literature prefer to use the terms *major incident, multiple casualty emergency, mass casualty incident, mass casualty event,* or *complex emergency.* There are also at least four definitions of *disaster medicine* widely used. We should therefore just remember that disaster medicine is the medical response when the needs for acute medical care exceed the immediately available resources.

Disaster medical planning for a sport event should be understood as the preparations and measures that need to be put in place in order to be able to respond to the medical needs of the sick and injured at the event should a disaster strike.

Disasters are usually divided in three large categories:

- Natural or environmental
  - Weather (i.e., extreme heat/cold/rain)
  - Earthquake
- Technological or man-made
  - Structural failure
  - Fireworks
  - Power failure
  - Hazardous materials (HAZMAT)
- Sociologic or man-conceived
  - Disorder (including alcohol or drugs)
  - Hooliganism
  - Terrorism

Disaster medical planning is a crucial aspect of the overall medical plan for any large sport event and the Event Physician (EP) should never neglect to address the issue. Having stated this, it should be very clear that the EP is not expected to be an expert in disaster medicine or play a leading role in the overall disaster planning.

What is expected though is that he or she should have basic knowledge about the issues involved and ensure that disaster medicine professionals are included in all phases of the disaster planning, as well as in the immediate response to any eventuality. In most cases, disaster medical planning should fall under the responsibility of local, provincial, or state health authorities that deal with medical emergencies on a daily basis, and the EP must ensure that the sport event plan is fully integrated into the overall disaster plan.

The EP should therefore have the following agendas regarding timeframes:

- *Before*: Always be part of the disaster planning process in order to contribute valuable knowledge about the sport, its rules, and other relevant sports medical information that other emergency responders may lack. Being a part of the process keeps one familiar with the overall disaster plan.

- *During*: Be an integral part of the coordination mechanism that will be in place for the event and maintain contact with the coordination heads of the other emergency services. It is crucial that the EP is linked to the operations network of the sport event at all times.

- *After*: Perform a critical review of the sports medical aspects and share this experience with all active participants in the disaster plan group.
- *Always*: Participate in the education of all stakeholders of the disaster plan group regarding the medical aspects of any sport event.

3.1 BEFORE

The *before* stage of any disaster plan can be further defined by

- Anticipation: Risk assessment
- Prevention: Actions to counter the results of the risk assessment
- Preparedness: Measures to respond to the residual risk (i.e., the risk that remains after prevention measures have been in place)

Risk assessment is usually analyzed in five steps:

- Look for the hazards (i.e., anything that can cause harm).
- Decide who can be harmed and how.
- Evaluate the risks (i.e., the chance, high or low, that somebody will be harmed by the hazard) and decide whether existing precautions are adequate or whether more should be done.
- Record your findings.
- Review your assessment and revise it if necessary.

Important factors to remember should include the following:

- Profile of the audience (e.g., number of persons, age groups, persons with special needs)
- Profile of the expected behavior of audience
- Profile of the sport hazards and risks
- Profile of the sport venue (e.g., open or closed structure, seating arrangements and number of exits, access of rescue vehicles)

Therefore, the EP should make sure that an overall all-hazards disaster plan from relevant and competent authorities (police, fire, and ambulance) is in place and that it includes a medical disaster plan with which he or she is fully familiar. The medical disaster plan should also include responses to the following issues:

- Activation of the medical response
- On-site organization
- Management of outside resources responding to disaster
- Evacuation of patients to health facilities

Obviously, the scale and magnitude of the sport event dictates the detail and complexity of such plans.

3.2 DURING

During the sports event, the EP should be in direct contact with the event coordination/command post either through a medical team representative or via direct communication (preferably radio, not mobile phone as the network may be down) in order to be informed of all events as they unfold and to be able to initiate a medical response as soon as possible.

The sports event venue is usually divided into two separate zones. The first zone is that which athletes, referees, officials, and support personnel utilize including the field of play (also referred to as *back of house*) while the second zone includes the spectator areas (the *front of house*). Depending on the event security measures, these two zones can be completely separate or loosely defined. It is the responsibility of the EP to ensure that medical personnel have unhindered access to both zones, especially if disaster strikes irrespective of the security measures in force.

The EP should be fully familiar with the venue location layout well in advance of the event. On the day of the event, he or she should ensure that the dedicated ambulance entry/exit points are not used for other purposes, blocked, or otherwise utilized and that free passage for a stretcher or a wheelchair is secured.

If disaster strikes, the EP should first ensure the safety and security of the medical personnel and should never initiate any medical response before competent authorities (in most cases, the police or fire brigade) allow entrance to the disaster-stricken area.

Another important item for immediate consideration is the delayed start, postponement, or abandonment of the event.

A medical care post should be established as soon as possible and as close to the disaster site as possible and all medical personnel from other medical posts should congregate there. Patient treatment should be based on the three Ts of medical disaster response:

- TRIAGE (sorting of patients) (Fig. 3.1).

- TREATMENT (lifesaving procedures and stabilization)

- TRANSPORT (to the nearest appropriate medical facility)

The Advanced Trauma Life Support Course (ATLS) from the Committee on Trauma of the American College of Surgeons defines triage as the "sorting of patients based on the need for treatment and the available resources to provide that treatment." The patients are usually divided in four color-coded categories:

- *Red*—patients in need of immediate treatment: A, B, or C is compromised

- *Yellow*—patients for whom treatment can wait: A, B, or C has been or can be compromised

- *Green*—ambulatory patients for whom treatment must wait: A, B, or C has not been and is not compromised

- *Black*—when the person is either dead or injured beyond salvation

A marker, usually in the form of triage tags or color tape, should be available to be placed on patients to identify their triage category. It is also helpful to have a numbering system for each color due to potential confusion with color-blind volunteers. It cannot be overly emphasized that triage is a dynamic process and patients should be retriaged at intervals as their medical condition may change.

Triaged patients should undergo treatment for lifesaving procedures and stabilization, remembering that ABC (A = airway, B = breathing, C = circulation) priorities apply to both injuries and illnesses alike. Follow accepted algorithms for treatment.

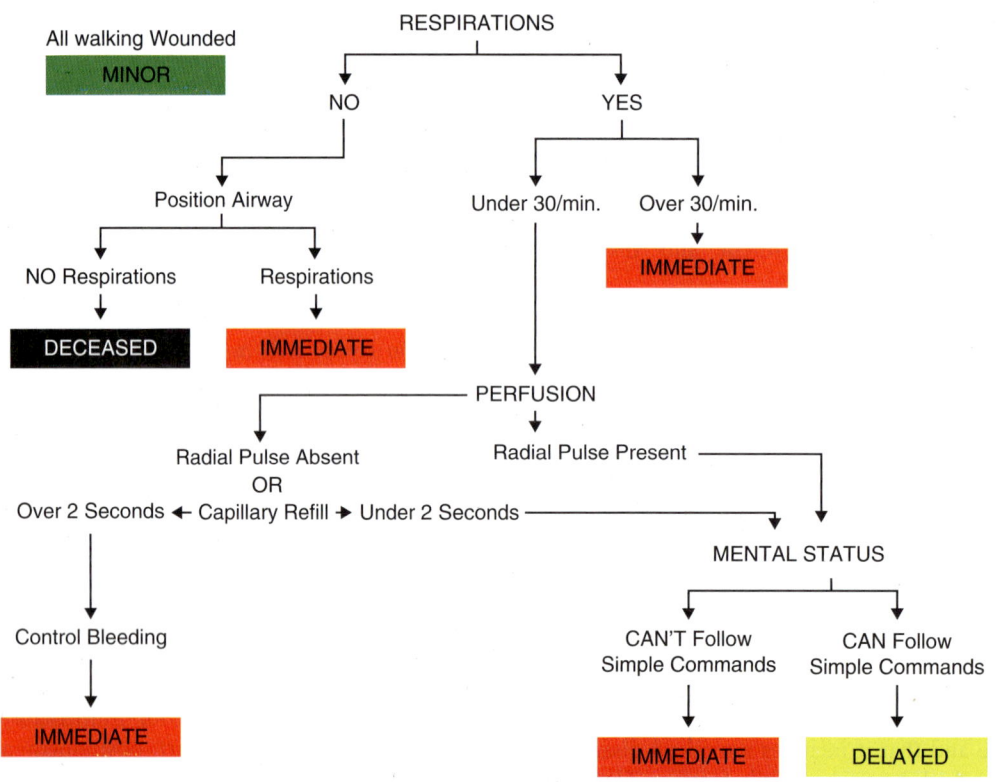

FIGURE 3.1. Detailed flowchart. (This diagram was created using copyrighted material developed by Newport Beach Fire Department. Used with permission.)

Finally, following treatment, patients should be retriaged based on their transportation priorities.

There are two rules that apply for transporting disaster victims:

- Transport each patient to the closest most appropriate facility able to treat all the patient's medical problems.

- Do not transport *all* patients from the disaster scene to *one* single hospital, as that would turn that hospital into a *disaster* site.

3.3 AFTER

Once all patients have been evacuated out of the venue, consider the need for psychiatric or psychological care for the responders, victims' relatives, and disaster witnesses.

Remember that the scene of the disaster event may also be a crime scene. Deceased patients should be covered with a blanket or a sheet of sorts. Without interfering with lifesaving treatment, which clearly takes precedence at all times, try to preserve the scene and evidence as much as possible.

In the following days, perform a critical medical review of the sport event. If the event was incident free, try to imagine what the response would have been had there been a large-scale incident. Share this knowledge with all active participants of the disaster plan group.

3.4 MEDIA

During a major incident, refer all press and media approaches to the police spokesperson. You have other things to do.

3.5 ALWAYS

The planning and execution of a disaster response should always be a team effort. Police, in most instances and in most countries, have the overall responsibility in dealing with disasters. The fire department may have the overall responsibility in fire incidents. Ambulance personnel have often been in situations where triage and rapid transport is required. The civil protection or civil defense entity in your country might also have a say in the disaster plan. Preevent cooperation with your emergency services partners will be a valuable plus should disaster strike. Remember to make available your sports medical expertise and endeavor to transfer your knowledge to all members of the disaster plan group.

Recommended Reading

American College of Surgeons, Committee on Trauma. *Advanced Trauma Life Support "ATLS®" Instructor Course Manual*. 6th ed. Chicago, IL: ACS; 1997. http://www.facs.org/trauma/atls/program.html. Accessed March 24, 2011.

de Boer J, Dubouloz M. *Handbook of Disaster Medicine*. Utrecht, The Netherlands: VSP; 2000.

Debacker M, Domres B, de Boer J. Glossary of new concepts in disaster medicine: a supplement to Gunn's, Multilingual Dictionary of Disaster Medicine. *Prehosp Disaster Med*. 1999;14(3):146–149.

Great Britain, Home Office. *Guide to Safety at Sports Grounds*. 4th ed. London, UK: The Stationery Office; 1999.

Gunn SWA. *Multilingual Dictionary of Disaster Medicine and International Relief*. Boston, MA: Kluwer Academic Publishers; 1990.

Pyrros DG. The Current State of Affairs Regarding Triage Tags in the European Union [EMDM thesis]. Republic of San Marino: European Centre for Disaster Medicine; Novara, Italy: University of Eastern Piedmont "Amedeo Avogardo"; and Leuven, Belgium: Catholic University of Leuven; 2001. Available at: http://ec.europa.eu/environment/civil/prote/pdfdocs/disaster_med_final_2002/d8.pdf. Accessed March 24, 2011.

Tsouros AD, Efstathiou PA. *Mass Gatherings and Public Health*. Copenhagen, Denmark: WHO Europe; 2007.

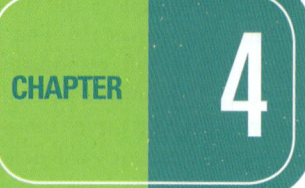

CHAPTER 4

Triage and Mass Casualty Incidents

Contributed by David McDonagh, Deputy CMO, Lillehammer 1994 Olympic Winter Games

Reviewers: Demetrios G. Pyrros, President, WADEM, Deputy CMO, Athens 2004 Olympic Summer Games; Mike Wilkinson, Deputy CMO, Vancouver 2010 Winter Olympic Games, Canada; and Johan Arnt Hegvik, NTNU, Trondheim, Norway

On rare occasions, mass casualty incidents at a sports event may unfortunately occur. On such occasions, the EP will be expected to participate in the rescue work and join in, or even initially lead, the rescue program. Such mass casualty events are unfortunately not uncommon and have usually occurred at large football stadia.

The cause of these events has almost always been twofold: an initial incident—a fight, panic, fire, structural collapse, etc.—followed by a stampede, resulting in spectators being crushed and trampled to death. Below is a list of some of the incidents that have befallen soccer stadia around the world.

- 1982, Moscow: 340 killed, Spartak Moscow versus Haarlem, police push fans down a narrow, icy staircase; late goal scored, fans reenter

- 1985, Bradford, England: 56 killed, cigarette stub ignites stadium's wooden terrace

- 1985, Brussels, Belgium: 39 killed, Heysel Stadium, riot and wall collapse

- 1987, Tripoli, Libya: 20 killed, panic after knife attack, wall collapse

- 1988, Katmandu, Nepal: 93 killed, 100 injured, hailstorm, stampede

- 1989, Sheffield, England: 95 killed, crush outside ground; police open gates to a full stadium, crush

- 1991, Orkney, South Africa: 40 killed, fight, panic, trampled or crushed along fences

- 1992, Bastia, Corsica: 17 killed, 1,900 injured, temporary grandstand collapse

- 1996, Lusaka, Zambia: 9 crushed, 78 injured, stampede

- 1996, Tripoli, Libya: 50 killed, riot

- 1996, Guatemala City, Guatamala: 78 killed, 180 injured, stampede

- 2000, Monrovia, Liberia: 3 killed, fans forced into an overcrowded stadium

- 2000, Harare, Zimbabwe: 12 killed, stampede; World Cup qualifier, South Africa versus Zimbabwe

- 2001, Johannesburg, South Africa: 43 killed, too many people turned up, entry stampede

- 2001, Lubumbashi, Congo: 8 killed, stampede

- 2001, Mazandaran, Iran: 3 killed, hundreds injured, roof collapse

- 2001, Ivory Coast: 1 killed, 39 injured, fight

- 2001, Accra, Ghana: 100 killed, riot, police fired tear gas, panic and stampede

- 2009, Ivory Coast: 22 killed, crowd turned up without tickets, push and crush injuries

As you can see, this is a long list. There is not a lot a physician can do to prevent such tragedies, but it is essential that the leading venue medical officer participates in meetings with other venue leaders when discussing and planning disaster medical plans. Prevention lies in the hands of the event organizers—in particular, security and police. Many things have improved over the years regarding stadium safety. All-seating stadia have become the norm. New stadia tend to have wider exits. Fencing has been removed from around the pitch so that spectators can spillover onto the field of play if necessary. Alcohol restrictions are common. Security staff are now more prevalent and police are more aware of the potential dangers.

Another issue is that of issuing prematch tickets. At the 2001 Kaizer Chiefs versus Orlando Pirates annual soccer derby game in Johannesburg, tickets could be purchased at the stadium. This resulted in a huge crowd descending on the stadium—far larger than the arena had capacity to accommodate. A wild rush for tickets ensued, resulting in the death of 43 people, including some children.

Death in such events is caused by being knocked over and trampled upon, and then subsequently being crushed under other bodies. Spectators may also be crushed up against walls or fences. The actual cause of death is usually asphyxiation, but head and neck injuries, thorax injuries, and even pelvic injuries have been seen.

4.1 TRIAGE

Step 1—WALKING

In such a situation, where there are multiple injuries but limited medical staff, priorities will have to be made. The primary goal is to identify those with life-threatening injuries and to offer them appropriate treatment. One should not attempt to resuscitate patients who are obviously dead. Neither should one use time on treating non–life-threatening conditions, at least not until a later time when it is more appropriate to do so. The goal is to save lives. In order to achieve this, a system for categorizing injury severity must be created—a triage must be conducted. On receiving information from the police that it is safe to enter the incident area, the initial medical responder enters the area, identifies himself or herself, and instructs all patients who can walk to leave the accident site and to gather and remain in a safe place (Fig. 4.1). These patients will be marked with green cards

and should be retriaged later, after more critical patients have been treated.

The initial responder briefly examines all patients not able to walk away from the accident scene. The physician should not use more than 30 seconds per patient. Patients have been traditionally classified into four groups:

1. *Red*—patients in need of immediate treatment: *A, B, or C is compromised.* Red tags should be used to label those who cannot survive without immediate treatment but still have a chance of surviving.

2. *Yellow*—patients for whom treatment can wait: *A, B, or C has been or can be compromised.* These patients may have serious injuries but are not in need of immediate lifesaving treatment. Their condition is stable for the moment and they can, or must, wait for treatment. Most of this group will still need hospitalization and would have been transferred immediately under less abnormal circumstances.

3. *Green*—ambulatory patients for whom treatment must wait: *A, B, or C has not been and is not compromised.* These are the "walking wounded" who will need medical attention at some point when other more critical patients have been treated and dispatched.

4. *Black*—when the person is either dead or injured beyond salvation.

Having thus classified patients, a color-coded card is placed on each individual (Fig. 4.2), which allows

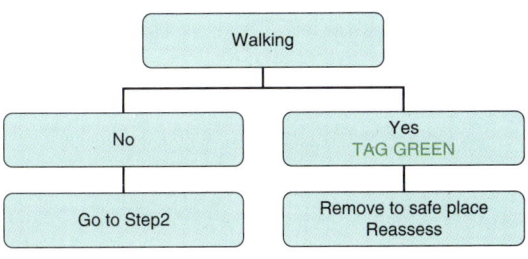

FIGURE 4.1. Step 1—Walking.

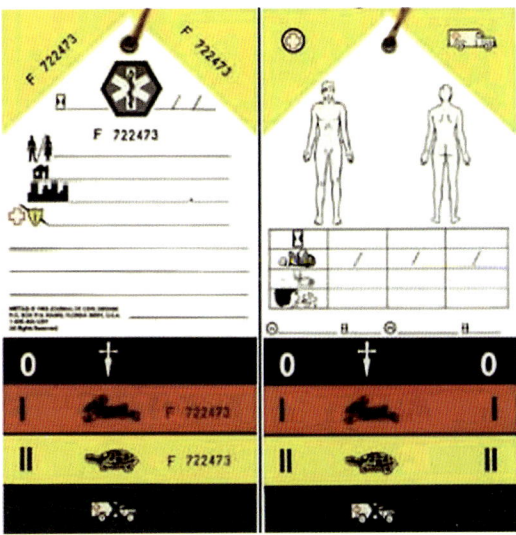

FIGURE 4.2. One of the commonly used triage tags.

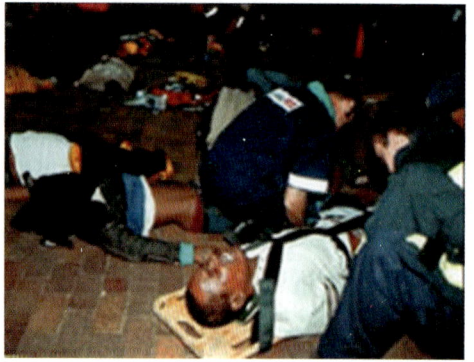

FIGURE 4.3. Victims from the Ellis Park disaster, Johannesburg, 2001, 43 people killed.

other medical staff to prioritize treatment according to color of the tag. As mentioned previously, there are several ways to conduct a triage, the most accepted being that of ATLS from the American College of Surgeons.

Evaluate nonambulatory patients where they are lying (Fig. 4.3).

Step 2—RESPIRATION

Are respirations normal, rapid, or absent?

If absent, reposition airway to see if breathing begins.

If respirations remain absent, tag BLACK. Do not perform CPR.

If the patient requires help maintaining an open airway or has a respiratory rate <8 or >30 rpm, tag

RED (attempt to use bystanders to hold position of the airway). Fix A before going on to B!

If respirations are normal >8 or <30 rpm, go to the next step (Fig. 4.4).

Step 3—CIRCULATION

Assess patient's circulation by palpating a radial pulse or carotid pulse. If the radial pulse is absent or difficult to find, palpate the carotid artery, being careful not to disturb a potentially injured neck. If there is still absent pulse, look for external bleeding, apply compression, and tag RED.

If radial pulse or carotid pulse is present, go to the next step, Step 4.

Any life-threatening bleeding should be controlled now (utilize nonmedical personnel for to hold pressure/bleeding control). In the presence of a grossly dislocated fracture, reduction may reduce bleeding (Fig. 4.5).

Step 4—MENTAL STATUS

Now assess the patient's mental status.

If the patient cannot follow simple commands, ask him or her to perform a simple task.

If patient cannot follow simple commands, then tag YELLOW.

If patient can follow simple commands, tag the patient YELLOW or GREEN depending on the condition (injuries will determine the priority

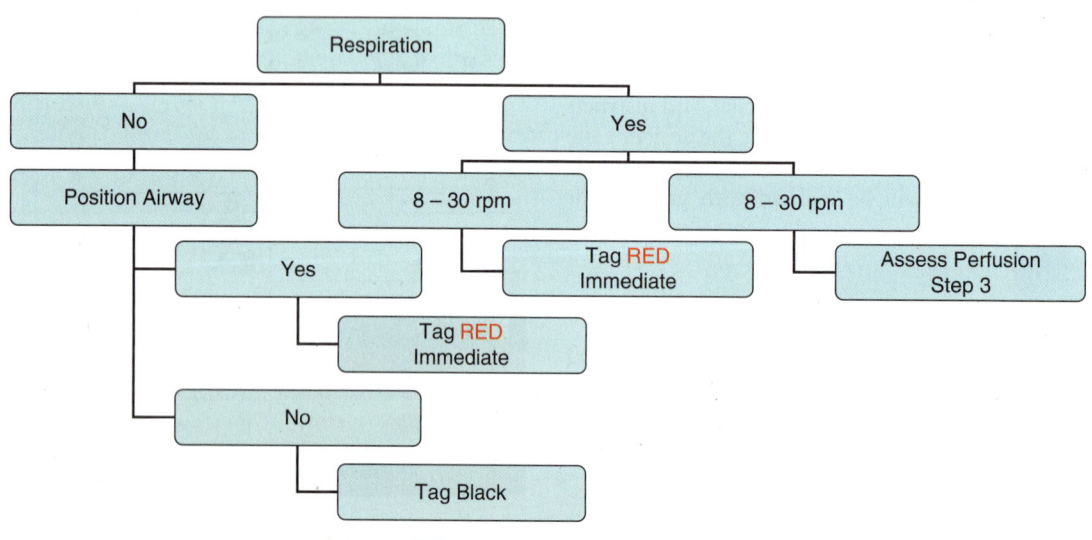

FIGURE 4.4. Step 2—Respiration.

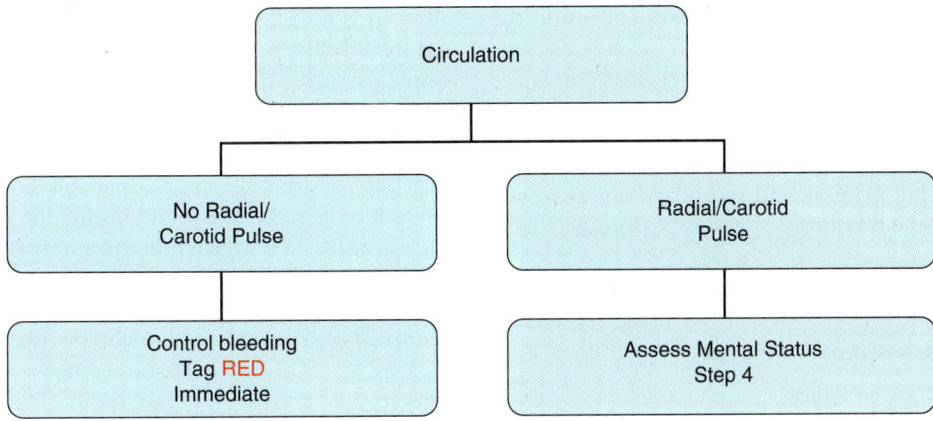

FIGURE 4.5. Step 3—Perfusion.

of yellow vs. green, i.e., multiple fractures would require a higher level of treatment than superficial lacerations) (Fig. 4.6).

Once this initial triage has been completed, the initial responder may choose to retriage the patients depending on the level of support that has arrived. By the time the initial triage has been completed, or whilst it is taking place, medical staff will have usually arrived and will usually have begun to treat the red-tagged patients. On completion of the primary triage, the initial responder should make a report to the police and the incident medical officer regarding the number of injured—*x* red, *y* yellow, *z* green, etc.—so that a decision can be made regarding the need to import further external medical resources as well as the need for patient transport. The medical disaster plan, which should be in place, must then be followed. If the initial responder is still alone and no other help has arrived, he or she should then set about treating the red-tagged patients most in need of immediate lifesaving treatment and most likely to survive. Try to treat as many patients as possible, concentrating only on airways, breathing, circulation, and cervical immobilization.

All patients must be reassessed often, as patients may suddenly deteriorate.

Do not begin a secondary survey on a patient if other red-tagged patients need basic ABC. Remember that the goal is to save as many lives as possible using whatever means are available.

The medical staff that arrives should treat red-tagged patients first, based on the following principles:

- Primary survey—based on ABCDE, followed by resuscitation
- Secondary survey
- Stabilization
- Transfer
- Definitive care

It is important to start resuscitation at the same time as making the primary survey.

Do not start the secondary survey until you have completed the primary survey.

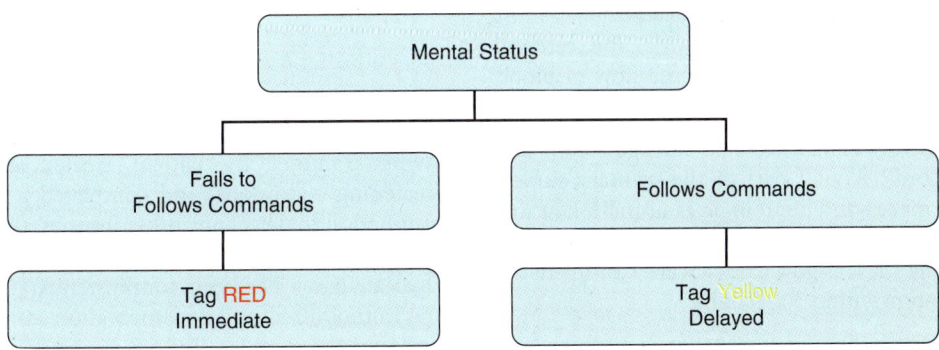

FIGURE 4.6. Step 4—Mental activity.

Do not start definitive treatment until the secondary survey is complete.

4.2 PRIMARY SURVEY

Make a full primary and secondary survey of any patient who is injured, especially patients who have

- Airway or respiratory distress
- Circulatory distress
- Glasgow Coma Scale < 13
- Penetrating injury
- >1 area injured

Or have a history of

- A fall > 3 m
- Net speed > 30 km per hour
- Thrown from a vehicle or trapped in a vehicle
- Pedestrian or cyclist hit by a car
- Been in an accident with fatality
- And/or on examination

ABCDE

A—Airway with cervical spine immobilization: The commonest cause of obstruction is when the patient is unconscious, in a supine position, when the tongue falls back, and the pharynx collapses. Other causes include neck trauma and foreign bodies. Remember to immobilize the cervical spine.

B—Breathing: May cease with severe head injury, hypoxia, mechanical, or circulatory arrest.

C—Circulation with major bleeding control: Common reasons for inadequate circulation include blood loss, pneumothorax, or hemopericardium. Shock and low blood pressure are particularly dangerous for all patients with head injury as this causes a vicious circle of hypoxia and cerebral edema, which, in turn, reduces the flow of blood to the brain.

D—Disability and neurologic damage (brain and spinal cord): A vital part of the primary survey. Do not make a full neurologic examination at this stage. Grade the patient's initial level of consciousness using the Glasgow Coma Scale. Complete the examination within 30 seconds.

E—Exposure: Remove the patient's clothing and examine the whole patient, front and back, but afterwards remember to cover the patient in order not to allow the patient to get cold. Examining the whole patient is the only way to be sure that you have not missed other injuries.

Immediately treat any life-threatening problems, such as obstructed airway, pneumothorax, or major bleeding, that are found during the primary survey—ABC. Less urgent problems, such as an arm fracture, must wait until the patient is stable; they will be picked up in the secondary survey and should be treated appropriately in the definitive care phase.

4.3 SECONDARY SURVEY

During the secondary survey, examine all systems and body parts, try to identify all injuries, and consider a treatment plan. Should there be any form of unexplained deterioration at any time, repeat the primary survey.
Examine:

- Thorax
- Abdomen
- Pelvis and limb injuries
- Head, neck, and spine
- Nervous system

After the secondary survey, document your findings as thoroughly as possible, including:

- Detailed history of the injury
- Previous medical history
- Medication
- Drug allergies
- Findings from primary and secondary survey:
- Results of any special investigations (e.g., glucose, urine)
- Details of treatment given and the patient's response

4.4 STABILIZATION

Having examined the patient, treated any life-threatening conditions, and completed a second examination to detect any other injuries, the management plan of the patient should now be clear. When analgesia has been administered, any fractures immobilized, and documentation completed, decide on the next level of treatment: Discharge, observe, or transfer to x-ray or hospital.

4.5 ESTABLISHING A TRIAGE AREA

Many books have been written on this topic and there are many variations from country to country, not to mention from civilian to military, and industry to industry. The principle of triage is to do the most good for most people. The triage site must be carefully chosen, so that injured victims can be removed to a safe but nearby place, where they can be registered, evaluated, sorted, treated, and eventually evacuated for further medical care. Obviously, ambulances should have access to this triage area.

Without going into great detail about the design of a triage area, it should contain

- An entrance area where patients are numbered

- A central sorting/treatment area where patients are triaged by color or tagged

- Four color zones: red zone, yellow zone, green zone, and black zone

- An exit area where a register is kept

- Ambulance zone, where exit victims are brought

4.6 TRANSFER

Decide the mode of transport and the level of priority transfer:

- Helicopter

- Ambulance with siren or without

- Level of ambulance care

- Taxi or other transport

Remember that the goal is to transport each patient to the nearest appropriate facility for the injuries and/or problems he or she is facing. Remember also not to export the disaster from the scene to the nearest hospital by transporting all or most patients to a single health facility.

Before referring a patient:

- Contact the referral center to ensure that they can help

- Anticipate what else may go wrong on the road and prepare

- Provide pain relief for the journey

- Arrange for a trained person to travel with the patient, if needed

- Red-tagged patients must be the first patients to be transferred

Before dispatching the patient, reassess both your primary survey and secondary survey in order to verify your triage categorization.

Try to assign the role of transportation officer to someone in order to keep a record of who is transported to which facility.

4.7 YELLOW-TAGGED PATIENTS

This group of patients may, in a worst-case scenario, all become red-tagged patients. By definition, they are seriously injured or ill patients, who do not require immediate lifesaving treatment. This group can include patients who have pneumothoraces, cerebral hematomas, internal bleeding, etc., and can at any time suffer respiratory or circulatory arrest. They should be continuously retriaged. Be prepared for an emergency intervention in this group. If you have responsibility for this group, ensure that all patients have free airways, that bleeding has been stopped and that circulation is being maintained.

4.8 GREEN-TAGGED PATIENTS

Once the critical patients have been transferred, it is now time to evaluate the "walking" green patients. Preferably, this group should have been retriaged on several occasions, as patients can, and often do, deteriorate. Go through a standard clinical examination to evaluate the need for further care. Discharge or refer these patients as appropriate. Consider the need for psychiatric or psychological care for responders, victims, relatives, and disaster witnesses. Designating someone (nonmedical) to be in charge of communication with relatives and walking wounded is helpful to keep patients flowing and to avoid chaos and congestion at the medical triage and stabilization area.

4.9 BLACK-TAGGED PATIENTS

Deceased patients should not be brought into the triage area. Patients who die in the triage area may be moved to the black zone. Do this when there is time or there are the resources to do so.

4.10 OTHER CONSIDERATIONS

Remember, a disaster scene may also be a crime scene, so without interfering with lifesaving treatment, try to preserve the scene and evidence as much as possible. Do not move the dead but do cover them.

Always consider the need for psychiatric or psychological care for responders, victims, relatives, and disaster witnesses.

4.11 REVIEW

Perform a critical medical review of the sport event. If the event was incident-free, imagine what the response would have been had there been a large-scale incident. Share this knowledge with all active participants of the disaster plan group.

CHAPTER 5

Ambulances

Contributed by David McDonagh, Deputy CMO, Lillehammer 1994 Olympic Winter Games

Reviewers: Johan A. Hegvik, Anesthetics Department, St. Olavs Hospital, Trondheim, Norway; and Mike Wilkinson, Deputy CMO, Vancouver 2010 Winter Olympic Games, Canada

There are many types of ambulances and not all are suited to the requirements of modern sports medical management. Organizers are often obliged by local municipal, national, international, IF, or IOC regulations to have one or more ambulances present at an event. Ambulance sophistication levels vary enormously, from complete mobile intensive care units to vans with seats. It is therefore a good idea for the event physician (EP) to check if the sporting federation has any special ambulance requirements regarding ambulance quality and then to check if the proposed ambulances meet these requirements. Should the ambulance not meet adequate quality requirements, then the EP should point this out to the event organizer. There are many types of ambulances and many ways to classify them.

- Emergency ambulances provide transport for patients with an acute illness or injury and have equipment onboard that allows one to conduct emergency lifesaving procedures.

- Mobile intensive care units are more sophisticated units containing equipment such as ventilators and are staffed by trained medical personnel.

- Patient transport ambulances are transport vehicles used for moving patients to, from, or between places of medical treatment, for nonurgent care. They usually have a limited amount of medical equipment onboard.

- Response unit is a vehicle containing advanced medical equipment (and often qualified medical staff) and is used to drive to the emergency site and provide on-site emergency care, but without the ability to transport the patient away from the scene. Response units may be backed up by an emergency ambulance or helicopter.

- Charity ambulance, a special type of patient transport ambulance, is provided by a charity for the purpose of taking sick children or adults on trips or vacations away from hospitals, hospices, or care homes where they are in long-term care.

All of these ambulances can be useful at a sports event; however, it is obvious that a patient transport ambulance alone is inadequate at a downhill skiing or diving event. Unscrupulous event managers may try to save expenses by hiring an elementary transport vehicle. If so, the onus then lies with the EP to demand a vehicle that allows for an appropriate level of care to be conducted. At the same time, it is often unnecessary to have a full mobile intensive care unit at every event. Hardly any of the International Sports Federations specify the standard of ambulance that should be present, so the potential for conflict between the EP and the event organizer is always present.

In Europe, ambulances have been classified by the CEN standard. In North America, the terms basic life support and advanced life support ambulances are used.

Ambulances can also be used as a warm-up location for both staff and patients. One has more privacy in an ambulance—if this is needed for "special situations."

Sirens and lights send two main messages: Here we are, and get out of our way. They are useful if there is heavy traffic, if there are unresponsive drivers in front of you, or if approaching traffic lights or entering areas with pedestrians, cyclists, etc. In an emergency situation, flashing lights can be used at all times, but sirens can be turned off if you are moving smoothly through the country-side or in low-traffic scenarios. There is no need to wake half the city at nighttime.

Reliable communication systems and equipment are essential in order to achieve safe and effective patient transfer and retrieval. Satellite navigation is great if available and affordable. Dedicated radio channels should be used.

Mobile phones are also useful and it is a good idea to have appropriate telephone numbers—hospital, ambulance, etc.—stored on the phone. The referring and retrieval physician should swap telephone numbers should there be a need to communicate at a later stage. Mobile phones must be properly charged.

One should try to develop a polite yet clear and concise communication style in order to optimize cooperation between various rescue personnel.

5.1 NUMBER OF AMBULANCES

Number of Ambulances: Many sports federations today require two ambulances to be present at televised sporting events, either due to the fact that many athletes are participating in high-velocity sports (most winter sports) and there is a risk of multiple injuries (e.g., bobsleigh, downhill skiing) or due to the fact that departure of an ambulance from the track may oblige the event organizer to stop the event due to Federation regulations.

A motorized buggy for athlete transport from the field can be useful, particularly when treating spinal or cardiac patients.

Also, services are often required for the spectators, as crowds can vary up to 100,000 people and more.

5.2 POSITIONING OF AMBULANCES

It is one thing to have ambulances present at a sporting event; it is another thing to position them correctly. It is usually pretty easy to decide on the positioning of ambulances at a stadium; the main concern is to ensure effective evacuation routes out of the stadium. This involves cooperation with police or traffic staff to ensure that a rapid departure from the arena is not hampered by large crowds of spectators and traffic. This usually works pretty well at the arena level, but problems often arise if the traffic outside the arena is heavily congested. Consider the use of helicopter transport, even in cities, if the patient is critically ill and if motorized transport will likely take longer than 30 minutes. At the Olympic Games, there are often accredited roads (to be used only by those with a special permit) that allow ambulances access to uncluttered roads.

At outdoor events that are spread over a large area—marathon, skiing, orienteering, cross-country running, equestrian events, etc.—it is not always easy to plan where ambulances should be positioned. It is important to have medical staff placed at sites along a course where injuries are to be expected (usually having had the experience of previous events) and to have that staff positioned so that injured or ill athletes can be reached in a relatively short period of time.

What is an acceptable period of time? It is impossible to give an answer to suit all scenarios, but it is obvious that staff should be present within minutes if an athlete is drowning. It is also obvious that you cannot cover the whole of the Paris-Dakar Rally and supply service within minutes.

The term "golden quarter" is still used by many in the emergency medical world and implies that emergency services must be able to arrive at a scene and initiate treatment within 15 minutes. This should, in my opinion, be the minimum standard for emergency sports medicine, but one should strive to have services available as quickly as possible.

Having positioned one's medical staff, one must decide if it is necessary to also have an ambulance in position at these posts or if it is more feasible to transport patients on sleds, buggies, etc. These decisions will be influenced by how accessible roads to the medical posts are (it is often difficult to find access roads at alpine skiing events), weather conditions, traffic issues (as in marathon), the size of the course, the number of competitors/spectators, and obviously budget issues.

Another thought to consider is that patient transfer from sled, buggy, boat, etc. to the ambulance should, if possible, take place in a secluded area free from the watching spectators and media, in order to protect the patient's privacy.

5.3 HELICOPTERS

Medical helicopters are now commonly used (or are available) at major sports events. They serve two functions: They can rapidly transport expert medical personnel and equipment to an accident site, and they can rapidly transfer a patient from the accident site to hospital. At a major sports event, there is usually an adequate number of well-qualified physicians present to treat most conditions. The need then for a helicopter is to transfer a patient to the hospital. The assumption is that helicopter transfer is speedier than ambulance transfer. This may or may not be the case. There are many articles written about the cost-benefit of helicopter transport and many have questioned if time is actually saved by using air transport instead of road transfer. Helicopter services have to be contacted, staff have to be scrambled (5 to 15 minutes, depending on local response time, helicopter type, etc.), and then there is flight time to the accident site to be considered. It takes some more minutes to prepare the patient before entering the helicopter and more minutes again to restabilize and secure the patient before evacuation. The receiving hospital should also have an appropriately located helicopter pad (many pads are 5 to 10 minutes away from the emergency department). All these minutes add up. It is very difficult to describe all situations, but in general, if a road ambulance can get an athlete from the sports arena to the hospital in 30 minutes, then helicopters are seldom necessary.

Helicopters Should Obviously Be Used If

- Road ambulances cannot access a site (e.g., alpine skiing), but as a rule major sporting events are not located in such isolated environments. (If the terrain is uneven, forested, or rocky, it may be impossible for the helicopter to land at the site. Therefore, the helicopter must be able to lift the stretcher or harnessed patient from the ground using a winch or rescue rope.)

- Road transport will take inordinately long time due to distance or traffic conditions.

- Transport time to hospital is absolutely essential for patient survival.

- The patient's condition is critical. Correct triage practices must be in place: Some papers show that up to 40% of patients transferred by helicopter are released from the emergency department.[1]

Obviously, conditions that require immediate surgical intervention (such as serious head injuries, penetrating thorax or abdominal injuries, amputations, major hemorrhage or aneurysms, etc.) or immediate medical intervention (cardiac infarctions, coma, diabetic or epileptic emergencies, etc.) need to get to a hospital quickly and the use of a helicopter should be considered. Similarly, most athletes with fractures do not need to be airlifted—even femur fractures (without femoral artery damage) can be safely transferred by road. Careful road transfer may be preferable and safe even with cervical injury.

If the CMO considers it necessary to have access to a helicopter, then a decision has to be made regarding the need for a dedicated on-site helicopter or if one can utilize local helicopter services (which may or may not be available at the precise time needed by the event organizer). Appropriate helicopter sites must be allocated before the event and ambulances must have easy access to this site.

Other aspects to be considered are those of safety routines regarding helicopter landings and patient transfer to the helicopter. Loose items and personnel must be removed from the dedicated landing area—helicopters blades are deadly. Nobody should approach a helicopter unless given permission by the helicopter crew.

Finally, another issue that has to be addressed is that of payment for helicopter services. While most civilized events will not charge an athlete for ambulance transport to a hospital, some athletes have been charged for helicopter transport, which may not be part of the organization's responsibility. These bills can be horrific, so have this in mind.

Conclusion

Before the event, calculate flight time to the venue, loading time, and flight time to the hospital. Allow for traffic complications. Consider the consequences of external helicopter services not being available at the precise moment that they are required. Evaluate the need for an onsite helicopter. Predefine the necessary medical criteria for helicopter transport. Check that the helicopters are allowed to and have the ability to fly at nighttime. Be prepared to have a backup evacuation resource in case helicopters cannot fly due to weather conditions, darkness or are otherwise occupied, etc.

5.4 OTHER TRANSPORT VEHICLES

Motor boats, ski patrols with sled, skidoos, beach buggies, motorbikes, and even bicycles can be used as these give rescue staff a greater flexibility in terms of terrain accessibility, traffic problems, mobility, etc. In the event of a major evacuation, it is always handy to have an array of rescue vehicles that can be kitted out with a limited amount of medical equipment.

5.5 PREDEFINED HOSPITAL, MEDICAL CENTERS, AND ROUTES

It may sound obvious, but it is important that ambulances know exactly where the various hospitals and medical facilities are. It is not unusual to use several hospitals during the Olympic Games. Not all hospitals may have all services (e.g., MRI, neurosurgeon), so make sure the ambulance is sent to the correct institution and that the ambulance staff knows how to get there. I have heard reports from athletes telling about ambulances stopping to ask for directions to a hospital. Also, if transporting to private medical centers, remember opening times, etc. This type of information should be disseminated well in advance of the event so that unfortunate and unnecessary trips can be avoided.

5.6 ATHLETE TRANSPORT TO HOSPITAL

Athlete Identification

As a rule, athletes in competition do not wear accreditation. On some occasions, athlete identification has been a problem, so always make sure you look for the athlete's starting number singlet or patch, if available. At a larger event, most athletes are numbered in some way. If medically acceptable, delay athlete transfer until the accreditation card is available.

Team Physician

It is extremely disheartening for a team physician to be denied the right to accompany his or her athlete from the venue to a hospital or clinic. Try to accommodate the team physician and allow him or her to travel by ambulance. Obviously, this may not always be practicable, particularly with helicopter evacuation.

Hospital Address and Telephone Number

The least one can do is to inform the team physician/manager of where the athlete is being taken to. This is usually possible even in the most urgent situations. Even better, write down the name of the hospital and the hospital's telephone number.

Information Routines

It is important that protocols are developed for what kind of information should be given to the media and the spectators. It is also a good idea to decide beforehand who should do the talking.

CHAPTER 6

Radios, Telephones, Walkie-Talkies and Other Symbols of Importance

Contributed by David McDonagh, Deputy CMO, Lillehammer 1994 Olympic Winter Games

Reviewers: Irene Skaget and Jørn-Terje Iversen, Vinje Ambulance Service, Trondheim, Norway

6.1 THE RADIO REPAIR MAN, OR "FIXER"

Equipment failure—particularly radio equipment—is one of the trials one has to endure as an event physician (EP). It is always important to know who can help you and where to get a hold of your radio expert. Radio equipment staff are often very busy at large events and are often called to fix communication crises. They are thus often not stationary and difficult to locate, particularly if your radio has failed.

At large sporting events, it is really important to be on good terms with the radio experts. Some small pieces of advice: Make friends with the guy in the radio office; he is your "fixer." GET his cell phone number, landline phone number, radio frequency, and any other information you can. Also, try to get an extra battery and charger for your radio phone in case of a flat battery. Give him a pin!

If you do not have a battery charger, remember to deliver in your batteries at the end of each day, otherwise you may have a flat battery the next day.

6.2 BATTERIES IN COLD CLIMATES

Batteries in laryngoscopes and ophthalmoscopes can go flat quite quickly. Instead of leaving batteries in equipment, it is often a good idea to place the batteries in warm pockets or close to the skin to prevent battery failure in extreme cold.

6.3 SEPARATE RADIO CHANNELS FOR MEDICAL STAFF

Medical staff must have their own dedicated radio channel. Only the medical director should, on occasion, be allowed to change the radio channel; if other members of the event organizing committee want to speak to the EP, then they can contact him on the medical channel and ask him or her to change over to another channel. If the matter is confidential (e.g., *can the athlete continue? Can the event continue?*), then the EP can ring from a cell phone, landline, or other radio channel. (Remember, less scrupulous journalists have radio sets that can be tuned into the organizers' radio network.)

Respect confidentiality.

6.4 INFORM OF ARRIVAL AND DEPARTURE

Inform the event organizer of your arrival and departure. Event organizers are usually grateful for this information. For example, "This is David, Venue Medical Officer. Two ambulances present and in place. Full staff today. No absentees. All staff in position. Time now is 9:00."

6.5 BANDIT RADIOS

One problem I have experienced is that different teams have their own sets of radios. On occasions, these teams disrespect the allocation of radio channels and use whatever channel they wish. This can be extremely irritating and potentially life threatening if the medical channel is blocked by irrelevant gibberish from, often foreign, teams. To ensure that this does not occur, the event organizing committee must delegate a channel to the teams and inform them of this. Fines can be imposed if teams do not respect this channel allocation.

Another area where problems can arise is with eavesdroppers. Some of these are just nosey amateurs, others have malignant intentions, and others are professional reporters. Be careful when giving personal information over a walkie-talkie—anonymize the patient wherever possible—personal information is seldom necessary at the warning phase. It is enough to say, "Dr. Tom X here. Team B at the corner of M Street and T Street. We have a serious injury involving a 35-year-old man. Broken femur. Closed fracture. No shock. Currently stable. Code Yellow. Need ambulance assistance." You do not say, "Hi, it's Tom. Guess who I got: Brad P, and boy is he in bad shape. Busted leg." Say something like that, and then just wait for the paparazzi to arrive. If necessary, use a cell phone.

6.6 SOUND AND RECEPTION CHECK BEFORE EVENT START

Before the start of an event, the EP should complete a cell phone and radio test to ensure that signals are available. This is important. This should be completed in good time before the event start.

6.7 KNOW HOW TO USE A RADIO

Not all EPs know how to use a radio. A radio—or portable, handheld, two-way radio transceiver—often has an array of confusing buttons and controls, the most elementary of which are the (Fig. 6.1)

- On–off/volume control knob
- Channel/frequency selector knob
- Push-to-talk button

Only one person can speak at any time. To speak, you have to press and hold in the push-to-talk button. Whilst pressing this button, nobody else will be heard.

6.8 NOISE LEVELS

At large and loud sporting events, noise is a major problem. It can be extremely difficult to get in touch with medical staff due to vocal spectators, loudspeakers, etc. The following are ways you can avoid problems:

- Medical staff should not stand near loudspeakers. Try to place teams at least 50 m away from the sound source.

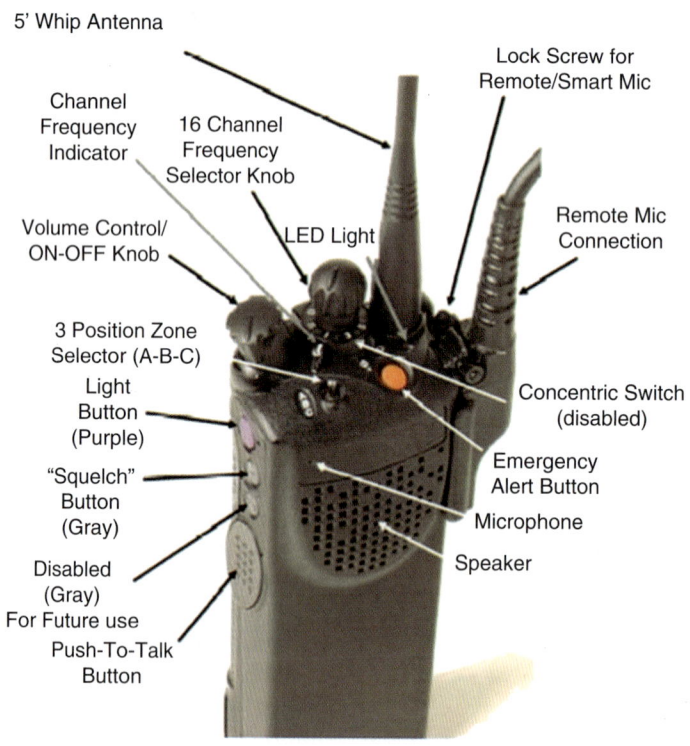

5' Whip Antenna

Lock Screw for Remote/Smart Mic

Channel Frequency Indicator

16 Channel Frequency Selector Knob

Volume Control/ ON-OFF Knob

LED Light

Remote Mic Connection

3 Position Zone Selector (A-B-C)

Light Button (Purple)

"Squelch" Button (Gray)

Disabled (Gray) For Future use

Push-To-Talk Button

Concentric Switch (disabled)

Emergency Alert Button

Microphone

Speaker

FIGURE 6.1.

- Use earpieces or headphones.

- Sometimes it is easier to use cell phones. Set the cell phones on buzzer, vibrating alert, and place the phone near to your skin, not in the outside pocket of a thick winter jacket.

- If possible, move to an area where there is less noise and better reception.

- Learn and use the NATO phonectic code.

6.9 HOW MANY PIECES OF EQUIPMENT SHOULD THE EP HAVE?

I have attended sport events where the EP carried two separate radios and two mobile phones, one with an earpiece. In certain circles, the number of radios hanging around one's neck is a status symbol—obviously, the owner is a person of great importance. However, the number of electronic appendages is usually inversely indicative of one's efficiency. The logic behind this telecommunications overload is the following:

- One radio set to the medical channel

- One radio set to the event organizers' channel

- One extra radio battery

- One cell phone from the event organizers

- The EP's own private cell phone

While there may be a rationale behind this, remember that most physicians have only two ears. It is extremely difficult to be able to listen to two radios at the same time, especially when an accident has occurred and medical staff are required. On top of all this, there may be 50,000 screaming supporters nearby; French, Dutch, or Mexican bands playing their hearts out; Welsh or Latvian choirs in full voice; hordes of screaming kids; fireworks displays; etc. The list is endless.

My advice is to use only one radio, with an earpiece, and one cell phone set on vibrate mode kept in an inside pocket.

6.10 GOOD RADIO PRACTICE

Over the years, good radio practice procedures have been developed and staff should be trained in these. Think about what you want to say before you initiate a conversation: Think, push, talk.

Start a conversation with the following:

- Press in the push-to-talk button

- Wait one second, otherwise parts of your message may disappear: "… David. Over!"

- Name of person you want to speak to

- Your own name

- Finish with "over." Always punctuate your conversation with "over."
  - Example: "John Smith, this is David McDonagh. Over."

- Wait for one minute. Repeat if no reply.

- Avoid unnecessary sentences, however polite.
  - Example: Jim: "Hello, meet you at the ambulance at 3 PM. Over."
  - EP: "OK, see you there. Over."
  - Jim: "Right. Bye for now. Over."
  - EP: "Bye. Over."

- When you have finished and the conversation has ended, say, "Out." That way, everybody knows the conversation is completed and the channel is available to others.
  - Example: EP: "Thanks Jim, message understood. Over and out."

- Never interrupt others' conversations unless it is really important. Do not interrupt other conversations until you have heard the word "out."

- If two people are blathering away about the weather or about what they intend to do after the event, the EP should interrupt and inform the conversationalists that they must cease talking and concentrate on their jobs.

The following are examples of bad radio practice:

- "Jim, can you hear me?" There may be several Jims, or Jim may be busy on a more important conversation. Also, Jim has no idea who is calling him.

- "Hello. Hello." Absolutely meaningless airway pollution.

Using radios in buildings and in towns can, on occasion, lead to problems in sending/receiving radio messages due to the reflection or lack of penetration of sound waves. If you have problems, change position. If that does not help, get in touch with the "fixer."

If the spelling of words is necessary, then the NATO phonetic alphabet (or military police alphabet) can be useful, though not all medical staff are fluent in this code.

A . . . . ALPHA	B . . . . BRAVO	C . . . . CHARLIE
D . . . . DELTA	E . . . . ECHO	F . . . . FOXTROT
G . . . . GOLF	H . . . . HOTEL	I . . . . INDIA
J . . . . JULIET	K . . . . KILO	L . . . . LIMA
M . . . . MIKE	N . . . . NOVEMBER	O . . . . OSCAR
P . . . . PAPA	Q . . . . QUEBEC	R . . . . ROMEO
S . . . . SIERRA	T . . . . TANGO	U . . . . UNIFORM
V . . . . VICTOR	W . . . . WHISKY	X . . . . X-RAY
Y . . . . YANKEE	Z . . . . ZULU	

Some languages have more letters than English (e.g., Danish) and extra letters are used.

CHAPTER 7

Doping Control and the Event Physician

Contributed by Peter Jenoure, IOC Medical Committee, Switzerland, and David McDonagh, Deputy CMO, Lillehammer 1994 Olympic Winter Games

After the advent of WADA, the responsibilities for doping control have moved away from physicians and are now mostly conducted by national antidoping organizations (NADOs), thus relieving physicians of this often difficult task. However, the event physician must be aware of several scenarios to facilitate efficient sports event management.

The first of these is, of course, the prescribing of medications in acute and nonacute situations.

Unless there is a medical emergency, physicians should avoid prescribing medications that are on the this list. It is therefore vital that the event physician (EP) is aware of the contents of this list. The EP should be comfortable with the list's contents and be aware of regular updates. The list is accessible at the WADA website. NADOs often have translations of the list on their websites.

7.1 THE DOPING CONTROL PROCEDURE

The athlete is notified after an event that he or she must be at the doping control station by a particular time, usually within 60 minutes of notification. The athlete signs the notification document, noting the time and date.

The athlete is then usually escorted by a doping control officer until he or she registers at the doping control station. The time of arrival at the station is noted.

The athlete must then give a urine or blood sample (urine is standard; blood is not—certain federations and certain countries require blood tests). The athlete must deliver an amount of urine—often 60 to 70 mL—before he or she may leave the station. Several attempts at urinating may be necessary—delivered urine being sealed in temporary bottles. When the athlete has delivered enough urine, the urine is tested for specific gravity. If this meets requirements and is not diluted, the urine is poured into two different bottles, the so-called A and B samples. Both samples are sealed, paperwork is completed, and the samples are then sent to a recognized WADA laboratory for testing.

7.2 THERAPEUTIC USER EXEMPTIONS

Should an emergency situation arise, and the EP is required to prescribe a medication, then he or she must remember that an athlete can be banned from sport if he or she has taken a listed medication. However, there is a system in place whereby an event physician may warn and seek approval from the appropriate anti-doping organization (ADO), National Federation (NF), or International Federation (IF).

The event physician must complete the appropriate documentation and apply for exemption—a so-called therapeutic user exemption (TUE). Documents are usually found on the Internet, usually at the NADOs or IF's Web site.

As often as not, we are talking about a retrospective approval of a medication given in an emergency situation. In such a situation, the event physician must inform the athlete that a listed medication has to be or has been administered and that the athlete must seriously consider if he or she wishes to further participate in the actual sports event.

Examples of this could be the following:

- An athlete has an acute asthmatic attack but no previous approval for the use of beta-agonists
- An athlete suffers an acute hyperglycemic reaction, again with no approval for the use of insulin
- Acute allergic response requiring the administration of an intramuscular steroid injection

There are good medical arguments for advising an athlete not to participate in further sporting activities that day, due to the danger of illness exacerbation.

Consultation with the athlete's team physician, if present, is advisable. If no team physician is present, then consult the athlete's coach/trainer.

If there is to be a planned in-competition doping control, then it is often a good idea to inform the team captains/coaches during their precompetition technical (i.e., nonmedical) meetings that antidoping controls will be carried out and that athletes with TUEs should have written documentation available at the time of control.

Some EPs also have the right, in certain sports and in certain countries, to deny an athlete the right to participate on the grounds of ill health. It is important that the EP is aware of IF and national rules if such a situation arises.

7.3 AWARD CEREMONIES

As well as being a medic, the EP is also a part of the event organizing committee. In televised events, or events with large amount of spectators, it is important to remember that medal or prize-giving ceremonies often take place 10 to 15 minutes after an event is concluded. If an athlete's treatment can wait, then let him or her experience the award ceremony or media interview and come for treatment afterwards.

The same is true of doping control. On several occasions, I have experienced athletes being escorted off to the doping control by overenthusiastic doping officials, thus denying the athlete the right to participate at a ceremony/interview.

On such occasions, I have spoken to the doping control officials, enquired about the time of notification and the time limits given. Often, the athlete has 60 minutes from notification to obligatory arrival at the antidoping station, thus giving adequate time to complete the award ceremony or media interview. Escorts can be provided to observe the athlete during the ceremony. I have, on occasion, volunteered as an impromptu escort, thus facilitating procedures.

7.4 DRINKS

Do not give drinks to notified athletes unless completely necessary. Drinks may include substances that may be controlled (e.g., caffeine), or forbidden and unnecessary problems may arise. Similarly, drinks may dilute the urine, thus elevating the specific gravity of the urine and delaying doping control procedures. If you have to give an athlete a drink, make sure it comes from a sealed bottle.

7.5 DOPING CONTROL ORGANIZATION

Often, at a major event, the chief medical officer or even the EP will also be asked to organize an in-competition doping control in conjunction with the event, even if there is quite little relation between medical care and this particular activity. This means that doping controls will be carried out on the same day as competition after the event has been completed.

Depending on the size of the event, it may be wise to share these responsibilities by nominating a colleague to deal exclusively with the antidoping affairs.

Steps:

- Number of tests: Decide how many tests are to be taken. Usually, if you have been asked to conduct tests by the event organizer then you will also be informed about the number of tests that are required. There may be obligatory requirements from the IF or from the NF regarding the number of tests to be carried out.
  - If no numbers are given, then it is not unusual to test the athlete/athletes in first, second, and third positions, as well as two random athletes.
- Localities—doping control room: Ensure that there are rooms available to carry out the test. You need at least one toilet (preferably two), a waiting room for the athletes and their accompanying trainer/doctor, and a room or area to conduct the paper work. Some organizations have clear recommendations regarding room size, etc, and it is a good idea to contact the IF or NF first regarding these structural requirements.

- Drinks: They must also to be provided for. They must come in sealed bottles and one should avoid drinks containing alcohol or caffeine.

- Doping escorts: There is often a problem getting enough assisting personnel. International antidoping regulations require that each athlete to be controlled is to be accompanied at all times from the moment of doping control notification to the moment he or she arrives at the doping control room. Female athletes should be accompanied by a female escort, and male athletes by a male escort. You must allow for at least one escort for each athlete to be tested. This can mean that you will need up to 5 to 10 or even more escorts. The escorts must be in place at least 30 minutes before the end of competition and must be available for one hour after the athlete has been notified. This means you need these people to work exclusively for you for at least 90 minutes and often longer. Ensuring that the right number of escorts are present is always a demanding task. (One suggestion: At large events, I often use the people from the ticketing department—the people who check your ticket on entry. Their work is often completed at the start of competition.)

- Budget: It is important to inform the organizing committee about the costs of doping control. Lab analysis of urine alone can cost $200 or more. Blood tests are even more expensive. The sealed doping samples must also be transferred to an accredited doping lab, which may include air transport.

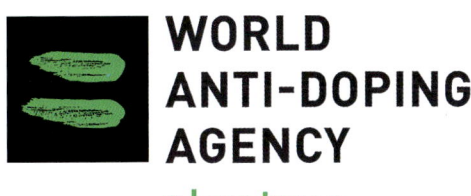

FIGURE 7.1.

Recommendation: The doping control procedure is a potential minefield for the uninitiated. I would strongly recommend that you outsource the whole doping control procedure to your national antidoping authority (NADO) or to a recognized commercial antidoping company. To save costs, you may have to supply doping control escorts, but believe me, it is tough enough being an event physician without having this extra responsibility. Outsource this work to experts. Define responsibility. Sign a contract. The costs must be added on to the budget.

The handling of these antidoping affairs can be a complex and difficult task. There is always the possibility of litigation and becoming famous for the wrong reason. Mistakes will be exploited by lawyers and the media.

There are several antidoping educational products available and I would refer to WADA's Web site (http://www.wada-ama.org). Antidoping Norway and Transform have produced an excellent antidoping educational program, Real Winner, to be found at http://www.realwinner.org

CHAPTER 8

The Event Physician and Antidoping Matters—A Legal Viewpoint

Contributed by Iain Higgins, In-house Sports Lawyer, International Cricket Council, Dubai, UAE

8.1 INTRODUCTION

In an era where athletes train longer and harder to build greater strength and endurance, seek to recover more quickly from injury, and embrace at every opportunity the latest training and nutritional programs, the potential for deliberate or inadvertent use of prohibited substances in sport is apparent. And sports physicians, because of their relationships with athletes and their access to prescribed medication, have a central role to play and important responsibilities across antidoping matters in sport.

This chapter explains how the World Anti-Doping Code (the "Code") impacts the manner in which physicians treat athletes who are subject to antidoping regulations. It highlights (in Sections 8.2, 8.3, and 8.5) the key documents that physicians need to be familiar with, including the Prohibited List and the International Standard for Therapeutic Use Exemptions, and goes on to highlight (in Section 8.4) the key antidoping rule violations, explaining how the conduct of physicians in treating athletes can be critical to an individual athlete's compliance with such regulations and the determination of sanctions that may be imposed against an athlete in the event of a breach (Section 8.6). It points out that the Code also applies directly to the physicians themselves, so that such individuals (and not just the athletes that they treat) may also be the subject of separate disciplinary proceedings. In addition, it highlights (in Section 8.7) the global movement toward state regulation of serious antidoping matters (over and above the Code), which by their very nature, often involve physicians or other "athlete support personnel."

Recent case law has shown that a physician's involvement in circumstances giving rise to an athlete's adverse analytical finding will often be investigated in great detail by a hearing panel, particularly as part of the assessment of the athlete's degree of fault. Although the author is not aware of any successful private law action having been brought by an athlete against his or her physician in relation to an antidoping matter, where the facts established by a hearing panel demonstrate, for example, that a physician has failed to check the Prohibited List correctly against the medication that was prescribed, and such conduct has resulted in the imposition of grave sporting and/or financial sanctions against an athlete, it is not inconceivable that athletes may consider bringing an action against the physician based upon the common law doctrine of negligence or its jurisdiction-specific equivalent.

With the above in mind, the author has set out (in Section 8.8) a "top-ten" list of practical tips and guidance for physicians to follow when treating sportsmen and women that are subject to antidoping regulation.

8.2 THE WORLD ANTI-DOPING CODE AND INTERNATIONAL STANDARDS

The World Anti-Doping Agency (WADA) was formally established on November 10, 1999, with a mission to coordinate and monitor the fight against doping in sport on a worldwide basis. Since its inception in 2003, the regulation of antidoping in sport has been governed by the adoption and implementation of the Code at international federation and national governing body levels.

A comprehensive process of consultation and review led, in November 2007, to the first set of revisions to the Code, which became effective on January 1, 2009.

The Code contains a number of specific antidoping rule violations (the most important of which are set out in Section 8.4), and physicians working in sport should familiarize themselves with the key violations and responsibilities so that they are best placed to minimize the risk that those athletes within their care and control do not commit antidoping rule violations (whether deliberate or otherwise).

However, the scope and application of the Code are not limited to participating athletes; it also extends to the "support personnel" of such athletes, including coaches, trainers, team staff, medical personnel, or any other person working with, treating, or assisting an athlete participating in or preparing for a relevant competition. In other words, it is important that physicians working in sport are aware that they too can be subject to antidoping regulations and can be the subject of disciplinary charges and hearings in relation to their conduct. Accordingly, since many of the substances on the list of prohibited substances and methods (see Section 8.3) can be found in common medications or prescriptions, physicians that recommend or prescribe the use of any form of medication by athletes must make sure that they take care to ensure that such medication does not contain any prohibited substances or that, where there is a medical justification for an athlete's use of medication containing such prohibited substances, an appropriate therapeutic use exemption (TUE) is sought prior to such use.

Sitting below the Code are the International Standards, which formalize different technical and operational areas within standard antidoping programs. The key International Standards of relevance to a sports physician are the Prohibited List (the cornerstone document containing the list of banned substances—see Section 8.3) and the International Standard for TUEs (which identifies the criteria to be used to determine whether there is medical justification for an athlete to be granted permission to use prohibited substances or methods, outlines the process to be followed in applying for a TUE, provides for the confidentiality of such process, and explains the type of evidence required to support an application—see Section 8.5).

NOTE: The new Code, Prohibited List, and International Standard for TUEs can all be found on WADA's Web site www.wada-ama.org

8.3 THE PROHIBITED LIST

The Code provides that WADA shall "as often as necessary and no less often than annually, publish the Prohibited List as an International Standard" and that all Code-compliant antidoping regulations must provide in their rules that the Prohibited List will come into effect within 3 months of such publication. Typically, the Prohibited List is reviewed on an annual basis and any amendments made to it are published on WADA's Web site in or around October of any given year, to take effect from 1 January of the following year. It is therefore vital that sports physicians familiarize themselves with the revisions to the Prohibited List each year and should never assume that the substances on the Prohibited List remain unchanged from year to year.

The Prohibited List distinguishes between substances banned at all times and substances that are only banned "in-competition." A substance or method that has masking properties and/or the potential to enhance performance in future competitions when used in training will be banned at all times, while other substances and methods will only be banned in-competition.

The categories of substances that are prohibited at all times include (i) anabolic agents, that is, agents that promote muscle growth and development, thus increasing endurance and shortening recovering time from injury; (ii) hormones and related substances, which include erythropoietin (EPO), human growth hormone (hGH), insulins, and gonadotrophins (such as luteinizing hormone [LH] and human chorionic gonadotrophin [hCG], which are prohibited in males only); (iii) beta-2-agonists, such as formoterol and terbutaline; (iv) hormone antagonists and modulators, that is, substances that antagonize and/or modulate hormone receptors, including aromatase inhibitors; (v) diuretics and other masking agents, such as epitestosterone and probenecid. Those methods that are prohibited at all times include (i) the enhancement of oxygen transfer (primarily blood doping, "including the use of autologous, homologous, or heterologous blood or red blood cell products of any origin"); (ii) chemical and physical manipulation (e.g., catheterization, urine substitution, and/or alteration, as well as intravenous infusions, save where used to treat an acute medical condition); and (iii) gene doping.

The categories of substances that are prohibited **only in-competition** are (i) stimulants, (ii) narcotics, (iii) cannabinoids, and (iv) glucocorticosteroids.

It is obviously important for physicians practicing in sport to be aware of the differences between the categories of substances on the Prohibited List, as well as to understand properly the nature of each athlete's sport and the athlete's particular participation commitments so that the physician might best be able to advise as to whether it may be necessary for an athlete to obtain a TUE prior to the use of a particular substance, which may only be prohibited in-competition.

8.4 THE KEY ANTIDOPING RULE VIOLATIONS AND APPLICABLE SANCTIONS

The Code sets out a number of different antidoping rule violations. To date, the most important of those violations has been the "presence" of a prohibited substance in a urine or blood sample provided by an athlete (Article 10.1 of the Code). The mandatory sanctions for such a violation are grave, although each athlete is given the opportunity to eliminate or at least reduce that ban if he or she can show how the substance came to be in his or her system and that he or she was not at fault or significant fault (Article 10.5 of the Code) or in certain circumstances did not intend to enhance his or her sports performance (Article 10.4 of the Code). Therefore, in order to help an athlete establish the circumstances surrounding the manner in which the prohibited substance came to be in his or her sample, the athlete will often look to rely on the evidence of the physician who recommended or prescribed a particular course of medication to that athlete. Often such evidence will be presented to a hearing panel by way of a sworn witness statement or affidavit and witnesses (including physicians) may well be required to attend a hearing and submit themselves to cross-examination on the content of their statement.

Moreover, physicians ought to be aware that in their capacities as "support personnel," they are potentially capable of committing (and therefore being the subject of separate disciplinary proceedings in relation to) any of the following antidoping rule violations:

Article 2.6.2 of the Code prohibits "possession" by an "athlete support personnel" of any prohibited method or substance, unless the "athlete support personnel" can establish that the possession is pursuant to a TUE granted to an athlete or other acceptable justification.

Article 2.7 of the Code prohibits "trafficking" or "attempted trafficking" in any prohibited method or substance. The Code defines "trafficking" widely so that it includes selling, giving, administering, transporting, sending, delivering, or distributing a prohibited substance or prohibited method (either physically or by any electronic or other means) to any third party, but includes various provisos and qualifications, for example, in relation to genuine and legal therapeutic uses.

Article 2.8 of the Code prohibits "administration" or "attempted administration" to any athlete of any prohibited method or substance or assisting, encouraging, aiding, abetting, covering up, or any other type of complicity involving an antidoping rule violation or any "attempted" antidoping rule violation.

To date, there have been few cases involving the range of conduct caught by such rule violations, although when Chinese swimmer Yuan Yuan and her coach Zhou Zhewen were discovered trying to smuggle large quantities of synthetic hGH into Australia for the 1998 World Championships, each of them was found guilty of trafficking in a prohibited substance and banned from participation in the sport for 15 years. And in 2006, the International Biathlon Union (IBU) banned a doctor for 2 years who had prescribed a medicine containing carphedon, a stimulant, to biathlete Olga Pyleva, causing her to test positive at the Turin Olympic Games.

The central premise of the Code is the harmonization and standardization of doping sanctions across all sports and athletes. This has been achieved through the creation of mandatory fixed sanction periods for certain antidoping rule violations, subject to reduction on grounds of mitigation (or increase in the case of aggravating circumstances) only in narrowly defined circumstances. For the key antidoping rule violations of Articles 2.1 (presence) and 2.6 (possession), the Code provides that the mandatory fixed sanction is for a **2-year** ban, while violations of Article 2.7 (trafficking) or Article 2.8 (administration etc) may attract a ban within the range of **a minimum of 4 years up to life**.

In addition, the basic rule provides that an antidoping rule violation in individual sports in an in-competition test automatically leads to disqualification of the individual result obtained in that competition with all resulting consequences, including forfeiture of any medals, points, and prizes won. And the Code moves beyond the competition or event at which the athlete tested positive to provide that all other competitive results obtained from the date a positive sample was collected, or other antidoping rule violation occurred, shall, "unless fairness requires otherwise," be disqualified with all of the resulting consequences. In team sports, there may be other sport-specific consequences for teams where individual team members commit antidoping rule violations.

8.5 THERAPEUTIC USE EXEMPTIONS

Through its International Standard for TUEs, WADA has established a process for the granting of TUEs to enable athletes who can satisfy the specified requirements to use substances or methods for therapeutic reasons that would otherwise be prohibited. In broad terms, a TUE may be granted where (a) the athlete would experience serious health problems without using the prohibited substance or method, (b) the therapeutic use of the substance would not produce significant enhancement of performance, and (c) there is no reasonable therapeutic alternative to the use of the substance or method. In order to obtain an appropriate TUE, an athlete must provide detailed supporting information (usually obtained from his or her physician) in relation to such factors.

To varying degrees, a physician will have an important role to play in the completion of a TUE application form, the filing of such form with the relevant authorities, and the ongoing management of the athlete's compliance with the terms of any such TUE granted. If an athlete holds a valid TUE for the source of the prohibited substance found in a sample, such TUE ought to be a complete defense to any antidoping rule violation brought against the athlete on the basis of such finding. However, if there is a TUE, it still needs to be established that the adverse analytical finding is consistent with that TUE, that is, the concentration of the substance found in the sample must be consistent with the therapeutic dosages covered by the exemption. Furthermore, physicians should note that a TUE must be for the specific substance found in the sample, and not for a substance in the same category of medication, even if it has the same therapeutic purpose and effect.

Most importantly, even if the athlete did not hold a TUE in advance for the medication in question, if that medication was given as part of medical treatment that was administered to the athlete on an emergency basis, then there is scope (narrow though it may be) to obtain a retroactive TUE to cover that use. Consequently, physicians ought to be familiar with the circumstances in which retroactive TUEs may be obtained.

8.6 MITIGATION BASED ON AN ATHLETE'S LACK OF FAULT

Where it is established that an athlete has committed an antidoping rule violation through the presence of an adverse analytical finding in his or her sample, the athlete has the opportunity to reduce the otherwise-applicable period of ineligibility that is to be imposed in accordance with the following fault-based provisions:

Where an athlete can establish how a "Specified Substance" entered his or her body **and** that such "Specified Substance" was not intended to enhance the athlete's sport performance or mask the use of a performance-enhancing substance, the period of ineligibility shall be eliminated or reduced based upon the degree of fault displayed by the athlete. In particular, the athlete must show that his or her degree of fault warrants a lesser period of ineligibility, and the degree of reduction warranted will depend on the relative lack of fault shown.

Where an athlete is able to show that he or she bears No Fault or Negligence for his antidoping rule violation, that is, that he or she "did not know or suspect, and could not reasonably have known or suspected even with the exercise of utmost caution, that he or she had used or been administered the Prohibited Substance," the hearing panel may **eliminate** entirely an otherwise-applicable period of ineligibility.

Where the athlete is able to show that he or she bears No Significant Fault or Negligence for his antidoping rule violation, that is, that his or her fault or negligence, "when viewed in the totality of the circumstances and taking into account the criteria for No Fault or Negligence, was not significant in relationship to the antidoping rule violation," the hearing panel may **reduce** an otherwise-applicable period of ineligibility by up to half.

Accordingly, in attempting to establish a low degree of fault or negligence, athletes will often point to the fact that he or she had been to see a sports physician or had medication prescribed to him or her by a physician for genuine therapeutic reasons. For example, in *ITF v Koubek*,[1] a tennis player went to a noted sports specialist doctor for treatment of a wrist injury. The player asked for assurance from the doctor that the proposed treatment would not cause any doping problems and was assured it would not. When he subsequently tested positive for the glucocorticosteroid contained in the drug injected into him, the hearing panel recognized those facts in reducing his sanction from the maximum 12 months allowable but still imposed a 3-month ban on the ground that he had failed to cross-check with other resources readily available to him, including a doping wallet card and drugs hotline supplied by the tennis authorities.

No Fault or Negligence

In the case of No Fault or Negligence, an athlete must show that the violation occurred notwithstanding his or her exercise of "utmost caution." According to the Court of Arbitration for Sport (CAS), this requirement of utmost caution means that the athlete must establish that he or she has done all that is possible, within the circumstances of the medical treatment, to avoid a positive testing result. So, for example, where an athlete is prescribed certain medicine by a physician, but does not take any steps to check if the medicine contains a prohibited substance, either on his or her own or by specifically asking the physician, the athlete cannot be said to have discharged the burden to exercise "utmost caution" and so cannot establish No Fault or Negligence.

For purposes of determining the extent to which the athlete complied with his or her duty of care, the Code fixes the athlete not only with his or her own acts or omissions but also the acts or omissions of his or her friends, associates, and physicians. As the commentary to the Code expressly states, "athletes are responsible for the conduct of persons to whom they entrust access to their food and drink." So, for example, CAS has attributed the failure of the athlete's chiropractor to check the packaging of glucose tablets he provided to an athlete for purposes of assessing the athlete's fault under this provision.[2] Such approach must be correct, since it would otherwise put an end to any meaningful fight against doping if an athlete was simply able to shift his or her responsibility with respect to substances that enter the body to someone else and avoid being sanctioned because they had no knowledge of that substance.

The author is only aware of a handful of cases where a hearing panel has accepted an athlete's plea of No Fault or Negligence and therefore eliminated completely the otherwise-applicable period of ineligibility to be imposed. In each case, **the role of the physician involved and the evidence provided by that individual was central to the athlete's defense:**

In *Pobyedonostsev v IIHF*,[3] the CAS accepted the athlete's plea of No Fault or Negligence where the source of the nandrolone metabolite found in a sample was an injection of Retabolil that had been administered to the athlete by a hospital emergency room doctor while the athlete was experiencing heart failure after crashing into the board on the side of the ice rink.

In *the Matter of Albert Garcia*,[4] a basketball player's sample had tested positive for nandrolone because of a one-time injection of Deca-Durabolin administered to the player in hospital to treat his severe back pain. The International Basketball Federation (FIBA) Commission decided, by a two to one majority, to accept the athlete's plea of No Fault or Negligence.

In *ATP v Perry*,[5] a tennis player had been granted a TUE for a beta-2 agonist, terbutaline, administered by inhaler to treat his asthma. At an ATP tournament, he showed his inhaler to an ATP tournament doctor and asked him for a refill, but the doctor instead gave him a refill for salbutamol, a different beta-2 agonist also used in bronchodilator medication and also included on the Prohibited List, without explaining to the player that he was giving him a different medication from the one requested or querying his TUE position, so that the player believed he had been given a terbutaline inhaler. The antidoping tribunal was satisfied on the face of such evidence that the player had been able to establish No Fault or Negligence.

Similarly, in *FISA v Olefirenko*,[6] where a rower had followed in good faith the advice of the team physician at the Olympic Games in order to deal with an accepted medical condition, she was found to have done all that could reasonably be asked of her and therefore to have displayed No Fault or Negligence for the adverse analytical result caused by the medicine the physician had prescribed. In that case, it was determined that the team's physician was significantly negligent and the physician was banned for 4 years.

8.7 NO SIGNIFICANT FAULT OR NEGLIGENCE

While it is unusual for an athlete to be able to establish the high standard of care required by No Fault or Negligence, athletes are more likely to be able to demonstrate the lower standard of No Significant Fault or Negligence, so as to reduce (but not eliminate) the otherwise-applicable period of ineligibility to be imposed. In many of those types of cases, in an attempt to minimize their own degree of fault for the commission of the antidoping rule violation, athletes often submit that they were simply following the instructions of their physician or doctor. Here again, **the role of the physician involved and the evidence provided by such individual will be central to the athlete's defense:**

In *Edwards v IAAF and USATF*,[7] an athlete established that her positive test for nikethamide, a banned stimulant, was caused by her ingestion of two glucose tablets bought for her by her physical therapist. CAS rejected her plea of exceptional circumstances on the basis that it was not reasonable to accept without query a product that was purchased while abroad, which was not available in the athlete's home country, and without examining the packaging and leaflet that came with the product, which indicated nikethamide as an ingredient and included an express antidoping warning (albeit in French).

In *ITF v Karic*,[8] an International Tennis Federation (ITF) antidoping tribunal rejected a wheelchair tennis player's plea of No Significant Fault or Negligence on the basis that the player took no steps whatsoever to check whether her medication infringed the applicable antidoping rules. The tribunal found that there was no evidence that the player had consulted any doctor with particular knowledge of sports medicine and antidoping rules. Nor had the player checked the prohibited list each year and there was no evidence that the player made any enquiry at all about whether she might have been taking prohibited substances. By failing to do so, the player was, without doubt, significantly at fault.

Similarly, in *USADA v Sahin*,[9] a tribunal found that it was not reasonable to take an unlabelled pill that did not come from its original package without at least trying to verify what was in the pill. It declared that it could not allow an athlete's lack of questioning and lack of investigation in relation to medication that the athlete ingested to become the standard by which athletes circumvent the antidoping rules.

The case of *WADA v Stauber*,[10] is particularly instructive to all physicians practicing in sport. In that case, a handball player tested positive in-competition for hydrochlorothiazide, a banned diuretic, as a result of his ingestion of Co-Diovan, as prescribed for him by his doctor to treat his high blood pressure. After the test, the player sought and was granted a TUE for Co-Diovan. CAS subsequently found that the player could not establish No Fault or Negligence but could establish No Significant Fault or Negligence, and reduced his ban to 12 months, that is, the maximum reduction permitted under the Code. Its reasoning went as follows:

35. All Athletes being responsible for that what they ingest … – whether within a medical treatment or not – the elimination of a period of suspension must not be found except in exceptional circumstances. In accordance with the constant jurisprudence of CAS, the Athlete cannot hide behind the potential misunderstanding of the anti-doping rules by his doctor to escape any sanction. The prescription of a medicine by a doctor does not relieve the Athlete from checking if the medicine in question contains forbidden substances or not. Indeed, the personal, strict and proactive duty imposed on the athletes by the anti-doping rules requires that an athlete who relies on third party advice (medically trained or trustworthy person) effectively raises the question whether a prohibited substance is contained or not.

36. In the present case – notwithstanding the fact that (a) the list of prohibited substance is published annually and therefore changed several times since 2003 and that (b) Mr Stauber changed twice doctors – he never made any check in connection with the original prescription or with the renewed prescription, either by himself or by asking questions to either one of the Doctors who prescribed the medicine.

37. Therefore, he has not exercised "the greatest vigilance" or "the utmost caution" and committed a fault. In addition, as a sporting elite, Mr Stauber has expressly undertaken in his declaration of submission to keep himself informed of the evolution of the rules and of the lists relating to the prohibited substances and methods. He should thus have known that the consummation of hydrochlorothiazide was forbidden. …

When considering the fault of the athlete for the purposes of determining No Significant Fault or Negligence, a hearing panel should consider to what extent there was more that the athlete could and should have done to avoid the doping offence in question. Numerous hearing panels have found that an athlete cannot come close to establishing No Significant Fault or Negligence where the athlete has taken no steps whatsoever to check whether medication prescribed to the athlete by a physician might have contained a prohibited substance.

It is well established that it is the personal responsibility of an athlete to ensure that no prohibited substance is present in his or her system. Hearing panels have consistently found that they would expect athletes, in discharging that responsibility, to take some or all of the following steps available to them: (a) use only a sports-specialist physician; (b) explain to the physician that they are subject to drug-testing regulations; (c) carry with them a copy of the Prohibited List at all times; (d) check the medication against the Prohibited List and/or ask the physician to do the same; (e) read the packaging and drug information leaflet enclosed with the medication; (f) check the Prohibited List each year to review any changes that may be of relevance; (g) check with their national antidoping organization and/or their national/international federation; and (h) utilize any other facilities made available to them, such as the 24-hour hotline provided to tennis players by the ITF or the information on various antidoping Web sites, such as the online drug information database (at www.didglobal.com).

It is worth highlighting that a typical doping control form will ask an athlete to declare any medications or supplements taken in the 7 days prior to the date of sample collection. While declaring a medication on the form does not excuse its use if it turns out to contain a prohibited substance, it may assist the athlete in credibly arguing that a metabolite may have come from something other than a prohibited substance or (if he or she is trying to mitigate sanction under the provisions discussed above) in identifying a medication or supplement as the source.

8.8 ANTIDOPING CONTROL BEYOND THE WADA CODE

Physicians should be aware that governments are increasingly adopting sports-specific antidoping legislation, providing for state-sponsored doping controls and for criminal investigation (including search and seizure), liability, and sanction. In such countries, national authorities (often the National Olympic Committee, but in some cases government agencies or even the police) have the right to conduct investigations into suspected drug abuse in sport (including carrying out drug testing), to bring disciplinary proceedings (directly or through the National Sports Federation) against transgressors, with lengthy bans from the sport among the possible sanctions, but also in some cases to bring criminal charges seeking criminal penalties (including imprisonment) against those that supply banned drugs to athletes and even against athletes that knowingly use such drugs.

Indeed, WADA has made it very clear that it expects government signatories to ensure that their respective national laws contain appropriate provisions that make it a criminal or regulatory offence to traffic, supply, and/or administer steroids, hormones, or amphetamines, either generally or specifically to athletes and athlete support personnel.

Most countries also carry a strong legislative and regulatory framework for controlling the use, possession, importing or exporting, production or sale of certain drugs in any event. However, such framework is often aimed at society as a whole, not sport in particular, and there is no necessary correlation between the same and the Code or the Prohibited List. In recent years, some of the biggest breakthroughs in the fight against doping in sport have been made by public authorities, exercising compulsory state powers under force of national law. Typically, they have involved physicians or other "athlete support personnel":

- 2003 BALCO: US law enforcement agents used noncompulsory techniques, such as Internet searches and garbage searches, followed by legally sanctioned search and seizure operations, to gather evidence against BALCO and its president, Victor Conte, who had been administering prohibited substances to a number of international athletes.

- 2006 Operation Puerto: In May 2006, federal drug agents raided the premises of Dr. Eufemiano Fuentes in Madrid and seized steroids, hormones, EPO, bags of frozen blood, and equipment for treating blood, as well as documents on doping procedures performed on athletes and lists with the names of top-level athletes who received blood transfusions.

WADA has called upon government signatories of the Code not only to ensure that their national laws are suitable to equip and incentivize law enforcement agencies to act effectively against trafficking and other violations involving substances and methods prohibited in sport but also to develop mechanisms for efficient and effective cooperation between the sports movement and such law enforcement agencies, to facilitate in particular the provision of information by such agencies to the sports movement of any evidence of the involvement of athletes and athlete support personnel in activities that may constitute antidoping rule violations under the Code.

In short, sports physicians need to be aware that any activity that constitutes an antidoping rule violation under the Code (e.g., administration, trafficking, etc.) may also contravene national criminal or regulatory laws and vice versa. The consequences of any such activity may therefore be more wide-ranging and punitive than the sanctions prescribed by the Code.

8.9 "TOP-TEN" TIPS AND GUIDANCE FOR PHYSICIANS

The author has put together the following list of the "top-ten" tips and guidance for physicians in order to help them best minimize the risk of (a) a patient committing an antidoping rule violation and/or (b) being subject to criticism in relation to the approach taken when prescribing a medication to a patient who is subject to antidoping regulation. Of course, there are many other steps that physicians could take in practice and the list is not designed to be exhaustive—it simply reflects the concerns raised by this chapter and the lessons to be learned from the relevant case law to date:

- Physicians must **familiarize themselves** with the Code, the Prohibited List, and the International Standard for TUEs.

- Physicians must have access **at all times** to a **current** Prohibited List.

- Physicians must check any medication (including all of its ingredients) against the substances on the Prohibited List **before** prescribing or recommending the use by an athlete of such medication.

- Physicians must not make any prescription or recommendation unless and until the physician is **100% certain** that the medication (including all of its ingredients) does not contain any of the substances on the Prohibited List.

- Physicians must be particularly diligent when advising in a **foreign country** where (a) there may be language difficulties and/or (b) common "brand names" may contain different ingredients.

- Where a physician is not 100% certain that the medication (including all of its ingredients) does not contain any of the substances on the Prohibited List, he or she ought to **undertake further research** (including by contacting WADA, the relevant NADO, International Federation, National Federation or otherwise).

- Physicians must explain to the athlete that under the Code it is the athlete's **personal responsibility** to ensure that no prohibited substances are present in his or her sample and that the athlete ought to take steps to independently verify that the medication (including all of its ingredients) does not contain any of the substances on the Prohibited List.

- Physicians must be careful **not** to recommend nutritional/dietary supplements to an athlete where the physician cannot be **100% certain** of the content of such nutritional/dietary supplements. Any athlete asking for advice in relation to nutritional/dietary supplements must be advised that (notwithstanding what is recorded on the list of ingredients) there is always a risk that such supplements may be contaminated with substances on the Prohibited List.

- Where a physician is asked to prescribe a medication pursuant to a TUE, he or she must be careful to prescribe to the athlete the precise substance and dosage consistent with **the conditions set out in the TUE**, irrespective of whether another substance or dosage might have a similar therapeutic effect.

- Physicians ought to **document clearly and concisely** the circumstances of any prescription of medication to an athlete that is subject to antidoping regulations, including by recording the details of any significant conversations or checks made.

Case References

1. *ITF v Koubek*, Anti-Doping Tribunal dated January 18, 2005.
2. *Edwards v IAAF and USATF*, CAS OG 04/003, award dated August 17, 2004.
3. *Pobyedonostsev v IIHF*, CAS/2005/A/990, award dated August 24, 2006.
4. *In the matter of Mr Albert Garcia*, FIBA Commission decision dated July 7, 2006.
5. *ATP v Perry*, Anti-Doping Tribunal decision dated November 30, 2005.
6. *FISA v Olefirenko*, FISA Commission decision dated February 9, 2005.
7. *Edwards v IAAF and USATF*, CAS OG 04/003, award dated August 17, 2004.
8. *ITF v Karic*, Anti-Doping Tribunal decision dated December 21, 2006.
9. *USADA v Sahin*, AAA Case No. 30 190 01080 04, decision dated March 25, 2005.
10. *WADA v Stauber & Swiss Olympic Committee*, CAS 2006/A/1133, award dated December 18, 2006.

CHAPTER 9

Injury Statistics

Contributed by Colin Fuller, Professor, University of Nottingham, England; Advisor, FIFA and the IRB

Information about the incidence, nature, and causes of acute and gradual onset sports injuries is built up from injury statistics collected in epidemiological studies. These injury statistics allow the injury burden within a sport to be defined, and they provide the evidence that enables

- Athletes to assess the risk of sustaining an injury within a sport
- Physicians to determine the range of medical facilities and personnel required to support athletes during competition and training
- Tournament medical officers to identify what additional specialist and emergency medical services may be required locally to support team physicians during competitions
- Governing bodies to define the baseline injury risks associated with their sports and to evaluate the impact of changes to the laws/regulations of the sport
- Stakeholders to identify, implement, and evaluate injury prevention strategies.

Major sport events provide the ideal opportunity to collect injury statistics; however, to ensure that the data collected provides meaningful information, it is essential to plan surveillance studies at these events thoroughly so that the data are collected effectively, efficiently, and consistently. In order to achieve this completely, injury surveillance studies should be supported and actively promoted by the tournament organizers and the appropriate sports governing bodies.

Irrespective of the size of the study or the data being collected, personnel involved in recording and reporting injury data must be thoroughly briefed on the following issues:

9.1 AIMS AND OBJECTIVES OF THE STUDY

- Who initiated the study (e.g., tournament organizer, sports governing body)?
- What the intended purpose of the study is (e.g., part of an ongoing injury surveillance philosophy within the sport or a study of a specific injury-related issue)?
- Who will be responsible for implementing the study (e.g., sports governing body)?
- What data will be collected (e.g., athletes' competition and/or training injuries or spectators' injuries and illnesses)?
- How will the injury surveillance study be reported (e.g., as an internal report to a governing body or as a peer-reviewed research publication)?

9.2 STUDY DESIGN AND SAMPLE POPULATION

- Prospective (preferred) or retrospective cohort
- All athletes (preferred) or a representative number of athletes

9.3 ATHLETES' BASELINE ANTHROPOMETRIC DATA AND INFORMED CONSENT

- Ethical considerations mean that, although organizers and governing bodies can insist that teams and countries participate in epidemiological studies at major tournaments, individual athlete participation must be on a voluntary basis.

- Athletes should be provided with a brief summary of the study before asking for their consent to be included.

- Athletes' consent to be included in the study must be obtained before injury data are recorded.

- Athletes' consent can be recorded on a form alongside their baseline information (e.g., stature, body mass, and age).

Injury definition and classification define what constitutes a recordable injury within the study; this definition should preferably agree with international consensus statements on epidemiological studies in sport unless the study specifically relates to a nonstandard investigation. Injury definitions will normally refer to sport-related injury events resulting in an athlete missing time from competition and/or training; injury classification systems should preferably follow a recognized recording system, but, as a minimum, the injury location, type, diagnosis, severity, and cause should be recorded.

Exposure Information

Competition Exposure: For most tournaments, recording the total exposure experienced by all athletes taking part in the tournament will be sufficient; this information is often accessible retrospectively from tournament records. However, if the study relates to athlete-specific risk factors, it will be necessary to record athlete-specific exposure data, which may be obtainable from tournament records, but if not, it must be recorded prospectively during the tournament

Training Exposure: This information will not be available from tournament records and must therefore be collected prospectively during the tournament by athletes/teams. This information can again be collected as a total grouped training exposure value unless the effects of athlete-specific risk factors are being investigated, in which case, athlete-specific training exposures must be recorded during the tournament.

Documentation for Recording Data

Specific forms should be prepared and used for recording athletes' baseline data, consent,

exposures, and injuries. Provide guidance on the specific categories that should be used for recording injury location, type, diagnosis, and causation. A computer database must be established to record and analyze the data collected.

9.4 REPORTING PROCEDURES

- Identify the study coordinator to whom the data should be sent.

- Communicate the timescales (e.g., daily, weekly, posttournament) and procedures (e.g., e-mail, telephone, fax) for reporting injury and exposure data to the study coordinator.

- Clarify the posttournament follow-up procedure that will be used to collect outstanding injury and exposure data.

- Provide the name and contact details of a person who will be available to give information and to answer questions about the study before, during, and after the tournament.

The information outlined above should ideally be communicated to medical personnel involved in the study in a tournament-specific guidance document that is prepared and distributed at least 1 month prior to the start of the tournament. It is beneficial if the guidance document also contains examples of how each form should be completed. If possible, time should be made available to brief medical personnel at a pretournament meeting.

Injury statistics provide a wealth of clinically relevant information, but to maximize their utility, it is essential to adopt recognized protocols when analyzing and reporting data. The person responsible for preparing the final study report should therefore aim to comply wherever possible with the following general guidelines:

- Data should be analyzed, assessed, and presented using internationally recognized and accepted categories for each variable.

- Incidence of injury should be reported as the number of injuries per 1,000 player-hours or number of injuries per event; severity of injury as the mean and median number of days absent from competition and/or training; and distributions of injury location, type, and causes as percentages of the total incidence of injury.

- All values of variables should be calculated and reported separately for competition and training injuries.

CHAPTER 10

Sports Medicine Ethics

Contributed by Michael McNamee, Professor, Centre for Philosophy, Humanities and Law, University of Wales, Swansea, Wales

In everyday sports medicine discourses, clinicians may refer in positive terms to colleagues whom they consider to be "good professionals," as opposed merely to good surgeons, good strength and conditioning trainers, good physiotherapists, and so on. What they typically mean is that they are "morally good" or "ethically admirable" practitioners. Another way of putting this is to say that they are principled professionals. One common way of thinking of moral action is to think of it as "principled action." Quite what this means is not straightforward. In this short essay, I offer some introductory remarks to the idea of ethics for event physicians (EPs). I show how one principled approach to sports medicine ethics can help to guide actions in the professional life of an EP but how the particularities of sports medicine can bring particular problems to the practitioner aiming to do the right thing. What I do not do—indeed what cannot be done—is to offer an *ethical algorithm* for all EPs in the dilemmas that form their daily work. Such a thing does not exist.

10.1 ETHICS, MORALITY, AND SPORTS MEDICINE ETHICS

The terms *morality* and *ethics* are often used interchangeably. Philosophers, however, tend to distinguish them in the following way: "ethics" is the local, particular, thick stuff of personal attachments, projects, and relations, while "morality," by contrast, is detached, general (even universal), impartial, thin rules or norms governing how you should treat others or be treated by them. Typically, "ethics" in this broad scheme of things is

fiercely contested. It is prefigured by the name of a particular group or institution: business ethics, feminist ethics, journalistic ethics, medical ethics, military ethics (if that is not an oxymoron), professional ethics, sports ethics, and, of present concern, sports medicine ethics (SME). How shall we understand SME and the actions that the good EP should demonstrate and embody?

In medical ethics, generally there have been several contenders to the question of how one ought to act when faced with apparently competing demands. Each claims that its precepts are authoritative. There are those who think that right action issues always from a proper consideration of duties, or rights of the patient. Adherents to this theoretical approach are usually referred to as "deontologists" (from the Greek word for duty: *deon*). Before acting, they consider what rules or principles apply in terms of moral duties or rights that can be known before one acts. These types of considerations are widely held among medical professionals, and they are fairly closely related to, but not synonymous with, legal considerations. Others, in sharp contrast, suggest that because such duties or rights can clash, and because they are somewhat intangible, only coherently measurable outcomes in terms of patient welfare ought to concern us. These professionals, who figure prominently in medical ethics, are called "utilitarians" after the founding idea of Jeremy Bentham in the 18th century that the utility of an action—in terms of its ability to produce more or less pleasure or pain, help or harm—justifies it in moral terms. Both these groups, though apparently opposed, share the belief that moral beliefs are principled, impartially applied, and ought to issue in action.

A third group thinks that there are no such universal guides to right action but that we should focus on the kinds of character traits (honest, reliable, trustworthy, and so on) that characterize the good professional. These theorists are typically called "virtue ethicists," and though there are prominent advocates for this approach following its advocacy by Aristotle, it has until fairly recently been something of a marginalized ethic in the sphere of medicine. Each of these theoretical approaches is not unified, but rather presents a more or less strongly connected family of theories.

There are others yet, who may be called antitheorists. When it comes down to it, they believe that there are neither reliable and authoritative guides to action—in which deontologists and utilitarians believe—nor that there is a sufficiently reliable idea of character immune from the stresses of every situation—in which virtue ethicists believe. So they plump for some kind of relativism or subjectivism. The right thing to do is, for these practitioners, either relative to their situation, to the ethos of the team, or to some other relevant social standard, or is simply a matter of subjective conscience. Clearly the subjectivitist and the relativist generate difficulties for sports medicine understood as a profession with ethical authority. In the relativist case, what happens to be the dominant norms—how people just get on with things—is said to be the right thing, whereas in the latter there is nothing beyond one's intuitions, which is an unreliable foundation for ethical conduct.

10.2 PRINCIPLED ETHICS FOR THE EVENT PHYSICIAN

In the field of medical ethics, of which the SME is a family member, the idea of a principled ethic has achieved widespread use. It is often referred to as the "principles" approach. This most famous and widely applied composite principled approach in applied ethics emerged largely as a response to publicly aired conflicts and problems in medicine during the 1960s and 1970s in North America. The response was formulated in *The Belmont Report*[1] and is given its most sophisticated expression in Beauchamp and Childress's text *Principles of Biomedical Ethics*.[2] First published in 1978, it is now in its sixth edition and has evolved in response to rigorous criticism of its approach. Beauchamp and Childress developed an approach to ethical reasoning and decision making comprising four moral principles that can be brought to bear on moral problems in all branches of healthcare and medicine. The basic principles operate as a framework rather than a method, which serve as guidelines for professional ethics[2]: (1) respect for autonomy; (2) nonmaleficence; (3) beneficence; and (4) justice. FIMS Code of Ethics makes reference in its general considerations to a version of the first three of these principles.[3] I shall briefly outline each of them before moving to three potentially problematic scenarios for the principled EP.

Respect for autonomy is central to medical practice. When in former days, trust in medical practitioners was absolute, it was not uncommon for the patient to think that the physician always and necessarily knew what was best for the patient. "Trust me, I'm a doctor" was a hackneyed expression, but it captured this truth. In contemporary times, against a background of paternalistic interference by physicians, it is a widely shared norm that the physician must request permission to treat the patient, and in so doing, must seek his or her authorization as to any treatment plan that is aligned to the patient's conception of what is good for him or her and not the physician. Many would argue more strongly that this is the foundational principle of the principles approach.[4] This can be a difficult principle to apply for the physician since he or she is armed with expertise that the patient typically lacks and can, in turn, lead them to know what is in the best interests of the patient. Respecting autonomy, however, entails that the physician must give priority to the patient's own conception of what is good for him or her in his or her own life. Acting in an autonomy-respectful way that is contrary to the patient's interest in normal, healthy functioning may be among the most difficult thing for physicians to do. Nevertheless, patients' right to shape their own lives—so long as they do not harm others in the commission of those choices—is a long-standing right in democracies. This principle is the ethical foundation of informed consent and the duty of the physician to tell the truth to their patients so that they can form their own plan of action. One important caveat here is that, while respecting autonomy is of the highest ethical importance in medical ethics, there are populations such as children or the temporarily incompetent, (whether through concussion or some other injury), who may not qualify as rationally autonomous. They may be thought, however temporarily, to be incapable of forming a rational picture of their own good. In this case, being nonautonomous (or at least lacking full autonomy), the physician is not necessarily obliged to respect their patient's wishes. Therefore, it will be among the first tasks of a physician to evaluate his or her patient's capacity to make decisions regarding treatment.

Secondly, the principle of beneficence directs physicians to aim at the patient's good or welfare. In the care of their patient, physicians must not privilege their own interests above those of the patient. Those who are in need of medical intervention are typically in a state of vulnerability, and it would be improper for physicians to use this condition to pursue their own agenda. I shall discuss such a case in Section 10.4 below. The principle of beneficence explains in large measure why physicians are trusted (there are, of course, others, such as their willingness to maintain patient confidentiality, and truth telling, which weave respect and beneficence together) and ought to interlock with their autonomy the respectful treatment of the patient.

Thirdly, and closely connected to the former, if the physician treats the patient in accordance with his or her autonomous wishes, aiming at his or her well-being, the physician will not harm the patient. This is what nonmaleficence, the principle that the physician will not harm the patient, amounts to. This principle extends into other areas of professional practice that are not obvious. Medical science progresses at a rapid rate and it is a duty of the doctor to maintain an appropriately up-to-date knowledge base in case previous best practice comes to be understood as contraindicated. It also means that there will be limits to the kinds of treatments that can be offered. One interesting case arises in the use of treatments that are simply designed to temporarily restore functional ability but that will mask ongoing problems or even exacerbate them, thus potentially harming the patient. I shall discuss the potential uses and abuses of corticosteroid injections in Section 10.5.

Fourthly, the principle of justice demands that all physicians are fair in their dealing with patients. This principle can extend over the lifetime of treatment with the patient and crucially as a norm between patients. Its most common application is in the allocation of resources across patients. This does not entail that we treat all patients in an identical way. Indeed to the contrary, the formal principle of justice says that physicians must treat equals equally and differences differently. So, the patient who is critically injured takes precedence over the trivially injured one. We treat them differently but in a just or fair way. There are several ways in which just actions can be justified; we may allocate resources (such as the EP's time and expertise) according to clinical need, according to who deserves it most, according to the social utility of the respective patients, or according to some right, say, based on who has waited longest, or indeed on who can or cannot pay for it. Determining which criterion should dominate is not always straightforward. I shall discuss a scenario of the just treatment of multiple trauma athletes in Section 10.6 below.

Beauchamp and Childress[2] argue that these basic principles are to be found in most classical ethical theories. Respect for autonomy is central to deontological medical ethics in terms of the gaining of informed consent and how that theory might serve to uphold nonmaleficence, while it is clear that utilitarianism is centrally concerned with beneficence in terms of the widespread promotion of welfare. Nevertheless, utilitarianism has historically been criticized for being rather unconcerned with justice or individual rights and duties at the expense of securing the greater good, while deontology has typically been thought silent on issues of balancing benefit and harm when duties are owed to many and resources are scarce. There is then some strong justification for Beauchamp and Childress's claim that their basic principles are already to be found in common morality, but applying them is always a matter of wise practical judgment, which is both a product of good role modeling, good advice and guidance, and—most critically—experience guided by these factors. I shall now turn to three problematic scenarios specifically encountered by the EP.

10.3 RESPECT FOR AUTONOMY: THE ATHLETE'S CHOICE COMES FIRST SO LONG AS HE OR SHE IS COMPETENT

There are many scenarios in which athletes are rendered unconscious by traumas: the knockout blow in boxing; a severe contact with the ground after a high catch by the wide receiver who is hit while high in the air; the racing driver upon contact with the safety barriers; a clash of heads between attacker and defender simultaneously going for the ball in soccer; a collapsed scrum in rugby. And of course, there are situations, such as crowd crushes, in which multiple serious injuries can occur on a very large scale. Having said that respect for autonomy is often thought to be the most important medical ethical principle, there will be particular challenges in applying this principle for EPs.

In cases such as these, the first ethical priority is to assess the potential harm to the patient, but it is also the case that his or her decision-making competence must be evaluated. In cases of concussion, this is rendered impossible. In other cases, it may be less than clear-cut. In situations such as these, the EP must either ask for proxy consent or assume paternalistic powers. In certain situations, such as boxing or football, there will be a group of coaches or trainers who will understand the athlete and can make informed judgments about his or her wishes in the absence of family members who can assist. Clearly, here, one can respect the autonomy of the athlete by way of proxy. In others, the EP is likely to make judgments based on clinical indicators. Here, the principles of beneficence and nonmaleficence should guide his or her judgment, although it will be connected with considerations of justice, as we shall see below.

There remains a further challenge to the principle in cases where, after acute trauma, the athlete rejects the treatment the physician determines to be in his or her best interests. The most widely discussed of these cases is when a Jehovah's Witness rejects blood transfusions on religious grounds. Where a patient has impaired autonomy, it is thought that the physician is ethically permitted, in the absence of any legitimate proxy decision maker, to make choices *for* the patient. This is usually called "weak" or "soft" paternalism.[5] It is to be contrasted with hard paternalism where the physician acts over and against the wishes of a competent adult or adolescent. There is widespread agreement that respecting the autonomy of a competent patient is of the highest moral importance even where the choices he or she makes, such as the refusal of blood transfusion, which he or she fully understands is necessary to save his or her life, is simply an unacceptable imposition of the nonmedical values and commitments of the physician over the patient whom he or she has pledged to save. This does not mean, however, that the physician cannot engage in rational, normative debate about the depth or wisdom of, say, the critically injured Jehovah's Witness athlete. It does mean, however, that attempts at persuasion ought not to go so far as to coerce the athlete into the treatment plan the EP considers the option that is in the patient's best interests. Watching a patient die for his or her beliefs while forsaking standard medical treatment may be the hardest thing the physician will ever have to do as a professional.

10.4 BENEFICENCE, NONMALEFICENCE, AND AUTONOMY: WHY THE EVENT PHYSICIAN MUST JUDGE THE BALANCE BETWEEN THE SHORT AND THE LONG OF AN ATHLETE'S BEST INTERESTS

For all serious athletes, whether professional or amateur, competing in sports matters deeply. While the variety of sports is so great it is difficult to generalize, we must accept that injury, pain, and suffering are part and parcel of an athletic way of life.[6,7] Coping with the competing motivations of continued performance and health is not an easy balancing act. And for elite athletes whose financial well-being is intimately tied into their continued athletic participation, this often means choosing to play while injured. To do so requires more or less powerful analgesia. It is widely known that professional athletes frequently and competently request corticosteroid/anesthetic injections. Their use is legally permitted and within the bounds of the WADA code. Most physicians agree, however, that a period of inactivity (or diminished activity in relation to competition levels) is desirable in order to prevent consequent ligamental or tendinous injuries, which are caused effectively because the athlete has masked the ongoing problem. Let us assume that the injection is therapeutic and not merely placebo in its effects and that it is ministered solely to put an athlete either back onto the field of play during a competition or immediately prior to it. To what extent is the event physician justified in ministering short-term therapy to the athlete?

First, it should be clear that acting in such a manner is against the FIMS Code of Ethics, Section 5, which states, "Sports medicine physicians should oppose training and practices and competition rules as they may jeopardize the health of the athlete," and also in Section 8 where it states, "Injury prevention should receive the highest priority."[3] It is, however, in cases such as these that the principled approach to sports medical ethics is open to critique. First, when ethics is conceived as a kind of rule book, one has to know which rules take precedence, when, and why. When the athlete is given all knowledge of the potential risks of an immediate return to competition after a corticosteroid injection, the EP is still in a position to refuse it, according to which principle is prioritized. Secondly, it calls into question the function of codes of ethics that operate at a distance from widespread practice.

10.5 JUSTICE ACROSS COMPETITORS: WHY MY TEAM FIRST MAY BE UNACCEPTABLE FOR THE EVENT PHYSICIAN

In many, and perhaps most, circumstances the EP may find himself or herself as the only qualified medical practitioner at the field of play. He or she may or may not be employed by the host team or club with certain contractual obligations to treat its athletes. When, however, there are multiple injuries it is highly likely that they find themselves in a practical dilemma regarding who ought to be treated first. It is often the case that head collision injuries present this scenario. While EPs will be familiar with the guideline that they ought first to treat thorax injuries, then abdominal injuries, then head injuries, etc, this is effectively a system of practical triage. And according to broader medical ethics considerations, the EP must effectively treat his or her capabilities as a scarce resource that ought to be distributed justly. It is not acceptable for him or her to privilege members of the host team merely in virtue of the fact of his or her employment or the close relations with them (see FIMS, 1997 Code of Ethics, Section 3).[3] Clinical need is properly thought to be the dominant norm to base the fair prioritization of time and effort.

10.6 SOME CONCLUDING REMARKS

In each of the cases presented above, two kinds of problems (among many) ought to be highlighted. There are times when the EP knows exactly the right thing to do but finds it hard to do it. This may be because of the situational pressures placed on the EP by the coach, other players, the team manager or the employer, the noise of the crowd, the importance of the occasion, and so on. And of course it may just be weakness of will: the EP cannot bring himself or herself to do what he or she knows to be right. Equally, there may be times when doing the right thing is not an option and doing the least harm may be the best option available. Little can assure right conduct in all cases—certainly not a code of conduct, nor a short instructional essay of this kind. Everything, though, will hang on the character of the EP. This, in part, will be part of the nature and values of the medical education he or she has received, the guidance given by senior and respected others within the sports environment, and the sports medicine profession generally. It may be said that the principled approach—respect autonomy, promote the welfare of the athlete and do no harm to them, and finally, act justly—is no more than an assembly of reminders. There is some truth to this. And medical ethics in practice is ambiguous, messy, and unclear. This is the nature of the beast. Matters of life and death, both in the literal sense and in the sense of athletic careers, often lie in the hands and hearts of EPs in decisions that may need to be made in split seconds. Nevertheless, the EP who considers these principles seriously is unlikely to go too far wrong.

References

1. The National Commission for the Protection of Human Subjects of Biomedical and Behavioral Research. *The Belmont Report: Ethical Principles and Guidelines for the Protection of Human Subjects of Research*. http://ohsr.od.nih.gov/guidelines/belmont.html. Published April 18, 1979. Accessed October 2, 2008.
2. Beauchamp T, Childress JF. *Principles of Biomedical Ethics*. 6th ed. Oxford, UK: Oxford University Press; 2009.
3. FIMS. *Code of Ethics*. http://www.fims.org/en/general/code-of-ethics/. Accessed October 2, 2008.
4. Gillon R. Ethics needs principles—four can encompass the rest—and respect for autonomy should be "first among equals." *J Med Ethics*. 2003;29(5):307–312.
5. Feinberg J. *Harm to self*, Oxford, UK: Oxford University Press; 1986.
6. Scranton PE. *Playing Hurt: Treating and Evaluating the Warriors of the NFL*. Washington, DC: Brassey's, Inc.; 2001.
7. Howe PD. *Sport, Professionalism and Pain*. London, UK: Routledge; 2003.

CHAPTER 11

Repatriation of Injured and Ill Athletes

Contributed by Lars Toft, Medical Director, SOS International a/s, the largest Nordic assistance organization, servicing more than 100 insurance companies and handling around 70,000 medical cases per year

I have asked the medical director of the largest Nordic assistance organization to write about how his company carries out these procedures. Other assistance providers may function differently. — Ed. David McDonagh

11.1 HOW DOES ASSISTANCE TAKE PLACE IN PRACTICE?

When a policyholder is hospitalized, he or she will be asked to provide an insurance card. If this insurance card refers to SOS International as the assistance provider, the treatment facility (hospital) usually contacts our emergency center relatively quickly. The treatment facility will ask SOS International for a guarantee of payment. The treatment facility must notify us of policy number, name of the policyholder and personal identification number, admission diagnosis, and name and contact details of the attending physician and treating hospital. SOS International can quickly establish whether the insurance cover stated is valid.

Once registration has been completed and verified, one of our coordinating physicians contacts the attending physician and collects necessary medical data. Our physician's goal is to ensure that the treating hospital has the optimal facilities and competence to treat the patient. If our physician is not certain that optimal treatment will be supplied, he or she will make sure that the patient is transferred to a hospital with suitable facilities.

Should our physician request a transfer to another place of treatment, he or she will define the demands that must be met by this other hospital. The SOS emergency centre, will by means of their international network or national business partner in the country in question, find a suitable place. Subsequently, transfer is usually arranged by air ambulance to the relevant treatment facility.

If the primary treatment facility is considered satisfactory, our physician will stay in regular contact with the attending physician until the patient is discharged for a planned return journey or repatriation.

Often, when the ill or injured person is an athlete, the team brings their own physician. In such cases, our physician, as well as the attending physician, will keep in regular contact with the team physician. As SOS International has several specialists at its disposal, the team physician can avail of our specialist advice if requested.

Should repatriation be necessary, the SOS International physician will determine the level of care that is needed. This may include

- Transport via a commercial airline, either seated (in first, business, or tourist class) or on a stretcher

- Air ambulance

- A medical escort, either physician or nurse (with specific specialty if necessary); in case of long distance repatriation, both physician and nurse may be required

- Extra medical equipment, in addition to the contents of a basic medical bag.

Our physician sets the time frame for transport. The SOS emergency center arranges all the practicalities of the repatriation, such as the booking of tickets, the ordering of the air ambulance, the provision of escorts and equipment, and also surface transportation to and from the airport, as well as hospitalization at the home destination.

11.2 TRANSPORT BY COMMERCIAL AIRLINER

Most repatriations take place by commercial airliner and most patients can travel as "seated sick." Many of these patients are seated in business class or first class. Many airlines have extremely comfortable seats (flat seats) on their international routes in these two classes. In order to be able to travel in these classes, a patient must be able to elevate the back of his or her seat to an upright position during takeoff and landing. If he or she cannot, he or she cannot travel as a sitting patient.

Patients with immobilized knees may be offered two seats. If a patient has received a circular plaster cast less than 48 hours before the flight, this should be split before the home journey. A transport plaster cast (rear plaster cast) will be often be applied before repatriation by the airline.

Another possibility is repatriation on a stretcher by commercial airliner. Not all, but most airlines can arrange stretcher transportation on commercial flights. Typically, this demands six to nine seats depending on the type of aircraft. The stretchers are arranged in tourist class. A curtain is arranged around the stretcher in order to allow the patient some modicum of privacy during the flight. Stretcher transportation requires an escort. On most airlines, urine bottles and a bedpan are available when a stretcher has been ordered. Oxygen and wheelchairs can be ordered in connection with boarding, with connecting flight transfers, and at the destination. Other equipment must be brought by the escort. Electronic equipment (monitoring equipment) must be approved for use during flight.

In most major airports, medical clinics are available to patients and their escorts where they can wait until the airport ambulance arrives to transport the patient to the aircraft. Most major airports have high-loaders, which can lift both the escort and the stretcher patient from ground level to board the aircraft.

Repatriation by commercial airliner is possible when the patient is stable and no actual treatment is expected during the flight. This is obviously in the patient's best interest but also for the sake of the other passengers.

When repatriation of a patient by commercial airliner is planned, a medical information form (MEDIF) has to be sent to the airline. This form is completed by the attending SOS physician, but in the repatriations we carry out, SOS International's physician will fill in the form.

The MEDIF form is the same for all airlines that are members of the International Air Transport Association (IATA). The form contains information about the date of diagnosis, operations, if any, vital signs, need for oxygen during transport, need for escort, and other information.

The MEDIF form is assessed in the medical department of the airline in question. If the transport seems medically sound, it will be approved, and medical clearance will be obtained. Further information may be requested. In some cases, the airline may deny medical clearance. The emergency center in question must then find an alternative mode of transportation, often by air ambulance.

11.3 WHO CAN BE REPATRIATED BY COMMERCIAL AIRLINER AND WHEN?

Not all patients can be repatriated by a commercial airliner. Patients who can expose other passengers to risk will under no circumstances be accepted. This may be due to the risk of contamination (even something as minor as chickenpox) or when there is a risk of a psychiatric patient disturbing other passengers. For more information regarding these regulations please refer to the *Medical Manual*, 1st edition, 2004, or access the major airlines' websites.

Many airlines will typically accept patients who have undergone uncomplicated laparoscopic appendicitis surgery on the fifth day postoperatively. Uncomplicated heart attack victims are accepted by most airlines 10 to 14 days after debut symptoms, thrombosis cerebri after 8 to 10 days, and open abdominal procedures 10 days after a return to normal peristalsis.

However, some airlines are more restrictive than others, so conditions should be checked with the medical department of the airline in question.

Stretcher transportation cannot be arranged on domestic flights in the United States. Air ambulance should be used when transporting the patient to the airport from which repatriation to an overseas final destination is to take place.

11.4 REPATRIATION BY AIR AMBULANCE

This transport form should be used for patients who are not medically fit enough to be transported by commercial airliner. However, air ambulances are also used for logistic reasons, such as if transfer by commercial airliner requires multiple airport transfers or if the necessary number of seats to allow for a stretcher are not available.

The air ambulances in use at our company are equipped as intensive care units. The medical crew is usually composed of an intensive care physician and nurse.

Air ambulances should also be used if a patient is to be transferred at sea level. This is not a common occurrence but may be necessary if, for example, a patient needs transport to have an ileus operation. The air ambulance flies low enough so that cabin pressure does not deviate from normal atmosphere pressure. However, this type of flying is often associated with turbulence and uses more fuel. During a normal commercial flight, cabin pressure is equivalent to that of pressure at an altitude of approximately 2,000 m.

When choosing air ambulance as a means of transportation, no MEDIF form should be filled in. No medical clearance is needed other than the approval of the responsible physician.

11.5 WHO IS TO BE TREATED LOCALLY AND WHO IS TO BE REPATRIATED FOR TREATMENT?

Usually, emergency treatment is supplied locally. In case of acute appendicitis, it may be riskier to repatriate the patient than to be operated locally. Obviously, acute joint dislocations should be treated on location. In other cases, it is often judicious to transfer/repatriate after the condition has been stabilized.

SOS International has a database containing information regarding the treatment capacity of hospitals around the world. If a hospital is unknown to us or to our business partner in the country in question, our coordinating physician must assess whether it is advisable to have the planned procedure performed locally.

However, there are a number of countries where we are prepared for rapid emergency evacuation.

Even if a patient is hospitalized in a unit with fully qualified treatment facilities, patients may demand or desire to be repatriated and operated upon in their home country. If the insurance company or another financial sponsor accepts this argument, repatriation will be arranged if transport can be arranged with no additional risk to the patient.

11.6 PLANNING OF MAJOR ATHLETIC EVENTS

If a major event is planned, it is important that venue treatment facilities are inspected and that the competence of the local staff is evaluated. Assistance providers such as SOS International may be of assistance with their detailed knowledge of treatment facilities.

It may also be wise to check that local blood banks are fully trustworthy and also to investigate how blood is tested and treated before being used for transfusion purposes.

As for legal responsibility: The physicians who work for SOS International are covered by professional liability insurance. Most private hospitals worldwide have taken out malpractice insurance; however, this is not always the case.

Recommended Reading

Cummin ARC, Nicholson AN, eds. *Aviation Medicine and the Airline Passenger*. London, UK: Arnold; 2002. www.kcl.ac.uk/biohealth/study/short/aviation/DAvMedprospectus112.pdf

IATA. *Medical Manual*. 1st ed. http://www.iata.org/ps/publications/Pages/medical-manual.aspx

Shroeder E, Taudorf U, eds. *Air Travel and Transportation of Patients: A Guide for Physicians*. 22d ed. Danish Armed Forces Health Services; 1997

CHAPTER 12

Medicolegal Aspects of Organizing a Sport Event

Contributed by Dominique Sprumont, Professor, University of Neuchâtel, Switzerland; and David Townend, Associate Professor, Maastricht University, The Netherlands

Reviewer: Wiltfried Ideema, VP Legal Affairs, FIBT, University of Den Haag, The Netherlands

The organization of sport events, especially at the international level, is a challenging adventure. Think of the marathon that is run by the administrators, politicians, financiers, and authorities for the prize of hosting the Olympic Games or a world championship. This process is run in the stadium of public opinion and before the media that waits not only to enjoy the resulting competition of human achievement but also to delight in the human failings that the staging of the event inevitably brings. It is not only international events that pose organizational challenges: Sport event management and planning require the same considerations and offer the same problems, whether the event is international, national, or local. The only differences are differences of scale, and scale does not necessarily relate to the scale of risk involved: Sport is physically and mentally risky—that is its very attraction to the competitor and public alike. The purpose of the event for the competitor will be to push himself or herself to achieve the very best performance, which for top athletes will be in the controlled environment of professional coaching. For those further down the competitive slopes, coaching advice and risk assessment may be lacking or absent. This presents a different sort of difficulty for the event organizer: Will the environment within which the event is played out not only be a success financially and in sporting terms, but will it respect the participants' and spectators' dignity?

Defining how to respect this dignity is very difficult. For the spectators, health and safety legislation requiring risk assessment and certification offers a framework for preparation—built on the lessons learned from previous events that have gone wrong—sometimes tragically wrong. For athletes, there is an equal duty on the organizers to ensure that equipment and the stadium meet the health and safety, and the particular sport's governing authorities, required standards. These standards are known within the soft-law framework of codes of guidance and norms within each sport. However, for the participant sportsmen and sportswomen, there is a further balance when calculating dignity: The autonomy of the participant must be respected; the desire to participate in the risk of participation must be allowed to flourish. But how far is it necessary for an event organizer to consider whether the participant is exercising free will in offering himself or herself for competition, either because of the pressures of others or from the pressures from within? How far is it a duty of the event organizer to protect the athlete from himself or herself? Again, this is a question that is more difficult to answer the further down the competition slope one travels: An Olympic athlete with his or her entourage of professional advisers could be assumed, by an official, to have a greater degree of informed consent than the amateur runner who has decided to participate in a local "fun run" of 5 km, possibly for a noble charitable cause, dressed in a chicken suit but carrying an undiagnosed heart condition. Emergency medical preparations that an event organizer must make are one issue, but what questions the organizer must ask before allowing this man to participate is another. It is a question that in part is answered by the law, but equally, it is a question for the morality of sport, motive, and autonomy.

This chapter addresses the legal question and leaves the moral question somewhat hanging. This is partly because we feel that the proper place for such a moral question to be considered is in a forum with the sport event organizers and their governing bodies. The law also sets a framework within which society has produced its current working answer to the question. This will, over time, undoubtedly change—not least in the face of social reaction to events that expose that legal balance as inadequate. Therefore, this chapter is offered in a number of ways. First, it seeks to point to current legal issues. It does not seek to examine the general law relating to a sport event, so we will not discuss the nature of contracts, health and safety for venues, and the like. This chapter will examine issues about medical law in relation to sporting events, particularly the legal need to involve medical practitioners in the planning and running of events. Equally, the chapter is not designed to answer legal issues but to make the reader aware that there are legal issues that need appropriate, specific advice in the planning of each event. Second, it seeks to provoke the question: Is this level of provision sufficient or excessive, both for the moral debate and the legal debate? The law is a social construct, and those involved in the processes regulated by law have a voice, and arguably a duty to participate in framing the law. Many may think that the law is an encumbrance to the planning of an event. However, one of the most important parts of sport events is public trust and confidence—trust that the rules of the games will be observed, that there is no cheating, that there is value for money, and that they will be safe. This goes for the participation of athletes as well. The law and lawyers offer to sport event organizers assistance to protect the greatest assets that the event organizer has—the integrity of the event and the support of the people.

In the first part of this chapter, we will discuss the general obligation of the sport event organizer in relation to the protection and promotion of the health of athletes, spectators, and volunteers. As we will see, depending on the importance of the competition, especially in terms of the number of participants and the potential risks linked to the sport, one key responsibility is to organize proper medical support before, during, and after the competition. In the second part, we will discuss more specifically the scope and nature of the required medical support. We will also analyze the legal questions raised by "preparticipation testing" that aims at identifying those athletes who are more at risk of injury or illness by their participation than others. The third part will address specifically the responsibilities of sport physicians in relation both to the athletes and to the sport event organizer. We will cover the most important issues at stake, not only in terms of liability, but also in terms of education and organization. This section will conclude with a list of basic thought-provoking points that both the event physician and event organizers should consider.

There are certainly other issues that could be covered. For example, what are IF's or NF's responsibilities in defining the rules that protect and promote athletes' health? What specific training should sports physicians undergo? How should the athlete's right of privacy and antidoping requirements be balanced? The scope of this chapter is focused on more specific questions directly linked to the organization of sport events from a medicolegal viewpoint. Once again, our objective is to give a broad overview of the main problems likely to be faced by organizers and sports physicians in a competition. We will refer when necessary directly to the Olympic Movement Medical Code (OMMC) as it reflects an international consensus in medical ethics and is a useful tool to guide the practitioner in his or her activities.

12.1 SPORT EVENT ORGANIZER'S GENERAL RESPONSIBILITIES

In principle, a sport event should be organized in a way that prevents the risks of physical injuries, illnesses or psychological harm to athletes and all involved, including spectators, based on the general legal obligation not to cause harm to others and to respect other's rights, welfare, and interests. Hurting someone deliberately or by negligence or lack of precaution is generally sanctioned by law, creating in the person responsible for the damage an obligation to indemnify the victim; in severe cases, the risk includes a criminal conviction and penalty.

There are several types of liability:

- Civil liability aims to compensate damages financially. For instance, the person responsible for a car accident will have to cover the cost of the victim's healthcare, the damage to his or her car and, perhaps, the loss of income suffered during treatment for the injuries or due to any incapacity following the accident. Second, through the

- Criminal law, by which the state sanctions more severe violations of private or public goods or interests, such as causing fatal or severe injury to another person or causing damage to another's property or privacy. The purposes of criminal sanctions are both punitive and preventive: The actual criminal pays a penalty for his or her wrongdoing and potential criminals are discouraged to act through fear of the severity of those penalties.

■ There can be administrative or professional consequences and sanctions. For instance, a physician who has broken his or her duty of professional secrecy by transmitting, without consent, a patient's file to his or her insurance company or to the media could lose his or her license to practice or be restricted in his or her activities.

■ There are also indirect labor law consequences, for example, an employee may be fired for having acted in violation of his or her professional or contractual duties.

These basic social expectations and constraints apply to sports, and are accepted by the governing bodies of sports. For example, according to the OMMC, "no practice constituting any form of physical injury or psychological harm to athletes is permissible." Because of these "internal" sporting community rules and the general external laws of society, necessary measures to minimize the risk of injuries and illness must be adopted. This obligation belongs to both the IFs and the NFs, but also for sport event organizers at whatever level of competition. As suggested in the OMMC, "the participation of sports physicians is desirable in the drafting of such measures." Even before addressing the potential need for medical support during competition, there are preventive measures that can be taken to avoid unnecessary risks, for instance, by assessing and improving the safety of the facilities.

This development of an understanding of what it is to produce an appropriate environment for sporting events is a continuing process in which the contribution of sports physicians and sports scientists is fundamental. There are strong examples as to how these discussions have played a part in the development of health and safety requirements. After the 1985 Heysel and the 1989 Hillsborough disasters, which cost the lives of 39 and 96 people, respectively, there have been major efforts made to improve the safety of sports facilities, including the obligation to provide a seat for each spectator and to remove barriers at the front of stands. One example that shows a greater involvement of sports

medicine practitioners is where the International Ice Hockey Federation (IIHF) imposes technical requirements on ice rinks used for official competitions. These include rules concerning the boards that "shall be constructed in such a manner that the surface facing the ice shall be smooth and free of any obstruction that could cause injury to the players," or the protective glass, at which interruption there "shall be protective padding to prevent the injury of the players." The IIHF Rules for Ice Rinks also prohibits smoking at indoor arenas "in the playing and spectator areas, as well as in the dressing rooms and all the facilities where the players are involved." A physician should usually be on-site during official competitions in ice hockey and should therefore remind the organizers of those requirements. Such warning should also be made in relation to the rules of game, and the rules of the game should not be underestimated as a source of medical protection: Studies have shown that breaking the rules of a game increases the risk of injuries. Reducing unfair activities during competition and training through enhanced enforcement of the sport's rules appears therefore to be a potentially efficient measure to reduce sport-related injuries. It is not the duty of the physician to implement those rules, but, by raising attention about them, he or she increases the responsibilities of the organizer to guarantee a safe environment during the sporting event. Therefore, there is a valuable contribution to be made by sports scientists and sports physicians in the preparation and running of an event. The sports physician is not directly responsible for this, but if he or she considers that some risks could be avoided, he or she could inform the organizer so that proper actions can be taken. (Indeed, if such a professional is involved, then he or she could be considered to be under a duty to inform the organizer both through his or her professional oath and the general law of negligence indicated above.) Further, this professional opinion is available to the organizer and we suggest it should be sought as part of due diligence.

12.2 SOME SPECIFIC REQUIREMENTS: MEDICAL SUPPORT AND PREPARTICIPATION SCREENING

Medical Support

Depending on the nature of the sport and the level of the competition, organizing a sport event may require the organizers to provide full

TABLE 12.1 **High-risk Sports and Events**

Athletics (marathon, 30-km walk, 50-km walk, and pole vault)	Judo
	Modern pentathlon (equestrian segment)
Boxing	Skating (figure, long track, and short track)
Diving	Skiing (alpine, freestyle [aerials] and jumping)
Canoeing (slalom)	Soccer
Cycling	Tae kwon do
Equestrian (3-d event, show jumping)	Triathlon
Fencing	Water polo
Field hockey	Weightlifting
Gymnastics	Wrestling
Handball	Ice hockey

medical support. The 2000 IOC Medical Manual proposes a classification of sports depending on the potential risk of injuries.[1] The first category covers sports or events that can be considered as presenting relatively high risk as they have the potential for serious or life-threatening injury (Table 12.1).

When organizing events for these sports, it is suggested that the range of medical professionals required to be present at the event must include a physician supported by a therapist or a nurse and an ambulance with its attendants: The number of such professional teams of healthcare providers, including physicians, to be present will depend on the number of athletes involved in each location. For winter sports, the range of professional skills necessary for the healthcare team must also include a ski patrol, while qualified lifeguards should be available for water sports. Provision 9.1 of the 2006 FIS Medical Guidelines even recommends, depending on the event needs, that a helicopter be present and that a Level I trauma center be available near the competition. Such requirement is also mentioned in other sports, for instance, in motor sport, according to provision 9.2 of Appendix H to the FIA International Sporting Code. This is not just common sense,

it is the way of creating a suitable and appropriate environment for the event: One must think of the reasonable level of provision for a prudent and properly run event, and then test this specific protocol with sports physicians and technologists, and with a sports lawyer, and one must document their advice and act on it. These considerations are for the competitors. The assessment must then go on to include an assessment of the emergency medical needs that are foreseeable for the spectators as well.

The second category includes moderate-risk sports and events where most injuries are only of minor or moderate severity (Table 12.2). In such cases, it is also advisable to have the skills of a physician and a therapist on-site but with

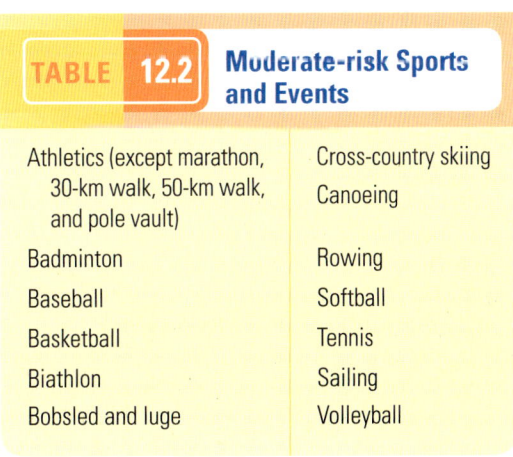

TABLE 12.2 **Moderate-risk Sports and Events**

Athletics (except marathon, 30-km walk, 50-km walk, and pole vault)	Cross-country skiing
	Canoeing
Badminton	Rowing
Baseball	Softball
Basketball	Tennis
Biathlon	Sailing
Bobsled and luge	Volleyball

---

[1] We are aware that those lists are controversial among sports physicians, but they illustrate that sports present various risks and therefore require specific medical support to prevent them.

the ambulance only on-call: Again, the size of the medical health team depends on the number of athletes in the given facility, and the due diligence work and evidence of advice also applies.

Other sports only present low risks, especially if they are not "contact sports." Here, the presence of a physician or a therapist may not be required at the venue, but one should make sure that healthcare providers are available on-call to provide assistance in a reasonable time in the event of an injury. In any case, first-aid attendants or other individuals qualified to provide basic support in case of accident should be present on-site with adequate first-aid kits. This basic support must reflect the likely injuries that could occur. Increasingly, the awareness of conditions leading to, for example, sudden cardiovascular death, is raising an expectation that such provision should include defibrillators available during competition. Technical progress has made this equipment such that almost anyone can use it. Arguably, when considering the statistical likelihood of such an attack on a competitor or a member of a large crowd during an event, such equipment should be standard in stadiums in the same way that fire extinguishers are required. Of course, one should also take into consideration the resources available and the local and national medical standards, especially when in the developing countries. But those issues of access to healthcare and the standard of care are beyond the scope of sports medicine.

This assessment of the level of support necessary must be made in the context of the whole event and not just in the provision for the competitors. An event will have a crowd of, one would hope, excited, emotionally charged spectators; the numbers of trained professionals should be appropriate to the size of the crowd. Therefore, while the categorization of sports as "low risk" may be appropriate, an adequate analysis must include the general question of the needs of the crowd, and that could raise the level of the provision required for the event.

Furthermore, when considering the provision for medical care, it is also recommended to have sufficient stewards and officials in place to guarantee proper emergency evacuation, to facilitate the work of the medical and paramedical personnel, or strategies to give the medical workers access to the injured. These procedures must be clearly understood and practiced in advance of the event, and increasingly, it is either considered good practice or a requirement to make the participants and spectators aware of the emergency exits at the start of the event.

In the absence of the proper medical support, a sport event organizer may be held liable in the case of an injury that is not treated properly and results in increased damage to the athlete. Following the comments made above, it would be fair to ask: Why *may* be held liable? First, it may be that a third party (not the organizer or the athlete) may be responsible for the injury. This would be a matter of evidence. Second, the responsibility may fall to the athlete, but this reopens the difficult question of the autonomy of the competitor to take a risk for himself or herself. The responsibility of the organizer will ultimately depend on the judgment of a court if the matter cannot be settled before litigation that the athlete himself is not responsible for the injury. The organizer could attempt to invoke the maxim *volenti non fit injura*. According to this legal principle, someone who knows and understands a danger and who voluntarily exposes himself or herself to that danger, without being negligent, is deemed to have assumed the risk and thereby to have lost the right to recover compensation for that injury from someone else (as no one else is responsible for the injury). In other words, the athlete could not recover compensation for an injury to which he has consented. The organizer would not have, in this case, an obligation to limit the risk, and even less to provide medical support. However, the success of such an argument may be limited.

The *volenti non fit injura* argument has been raised not only in cases of sport-related injuries but also in medical liability cases. In medical law, it has had a limited impact, at least in Europe, because the fiduciary nature of the doctor–patient relation imposes high duties on the physician to act in the patient's best interests. Consent of the weaker party, namely, the patient, constitutes a fragile defense for the physician as the bearer of a fiduciary obligation. We will come back on this issue in Section 12.3. In sport law, there are also several arguments leading to the same conclusion, suggesting that a *volenti* argument may be weak. First, the provision of medical support during a game or a competition is often required by the IF or the NF, at least for official events. Athletes are therefore entitled to expect that such support is available and their consent to the risk involved in the competition does not come into consideration.

Second, there is a contractual relationship between the participants and the organizer, either directly or indirectly (through the athletes' club or federation), that imposes an obligation to prevent risk and provide necessary care in case of injury. This is also supported by the fact that the organizer is expected to act according to the state of the art in the sport, and that his or her negligence will be weighted in view of the applied standards in the field, particularly to provide medical support as requested by the sports federations.

Third, sport events, at least major ones, usually require an authorization from the competent authorities demanding that protective measures have been taken in favor of the participants and the public. Such authorization often includes specifically the need to provide adequate medical support depending on the number of participants and the public's size. Even where the *volenti* argument could be possible, it could equally involve costly litigation requiring a detailed analysis of the representations made by both sides both before and during the whole event—costly financially, in time, and, perhaps most damagingly, in reputation, even if the argument is successful for the organizer.

As we have seen, providing medical support according to the risk of injury presented by the sport and the circumstances of the competition is standard practice according to IF and NF rules, but it may also be required for liability reasons by law. Yet it does not suffice to have any physician with an ambulance on-site. The sport event organizer should make sure that the physician has the appropriate level of expertise to deal with the potential injuries that could occur during the competition. In a recent case in the United Kingdom, the British Boxing Board of Control Limited (BBBC) was ordered to pay £1 million to a boxer who suffered irreversible brain damage, leading to the paralysis of one side of his body, after being injured during a fight. The court found that the BBBC owed the boxer a duty of care and that it breached that duty by not providing the required medical equipment and making sure that the physicians on-site had the proper expertise. According to the court, the severe head injuries would not have had such dramatic consequences if treated in time and with the proper equipment, drugs, and skills. It is therefore necessary to consider not only the scope of the medical support but also the required level of medical expertise according to the sport and the event. Indirectly, this may also have consequences for the liability of a physician who lacks the necessary expertise, but who, knowing his or her inadequacy, nevertheless accepts the invitation to provide support during a particular event. It is strongly recommended that his or her

liability be clearly defined before the competition. We will come back to this issue.

Preparticipation Screening

Another important measure often cited in injury prevention is preparticipation screening programs. Such screening is now recommended in particular to detect athletes at risk of sudden cardiovascular death. The IOC Medical Commission published recommendations on this issue in 2004: The so-called Lausanne Recommendations. Despite these recommendations, there are diverging opinions on the scope and nature of the preparticipation examination to be performed. For instance, US physicians fear that a too detailed list of tests to be conducted, namely, a 12-lead ECG, would increase their risks of being held liable for the death of an athlete who underwent such tests but was undetected as being at risk and then subsequently died from the condition. Yet, the objective of such preparticipation screening remains the same. Prevent injuries by identifying athletes whose conditions increase the likelihood that they will be injured or become ill during competition. In some countries, such as France or Italy, all athletes have to undergo a detailed preparticipation screening by law. In other countries, such testing will be requested for liability insurance issues in professional sports, and also in college or university sport.

Preparticipation testing poses two sets of questions: First, the liability of the physician who tests the athlete, and second, the liability for the event organizer. There is a third question, namely, "which events should have testing?" But this is a more political question, which is not for us to address here. In some sports, athletes have to provide a medical certificate testifying that they are fit to compete; in other cases, the test may be voluntary. Physicians should be careful in making such a certification, as the fitness to participate will not only depend on the athlete but also on the nature of the sport and the level of competition. It is hard to define *in abstracto* if someone is fit to participate in a sport event without knowing precisely the risks at stake. A physician who is asked to provide such a medical certificate should take a good case history from the patient about the competition in which he or she wishes to participate and it is recommended that he or she obtains further information from relevant sports physicians about which tests to conduct and under which standards; it is also recommended that one retains evidence of these enquiries. In any case, physicians should be cautious in providing a "fit to participate" medical certificate, as it could engage their legal responsibility in case of injury. Both the athlete and the organizer could argue that they were mislead by the certificate and therefore suffered damages. At least, instead of certifying that someone is fit to participate, it is more appropriate to indicate that the athlete does not have any apparent contraindications to participate in a competition. Such wording is compatible with provision 8.2 of the Olympic Movement Medical Code and is also used in national regulation such as in France.

It must be stressed that preparticipation screening, especially for sudden cardiovascular death, never completely excludes the risk of sudden death on the field of play. Preparticipation testing is only one of many measures created to safeguard the athlete. Even the most rigorous preparticipation screening will not replace the need for adequate medical support at the event, as discussed above. Preparticipation screening is available, however, and that opens the very difficult question of how far the event organizer should go to protect the athlete from himself or herself. Consider, again, the organizer of a local "fun run" for charity, where many unfit or poorly trained participants will attend. There is a dilemma here for the organizer. How far is it legitimate for the organizer to expect that individuals have the autonomy only to present themselves if they are fit to participate, or, indeed, to assume that such adults assume the risk for themselves even if they are not? It may be sufficient, in jurisdictions where the law does not require organizers actively to test participants prior to their participation in the event, to draw the potential athlete's attention to foreseeable risks that participation may entail with the very strong recommendation that the participant should seek medical advice before participating. It may also be possible, in particular jurisdictions, to limit the liability to participants by such information, effectively ensuring that the participant is offering himself or herself for participation with informed consent, and thus accepting the risk. Equally, such a contractual arrangement may be interpreted as ineffective in some jurisdictions: This is a matter that does vary, and unfortunately, we can only conclude that it is a matter upon which very specific legal advice must be taken in the relevant jurisdiction.

The position where the event includes child participants raises the responsibility question even further, as the capacity to give informed consent in the best interests of the child are held by parents or guardians. However, how far should the organizer be aware that in sports it is not impossible that the parent's view of the child's welfare is influenced by other considerations (i.e., the pushy parent)? Again, this is a matter for very specific, country-dependent legal advice. The question of consent and autonomy is considered below.

12.3 SPECIFIC RESPONSIBILITIES OF SPORT PHYSICIANS AND PHYSICIANS INVOLVED IN A SPORT EVENT

As stated in Provision 1.1 of the OMMC, "athletes are entitled to the same fundamental rights as all patients." In the same spirit, Provision 6.1 reminds that "the same ethical principles that apply to the current practice of medicine apply to sports medicine." The mere fact of being involved in a sport event or of treating an athlete does not modify fundamentally the ordinary responsibility of a physician. Yet the nature of competition and the specific profile of athletes have to be taken into consideration. Provision 6.2 of the OMMC stresses that sport physicians "have a duty to understand the physical and emotional demands placed upon athletes during training and competition, as well as the commitment and necessary capacity to support the extraordinary physical and emotional endurance that sport requires." As a consequence, athletes, perhaps more often than any other patients, push themselves to the limits, waiting until the last minute before consulting a physician in case of injury or fatigue, and asking the physician to suggest a shortcut to get back to the field, even at cost for their health. This is, of course, for legitimate athletes; doping opens a further set of questions around the involvement of physicians in illegal and illegitimate acts in sport.

When collaborating in the organization of a sport event, physicians have a dual role. First, they should act with the athletes as they would for their own patients, caring for their health and in their best interests, both in preventing injuries and treating injured athletes. Second, physicians may have a duty to advise the organizer on health-related issues, setting up a preparticipation screening program, assessing the safety of the facilities and equipment to limit the risks of injury, and organizing the necessary medical support. We will review the specific rights and duties of the physicians in each case.

The Doctor–Patient Relationship during Sport Events

Basically, a physician has the same rights and duties during a competition or when caring for athletes in general as they do with all their other patients. Yet physicians should be aware that athletes often have different priorities from their "ordinary" patients. Sports physicians (or physicians who deal with sports men and women) are also bound to respect specific rules in terms of healthcare, namely, the antidoping regulations. This imposes increased responsibilities in terms of informed consent, knowledge of antidoping regulations, and liability.

The need to obtain the patient's consent is now well established. It is not only a medical and ethical requirement, but is also a legal obligation. To be valid, the consent needs to be informed. This means that the patient must have received all the necessary information in a way that is understandable by him or her in order to exercise his or her autonomy and choose the treatment that fits best with his or her needs and interests. Failure to provide the proper information makes the physician liable for any damage that could result to the patient. It is therefore of particular importance for the physician to act in the most transparent way and to engage with the patient in an open dialogue. Beside this duty of information, the rule of informed consent also requires that the patient be legally competent to give his or her consent. This raises a problem when acting with minors. Normally, consent should be sought from their parents. Yet most national laws admit that a particular minor may also have the maturity to consent for himself or herself. In general and in many jurisdictions, children under 10 years of age should be presumed to be incompetent, while their capacity should be presumed above the age of 15. These are rules of thumb: Between the ages, one must determine the question of capacity to consent according to the particular child—but equally, outside the ages, one should be open to evidence of the particular case. During sport events and when caring for child athletes, physicians should be careful when informing their patients, as they must with all athletes in their care, on the specific risks connected to their participation in the competition.

In the general doctor–patient relationship, there are well-established expectations concerning privacy. In relation to the doctor–athlete–patient relationship, it must be made clear to the athlete that there may be legal requirements placed upon the doctor to disclose certain opinions about the athlete to governing bodies or event organizers (as discussed above). For example, when performing a preparticipation screening, the athlete should be made clear on the purpose of the test and that, even if the specific results of the test will be only communicated to the concerned athlete, his or her fitness-to-participate status will be given to the organizer, who could then refuse his or her participation. In no circumstance should a physician provide information on the specific health condition of an athlete beyond his or her fitness or unfitness to compete without the consent of that athlete. Without that informed consent, this would be a breach of confidentiality for which the physician could be held liable. Equally, the physician must make any duties to give opinions to others absolutely clear to the athlete to ensure that he or she is fully informed before giving this consent. Further, when approached for disclosures of opinion, the physician must ensure that he or she has the informed consent of the patient to make such disclosures, unless the physician is compelled to do so by a law that requires such disclosure without consent (e.g., in case of epidemic).

When dealing with athletes, the physician should also inform about doping issues. This means that the physician must make himself or herself aware of the list of prohibited substances in order to give appropriate advice, and must control carefully that the athlete is not prescribed such drugs unless they fall under a therapeutic use exemption (TUE). According to the World Anti-Doping Code, it is the responsibility of the athlete to avoid taking any prohibited substances. Under the strict liability rule, the mere fact that a test demonstrates the presence of a prohibited substance in the athlete's body or fluids suffices to prove the offense and to sanction him or her. The argument that the athlete ignored how this substance came into his or her body or that it has been prescribed by a physician, a coach, or someone else from his or her entourage is not considered a valid excuse to absolve the athlete from the offense. Yet even if in sport law it is the athlete's responsibility to avoid taking any prohibited substance, his or her physician could be held liable in an action for not having provided the proper information to the athlete or, worse, for having misled the athlete to take such substance either voluntarily or by negligence. When dealing with athletes, it is, therefore, highly recommended to keep in mind antidoping regulations and to take the necessary measures to prevent that an athlete could, even by accident, take a prohibited substance. A physician who fails to do so risks being held liable for negligence.

On the issue of liability, the physician should clarify with the organizer exactly who has the principal responsibility, and this should be based on legal opinion. In principle, the organizer should take the necessary action to cover the risks of damages, for instance, by purchasing liability insurance for the physician during the length of the competition and for all activities in connection with it. If this proves impossible, especially for nonprofessional events or "sport-for-all" competitions, physicians often offer support on a voluntary basis. In such circumstances, it is important for all parties involved to verify beforehand that the physician's professional liability insurance will cover his or her activities during and in relation to the sport event. As discussed earlier, it could also be useful to explore the possibility of asking athletes and other participants to sign a waiver of responsibility for their participation, a waiver that would include the risks of damages in relation to medical care. This goes back to the issue of "assumption of risks" that we mentioned before, concerning the legal maxim *volenti non fit injura*. Under limited circumstances, a physician could use as a defense the fact that the athlete fully appreciated and understood the risks and, based on this understanding, knowingly and voluntarily accepted to participate in the competition in any case. However, as indicated before, due to the fiduciary duty of the physician, courts may consider such waivers as invalid, especially when physicians acted negligently or in violation of a public policy. And, as discussed previously, the process of testing this liability in a court could be very costly in time, money, and reputation.

Concerning the liability issue, it should also be mentioned that in some jurisdictions there are legal provisions that immunize volunteer sports physicians from negligent liability when they provide emergency medical care to athletes. There are also other places that have enacted so-called Good Samaritan laws that protect physicians from litigation when they act in emergency situations or offer their assistance freely to someone who is injured. However, even those laws have a limited scope and do not cover situations where a physician acts with gross negligence or where there is no emergency.

The Relationship between the Physician and the Sport Event Organizer

As we have seen, sport event organizers have a duty to guarantee a safe and healthy environment for athletes and the public. In specific cases, they also have to offer proper medical support and to coordinate emergency rescues. This requires close collaboration between organizers and physicians. It is therefore recommended that the health issues be raised at an early stage of the event's planning. Issues to be addressed include, for instance, ensuring that the local hospital is informed about the competition and is ready to accept patients in an emergency. A direct contact with the emergency unit is, therefore, highly recommended as this will most likely save time and allows one to give first-hand information to the care provider. The contribution of the physician should be understood as a way to minimize the risk of litigation and improve the level of safety of the competition, as well as caring for the people involved in the event. In medical terms, this should be seen as a public health issue where the target is to introduce preventative as well as health promotion measures.

The organizer has responsibilities for the health of the participants and ensures that a physician is present to discharge these duties. The physician's role is in one part to act as a professional on behalf of the organizer at all points in the process—to assess the health of the athletes through a preparticipation screening program, providing support before and during the competition, and intervening in case of injuries or illness of the athletes—all this on behalf of the organizer. However, despite the relationship between the physician and the organizer, the physician must maintain his or her primary role of healer, looking after the athletes' health. When an athlete's or other's health is at risk, the question arises whether a physician has the right or even the duty to inform the organizer of the athlete's ability to participate in the competition. According to Provision 6.4 of the OMMC, "in the case of serious danger to athlete, or when there is a risk to third parties (players of the same team, opponents, family, the public, etc.) health care providers may also inform the competent persons or authorities, even against the will of the athlete, about their unfitness to participate in training or competition." It is clearly in the interests of the organizer to follow such advice. However, such rules raise concerns not only in terms of privacy and data protection, but also in terms of liability. There is a growing pressure from athletes and their entourage to challenge return-to-play medical decisions. This is linked to the fact that athletes are more likely than other patients to take risks to remain in competition due to prestige, the timing of the event in his or her career, and, crudely, financial gain. We have already covered this question in relation to the issue of waiving liability.

When an athlete is willing to return to competition against the advice of his or her physician, the latter should insist on explaining the foreseeable risks to the athlete and his or her advisers. If the athlete has no change of mind, then the physician should ask him or her to confirm this decision in writing and also the fact that he or she has been clearly informed on the situation. Such a waiver could be acceptable only to the extent that the physician is not asked to provide a medical certificate or to conduct, on behalf of the organizer, a medical examination to assess the fitness of the athlete. In no case should a physician issue such a certificate if he or she believes the contents to be untrue. In some criminal law, it is a specific offense for a physician to issue a false medical certificate: One would argue that it is always a breach of medical ethics to bear false witness in these circumstances. At this point, the issue of allowing the athlete to return to the competition returns to the organizer. The athlete wishes to continue; the physician has given expert opinion of the risk. The physician is not required to force the outcome—that is the responsibility of the organizer, and again it is a decision that should be taken mindful of the legal liabilities involved. On the one hand, the risk is that the injury causes the damage predicted and the organizer is sued for allowing continued participation; on the other, the athlete could sue on the basis that an opportunity was removed by an overcautious decision. This is, again, a matter for evidence (which must be meticulously gathered and preserved) and the opinion of the reasonable decision maker.

It is also likely for a physician to be asked to assist in antidoping tests. This requires that the physician is fully informed about the correct procedures to follow, especially in terms of collecting and handling samples. Again, the rights of the athlete as a patient should be preserved and under no circumstances should an athlete be forced to provide a urine sample or have blood collected. Such refusal to collaborate in an antidoping procedure should not affect the doctor–patient relationship.

Of course, athletes should be made aware of the consequence of such refusal in sporting terms, but it is not directly the physician's responsibility to enforce the antidoping rules.

12.4 CONCLUSION

We have covered the most pressing medicolegal issues linked to organizing sport events. It is important that before any competition there is a careful assessment of the specific health hazards for both athletes and spectators, allowing an assessment of what preventive measures should be taken, the nature and scope, if any, of the medical support to be provided at the event, the procedures to follow in case of emergency, and the collaboration in the fight against doping, etc. A key element is that a sports physician remains a physician before everything else, and that he or she must remain independent even when acting on behalf of the organizer, for instance when performing preparticipation screening. This requires having the proper training to fulfill correctly these responsibilities. Sports medicine is more and more recognized as a specialty for which physicians can and should obtain specific training. There are many different skills and experiences that need to be acquired—personal experience of the actual sport usually gives the physician and organizer insight into the issues at hand—but this must be measured against wider views and evidence to make sure that the involved physician has a clear and balanced understanding of the specific medical training he or she needs. It is recommended, in any case, that a physician understands the sport's specific athlete issues and that he or she seeks full information on the specificities of participating in the particular sporting event, both in the literature and also by identifying and contacting the competent professional associations and experts in the field. The physician should make sure that he or she has the right to practice in such settings, especially when going abroad, and that he or she has the necessary liability insurance coverage to protect himself or herself in case of litigation. Yet even if there is a risk of litigation, participating in a sport event should be considered as an integral part of a physician's activities, as it contributes to a better health for the athletes. Last but not least, it is a source of joy and pleasure for the physician and therefore should be strongly recommended for his or her own good health and wellbeing.

Likewise, the event organizer should regard these medical laws in the same way as the laws of the particular sport. Medical laws have been created to ensure safety and to maximize fair competition. It is so often the case that professionals—be they physicians, paramedics, accountants or lawyers—have been drawn to providing specialist advice because they also share a passion for sport. The law is daunting for any event involving risk takers and the public; awareness of responsibilities and liabilities, both legal and moral, and effective planning and precaution make for better events and contribute to the advancing of the sport.

Recommended Reading

Collins CL, Fields SK, Comstock RD. When the rules of the game are broken: what proportion of high school sports-related injuries are related to illegal activity? *Inj Prev.* 2008;14(1):34–38.

Michael Watson v British Boxing Board of Control Limited (BBBC) (High Court of Justice, UK, 2000).

CHAPTER 13

2006 and 2009 Olympic Movement Medical Code—with Introduction

Abstract from Chapter 1 of the Sport Medicine Manual of the IOC Medical Commission. It provides an introduction to the 2006 version of the Olympic Movement Medical Code and does not take into account the 2009 revision of the OMMC. Yet, two major changes have been introduced at this occasion:

1. The 2009 version is expressed in terms of general goals and objectives as opposed to formal legal obligation;

2. In relation, the clause regarding the complaint procedure (section 12 of the 2006 version) has been delayed.

For more details, consult the 2009 OMMC cover letter at http://www. olympic.org/PageFiles/61597/Olympic_Movement_Medical_Code_Cover_ Letter_eng.pdf (last consultation: June 08, 2011).

INTRODUCTION

As stated in its preamble, the Olympic Movement Medical Code "recalls the basic rules regarding best medical practices in the domain of sport and the safeguarding of the rights and health of the athletes. It supports and encourages the adoption of specific measures to achieve that objective. It complements and reinforces the World Anti-Doping Code and reflects the general principles recognised in the international codes of medical ethics". It is an integral element of the Olympic Games, and is open for signature by all members of the Olympic Movement, in particular the International Federations and the National Olympic Committees.

This document has been adopted in order to reinforce the current measures relating to the promotion and protection of athletes' health. It is based on the fundamental principle that athletes, physicians and other health care providers all have the same rights and the same obligations within the scope of sports medicine as in medical practice in general. The rules established by the Code thus correspond to the general instructions applicable to physicians and health care providers in accordance with professional ethics. The aim of the Code is to make those rules directly accessible to the persons concerned within the domain of sport, in order to encourage dialogue between each of them. It is integral to the philosophy of Olympism, which is to place sport at the service of the harmonious development of man by preserving human dignity.

The Medical Code is structured into four chapters, with a preamble: Chapter 1 covers the relationship between athletes and health care providers, Chapter 2 deals with the protection and promotion of the athletes' health during training and competition, Chapter 3 regulates issues relating to the adoption of, compliance with and monitoring of the Code, and Chapter 4 stipulates its scope, entry into force and the procedure for amendments. The principal measures of interest to physicians and health care providers are therefore to be found in Chapters 1 and 2: the first more specifically concerns athletes' rights, the second the role of physicians and health care providers in defining healthy practice of sport in collaboration with the different people and groups involved in the sporting world, notably the federations, clubs and organizers of sporting events.

With regard to patients' rights, Chapter 1 sets out 6 main themes:

- general principles,
- information,
- consent,
- confidentiality and privacy,
- care and treatment, and
- the rights and duties of health care providers.

At the heart of this chapter lies the principle of mutual respect between athlete, personal physician, team physician and other health care providers. The point is to guarantee the pre-eminence of the athlete's interests and health over other interests, linked, for example, to competition, to the economy, to the law or to politics. The protection and promotion of athletes' health appears to take precedence over all other considerations (1.2.).

This objective is achieved in particular by guaranteeing transparency in the athlete-health care provider relationship, the corollary to which is the athlete's right to information. It will be noted that in principle, the latter has the right to obtain specific information about the effects on his or her return to training and competition of a treatment, or absence of treatment, as well as rehabilitation measures (2.). Top sportsmen in particular are in fact often motivated to follow a shorter course of treatment, even if the risks and difficulties involved may be greater. The question that therefore arises is whether the athlete is truly free to express his or her own choices. That is why the Medical Code stresses the precautions to be taken by health care providers to prevent pressures from the entourage and to guarantee an athlete's true freedom of choice (3.2.). Athletes' autonomy is also protected by strictly respecting the confidentiality of data concerning them, as well as their privacy. In principle, no information concerning the athlete's health may be transmitted to third parties without his or her consent (4.1.). This rule is reinforced by the fact that when health care providers are acting on behalf of third parties (employer, organizer, etc.), they must in principle restrict themselves to indicating an athlete's fitness or unfitness to resume his or her sporting activities and participate in training or in competition (6.7.). Finally, with regard to data protection, the Medical Code reiterates the athletes' right of access to their complete medical record (4.4.).

"Athletes have the right to receive such health care as is appropriate to their needs, including preventive care, activities aimed at health promotion and rehabilitation measures" (5.1.). While the right of access to care may be limited, depending on the resources available, any form of discrimination and violation of human dignity is intolerable. In particular, it is important to offer optimal, quality treatment according to the circumstances, and in compliance with the rules of the profession. Particular attention must be paid to this when traveling, especially abroad (5.3.). As far as possible, the right to health care implies that an athlete is free to choose a health care provider.

The relationship between the athlete and his or her attending physician must in particular be preserved (5.4.). Moreover, it is advisable to consider the culture, traditions and values of each in implementing the general rules set out in the Medical Code (5.5.). As part of the health care provision, management of an athlete's suffering creates a number of sensitive problems. Special precautions must be taken to limit the risk of the athlete's health being undermined (5.6.).

According to point 6.1. of the Code, "The same ethical principles that apply to the current practice of medicine apply to sports medicine". Nevertheless, athletes find themselves in a special environment, which often pushes them into exceeding their own limits, and which sometimes exposes them to pressure from outside to pursue their activities, especially in competition, beyond what is desirable and tolerable for their health. It is important for the health care provider to appreciate this particular reality (6.2.) and, as mentioned above, to do everything possible to limit external pressures (3.2.). That means refusing to prescribe treatments that are not medically justified, even at the request of the athlete or another health care provider, as well as refusing to supply medical certificates that are untruthful. In certain exceptional circumstances, where the physician is responsible for the security of a team or an event, the physician may be induced to inform responsible third parties (team management, competition organizer, authorities) if athletes are unfit to take part in training or the competition because they represent a danger to themselves or to others.

Point 6.5. relates specifically to the protection of children, adolescents and young athletes, whose sporting activities must not pose any risk to their health or development. Even more than for adults, it is important to promote the healthy practice of sport by making the protection of a child's health and interests a priority over any other interests. Special attention must be paid in this case to preventing pressures from the entourage.

In principle, within a competition, the decision to continue or resume an activity falls under the competence of the team or event physician (6.8.). In any case it is necessary to clearly identify where this responsibility lies by stipulating that it may not be delegated to non-physicians. The essential point remains that this decision must not be dictated by the outcome of the competition; the interests and health of the athlete are paramount.

Chapter 2 of the Medical Code is intended more for members of the Olympic Movement who must guarantee the protection and promotion of the athletes' health. This key objective primarily involves guaranteeing a general framework which limits the risks of illness and accident and which benefits the athletes' physical and mental stability equilibrium (7.1.). It would evidently seem useful to involve physicians in defining these measures. For each discipline, but also for each category of sportsmen, it is advisable to establish minimum safety requirements to protect both the athletes and the public. These requirements relate in particular to sports venues, equipment, the general environment for the practice of the sport (for example, air quality, temperature, etc.), but also cover training and competition programs and rules of the game which can have a direct impact on the athletes' health (7.2.). A careful assessment of the situation is necessary for each sport. Physicians can provide useful support in this regard.

Sports medicine must be based on the latest recognised medical knowledge. That encourages in particular the continuation of research in this domain, including research involving the athletes themselves. The Medical Code refers to this subject in the Helsinki Declaration of 2000. The key point is that research into sports medicine complies with the same basic rules as any biomedical research, in particular the rule covering participants' voluntary, express and informed consent (7.5.). It is also important to share scientific and technical knowledge that may contribute to the protection and promotion of health (7.6.).

In most cases, a sport can be practiced without having to undergo a medical examination beforehand, even a basic one. At the end of the day, scientists accept that reasonable physical activity is generally beneficial for health, without a physician having to intervene. There are, however, certain instances, for example where there is a family medical history or where there are known symptoms, when a medical consultation is advisable, even within the scope of sport for all (8.1.). For active athletes, the demands increase in proportion to the competition. For some of them, a fitness test is necessary at the start of competition, while for others, follow-up tests have to be done on athletes on a regular basis (8.2. and 8.3.). It will be noted that the Medical Code regards any genetic test as a medical test that can only be performed under the responsibility of an appropriately specialized physician (8.4.). This arrangement is intended to prevent abuse by certain companies offering genetic tests supposedly indicating which sport, or what type of competition a person, even a young person, might be best suited for. Such practices are contrary to medical ethics and to the ethics of sport,

because the tests in question are not based on reliable, recognised research. It is therefore a matter of preventing the risk of abuse and of discrimination.

Finally, the Medical Code broaches the question of medical support within training and in competition (9.1.). Minimum requirements should be defined for each discipline, taking into account the resources available and the nature of each sport. It must be stressed that there is already a classification of sports based on the level of risks they pose (see Chapter 17 of the present Medical Manual). This classification offers a useful indication of the levels of support required. It is therefore obvious that a downhill alpine ski race and a table tennis championship are different situations. In each case, the necessary medical supervision has to be assessed by taking all of the parameters into account.

With regard to the protection and promotion of athletes' health, the Code recommends setting up databases listing all injuries sustained during training or in competition (9.3.). Such databases should permit the development of research on this issue, and thus enable more effective protective measures to be perfected.

In principle, the Medical Code does not aim to interfere with the current regulations on the practice of health care professions, especially of physicians. The principles established by the regulations simply reiterate those already applied in medical ethics. To guarantee the effectiveness of the Code, there is nevertheless provision for a complaints procedure for all those men and women who consider themselves victims of a violation of one of the rights recognised by the Code (12.1.). That can be of concern equally to an athlete claiming an infringement of his or her rights as a patient by a physician or other health care provider, or to a physician whose activity is unjustly restricted by a federation, the management of a team or the organizer of a sporting event. Every signatory to the Code has to formally establish the procedure to be followed in such a situation. It must be stressed that the Code clearly encourages collaboration with the professional associations concerned, as well as with the competent authorities (11.1.). In certain cases, it actually seems more effective and pertinent to report the case to the competent official body so that it may investigate the matter itself and adopt whatever sanctions may be necessary.

The Code came into effect on 1 January 2006, and applies to all Olympic Games. It has already been adopted by several International Federations, and others are about to do so, not to mention the National Olympic Committees. It is therefore important to ascertain on each occasion whether the Code is directly applicable and, if need be, what the complaints procedure is. Notwithstanding its adoption by a particular federation, or by a National Olympic Committee, in all cases it remains applicable and must be complied with as an expression of medical ethics in sport. All health care professionals, especially physicians, who wish to practice sports medicine are therefore strongly encouraged to familiarize themselves with it, study it and master it. It is a matter of keeping a critical and open eye on sports medicine with the greatest respect for all partners, with the athlete and his or her health as their central concern.

2006 OLYMPIC MOVEMENT MEDICAL CODE (OMMC)

Chapter 1: Relationships Between Athletes and Health Care Providers

Chapter 2: Protection and Promotion of the Athlete's Health During Training and Competition

Chapter 3: Adoption, Compliance and Monitoring

Chapter 4: Scope, Entry into Force and Amendments

Preamble

"Fundamental Principles of Olympism

1. *Olympism is a philosophy of life, exalting and combining in a balanced whole the qualities of body, will and mind. Blending sport with culture and education, Olympism seeks to create a way of life based on the joy of effort, the educational value of Good example and respect for universal fundamental ethical principles.*

2. *The goal of Olympism is to place sport at the service of theharmonious development of man, with a view to promoting a peaceful society concerned with the preservation of human dignity."*
   —Olympic Charter, September 2004

1. The Olympic Movement, in accomplishing its mission, should take care that sport is practised without danger to the health of the athletes and with respect for fair play and sports ethics. To that end, it takes the measures necessary to protect the health of participants and to minimise the risks of physical injury and psychological harm. It also protects the athletes in their relationships with physicians and other health care providers.

2. This objective can be achieved only through an ongoing education based on the ethical values of sport and on each individual's responsibility in protecting his or her health and the health of others.

3. The present Code recalls the basic rules regarding best medical practices in the domain of sport and the safeguarding of the rights and health of the athletes. It supports and encourages the adoption of specific measures to achieve that objective. It complements and reinforces the World Anti-Doping Code and reflects the general principles recognised in the international codes of medical ethics.

4. The Olympic Movement Medical Code is intended to apply to the Olympic Games, the various championships of the International Federations and all competitions to which the International Olympic Committee (IOC) grants its patronage or support, and to all sport practised within the context of the Olympic Movement, either during training or during competition.

Chapter 1: Relationships Between Athletes and Health Care Providers

1. General Principles

1.1. Athletes are entitled to the same fundamental rights as all patients in their relationships with physicians and health care providers, in particular the right to respect for:

a. their human dignity;

b. their physical and mental integrity;

c. the protection of their health and safety;

d. their self-determination; and

e. their privacy and confidentiality.

1.2. The relationship between athletes, their personal physician, the team physician and other health care providers must be protected and subject to mutual respect. The health and the welfare of athletes must prevail over the sole interest of competition and other economic, legal or political considerations.

2. Information

2.1 Athletes have the right to be informed in a clear and appropriate way about their health status and their diagnosis; preventive measures; proposed medical interventions, together with the risks and benefits of each intervention; alternatives to proposed interventions, including the consequences of non-treatment for their health and for their return to sports practice; and the prognosis and progress of treatment and rehabilitation measures.

3. Consent

3.1. The voluntary and informed consent of the athletes is required for any medical intervention.

3.2. Particular care should be taken to avoid pressures from the entourage (e.g., coach, management, family, etc.) and other athletes, so that athletes can make fully informed decisions, taking into account the risks associated with practising a sport with a diagnosed injury or disease.

3.3. Athletes have the right to refuse or to interrupt a medical intervention. The consequences of such a decision must be carefully explained to them.

3.4. Athletes are encouraged to designate a person who can act on their behalf in the event of incapacity. They can also define in writing the way they wish to be treated and give any other instruction they deem necessary.

3.5. With the exception of emergency situations, when athletes are unable to consent personally to a medical intervention, the authorisation of their legal representative or of the person designated by the athletes for this purpose is required, after they have received the necessary information. When the legal representative has to give authorisation, athletes, whether minors or adults, must nevertheless assent to the medical intervention to the fullest extent of their capacity.

3.6. The consent of the athletes is required for the collection, preservation, analysis and use of any biological sample.

4. Confidentiality and Privacy

4.1. All information about an athlete's health status, diagnosis, prognosis, treatment, rehabilitation measures and all other personal information must be kept confidential, even after the death of the athlete.

4.2. Confidential information may be disclosed only if the athlete gives explicit consent thereto, or if the law expressly provides for this. Consent may be presumed when, to the extent necessary for the athlete's treatment, information is disclosed to other health care providers directly involved in his or her health care.

4.3. All identifiable medical data on athletes must be protected. The protection of the data must be appropriate to the manner of their storage. Likewise, biological samples from which identifiable data can be derived must be protected.

4.4. Athletes have the right of access to, and a copy of, their complete medical record. Such access excludes data concerning or provided by third parties.

4.5. Athletes have the right to demand the rectification of erroneous medical data.

4.6. An intrusion into the private life of an athlete is permissible only if it is necessary for diagnosis, treatment and care, and the athlete consents to it, or if it is legally required. Such intrusion is also permissible pursuant to the provisions of the World Anti-Doping Code.

4.7. Any medical intervention must respect privacy. This means that a given intervention may be carried out in the presence of only those persons who are necessary for the intervention, unless the athlete expressly consents or requests otherwise.

5. Care and Treatment

5.1. Athletes have the right to receive such health care as is appropriate to their needs, including preventive care, activities aimed at health promotion and rehabilitation measures. Services should be continuously available and accessible to all equitably, without discrimination and according to the financial, human and material resources available for such purpose.

5.2. Athletes have the right to a quality of care marked both by high technical standards and by the professional and respectful attitude of health care providers. They have the right to continuity of care, including cooperation between all health care providers and establishments which are involved in their diagnosis, treatment and care.

5.3. During training and competition abroad, athletes have the right to the necessary health care, which if possible should be provided by their personal physician or the team physician.

They also have the right to receive emergency care prior to returning home.

5.4. Athletes have the right to choose and change their own physician, health care provider or health care establishment, provided that this is compatible with the functioning of the health care system. They have the right to request a second medical opinion.

5.5. Athletes have the right to be treated with dignity in relation to their diagnosis, treatment, care and rehabilitation, in accordance with their culture, tradition and values. They have the right to enjoy support from family, relatives and friends during the course of care and treatment, and to receive spiritual support and guidance.

5.6. Athletes have the right to relief of their suffering according to the latest recognised medical knowledge. Treatments with an analgesic effect, which allow an athlete to practise a sport with an injury or illness, should be carried out only after careful consideration and consultation with the athlete and other health care providers. If there is a long-term risk to the athlete's health, such treatment should not be given. Procedures that are solely for the purpose of masking pain or other protective symptoms in order to enable the athlete to practise a sport with an injury or illness should not be administered if, in the absence of such procedures, his or her participation would be medically inadvisable or impossible.

6. Rights and Duties of Health Care Providers

6.1. The same ethical principles that apply to the current practice of medicine apply to sports medicine. The principal duties of the physicians and other health care providers include:

a. making the health of the athletes a priority;

b. doing no harm.

6.2. Health care providers who care for athletes must have the necessary education, training and experience in sports medicine, and must keep their knowledge up to date. They have a duty to understand the physical and emotional demands placed upon athletes during training and competition, as well as the commitment and necessary capacity to support the extraordinary physical and emotional endurance that sport requires.

6.3. Athletes' health care providers must act in accordance with the latest recognised medical knowledge and, when available, evidence-based medicine. They must refrain from performing any intervention that is not medically indicated, even at the request of the athletes, their entourage or another health care provider. Health care providers must also refuse to provide a false medical certificate concerning the fitness of an athlete to participate in training or competition.

6.4. When the health of athletes is at risk, health care providers must strongly discourage them from continuing training or competition and inform them of the risks. In the case of serious danger to the athlete, or when there is a risk to third parties (players of the same team, opponents, family, the public, etc.), health care providers may also inform the competent persons or authorities, even against the will of the athletes, about their unfitness to participate in training or competition.

6.5. Health care providers must oppose any sports or physical activity that is not appropriate to the stage of growth, development, general condition of health, and level of training of children. They must act in the best interest of the health of the children or adolescents, without regard to any other interests or pressures from the entourage (e.g., coach, management, family, etc.) or other athletes.

6.6. Health care providers must disclose when they are acting on behalf of third parties (e.g., club, federation, organiser, NOC, etc.). They must personally explain to the athletes the reasons for the examination and its outcome, as well as the nature of the information provided to third parties. In principle, the athlete's physician should be informed.

6.7. When acting on behalf of third parties, health care providers must limit the transfer of information to what is essential. In principle, they may indicate only the athlete's fitness or unfitness to participate in training or competition. With the athlete's consent, the health care providers may provide other information concerning the athlete's participation in sport in a way compatible with his or her health status.

6.8. At sports venues, it is the responsibility of the team or competition physician to determine whether an injured athlete may continue in or return to the competition. This decision may not be delegated to other professionals or personnel. In the absence of the competent physician, these individuals must adhere strictly to the instructions that he or she has provided. At all times, the priority must be to safeguard the health and safety of athletes. The outcome of the competition must never influence such decisions.

6.9. When necessary, the team or competition physician must ensure that injured athletes have access to specialised care, by organising medical follow-up by recognised specialists.

Chapter 2: Protection and Promotion of the Athlete's Health during Training and Competition

7. General Principles

7.1. No practice constituting any form of physical injury or psychological harm to athletes is permissible. The members of the Olympic Movement ensure that the athletes' conditions of safety, well-being and medical care are favourable to their physical and mental equilibrium. They must adopt the necessary measures to achieve this end and to minimise the risk of injuries and illness. The participation of sports physicians is desirable in the drafting of such measures.

7.2. In each sports discipline, minimal safety requirements must be defined and applied with a view to protecting the health of the participants and the public during training and competition.

Depending on the sport and the level of competition, specific rules are adopted regarding the sports venues, the safe environmental conditions, the sports equipment authorised or prohibited, and the training and competition programmes. The specific needs of each athlete category must be respected.

7.3. For the benefit of all concerned, measures to safeguard the health of the athletes and to minimise the risks of physical injury and psychological harm must be publicised in order to benefit all those concerned.

7.4. The measures for the protection and the promotion of the athletes' health must be based on the latest recognised medical knowledge.

7.5. Research in sports medicine and sports sciences is encouraged. It must be conducted in accordance with the recognised principles of research ethics, in particular the Helsinki Declaration adopted by the World Medical Association (Edinburgh, 2000), and the applicable law. It must never be conducted in a manner which could harm an athlete's health or jeopardise his or her performance. The voluntary and informed consent of the athletes to participate in such research is required.

7.6. Advances in sports medicine and sports science must not be withheld, and must be published and widely disseminated.

8. Fitness to Practise a Sport

8.1. Except when there are symptoms or a significant family medical history, the practice of sport for all does not require undergoing a fitness test. The choice to undergo such a test is the responsibility of the personal physician.

8.2. For competitive sport, athletes may be required to present a medical certificate confirming that there are no apparent contraindications. The fitness test should be based on the latest recognised medical knowledge and performed by a specially trained physician.

8.3. A pre-participation medical test is recommended for high level athletes. It should be performed under the responsibility of a specially trained physician.

8.4. Any genetic test that attempts to gauge a particular capacity to practise a sport constitutes a medical evaluation to be performed solely under the responsibility of a specially trained physician.

9. Medical Support

9.1. In each sports discipline, guidelines must be established regarding the necessary medical support depending on the nature of the sports activities and the level of competition.

These guidelines must define, but not be limited to, the following points:

- the medical coverage of training and competition venues and how this is organised;
- the necessary resources (supplies, premises, vehicles, etc.);
- the procedures in case of emergencies;
- the system of communication between the medical support services, the organisers and the competent health authorities.

9.2. In the case of a serious incident occurring during training or competition, there must be procedures to provide the necessary support to those injured, by evacuating them to the competent medical services when needed. The athletes, coaches and persons associated with the sports activity must be informed of those procedures and receive the necessary training for their implementation.

9.3. To reinforce safety in the practice of sports, a mechanism must exist to allow for data collection with regard to injuries sustained during training or competition. When identifiable, such data must be collected with the consent of those concerned, and be treated confidentially and in accordance with the recognised ethical principles of research.

Chapter 3: Adoption, Compliance and Monitoring

10. Adoption

10.1. The Code is intended to apply to all the members of the Olympic Movement, in particular the IOC, the International Sports Federations and the National Olympic Committees (hereafter the Signatories). Each Signatory adopts the Code according to its own procedural rules.

10.2. The Code is first adopted by the IOC. It is not mandatory but desirable that the other members of the Olympic Movement adopt it.

10.3. A list of all Signatories will be made public by the IOC.

11. Compliance

11.1. The Signatories implement the applicable Code provisions through policies, statutes, rules or regulations according to their authority and within their respective spheres of responsibility.

They undertake to make the principles and provisions of the Code widely known, by active and appropriate means. For that purpose, they collaborate closely with the relevant physicians' and health care providers' associations and the competent authorities.

11.2. The Signatories ensure that the physicians and other health care providers caring for athletes within their spheres of responsibility act in accordance with this Code.

11.3. Physicians and other health care providers remain bound to respect their own ethical and professional rules in addition to the applicable Code provisions. In the case of any discrepancy, the most favourable rule that protects the health, the rights and the interests of the athletes shall prevail.

12. Complaints Procedure

12.1. Each Signatory designates a competent body to deal with complaints concerning alleged violations of the applicable Code provisions and with all other situations brought to its attention concerning the implementation of the Code. This body must have the power to take sanctions against the person or organisation at fault or to propose sanctions or the necessary measures to other authorised bodies.

12.2. The IOC Medical Commission designates a committee (hereafter: Complaints Committee), composed of three of its members, to deal with all cases of alleged violations of the applicable Code provisions occurring during the Games. This Committee also acts as a body to review decisions taken by the competent bodies of the Signatories pursuant to the Code. A request for a review may be submitted to this Committee by the person or organisation sanctioned, as well as by the claimant.

12.3. Decisions taken by the Complaints Committee in the first instance may be submitted to the IOC Executive Board for review. Decisions taken by the Complaints Committee as a review body and those taken by the IOC Executive Board are final.

12.4. The Signatories establish the necessary procedural rules, including the applicable sanctions in the event of a violation of the applicable Code provisions. The competent bodies of the Signatories and the Complaints Committee have the power to act upon the filing of a complaint or under their own authority.

13. Monitoring

13.1. The IOC Medical Commission oversees the implementation of the Code and receives feedback relating to it. It is also responsible for monitoring changes in the field of ethics and best medical practice and for proposing adaptations to the Code.

13.2. The IOC Medical Commission may issue recommendations and models of best practice with a view to facilitating the implementation of the Code.

Chapter 4: Scope, Entry into Force and Amendments

14. Scope

14.1. The Code applies to all participants in the sports activities governed by each Signatory, in competition as well as out of competition.

14.2. The Signatories are free to grant wider protection to their athletes.

14.3. The Code applies without prejudice to the national and international ethical, legal and regulatory requirements that are more favourable to the protection of the health, rights and interests of the athletes.

15. Entry into Force

15.1. The Code enters into force for the IOC on 1 January 2006. It applies to all Olympic Games, starting with the 2006 Games in Turin.

15.2. The Code may be adopted by the other members of the Olympic Movement after this date. Each Signatory determines when such adoption will take effect.

15.3. The Signatories may withdraw acceptance of the Code after providing the IOC with written notice of their intent to withdraw.

16. Amendments

16.1. Athletes, Signatories and other members of the Olympic Movement are invited to participate in improving and modifying the Code. They may propose amendments.

16.2. Upon the recommendation of its Medical Commission, the IOC initiates proposed amendments to the Code and ensures a consultative process, both to receive and respond to recommendations, and to facilitate review and feedback from athletes, Signatories and members of the Olympic Movement on proposed amendments.

16.3. After appropriate consultation, amendments to the Code are approved by the IOC Executive Board. Unless provided otherwise, they become effective three months after such approval.

16.4. Each Signatory must adopt the amendments approved by the IOC Executive Board within one year after notification of such amendments. Failing this, a Signatory may no longer claim that it complies with the Olympic Movement Medical Code.

(Adopted by the IOC Executive Board in Lausanne on 27 October 2005)

2009 OLYMPIC MOVEMENT MEDICAL CODE

Adopted by the IOC Executive Board in Lausanne on 16 June 2009.

Preamble

"Fundamental Principles of Olympism

1 Olympism is a philosophy of life, exalting and combining in a balanced whole the qualities of body, will and mind. Blending sport with culture and education, Olympism seeks to create a way of life based on the joy of effort, the educational value of good example and respect for universal fundamental ethical principles.

2 The goal of Olympism is to place sport at the service of the harmonious development of man, with a view to promoting a peaceful society concerned with the preservation of human dignity."

—Olympic Charter, July 2007

1. The Olympic Movement, in accomplishing its mission, should encourage all stakeholders to take measures to ensure that sport is practiced without danger to the health of the athletes and with respect for fair play and sports ethics. To that end, it encourages those measures necessary to protect the health of participants and to minimize the risks of physical injury and psychological harm. It also encourages measures that will protect athletes in their relationships with physicians and other health care providers.

2. This objective can be achieved mainly through an ongoing education based on the ethical values of sport and on each individual's responsibility in protecting his or her health and the health of others.

3. The present Code supports the basic rules regarding best medical practices in the domain of sport and the safeguarding of the rights and health of the athletes. It supports and encourages the adoption of specific measures to achieve those objectives. It complements and reinforces the World Anti-Doping Code as well as the general principles recognised in international codes of medical ethics.

4. The Olympic Movement Medical Code is directed toward the Olympic Games, championships of the International Federations and competitions to which the International Olympic Committee (IOC) grants its patronage or support, and to all sport practiced within the context of the Olympic Movement, both during training and competition.

Chapter I: Relationships Between Athletes and Health Care Providers

1. General Principles

1.1. Athletes should enjoy the same fundamental rights as all patients in their relationships with physicians and health care providers, in particular, respect for:

   a. their human dignity;

   b. their physical and mental integrity

   c. the protection of their health and safety;

   d. their self-determination; and

   e. their privacy and confidentiality.

1.2. The relationship between athletes, their personal physician, the team physician and other health care providers should be protected and be subject to mutual respect. The health and the welfare of athletes prevail over the sole interest of competition and other economic, legal or political considerations.

2. Information

2. Athletes should be fully informed, in a clear and appropriate way, about their health status and their diagnosis; preventive measures; proposed medical interventions, together with the risks and benefits of each intervention; alternatives to proposed interventions, including the consequences of non-treatment for their health and for their return to sports practice; and the prognosis and progress of treatment and rehabilitation measures.

3. Consent

3.1. The voluntary and informed consent of the athletes should be required for any medical intervention.

3.2. Particular care should be taken to avoid pressures from the entourage (e.g., coach, management, family, etc.) and other athletes, so that athletes can make fully informed decisions, taking into account the risks associated with practicing a sport with a diagnosed injury or disease.

3.3. Athletes may refuse or interrupt a medical intervention. The consequences of such a decision should be carefully explained to them.

3.4. Athletes are encouraged to designate a person who can act on their behalf in the event of incapacity. They may also define in writing the way they wish to be treated and give any other instruction they deem necessary.

3.5. With the exception of emergency situations, when athletes are unable to consent personally to a medical intervention, the authorization of their legal representative or of the person designated by the athletes for this purpose should be required, after they have received the necessary information.

When the legal representative has to give authorization, athletes, whether minors or adults, should nevertheless assent to the medical intervention to the fullest extent of their capacity.

3.6. Consent of the athletes is required for the collection, preservation, analysis and use of any biological sample.

4. Confidentiality and Privacy

4.1. All information about an athlete's health status, diagnosis, prognosis, treatment, rehabilitation measures and all other personal information should be kept confidential, even after the death of the athlete and all applicable legislation should be respected.

4.2. Confidential information should be disclosed only if the athlete gives explicit consent thereto, or if the law expressly provides for this. Consent may be presumed when, to the extent necessary for the athlete's treatment, information is disclosed to other health care providers directly involved in his or her health care.

4.3. All identifiable medical data on athletes should be protected. The protection of the data will normally be appropriate to the manner of their storage. Likewise, biological samples from which identifiable data can be derived should be protected from improper disclosure.

4.4. Athletes should have the right of access to, and a copy of, their complete medical record. Such access should normally exclude data concerning or provided by third parties.

4.5. Athletes should have the right to demand the rectification of any erroneous medical data in their files.

4.6. Intrusion into the private life of an athlete should be permissible only if necessary for diagnosis, treatment and care, with the consent of the athlete, or if it is legally required. Such intrusion is also permissible pursuant to the provisions of the World Anti-Doping Code.

4.7. Any medical intervention should respect privacy and be carried out in the presence of only those persons necessary for the intervention, unless the athlete expressly consents or requests otherwise.

5. Care and Treatment

5.1. Athletes should receive such health care as is appropriate to their needs, including preventive care, activities aimed at health promotion and rehabilitation measures. Services should be continuously available and accessible to all equitably, without discrimination and according to the financial, human and material resources available for such purpose.

5.2. Athletes should have a quality of care marked both by high technical standards and by the professional and respectful attitude of health care providers. This includes continuity of care, including cooperation between all health care providers and establishments involved in their diagnosis, treatment and care.

5.3. During training and competition abroad, athletes should receive the necessary health care, which if possible should be provided by their personal physician or the team physician. They should also receive appropriate emergency care prior to returning home.

5.4. Athletes should be able to choose and change their own physician, health care provider or health care establishment, provided that this is compatible with the functioning of the health care system. They should have the right to request a second medical opinion.

5.5. Athletes should be treated with dignity in relation to their diagnosis, treatment, care and rehabilitation, in accordance with their culture, tradition and values. They should enjoy support from family, relatives and friends during the course of care and treatment, and to receive spiritual support and guidance.

5.6. Athletes should enjoy relief of their suffering according to the latest recognised medical knowledge. Treatments with an analgesic effect, which allow an athlete to practice a sport with an injury or illness, should be carried out only after careful consideration and consultation with the athlete and other health care providers. If there is a long-term risk to the athlete's health, such treatment should not be given.

Procedures that are solely for the purpose of masking pain or other protective symptoms in order to enable the athlete to practice a sport with an injury or illness should not be administered if, in the absence of such procedures, his or her participation would be medically inadvisable or impossible.

6. Health Care Providers

6.1. The same ethical principles that apply to the current practice of medicine should apply equally to sports medicine. The principal duties of physicians and other health care providers include:

    a. making the health of the athletes a priority;

    b. doing no harm.

6.2. Health care providers who care for athletes should have the necessary education, training and experience in sports medicine, and keep their knowledge up to date. They should understand the physical and emotional demands placed upon athletes during training and competition, as well as the commitment and necessary capacity to support the extraordinary physical and emotional endurance that sport requires.

6.3. Athletes' health care providers should act in accordance with the latest recognised medical knowledge and, when available, evidence-based medicine. They should refrain from performing any intervention that is not medically indicated, even at the request of the athletes, their entourage or another health care provider. Health care providers must also refuse to provide a false medical certificate concerning the fitness of an athlete to participate in training or competition.

6.4. When the health of athletes is at risk, health care providers should strongly discourage them from continuing training or competition and inform them of the risks.

In the case of serious danger to the athlete, or when there is a risk to third parties (players of the same team, opponents, family, the public, etc.), health care providers may also inform the competent persons or authorities, even against the will of the athletes, about their unfitness to participate in training or competition, subject to applicable legislation.

6.5. Health care providers should oppose any sports or physical activity that is not appropriate to the stage of growth, development, general condition of health, and level of training of children. They should act in the best interest of the health of children or adolescents, without regard to any other interests or pressures from the entourage (e.g., coach, management, family, etc.) or other athletes.

6.6. Health care providers should disclose when they are acting on behalf of third parties (e.g., club, federation, organizer, NOC, etc.). They should personally explain to the athletes the reasons for the examination and its outcome, as well as the nature of the information provided to third parties. In principle, the athlete's physician should also be informed.

6.7. When acting on behalf of third parties, health care providers should limit the transfer of information to what is essential. In principle,

they may indicate only the athlete's fitness or unfitness to participate in training or competition. With the athlete's consent, the health care providers may provide other information concerning the athlete's participation in sport in a manner compatible with his or her health status.

6.8. At sports venues, it is the responsibility of the team or competition physician to determine whether an injured athlete may continue in or return to the competition. This decision should not be delegated to other professionals or personnel. In the absence of the competent physician, such professionals or personnel should adhere strictly to the instructions that he or she has provided. At all times, the overriding priority should be to safeguard the health and safety of athletes. The outcome of the competition should never influence such decisions.

6.9. When necessary, the team or competition physician should ensure that injured athletes have access to specialized care, by organizing medical follow-up by recognised specialists.

Chapter II: Protection and Promotion of the Athlete's Health During Training and Competition

7. General Principles

7.1. No practice constituting any form of physical injury or psychological harm to athletes should be acceptable. Members of the Olympic Movement should ensure that the athletes' conditions of safety, well-being and medical care are favorable to their physical and mental equilibrium. They should adopt the necessary measures to achieve this end and to minimize the risk of injuries and illness. The participation of sports physicians is desirable in the drafting of such measures.

7.2. In each sports discipline, minimal safety requirements should be defined and applied with a view to protecting the health of the participants and the public during training and competition. Depending on the sport and the level of competition, specific rules should be adopted regarding sports venues, safe environmental conditions, sports equipment authorized or prohibited, and the training and competition programs. The specific needs of each athlete category should be identified and respected.

7.3. For the benefit of all concerned, measures to safeguard the health of the athletes and to minimize the risks of physical injury and psychological harm should be publicized for the benefit all concerned.

7.4. Measures for the protection and the promotion of the athletes' health should be based on the latest recognised medical knowledge.

7.5. Research in sports medicine and sports sciences is encouraged and should be conducted in accordance with the recognised principles of research ethics, in particular the Declaration of Helsinki adopted by the World Medical Association (last revised in Seoul, 2008), and the applicable law. It must never be conducted in a manner which could harm an athlete's health or jeopardize his or her performance. The voluntary and informed consent of the athletes to participate in such research is essential.

7.6. Advances in sports medicine and sports science should not be withheld, and should be published and widely disseminated.

8. Fitness to Practice a Sport

8.1. Except when there are symptoms or a significant family medical history, the practice of sport for all does not require undergoing a fitness test. The recommendation for an athlete to undergo such a test is the responsibility of the personal physician.

8.2. For competitive sport, athletes may be required to present a medical certificate confirming that there are no apparent contraindications. The fitness test should be based on the latest recognised medical knowledge and performed by a specially trained physician.

8.3. A pre-participation medical test is recommended for high level athletes. It should be performed under the responsibility of a specially trained physician.

8.4. Any genetic test that attempts to gauge a particular capacity to practice a sport constitutes a medical evaluation to be performed under the responsibility of a specially trained physician.

9. Medical Support

9.1. In each sports discipline, appropriate guidelines should be established regarding the necessary medical support, depending on the nature of the sports activities and the level of competition.

These guidelines should address, but not be limited to, the following points:

- medical coverage of training and competition venues and how this is organized;

- necessary resources (supplies, premises, vehicles, etc.);

- procedures in case of emergencies;

- system of communication between the medical support services, the organizers and the competent health authorities.

9.2. In case of a serious incident occurring during training or competition, there should be procedures to provide the necessary support to those injured, by evacuating them to the competent medical services when needed. The athletes, coaches and persons associated with the sports activity should be informed of those procedures and receive the necessary training for their implementation.

9.3. To reinforce safety in the practice of sports, a mechanism should be established to allow for data collection with regard to injuries sustained during training or competition. When identifiable, such data should be collected with the consent of those concerned, and be treated confidentially in accordance with the recognised ethical principles of research.

Chapter III: Adoption, Compliance and Monitoring

10. Adoption

10.1. The Code is intended to guide all members of the Olympic Movement, in particular the IOC, the International Sports Federations and the National Olympic Committees (hereafter the Signatories). Each Signatory adopts the Code according to its own procedural rules.

10.2. The Code is first adopted by the IOC. It is not mandatory, but desirable, that all members of the Olympic Movement adopt it.

10.3. A list of all Signatories will be made public by the IOC.

11. Compliance

11.1. The Signatories implement the applicable Code provisions through policies, statutes, rules or regulations according to their authority and within their respective spheres of responsibility. They undertake to make the principles and provisions of the Code widely known, by active and appropriate means. For that purpose, they collaborate closely with the relevant physicians' and health care providers' associations and the competent authorities.

11.2. The Signatories encourage the physicians and other health care providers caring for athletes within their spheres of responsibility to act in accordance with this Code.

11.3. Physicians and other health care providers remain bound to respect their own ethical and professional rules in addition to the applicable Code provisions. In the case of any discrepancy, the most favorable rule that protects the health, the rights and the interests of the athletes should prevail.

12. Monitoring

12.1. The IOC Medical Commission oversees the implementation of the Code and receives feedback relating to it. It is also responsible for monitoring changes in the field of ethics and best medical practice and for proposing adaptations to the Code.

12.2. The IOC Medical Commission may issue recommendations and models of best practice with a view to facilitating the implementation of the Code.

Chapter IV: Scope, Entry into Force and Amendments

13. Scope

13.1. The Code applies to all participants in the sports activities governed by each Signatory, in competition as well as out of competition.

13.2. The Signatories are free to grant wider protection to their athletes.

13.3. The Code applies without prejudice to the national and international ethical, legal and regulatory requirements that are more favorable to the protection of the health, rights and interests of the athletes.

14. Entry into Force

14.1. The Code enters into force for the IOC on 1 October 2009. It applies to all Olympic Games, beginning with the 2010 Vancouver Olympic Winter Games.

14.2. The Code may be adopted by the other members of the Olympic Movement after this date. Each Signatory determines when such adoption will take effect.

14.3. The Signatories may withdraw acceptance of the Code after providing the IOC with written notice of their intent to withdraw.

15. Amendments

15.1. Athletes, Signatories and other members of the Olympic Movement are invited to participate in improving and modifying the Code. They may propose amendments.

15.2. Upon the recommendation of its Medical Commission, the IOC initiates proposed amendments to the Code and ensures a consultative process, both to receive and respond to recommendations, and to facilitate review and feedback from athletes, Signatories and members of the Olympic Movement on proposed amendments.

15.3. After appropriate consultation, amendments to the Code are approved by the IOC Executive Board. Unless provided otherwise, they become effective three months after such approval.

15.4. Each Signatory must adopt the amendments approved by the IOC Executive Board within one year after notification of such amendments. Failing this, a Signatory may no longer claim that it complies with the Olympic Movement Medical Code.

CHAPTER 14

Sport-Specific Management Issues

Contributed by David McDonagh, CMO, World Skiing Championships, Oslo, 2011

For the event physician, good local knowledge is essential. If you and your team have drilled thoroughly before the event, then many stressful and potentially dangerous situations can be avoided.

Knowledge of the arena is a basic demand and staff should know exactly where the different arena zones are (*cardiac arrest, come to area Q 28 immediately*) and where the access routes for stretchers and ambulances are (*you do not want to be driving ambulances in a crowd, or worse, in the opposite direction of crowd flow*), have paramedics/first aid responders situated above the spectators if possible (*it is easier to run down steps than to run up, particularly if carrying a patient*), and plan exit routes for stretchers at levels below the site of injury (again, it is easier to carry a patient down a level than up).

It is important to know where the doping rooms are located (*an athlete is receiving treatment and suddenly remembers that he has 5 minutes to make it to the doping room, but where is the doping room?*). What do you do? First, ring the doping room or the doping control team and inform them of the situation and the athlete's whereabouts and ask the doping control officer to make a log of the telephone call—you need their telephone number, so get it before the event starts! Secondly, ask to speak to the leader of the doping control team. Ask the doping control team to come to the medical treatment room or offer to escort the athlete to the doping control room.

14.1 OUTDOOR ARENAS

Many outdoor arenas can cover large areas and are potentially more difficult to "manage" medically. Cross-country running/skiing events are notoriously difficult, as they often go through unnamed areas or access routes. The medical staff should have maps supplied by the event staff and review landmarks and access routes so that transport to the accident site can be quick and effective.

Everyone who has worked in emergency medicine knows the importance of obtaining correct and precise information from the "caller."

(*Come to the corner of that big street near the food store. There is a guy bleeding from his head!*) or (*Someone has broken his leg on the road beside the hill with the trees—which is fine if you are in Iceland [hardly any trees] but awful if you are in Finland [only trees]*).

The person ringing in the emergency call is probably an event staffer—how else would he know your number? Ask him to give precise directions from known vantage points. Always ask about access. Can an ambulance drive to the location, and do you have to use a motorbike, buggy, snow scooter, boat? Can an ambulance drive on from the accident site, or does it have to turn? Can it turn, or should some other form of rescue vehicle be dispatched instead (e.g., helicopter)? Do you have to stop the race or event?

As you can see, there are many, many considerations to be taken into account. The only way to prepare for these scenarios is to prepare contingency plans, know your access routes, and know where your staff is located and what equipment and competence they possess.

Once, during the cross-country skiing World Championships, the medical command center received three different phone calls in the space of 4 minutes: (1) a man has fallen over and is unconscious, (2) a man has fallen and broken a leg, and (3) a man has been found lying in the snow. Three calls from almost the same location—within a kilometer of each other. What to do—send three ambulances? It turned out that all three callers were describing the same incident, but all gave different locations and different descriptions. Not easy. It is impossible to plan for all eventualities, but site knowledge can really help.

It is important that before an event the EP communicates with other track/site workers and that everyone has the same reference points.

14.2 WATER ENVIRONMENTS

Contributed by Margo Mountjoy, Chair, FINA Medical Committee, Guelph, Canada

Open Water Swimming

Due to the diversity of open water swimming venues, great demands are placed on the medical staff, and a close relationship with the event organizers is essential. The appointment of a medical officer is mandatory and The Fédération Internationale de Natation (FINA) guidelines must be followed.

Briefly there are two main areas of medical concern:

1. Environmental conditions
2. Swimmer health and safety

Environmental Conditions: Firstly, the venue and course are subject to the issue of a certificate of suitability issued by the appropriate local health and safety authority. FINA regulations demand a minimum depth of 1.4 m and a water temperature of no less than 16°C, checked at specified times and depths by a designated commission. The results of these measurements must be verified by the medical officer, who must also ensure the absence of other course hazards including aquatic flora and fauna or the potential for any form of pollution from industrial, biochemical, or bacteriological sources.

Where applicable, swimmers should be encouraged to apply ultra violet light (UVL) protection and the organizers should ensure adequate protection from natural elements at the conclusion of the event.

Swimmer Health and Safety: During the event, the surveillance of swimmers by accompanying craft is mandatory for safety reasons. Swimmers in obvious distress and those deemed to be incapable of continuing should be removed expeditiously from the water and assessed with appropriate urgency by a doctor.

Rendering assistance to swimmers in such situations should always supersede official rules of disqualify through "intentional contact" with a swimmer.

Adequate sustenance should be available to swimmers during the event. Swimmers are encouraged to hydrate well prior to and following the event.

A member of the medical staff should be positioned to observe all competitors at the completion of the event and administer medical support as required.

An appropriately equipped first aid post and medical center is mandatory.

In the event of a medical emergency, there must be an adequate system of rapid transfer to secondary or tertiary medical services. This will demand access for motorized ambulance service and clear communication with a receiving hospital.

Nutrition and Fluid Balance: Competing in open water swimming events is a major physical effort, for which all competitors should have adequately trained. Swimmers can expect to be in the water for 2 to 4 hours for events up to 8 km and 6 to 8 hours for an event over 25 km. It is therefore important to recognize that the body has a finite reserve of carbohydrate and liquid and that the frequent intake of nutritional substances is essential.

It is not appropriate for swimmers to wait until they feel their energy levels decreasing before stopping for nutrition. Rather, swimmers should aim to complete the event with "half a tank full" of energy. This will require frequent stops over the longer events exceeding 25 km even though they may feel their energy reserves are adequate.

It is recommended that approximately 200 to 400 mL of a balanced carbohydrate/electrolyte solution is ingested every half hour. This will also help in reducing cramps that are due to electrolyte depletion. Food may also be ingested, but it will be difficult to chew with a fast heart rate. Chopped-up banana, peach, or fruit salad are recommended. Ingested substances should not be icy cold. It is important to limit the duration of each break in order to reduce the risks of hypothermia (getting too cold) and muscle stiffness.

Hypothermia: Prevention of hypothermia is essential. Wool fat (anhydrous lanolin) can be applied and will also help to lubricate the skin, especially around the neck, groin, and armpit. Double bathing caps should be worn because a large amount of body heat is lost through the head. As body temperature is reduced, the blood vessels in the skin constrict and a disproportionately larger amount of heat is lost through the head and neck rather than through the rest of the body.

Nutrition stops should be brief because exercise increases the amount of blood flow through the skin, thereby increasing heat loss. While active exertion is taking place, this is balanced by the increased muscle activity, but when the swimmer stops, the increased flow through the skin results in further heat loss while muscular heat production is reduced. Prolonged stops are an easy formula for the development of hypothermia.

Swimmers who begin to feel cold should ingest more food by taking more stops of short duration. Food increases the body temperature because heat is produced by digestion and because the muscles require high levels of nutritional substances for maximum efficiency including heat production.

Escort crews should always be on the lookout for the development of hypothermia in their swimmers. Early symptoms consist of uncoordinated swimming movements and continual veering off course. When a swimmer stops, his or her mental processes may be dulled and the swimmer may appear vague. If a swimmer is unable to raise his or her arms above the head, obey other commands, or answer questions appropriately, then he or she should be retrieved from the water.

Hypothermia casualties should be handled gently. They should be dried thoroughly and wrapped on all sides with thick blankets. Towels, etc. may be wrapped around the scalp and the sides of the neck. They should be protected from the wind with either windproof jackets or large green plastic bags. Food and fluids should be encouraged frequently in small amounts, but alcohol is strictly to be avoided.

The medical officer for the event should see the patient retrieved from the water on account of hypothermia.

Exhaustion: Exhaustion occurs because of lack of energy from inadequate nutritional intake and from the effects of hypothermia. Its recognition and management are similar to hypothermia.

Pain: Approximately 15 km into a swim, many swimmers develop pain, especially in the shoulders. They may become abusive but can obey commands and answer questions. Support crews will require considerable tolerance in this situation but should encourage their swimmer to continue.

Sunburn: This is a real risk despite the water. As a minimum, Sports Blockout 15+ should be applied 15 minutes prior to wool fat. It is important to include the area behind the ears, the back, the back of the legs, and the bottom of the feet. Fair-skinned persons should reapply sunblock every 2 hours to any area of their body not covered by wool fat.

Jellyfish Stings: These could be a problem for those people susceptible to stings. Wool fat will help to prevent them, but Vaseline is far less effective because it melts off. The main problem with jellyfish stings is pain, although if there are multiple contacts, the pain may be severe and systemic symptoms such as nausea and vomiting may develop. Pain is often soothed by the coolness of the water. Persistent severe pain should be reported to the medical officers.

Swallowed Salt Water: Salt water is approximately 3% sodium chloride that is three times more concentrated than the body's internal fluids. Ingestion often results in vomiting. Treatment includes reassurance in the first instance, but persistent vomiting may require withdrawal.

Trauma: Shark attack is unlikely. A significant risk however exists from escort boat propellers and extreme care must be taken when maneuvering near swimmers.

Removal from Open Water: Removing the athlete from the open water requires personnel experienced in water rescue. It is important that the rescue boat does not interfere with the remaining swimmers. The boat should be stabilized so that it does not capsize while rescuing the swimmer. The swimmer should be removed by grasping the swimmer under the axillae and lifting with the legs. The athlete should have his or her back against the side of the boat. Two rescuers may be needed depending on the size of the athlete. Once in the boat, the athlete should be protected from the environment, and emergency first aid can be administered. In particular, an assessment of airway, breathing, circulation, and cognitive state is essential. Laying the swimmer in the semiprone position if possible in the vessel is appropriate. Quick removal to a medical station on land is advantageous.

Aquatic Events in the Swimming Pool

Swimming, water polo, diving, and synchronized swimming occur exclusively in a swimming pool. There are specific concerns and requirements that medical officers should attend to when supplying the medical care for the athlete in the swimming pool.

Environmental Conditions: The safety of the pool environment is the responsibility of the event physician. The physician should ensure that the local public health guidelines are followed to ensure adequate sanitation and pool water safety standards are met. The external pool environment should also be evaluated for any obvious hazards such as exposed electricity, obstructing objects, or other environmental hazards. As with all swimming events, the pool environment should be smoke free.

Swimmer Health and Safety: All aquatic events should have a qualified and experienced lifeguard staff present during competitive and training sessions. A medical station should be located close to the pool deck for easy access in case of an emergency. For diving and water polo events, a poolside medical station is recommended.

The medical station should be equipped to manage primary first aid. It should contain a spinal board (floatable), automatic external defibrillator, oxygen, IV equipment, ECG, and first aid equipment. A clear and easily accessed evacuation path for ambulance removal to a tertiary care emergency center should be predetermined in case of emergency. The most common injuries in aquatic sports are overuse injuries. As such, the event physician should be experienced in the management of chronic overuse injuries. In addition, familiarity with general practice presentations such as gastroenteritis, dermatology, respiratory infections, etc. is recommended.

The on-site pool deck emergency station for water polo and diving should include a floatable spinal board and emergency first aid equipment. Water polo event physicians should be prepared to manage lacerations, contusions, head injuries, facial injuries, and dental injuries. Other traumatic injuries can be seen in water polo. The bleeding athlete should not be allowed to enter the water; hemostasis is required prior to reentry to competition. Quick-drying skin glue and/or Steri-Strips are useful in managing lacerations in the water polo player to allow fast return to play. The event physician should be familiar with the latest recommendations for the management of concussion as concussion is one of the most common injuries in water polo.

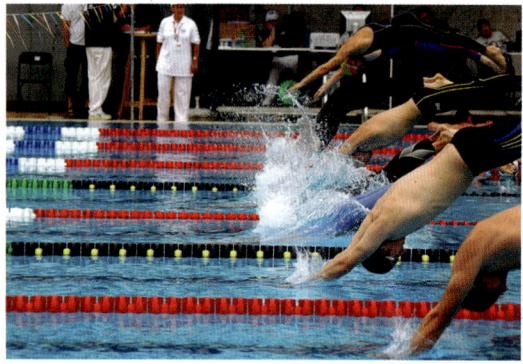

Traumatic injuries in diving are very rare; however, they can be serious upon occurrence. Falls from the 10-m tower can result in pneumothorax, ear perforations, head injuries, and cervical spine injuries. Traumatic collision with the board/tower can result in contusions, abrasions, and, more rarely, catastrophic injuries. Event medical staff should be trained in deep water cervical spinal removal procedures. These procedures should be rehearsed on a regular basis. Maintenance of cervical stability during the rescue is mandatory. Techniques to provide ventilation during cervical stabilization should also be practiced. Upon removal from the pool, attention should be paid to maintaining body temperature while providing emergency first aid.

14.3 WORKING IN DRY/HOT ENVIRONMENTS

Contributed by Andreas Michael Niess, Professor, University of Tübingen, formerly with German National Athletics Team, Germany

Race Organization

Race organizers should be aware of the local weather history and not plan prolonged endurance events in months with a higher risk of extreme conditions. During the summer season, scheduling races in the morning or evening may help to prevent extreme heat stress. It should be taken into account that the first hot days in spring pose an increased risk for heat illness, as most of the athletes are still not sufficiently acclimated.

For long-distance or endurance events, many organizations require athletes to inform them about possible medical problems, risk factors, etc. (especially with respect to heat illness), when they complete the competition registration papers. In order to prevent heat-related health problems, it is often useful to provide athletes with practical information regarding heat acclimatization, fluid intake, and clothing both on registration and before the event.

Prior to the start of an event, the medical director should inform the participants about the current and predicted weather conditions and the risk of heat illness and give preventative tips regarding clothing, etc.

Monitoring of actual weather conditions before, during and after the event is recommended and is often mandatory at large events, to allow medical staff to assess the extent of heat stress.

As a minimum, dry-bulb temperature and relative humidity should be measured. More precise information is gained from assessing the wet-bulb globe temperature (WBGT) index, which is easily determined using portable devices. For continuous activity or competition, a WBGT of 27.8°C is defined as a threshold level. Cancelling exercise or a sporting event for an athlete should be considered if levels are higher than this. Under certain circumstances, especially if exercising athletes are well trained and heat acclimatized, this limit may be exceeded. However, it is important to remember that there is still an increased risk of heat illness for these acclimatized and well-trained athletes.

Medical staff should be trained to recognize symptoms and signs of dehydration and heat illness. Persons with lower fitness and/or low acclimatization levels should be carefully watched. In addition, athletes competing in multistage events are at increased risk of dehydration.

In order to allow sufficient athlete hydration, but also prevent hyponatremia due to excessive fluid intake, in events in the heat, placing fluid stations every 2.5 km seems to be a reasonable compromise to address both issues.

Organization of Medical Facilities

Sufficient medical staff and facilities should be carefully planned, especially during events under elevated ambient temperatures. (For more detailed information, see Chapter 69.)

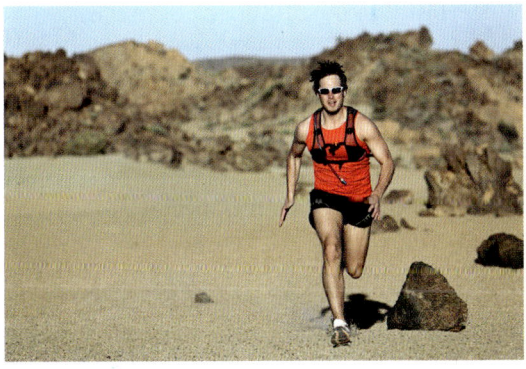

Medical Staff: In large endurance competitions such as triathlon, cycling, or running, the ACSM position statement recommends 1 to 2 physicians, 4 to 6 podiatrists, 1 to 4 emergency medical technicians, 2 to 4 nurses, 3 to 6 physiotherapists, 3 to 6 athletic trainers, and 1 to 3 assistants per 1,000

participants. The medical staff should be well trained for instituting appropriate medical aid. The team should be familiar with handling heat illness. Importantly, the medical staff must have the official allowance to exclude participants who show signs of heat illness from the race.

Medical Facilities: The primary medical aid station, including approximately 75% of the medical personnel, should be located in the finish area. Besides the common medical aid equipment cooling devices such as fans, crushed ice in plastic bags, small pools for cool or cold (ice) water immersion should be available. As hyponatremia may occur during such events, an important diagnostic tool would be onsite analysis of serum or plasma sodium concentrations.

In running events over 10 km, further medical stations should be placed along the route, ideally at 2- to 3-km intervals. A mobile emergency ambulance should be located near the finish. Further mobile ambulances can help transport participants with heat illness.

Communication: Sufficient communication using mobile phones or two-way radio devices should be guaranteed between the leading medical personnel and each individual staff member located on course. Furthermore, the local hospital(s) have to be informed timely about the date of the event and the estimated number of participants.

Medical Staff Needs: Don't forget that medical staff, who may also have to spend long hours in the sun, can also be exposed to heat-related illnesses. They also need protective clothing, sunglasses, shade, food, and hydration. Always keep your staff happy!

Recommended Reading

Armstrong LE, Epstein Y, Greenleaf JE, et al. ACSM position stand: the female athlete triad: heat and cold illness during distance running. *Med Sci Sports Exerc.* 1996;28(10):139–148.

14.4 WORKING IN A COLD ENVIRONMENT

Contributed by David McDonagh

Never an easy task, working in cold environs requires careful planning. During the Winter Olympics in Lillehammer, outdoor temperatures at the downhill skiing events went down to −30°C and medical personnel were obliged to stand outdoors for up to three hours. It is important to be able to offer outdoor staff warm drinks, the option of warming up in a heated tent, special heat packs, and, of course, proper clothing. Volunteers with cardiac or respiratory problems were given jobs at other indoor stadia.

Clothing

Traditionally, cold climate clothing has been heavy and cumbersome and has made working in cold climates extremely difficult. Many have seen volunteer staff hulking to the injury location looking more like waddling cuboid giants than lithe first responders. Modern winter clothing is expensive but well worth investing in.

The clue to winter clothing is to have an outer layer that is water and wind resistant, an insulating layer to prevent heat loss, and an inner moisture barrier to prevent body moisture from condensing and freezing to the insulation. Wet clothes have reduced insulation quality. Adjust your clothing during the day to avoid sweating. This can be done by partially opening your jacket, by removing an inner layer of clothing or heavy outer mittens, or by changing to lighter headgear. The head and hands can be efficient in dissipating heat. Avoid plastic directly on the skin: this causes sweating even in the coldest weather. Alternating between sweating and freezing is uncomfortable, not good for morale, and often as not ends up with staff feeling sick. Modern clothing can compensate somewhat—a minimum requirement is to have a lightweight sweat-absorbent layer against the skin to allow some water movement away from the skin. Having several layers of clothing also creates a fabric/air interface at different levels, thus allowing for greater insulation and warmth, but also allows easier body movement.

Gloves and Boots

Gloves must be water resistant, thermally insulated and preferably have rubberized grips on the palms to facilitate working with metal and rough objects. In extreme cold, I recommend the use of two pairs of gloves: a thin insulated inner set as well as heavy outer gloves. Gloves are necessarily thick to retain heat, but it is extremely difficult to insert a cannula or intubate with thick gloves on. For a procedure that takes a short period of time, I usually remove all gloves and dry my hands, particularly if I am using metal instruments.

Finding a vein is often exceptionally difficult and one should always have a venous tourniquet available and preferably a small heat pack that can be placed over the puncture site (e.g., cubital fossa). In extreme situations the use of an intraosseous cannula must be considered. The midanterior tibial region gives good access.

Boots should be water resistant, thermally insulated, and have soft(ish) rubberized soles with good grip. Boots must not be too tight and should be at least one size larger than your normal shoe size to allow for two pairs of socks. In extreme cold, I have a thin inner layer of socks inside a heavier outer pair. Some practical problems:

- Equipment made of plastic becomes stiff in extreme cold. Normally pliable objects like cervical collars and endotracheal tubes become stiff and brittle and difficult to use. Try to keep these in the nearest, warmest place.

- Equipment made of metal is also difficult in such an environment in that it tends to freeze to the skin causing tears and burns if pulled away from the skin.

- Saline solutions and other intravenous solutions may also freeze, so again, try to keep these in the nearest, warmest place.

14.5 HIGH-ALTITUDE SICKNESS

Contributed by David McDonagh
Reviewer: Richard Budgett, IOC Medical Committee, Chief Medical Officer, London 2012 Olympic Summer Games

If you are predisposed to developing altitude sickness, then symptoms can arise as low as 2,400 m. Major competitions are seldom organized at these heights, though on some occasions, Olympic Games and World Championships are held at altitude (e.g., Mexico City at 2,240 m). This can cause problems for visiting lowland athletes. In an attempt to adapt to the lower barometric oxygen pressure, breathing becomes faster and deeper, particularly during exercise, leading to lower pCO_2 levels. Changes in pO_2 and pCO_2 levels and acid-base balance will then affect the respiratory center and respiration rate. Athletes may experience unusual breathing patterns, particularly at nighttime, with cycles of normal breathing, slower breathing, and breath-holding, followed by a recovery period of accelerated breathing. Breath-holding may last for up to 15 seconds, but in the absence of other symptoms is usually not a cause of concern. Most agree that this is not altitude sickness, but more a symptom of being at altitude that will resolve on descent.

Normal physiologic changes are

- Hyperventilation (breathing faster, deeper, or both)
- Dyspnea on exertion
- Nocturnal respiration rhythm and rate changes
- Poor night sleep, awakening often
- Increased urination

Terminology can be a bit confusing here, but the term *altitude sickness* includes at least three recognized conditions:

- Acute mountain sickness (AMS), or the more serious
- High-altitude cerebral edema (HACE) and
- High-altitude pulmonary edema (HAPE).

Symptoms of mild altitude sickness are more pronounced than in the normal physiologic reaction with malaise, tiredness, vomiting, and weakness during exercise. Symptoms of severe altitude sickness include respiratory and cerebral symptoms such as dyspnea, disorientation, hallucinations, and psychotic behavior.

Acute Mountain Sickness

AMS may present with a number of symptoms, but as a rule there must be at least two symptoms present: Headache + one of the following:

- Loss of appetite, nausea, or vomiting
- Fatigue or weakness
- Dizziness or light-headedness
- Difficulty sleeping

All of these symptoms may vary in intensity from mild to severe (grading system: Lake Louise Consensus on the Definition of Altitude Sickness). Most experts believe that one's predisposition to develop AMS is independent of age, gender, physical fitness, or previous altitude experience. Some people acclimatize quickly, some do not. The same person may react differently on different occasions. High-altitude cough can occur, often with a dry persistent cough, without fatigue or dyspnea. This is often a stand-alone condition.

High-altitude Cerebral Edema

A severe form of altitude sickness can develop with a life-threatening cerebral edema. Experts describe behavioral changes, lethargy, cognitive changes, confusion, and a classic ataxia (the "mountain drunk"), which constitute an emergency situation. If you suspect HACE, the athlete should desist all activities, rest on a stretcher, and be given oxygen (preferably hyperbaric) and IV fluids, and emergency evacuation is required—preferably by helicopter—as soon as possible. The recovery rate is good if rapid descent is enacted.

High-altitude Pulmonary Edema

Altitude-induced edema can also affect the lungs and can occur concomitantly with HACE.

Symptoms include

- Fatigue and tiredness
- Dyspnea at rest and worsened by exertion, increased respiratory rate
- Cough, with or without pink, frothy sputum
- Cyanosis
- Chest pain, discomfort

Again, this should be treated as an emergency and managed with rest, oxygen, IV fluids and immediate descent by helicopter. HAPE frequently occurs at night and patients can often develop HACE, so early symptoms must be recognized and taken seriously.

CONCLUSION

The key to good medical care is early symptom detection and early athlete removal from altitude. If the athlete is training in conditions under 2,400 m, it is unlikely that AMS is the cause of symptoms, so symptoms are either due to acclimatization or they may be due to other less exotic conditions, such as sinusitis, etc.

If you are higher than 2,400 m, the detection of headache is important, and headache combined with other symptoms may indicate the presence of mild AMS.

The presence of cerebral problems demands immediate action.

Respiratory problems may be less easily diagnosed, but if in doubt, remove the athlete from altitude. Only in extreme cases is dexamethasone indicated, that is, cerebral or respiratory edema. Treatment of AMS is rest, fluids, and descent from altitude.

It may be difficult to decide if headache is due to other causes—if altitude is less than 2,400 m, then it probably is. If over 2,400 m, my advice is to treat as AMS.

Acetazolamide (Diamox) and Dexamethasone Require TUEs

Acetazolamide (Diamox) is a tried and tested drug for altitude sickness prevention and treatment. Its purported effect is due to increased urinary excretion of bicarbonate, thus lowering blood pH and thus correcting the acid-base imbalance. Some athletes will take prophylactic doses of 250 mg twice daily for 1 or 2 days before traveling to altitude and continuing until 3 days after the highest altitude has been reached. As far as treatment for AMS is concerned, acetazolamide 250 mg × 2 to 3 daily does seem to reduce symptoms such as headache, nausea, shortness of breath, dizziness, drowsiness, and fatigue. However, acetazolamide is a prohibited substance and is on the WADA Prohibited List—an S5 diuretic and masking agent. A TUE is required if it is to be used. To avoid AMS, gradual ascent is the best option. Side effects of acetazolamide are excessive urination and tingling of the fingers and toes.

Dexamethasone is an effective drug that can be used if an athlete has a respiratory or cerebral edema. This is an emergency situation and the athlete must be sent to a lowland hospital as soon as possible. Obviously, the athlete will take no further part in sports activity. Dexamethasone is a glucocorticosteroid (S9) and is prohibited when administered orally, rectally, intravenously, or intramuscularly. Its use by these routes requires a TUE approval. If an athlete returns to play having received dexamethasone, he or she must first produce a TUE from his or her NF or national antidoping organization before reparticipating.

Recommended Reading

Auerbach P, ed. *Wilderness Medicine: Management of Wilderness and Environmental Emergencies.* 4th ed. St. Louis, MO: Mosby; 2001.

Ward MP, Milledge JS, West JB. *High Altitude Medicine and Physiology.* 3rd ed. London: Arnold; 2000.

Pollard AJ, Murdoch DR. *The High Altitude Medicine Handbook.* 2nd ed. Oxford: Radcliffe Medical Press, 1998.

Forgey WW. *Wilderness Medical Society Practice Guidelines for Wilderness Emergency Care.* 2nd ed. Guilford: Globe Pequot Press; 2000.

14.6 LIGHTNING

Contributed by David McDonagh

The EP should be aware of the dangers posed by lightning and, although relatively rare (28 registered deaths in the United States in 2008), some deaths and injuries can be avoided by taking simple safety procedures. Here is some advice from the U.S. National Weather Service:

- Have a plan in case of lightning storms
- Check the weather forecast
- Evacuate outdoor athletes to safe houses (solid, insulated, roofed structure) OR
- Evacuate to fully enclosed metal vehicles (not soft tops or roofless vehicles)
- Once inside a safe house, stay away from electrical appliances (telephones, PCs, TVs, etc.), electric cables, and plumbing pipes
- Bicyclists should get off the bicycle, leave it, and go to a safe house or vehicle
- Golfers should leave their clubs and head for the clubhouse
- Avoid standing in groups, in open fields, or under solitary trees
- Swimmers should leave the swimming pool and find a safe shelter
- If at sea in a small boat, try to get back to land, but avoid being at sea in the first place by checking the weather forecast
- Do not go outdoors until 30 minutes after the last sign of lightning or thunder

Event organizers should have a plan for what to do during a lightning storm. Teams and officials should be informed of this before the event. It is much easier to stop a football game or sports event if everybody knows the rules. Difficulty arises if there is a major tournament with many teams present (e.g., the Norway Cup, a soccer event with over 30,000 participants, all between the ages of 13 and 19 years), or if there is a terrain event over a long and remote course. If lightning is common in your area, then local procedures have probably been developed. Discuss these with the local rescue services.

If an athlete is struck by lightning, then injury can be caused by the lightning itself, by the fall to the ground, or by falling structures such as heavy tree branches (primary, secondary, and tertiary injuries). Such scenarios obviously demand an immediate medical response with patient resuscitation, stabilization and rapid transfer to hospital. One must however consider one's own safety before exposing oneself or other rescue colleagues to potential danger. Lightning injuries primarily affect the nervous system with damage to peripheral and central nerves, the brain, and, of course, the heart. Patients can be knocked unconscious but may also suffer cardiac arrhythmias or asystole. Treatment includes airways management, ventilation and circulation support. An ECG should be taken as soon as possible. Cardiac defibrillation may be necessary and should be used if indicated. Treatment is supportive.

Remember the adage "When thunder roars, go indoors," by Dr. Mary Ann Cooper, director of the lightning injury research program, University of Illinois at Chicago. For more information on lightning, look up the U.S. National Weather Service at http://www.lightningsafety.noaa.gov/overview.htm.

14.7 FALLS

Contributed by Lars Kolsrud, Team Physician, Norwegian Ski Jumping Team, Norway

The types of injuries seen in free falls in sport are dependent on several factors: the speed the athlete had before falling, the height of the fall, the ability of protective equipment to absorb energy, the nature of the landing surface, the presence of objects on the landing surface, and the athlete's state of health (preexisting injury, splenomegaly, etc.). Other determinants include the athlete's age and weight and the position at landing. Bone, joint, and soft tissue injuries are usually determined by the athlete's position at landing. Deceleration forces may cause damage to the brain and viscera (liver, spleen, lung, even heart and aorta, if the speed or fall height are great enough). Falls from great height are not that common in sport, as most sports are on or near to the ground. Non-Olympic sports such as mountain climbing and parachuting do of course have this potential, whereas only diving, pole vault, and gymnastics have falls from height in the summer Olympic sports and ski jumping, snowboard, and freestyle skiing, among the winter Olympic sports. Falls at high speed can occur in almost all winter sports, such as downhill skiing, bobsleigh, skeleton, luge, ice hockey, and ice skating, whereas in summer sports, great speeds are not achieved.

The surface one lands upon is also of consequence, so that falls onto softer surfaces, including water, are better tolerated.

The extent of injury is often determined by

- What one lands upon:
  - Soft—snow, grass, water
  - Hard—concrete, wood, water

  - Jagged surfaces—fences, metal poles, glass, etc.
- The body's position or angle of contact:
  - Children often land on their heads due to increased head weight
  - Children and elderly often injure the forearm or wrist
  - If a body part is rotating on impact, injuries can be exaggerated
- The amount of the body that absorbs contact:
  - The greater the contact area, the greater the ability to absorb forces
- Patient's general condition: A healthy patient tolerates more. The result of a fall can be much worse if there are underlying spleen, liver, cardiac, skeletal conditions, etc.

Types of injury mechanisms:

- Direct impact injuries are associated with
  - Landing on the feet—calcaneus fractures, compression fractures of the thoracic and lumbar vertebrae
  - Landing on the knee—patella, femur shaft, or acetabulum fractures
  - Landing on the elbow—elbow, humerus, glenoid, acromion, and clavicular fractures
  - Landing on the hand—distal radius, greenstick, and scaphoid fractures
- Vertical deceleration
  - Head injuries, neck injuries
  - Rib fractures, pneumohemothoraces, lung contusions
  - Splenic injury/rupture, liver injury/rupture
  - Fractures—pelvis/femur/tibia/calcaneus fractures, radius fractures
- Rotational forces—greenstick fractures, spiral fractures in the arms and legs

14.8 THE MARATHON EVENT: MEDICAL MANAGEMENT

Contributed by James MacDonald, Team Physician, University of California, Santa Cruz, and Pierre d'Hemecourt, Children's Hospital, Boston; Team Physician, Boston College and Boston Marathon

Overview

The marathon is an exacting endurance event with increasing numbers of runners around the world participating. Planning and delivering effective medical management of these events is increasingly becoming the responsibility of sports medicine clinicians. Some of the unique demands of the marathon—the intensity of the event, the varying skill levels of the participants, the injury patterns, the risks of environmental exposure, the logistics of managing injuries that can take place over 26.2 mi., the increasing popularity and numbers of runners—require similarly unique skills of sports clinicians covering these events. These skills have not always been acquired in the typical training of a team sports clinician. This chapter will attempt to give an up-to-date perspective on achieving high quality medical management of marathons.

General Administrative Principles

The following general principles should be adhered to in planning to provide medical services at a marathon:

- Establish a multidisciplinary medical team that will allow for reasonable medical coverage of participants and possibly spectators at the event.

- Establish appropriate stocking of medical supplies at medical tents and appropriate fluid and energy replacement supplements at stations on the race course.

- Management of injuries should include triage, treatment (first aid or more extensive, as determined by the medical director), transfer, and follow up.

- Develop medical protocols that will be followed by the medical staff. This will always include good communication among staff and may require education of staff.

- Develop a comprehensive data collection system (medical records) that will allow for appropriate real-time medical care and for follow-up of transfers from the medical tent and one that will protect athlete/patient privacy.

- Assist local medical care facilities, emergency medical personnel and other first responders in establishing appropriate
  - Transport of injured runners
  - Communication among geographically dispersed units, such as medical tents, staff on the course and local medical facilities
  - Disaster management and mass casualty event protocols

- Address access issues for medical staff to arrive in a timely fashion to assigned work stations.

Intelligent and informed anticipation of issues (ranging from parking to availability of access passes for staff) will avoid an administrative mess on race day.

Organization

Owing to the physical layout of an event that covers 26.2 mi. (42.2 km), the logistics of achieving the above-stated principles can pose unique challenges to organizers of a marathon. In addition, the sheer number of runners needing services can literally overwhelm a medical staff if inadequately prepared. The year 2006 set a record as the largest 100 US marathons produced 360,597 finishers or a 3,606 average per marathon. Five marathons in the world that year had over 30,000 participants. Finally, the medical management team is often also expected to participate in injury prevention before the race, and to establish protocols for medical care and disaster management for spectators as well as runners. A team approach to care is clearly required.

A medical director(s) should be chosen with an eye on experience managing similar mass participation events. Skill and knowledge are important, but so too are administrative deftness and good interpersonal skills. Ideally, the medical director will serve on the board of the race committee and be intimately involved in all of the planning stages for a race. A precise chain of authority should be developed, both between the director and his or her medical staff and between the director and other executive-level organizers of the event. Ideally, prerace and race-day medical decisions will be made by the medical director as final arbiter, without undue influence or pressure from corporate sponsors or race directors.

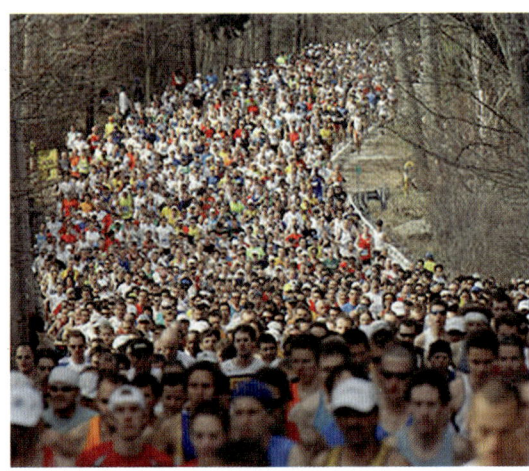

Photo courtesy of Dr. d'Hemencourt.

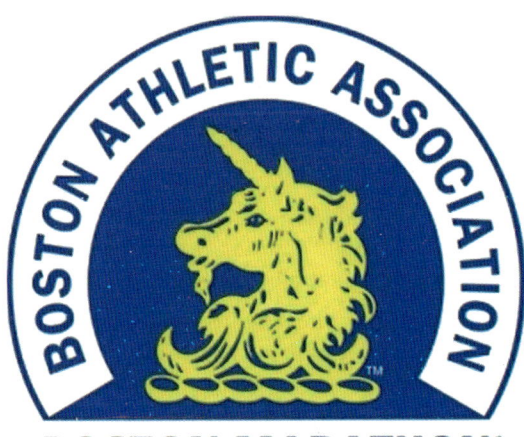

Image courtesy of Dr. d'Hemencourt.

When staffing a mass participation event such as a marathon, it is important that the medical director have some expectation of how many runners may have to be treated at each medical tent. Ideally, this could be extrapolated from historical data unique to each event. Alternatively, data obtained from other marathons might be used to calculate prospectively how many medical encounters might be expected. A 12-year profile of medical injury and illness for the Twin Cities Marathon in Minnesota (which takes place in early October, at a typically cooler time of year in North America) found that finish line medical encounter rates were 18.3/1,000 entrants and 25.5/1,000 finishers. It would be expected that these numbers might be more in events conducted in more extreme environmental conditions. It has been estimated that a medical team caring for an endurance event of 1,000 competitors should number 20, of which at least a third should be physicians.

It is likewise of great importance for the medical director, in consultation with other race organizing staff, to have an intimate knowledge of the unique course the race uses. The layout and terrain of the course both have significant impact on the placement of medical facilities. The approach to a point-to-point course, with medical needs dispersed literally along the entire 26.2-mi. course, will be different than that needed in an "out and back" course, or one that loops several times. The exact placement of tents and their orientation (which end will see intake of patients and which end will see discharge) is dictated by transport needs and the physical space surrounding the finish line.

The length of a marathon often traverses multiple jurisdictions. Coordination with all of the local hospitals/emergency medical personnel is of paramount importance, and, once again, is an issue requiring close communication among the medical director, race organizers, and local medical care professionals. Attention should be directed toward the following issues:

- Level of care that will be instituted in the medical tent. For instance, if a patient requires rehydration with intravenous fluids, will this be done in the tent or require medical transfer? To what extent will hyperthermic illnesses be addressed within the medical tent? Hyperthermic strokes must be addressed promptly on site with direct cooling methods using ice water tubs. Laboratory evaluation of serum sodium levels and glucose are very useful with the altered mental status patients. What if any medicines will be stocked and available? These and other such important questions will need to be determined by the medical director.

- Logistics of transportation. How will EMT personnel access injured runners from the tents to transport them to local hospitals? What route will they take that will not interfere with the marathon event route itself? Will sweep buses be provided to gather the participants that cannot finish?

- The medical director needs to maintain a plan of evacuation of the runners from the route in the event of extreme weather or other conditions. This will often involve local shelters and transportation. Communication to the runners during the race may be accomplished with flagging systems or at the water stations.

Staff

Provision of excellent medical care at a marathon results from a multidisciplinary team that is well educated, appropriately staffed, and working in concert. Physicians, nurses, athletic trainers, physical therapists, massage therapists, allied medical professionals (such as chiropractors), and medical assistants all play vital roles at the designated medical service areas along a marathon course. In addition, EMT personnel will be vital to the effective and safe transport of runners from medical tents or the course to local hospitals.

It is ideal that the medical team meet prior to race day, to review administrative and logistical issues and up-to-date medical protocols to treat the expected injuries. The medical director is responsible for this education of the rest of the staff.

Duties assigned to staff by the medical director are expected to remain within the individual's scope of practice.

Physicians will be primarily responsible for true medical emergencies as well as more routine medical issues. Nurses will play a vital role in terms of triage, medical documentation and delivering medical care in conjunction with physicians. It is very useful to have an experienced medical person stationed at triage to determine the athletes who require the most intensive care. Assistants will be helpful in transporting individuals to medical tents and assisting medical professionals in obtaining equipment. Certified athletic trainers, physical therapists, massage therapists and chiropractors can be invaluable in terms of massaging, stretching, and providing medical modalities (such as ice) that will represent the bulk of the needs required by runners in a tent. Podiatry, too, can be invaluable to care for the large volume of foot and ankle complaints, ranging from blisters to sprains, that will present.

At most larger marathons, it will be expected to have

- A finish line staff to make immediate emergency medical assessments

- A finish line medical tent(s), which will typically require the largest investment of medical staff and material and see the vast majority of medical injuries

- A starting line tent to address prerace issues. After race start, the tent staff can be divided up and team members transported to other locations.

- On-course first aid stations with staff and/or sweep vehicles combing the course keeping an eye out for injured or ill runners.

Two-thirds of the team should be at the finish medical tent; the remaining members of the team should be distributed in roughly equal numbers between the finish line itself, on the course (either at first aid stations or in sweep vehicles combing the course for injured runners), and at the starting line.

Medical Care Protocol

Medical staff should be familiar with care levels required for the expected injuries seen at a marathon, including

- Exercise-associated collapse

- Sudden cardiac death

- Thermal injury (including hypothermia and hypothermic illnesses: heat exhaustion and heat stroke)

- Hyponatremia

- Muscle cramps

- Accidental injuries such as ankle sprains or bony/soft tissue injuries from falls, such as abrasions, lacerations, or fractures

It is the medical director's responsibility to conduct prerace education of medical staff regarding diagnosis and treatment of these conditions. It is also the medical director's responsibility to establish the overall medical strategy and subsequent protocols to address these pathologies when recognized. As mentioned earlier in this chapter, all staff should be well versed in the extent to which medical care will provided in the tent versus that which will require transport.

The details of the care for these individual pathologies are beyond the scope of this chapter and are dealt with by other authors in this manual.

Hydration/Energy Replacement Needs for Marathons

Marathons are demanding long-distance events that require real-time, on-course replacement of fluids and nutrients. The medical director and staff will be involved in determining issues related to course management of fluid and energy replacement stations.

It is generally accepted that both water and dilute carbohydrate/electrolyte replacement fluids should be liberally available on the marathon course. Ideally, the fluids will be cooled to 15°C to 22°C for optimal palatability and absorption. The ideal carbohydrate/salt solution is 25 to 50 mmol/L sodium and 2% to 8% carbohydrate on the course. There is some controversy over the ideal spacing of fluid stations that revolves around attempts to provide liberal availability to fluid while reducing risk of hyponatremia. Spacing of stations is generally found to range from every 3 to 5 km.

There is increasing effort to address hyponatremia seen in marathon runners. Salty snacks, such as pretzels, and salty fluids, such as broths (with 50 to 100 mmol/L sodium) should be available at race end for participants both in and out of the medical tent.

Runners should also have available to them carbohydrate replacement containing a medium-chain sugar polymer, such as fruit, bagels, pretzels, or various commercial products often supplied by race sponsors (supplements, bars, goos, and the like).

Prevention

Ideally, the medical director will be intimately involved in race-day planning. This would include decisions associated with the timing of the event, to reduce risk for thermal illness. This also would include same-day decisions to modify or cancel events if there are severe environmental risk factors present on race day, ranging from extreme wet bulb globe temperatures to severe wind chill to lightning.

It is increasingly recognized that well-educated marathoners can do a lot to prevent injury. This of course begins with how the runner trains for the event, a key aspect to injury prevention over which race medical organizers might have little influence. However, communications from race staff to participants in the weeks and days just before an event can have a profound influence on runner safety. This can often times be accomplished via e-mail bulletins (obtaining e-mail addresses at registration) or Internet Web site postings. Updates on expected race day environmental conditions and ongoing education about proper fluid management can be sent out to participants prior to the race itself. It is also vital to remind participants to wear, if pertinent to the individual, medical alert braces.

Recommended Reading

ACSM. Mass participation event management for the team physician: a consensus statement. *Med Sci Sports Exerc*. 2004;36(11):2004–2008. Available on line at www.aafp.org and www.acsm.org.

Binkley HM, Beckett J, Casa DJ, et al. National Athletic Trainers' Association Position Statement: Exertional heat illnesses. *J Athl Train*. 2002;37(3):329–343.

Green GB, Burnham G. Health care at mass gatherings. *JAMA*. 1998;279(18):1463–1468.

Hew-Butler T, Ayus JC, Kipps C, et al. Statement of the second International Exercise-Associated Hyponatremia Consensus Development Conference, New Zealand, 2007. *Clin J Sports Med*. 2008;18(2):111–121.

International Association of Athletics Federations. *Competition Medical Handbook for Track and Field and Road Racing: A Practical Guide*. Available at http://www.iaaf.org/mm/Document/imported/41614.pdf.

Noakes T. Medical coverage of endurance events. In: Brukner P, Khan K, eds. Clinical Sports Medicine. Australia: McGraw-Hill Companies, Inc., 2006.

Roberts WO. A 12-year profile of medical injuries and illnesses for the Twin Cities Marathon. *Med Sci Sports Exerc*. 2000;32(9):1549–1555.

Hew-Butler T, Ayus JC, Kipps C, et al. Exercise-Associated Hyponatremia Consensus Panel, *Clin J Sports Med*. 2008;18:111–121.

14.9 COVERING TERRAIN SPORTS

Contributed by Ken Wu, Constantine Au, and HF Ho, Accident and Emergency Department, Queen Elizabeth Hospital, Hong Kong; and Tai-wai Wong and Pamela Youde, Nethersole Eastern Hospital, Hong Kong

Introduction

In a traditional sporting event, athletes compete against each other under controlled circumstances. In recent years, adventure racing in the open has become popular. The racing is often nonstop, 24 hours a day, over a rugged course, involving disciplines such as trekking, whitewater canoeing, horseback riding, sea kayaking, mountaineering, and mountain biking etc. These expedition style ultraendurance events usually attract well-trained athletes.

Nonprofessional athletes of different levels of fitness can participate in charity sport events such as the Oxfam Trailwalker (OTW). Hong Kong organized the first Trailwalker event in the world and was then followed by other countries, including the United Kingdom, Australia, New Zealand, Japan, and Belgium.

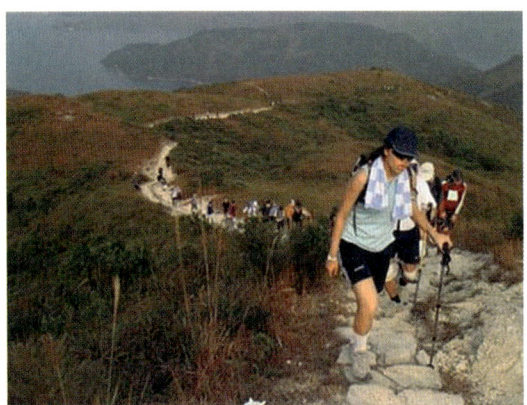

Photo courtesy of Dr. Wu.

In Hong Kong, the event is held annually on the MacLehose Trail, a 100-km hiking trail across mountain ranges. There are altogether 11 checkpoints, including start and finish points. Every year, about 1,000 teams participate in the event. Support teams and other voluntary workers provide different services, making up a few thousand people in all, often moving along the trail as the event unfolds. Some participants will take the event as an ultraendurance race, while some use it as an opportunity to challenge themselves physically and mentally, and some just take it as an opportunity to walk in the countryside. Therefore, the disparity of participant physical ability can be great. This is a real challenge for the EP.

A well-organized medical coverage plan is required to support a mass event. The medical coverage includes prevention of mass casualties, on-site triage and treatment, evacuation plan, and injury surveillance. The EP needs to coordinate with other supporting agencies, including the police, fire services, auxiliary medical services, physiotherapists and podiatrists, and other voluntary agents.

Medical Issues

The major concerns from the organizer's perspective are listed in Table 14.1. With such a big crowd at different levels of fitness, all sorts of medical problems are expected, with musculoskeletal injuries of the limbs being the most frequent complaints. More serious injuries such as cervical spine fractures, though rare, also need to be prepared for. Medical emergencies are often related to preexisting conditions such as epilepsy or coronary artery disease or can be environmentally related, for example, heat stroke, dehydration, or altitude sickness. The event physician must also take into account any specific climatic conditions or specific participant groups, for example, senior citizens or children.

The Role of the Event Physician

The EP should be involved in all phases of planning, right through to the execution of the medical coverage. The EP should be a member of the event organizing committee and should be involved in all major decisions with respect to medical services. Funding for medical preparedness must be set aside from the overall budget. The EP should chair the medical subcommittee if such a level of organization exists and should be empowered to delineate responsibilities among all paramedical/medical/nursing personnel, to take charge of contingency planning, to mobilize medical resources, and to act as the final judge of return-to-play issues. In order to fulfill these roles, the EP should be fairly familiar with the event, understand the logistics and irregularities of past events, and, last but not least, communicate with people at different levels.

On the date of the event, the EP must alert the organizer of any actual and potential hazards such as an unexpectedly high number of injuries, change in weather conditions etc. Weather surveillance

---

TABLE 14.1 Major Medical Issues in a Mass Sports Event

Major Concerns	Incidents in OTW
Sudden cardiac death/collapse	2001, severe asthmatic attack.
	2005, a young male walker collapsed to heart attack; helicopter evacuation; coronary artery abnormalities; no death was recorded in OTWs.
Trauma—acute or chronic	Out of the 1,639 medical contacts in OTW, 2006, there were 1,532 muscle cramps, 650 foot blisters, 146 wounds, 142 ankle sprains
Insect bites/snake bites/attacks by wild animals	Every year, there were some cases of bee stings. Some walkers were attacked by monkeys.
Mass casualty	Luckily, none.
Weather: extreme condition or sudden change (e.g., heavy rain, hyper-/hypothermia)	In OTW, 2006, five walkers were sent to the hospital due to heat illnesses, despite on-spot treatment.
Terrorist activities	Luckily none, but not everyone welcomes the event.
Natural disaster	In OTW, 2003, the event was temporarily suspended due to heavy rainfall.
Outbreak of infectious disease	No massive outbreak was ever recorded. Some walkers had diarrhea and vomiting. Massive outbreak is possible if the stool and vomitus are not handled properly.

includes temperature, relative humidity, ice, snow, and rainfall. Heat index that combines air temperature and relative humidity is a good index. The EP can also take part in participant education so as to prevent/reduce common problems like muscle cramps, foot blisters, etc.

Preevent Preparation

Demand: The single most important factor to predict the casualty load is the number of participants. The number and nature of casualties can usually be estimated from statistics from previous events. The pattern of medical problems is affected by factors related to the nature of activity, number and background of participants, and environmental conditions. For an outdoor endurance event, one needs to prepare for traumatic injuries, metabolic disturbances such as hyponatremia or hypoglycemia, environmental emergencies such as hypothermia or hyperthermia, preexisting medical illnesses such as exercise induced asthma (EIA) or epileptic seizures, and even sudden cardiac death.

Personnel Training: Experienced staff is the most important asset in the medical coverage of mass events. EPs should be well versed in emergency care for both traumatic and medical conditions. Training in wilderness medicine is an advantage, as improvisation is often needed when resources are limited in remote areas. They will also need to oversee care provided by other members of the medical team (e.g., first aiders, nurses). Adequate number, training, and experience of care providers are essential. On-site staff should be competent in performing cardiopulmonary resuscitation (CPR) and in the use of the automated external defibrillator (AED). BTLS skills (e.g., spine immobilization) should also be a minimum requirement. In addition to medical cover at the checkpoints, mobile teams of more experienced doctors/nurses/paramedics need to be organized and deployed with appropriate transport to cover the event in a long trail. Apart from providing on-site medical/nursing advice to checkpoint medical providers, they should also be equipped with ALS instruments and medications for medical emergencies. Lead time for transport of critically ill participant from terrain to hospital can be prolonged and significantly affect survival. The level of expectation from the public is understandably high when an on-site physician is available.

Supplies: The equipment and supplies need not be equally distributed among checkpoints. They are distributed according to previous injury records (i.e., according to perceived demands). All the medications must comply with Wada guidelines. The equipment and drug list available in the medical tent is shown in Table 14.2. Mobile nurses, doctors and paramedics should carry ALS equipment, such as an airway management set and an AED, in addition to first aid equipment. The logistics of maintenance and protection of equipment and supplies need to be carefully planned as they will be subject to heat, cold and rain in the wilderness. Some medicines must be stored in a controlled environment (e.g., succinylcholine in low temperature). Replenishment of medical supplies at checkpoints needs planning in advance. Backup medical supplies need to be stored at strategic sites with a rapid response team in place for timely delivery. For terrain activities involving movement of crowds in one direction, unused medical supplies at deserted checkpoints can be delivered to subsequent checkpoints to save costs.

Evacuation Plans: Routes and methods of evacuation of injured athletes should be planned in consultation with experts familiar with the terrain geography and with due considerations to possible weather conditions. Site visits along the trail should be done. Injured athletes are usually transported to the nearest checkpoint or nearest land transport accessible location for further management and delivery to hospital. Ambulances, being scare resources, should be placed at strategic locations to cover most parts of the terrain sport venue. Ambulances may move to other strategic locations when the crowd advances. A helicopter may be needed in areas of the trail that are poorly accessible. Helicopter landing sites need to be planned with pilots in advance. CASEVAC command should be centrally coordinated with input from the EP. Minor injuries should be managed on-site. Abuse of land ambulance or even helicopter is not uncommon in terrain sports when a physically and psychologically fatigued athlete decides to quit and desires to be transported back to the civilized world as soon as possible. Prior communication with hospitals destined to receive casualties is desirable and facilitates subsequent follow-up actions.

Communication: Communication in a mass event stretching over 100 km is always a challenge. Normal, everyday communication tools such as mobile phones or pagers may not work properly in the wilderness. Satellite phones and high-power radio should be considered as alternative means of communication. Radio transmitters set up at strategic locations along the trail is one way to provide seamless communication. The global positioning system (GPS) may better locate walkers in need of medical help. With the development of 3G phones and Wi-Fi Internet, telemedicine may be an option. Nevertheless, the usefulness of fixed-line phones cannot be underestimated, as they provide a reliable means of communication. Telephone lists should be compiled and distributed to all relevant personnel to facilitate communication. Mobile team members should ensure connectivity of their mobile phones and forward to the nearest fixed-line phone when entering an area of absent signal. Backup contingency fixed-line phone numbers should be announced to all participants. High-speed broadband Internet communication between computer terminals, mobile phones and pagers further enhances the group dispatch of important messages.

Prevention: Participant Education: Many of the medical problems encountered in terrain sport events are preventable. Regular training and good preparation of athletes are the cornerstones of prevention (e.g., hikers with appropriate training and adequate rehydration routines can prevent muscle cramps). Appropriate footwear, padding, and prophylactic the use of Vaseline can reduce friction blister formation. Iliotibial tract syndrome can be prevented by an appropriate knee brace and the use of a hiking stick, especially when going downhill. Ankle sprains can be reduced with good ankle support and regular stretching and exercise. Skin abrasions can be reduced with the use of prophylactic emollient. Regular training under competition climate leads to good temperature acclimatization. Appropriate team support should be arranged to provide change of clothing during both day and nighttime, when the temperature gradient can be steep. Careful planning of meal and rest times can prevent problems like hypoglycemia. The shared use of utensils for food and drinks should be avoided, as infectious gastroenteritis can spread widely and quickly among athletes. Inadequate lighting can be problematic in terrain sports at nighttime. Athletes should ensure adequate lighting through use of appropriate headlamps. Overexcitement and/or ingestion of alcohol at the finish point frequently cause problems such as vasovagal attacks, postural hypotension and related injuries as a result of a fall. The organizer might need to impose certain precautionary measures or even prohibition of alcoholic products for athletes at the finish point. The EP can assist the event organizers in educating participants before the event.

Information can be provided on the event website, in an event brochure, or through seminars.

Event Coverage

The EP should assume overall coordination of all medical services for the event. The EPs are stationed either at the command center or at the high-risk areas, or are mobile to meet emergencies on the trail. The physician who acts as the medical director should maintain communication with other physicians, nurses, and partners on issues related to evacuation, suspension of event, etc. It would be ideal if all the other section commands of the event are stationed together at the finish point for easy communication and updates. Anticipation is the key to preventing problems. Ensure the planned medical and nursing manpower at each location is in place through frequent monitoring, particularly during times of shift changes. The level of medical supplies should be checked at intervals and replenishment arranged before level runs too low. An unusual surge of athletes attending medical first aid stations, both in number and/or specific nature, should be reported to medical command for investigation and ad hoc management. Sudden weather change may impose safety issues to athletes such as change in competition route condition, abrupt temperature change, lightning, etc. Serious injuries or illnesses of athletes must be reported to medical command for subsequent follow-up of outcome and possible media enquiries.

On-site Treatment: Participants with minor injuries will usually present at the checkpoints. It is essential to allocate experienced staff to deal with emergencies at each checkpoint. Accurate information of the location of the injured on the trail is important for the deployment of the mobile team. The method of transport will depend on the terrain and weather. Physicians can give instructions on medical issues over the phone if they are not at the scene, and can make decisions on treatment or whether evacuation is necessary. The EP may need to be positioned at specific high-risk locations based on experience from previous competitions.

Multiple Injury Incidents: An incident with injuries affecting more than one victim could occur (e.g., in lightning accidents or flash flood). The priority should be safety of the rescuer. A plan for field triage should be in place. A method for the mobilization of backup resources for treatment and evacuation should be ready for deployment, and the establishment of one or more rapid response teams might serve the purpose. The EP should warn the organizer of such possibilities given the environmental conditions during the race. A close liaison with government agencies—such as fire services, mountain rescue, and emergency medical services—is required as the demand for medical attention may overwhelm the capacity of the organizer.

Athlete Collapse: The worst-case scenario is full cardiac arrest (e.g., as a result of acute myocardial infarction). Timely defibrillation may not be available unless the collapse occurs near a checkpoint with a medical tent. Bystander CPR should be encouraged and medical guidance through telecommunication may be helpful. Other causes of collapse that require quick medical action include heat stroke or hypoglycemia. Rapid cooling and glucose supplement should be applied as soon as possible. Epileptic convulsion can occur in an athlete with a history of epilepsy, particularly when there is an electrolyte imbalance such as hyponatremia due to overhydration by water alone. Most attacks are self-limiting. Common first aid techniques such as a lateral-lying posture to prevent aspiration and removal of the athlete to a safe place usually suffice. Exercise-associated collapse often occurs at the finish line, and the athlete usually responds to elevation of the lower limbs. Alcohol ingestion may precipitate the syncopal attack through its vasodilatory effect. Sometimes, the cause of collapse may not be obvious on-site; it would be safer to plan for evacuation to a hospital as soon as possible.

Major Trauma: The severity of the trauma should be assessed based on the mechanism of injury, physiologic parameters, and clinical assessment. Examples of major injuries that warrant early evacuation to a medical facility are:

- Head injury with loss of consciousness
- Neck or back injury with neurologic signs or symptoms
- Torso injury with abnormal vital signs
- Compound fracture of long bones

Immobilization of the injured parts should be achieved before transfer. Life support measures (e.g., maintaining a patent airway) should have priority. More invasive interventions (e.g., intubation, chest drain insertion) may not be feasible at the scene unless a skilled EP is at hand with the appropriate equipment.

Closed dislocations and fractures of the limbs alone are usually not life threatening. Closed reduction at the scene is not a must if there are no neurovascular complications. Immobilization and evacuation can be planned in a less hurried fashion.

Common Medical Problems: The most common medical encounters for terrain sport are related to ailments of the lower limbs.

- Muscle cramps are the results of muscle fatigue, disturbance of electrolytes, and dehydration. Rest, stretching, and appropriate rehydration are the mainstay of treatment. Continuation is almost always possible. It must be noted that muscle cramps can be a protective mechanism of joint injuries. Examination of nearby joints should be carried out.

- Ankle sprain is classified into three grades depending on joint stability. The on-site examination includes evaluating joint stability and gait. If the joint is stable and the walker can walk with a normal gait and without pain, continuation is allowed. Otherwise, further treatment with rest, ice, compression, and elevation are needed. Continuation may not be possible.

- Knee pain in a hiking event can be due to muscle pain in the quadriceps or the iliotibial band syndrome (ITBS). The iliotibial band causes pain in the lateral aspect of the knee and is aggravated when walkers go downhill. A knee brace or strapping may help. Stretching with the help of a physiotherapist is often necessary. Prevention is better than first aid treatment. The use of hiking sticks may help to relieve pain and prevent premature occurrence of the syndrome.

- Skin abrasion is the result of friction between the skin and the clothing. It usually takes place on the inner thigh. Dressings and use of Vaseline are the mainstay of treatment

- Blisters (friction blisters) occur when the foot rubs against the sock. The fluid inside a blister can be clear or filled with blood, or even pus. Small blisters are often left alone. They are cleaned and covered with an adhesive hydrocolloid wound contact dressing. Large blisters are aspirated and then dressed with an adhesive hydrocolloid wound contact dressing or strong adhesive elastoplast to act as a temporary false skin. Dry, nonadherent dressings should not be put on blister wounds, as the friction created during weight bearing will cause further damage and pain. Athletes must be warned not to remove the dressing too soon, as the dressing may tear out the underlying skin. The dressing should be left over for days. They can easily be peeled off once the new skin has been generated. The injection of a tincture benzoic compound into the blisters after aspiration previously practiced by the military is no longer recommended due to the possibility of a chemical burn to underlying tissue causing excruciating pain.

Evacuation of Patient

Ambulances should be stationed at different checkpoints along the trail and moved to other checkpoints dependent on crowd movement. Arrangement should also be made for helicopter transport. Landing sites should be identified with the flying service beforehand. The capability of the helicopter service should be ascertained during the planning phase. Volunteer or professional mountain rescue teams should be available to manage injured athletes in a difficult terrain. They can provide first aid treatment and, if required, carry injured athletes to nearby checkpoints for further treatment or stay with the injured athletes until conditions become favorable for airlift or other mode of transportation.

When evacuation of the victim has been decided, safety of the victim and the rescuers is paramount. Choosing the mode of transport can sometimes be difficult. Land evacuation should be employed as far as possible. Victims can be carried off the terrain by mobile teams (mountain rescue team) to a safe area where an ambulance or helicopter can stop. If helicopter transport is chosen, the EP or another appointed functionary should communicate with the pilot if possible to discuss the availability of a landing site, if winching is required, and what the weather conditions are.

For critical patients, the on-site nurses/ paramedics should be given the power to order transfer to hospitals. This "act first and report later" policy is important in terms of patient management. For less critical patients, on-site nurses are encouraged to discuss means of transport use with the medical command first. As the event is usually in a rural area, ambulances are rare resources and must be used with caution. In many cases, walkers can wait and be sent out as a group. Sometimes, transport vehicles other than ambulances can also be used.

Surveillance

The EP who acts as the medical director will benefit from surveillance of the number and pattern of injuries and/or medical illnesses at different checkpoints in order to reinforce support and replenish medical supplies. Surveillance of the use of medicines at checkpoints is essential as unintentional drug overdose may occur when an athlete is prescribed with analgesia repeatedly at each checkpoint.

Crowd movement surveillance has been used in the Oxfam Hong Kong Trailwalker.

Each walker wears a bar-coded wristband, and a computer can monitor dropouts and crowd movement. This is important, as the movement of the crowd affects medical supplies usage. A slow-moving crowd may suggest unexpected adverse conditions and predict a high number of casualties. A fast-moving crowd may suggest more than favorable conditions, but overexertion can be a problem to selected athletes. Crowd movement patterns in past events could also be used to guide the allocation of manpower and supplies.

Documentation

Medical logs and incident logs are kept and reviewed after the event. To reduce the workload of on-site workers, the medical log is set out in a table format. Common medical problems such as muscle cramps and blisters are listed on the top. Simple treatments like stretching and wound dressings are listed as well. Nurses simply tick the appropriate boxes. To reduce the workload of recording and also to protect walkers' privacy, only the walker number is recorded.

Another log sheet is dedicated for drug use, which may give better documentation of drug allergy and possible drug overdose. For example, a walker can suffer from paracetamol overdose if he takes two tablets of 500 mg paracetamol from each medical tent. A separate sheet allows easy checking. A nurse can call the nurse of the preceding medical tent for previous drug use.

An ambulance dispatch log sheet should also be kept so that medical conditions of hospitalized athletes can be followed. Backup transport may be required if another athlete requires hospital transfer before the ambulance returns.

All these logs are useful not only for the immediate and follow-up care of an individual athlete but also for future event planning purposes. The data can also be used for research purposes provided that ethical approval is sought from an educational institute and the organizer.

Postevent

Unused medical supplies need to be collected, sorted out, checked for integrity, categorized, and stored up for reuse if possible. Some can be returned to suppliers for reimbursement in order to cut costs. Log sheets need to be collected for evaluation and planning purpose for subsequent events. Debriefing among medical personnel and other agencies is required for continuous improvement. Outcome of hospitalized athletes should be followed up. Medical preparedness may need to be modified accordingly. A formal evaluation survey can be carried out among medical service providers and/or sport participants. Finally, a financial report on the cost of the medical provision needs to be submitted to the organizer for record purpose and cost-benefit analysis.

Conclusions

Medical coverage of events in rough terrain is challenging. Thorough preparation, especially in communication and coordination of the different parties, is the key to success. The EP should be personally familiar with the sport and able to anticipate the needs of and the potential dangers to the athletes. He or she needs to be versatile and resourceful in on-site triage and treatment of injured athletes. He or she should be cooperative and collaborate with other agencies, yet put the safety of athletes as the primary concern.

Recommended Reading

Luke A. Mass participation sports and events. In: Mellion MB, Putukian M, Madden CC, eds. *Sports Medicine Secrets*. 3rd ed. Philadelphia, PA: Hanley & Belfus; 2003.

14.10 CROSS-COUNTRY EQUESTRIAN SPORTS

Contributed by Craig Ferrel, Chair of FEI MC, USA; and Stefano Dragoni, Team Physician, Italian Olympic Team

In equestrian sports, the cross-country test is one of the most dangerous, from an injury point of view. For this reason, it is important to plan the event carefully. We recommend

- Preliminary meetings in which roles and tasks are assigned

- Radio and communication contact at all locations on the course

- That qualified personnel are in attendance

- Availability of adequate equipment

Preliminary Meetings in Which Roles and Tasks are Assigned

The organizing committee must nominate a chief medical officer (CMO) with sufficient trauma experience, a good knowledge of the discipline in question, and good local geographical knowledge of the track and surrounding amenities.

The CMO should develop a rescue plan that places necessary personnel and vehicles in locations that allow for quick and efficient intervention, irrespective of weather, local geography, or the type of event.

A map of the cross-country course should be drawn, indicating jumps and access routes for rescue vehicles, along with exit routes to the medical room or hospital. The course should be divided into sectors; each sector should have its own dedicated emergency team and vehicle (ideally four or five jumps in each sector). Preliminary meetings, with map distribution, access route demonstrations, and action plan discussions, are of the utmost importance.

In the days leading up to an event, the local hospital administration office should be informed of the precise dates and times of the event, so that they can make their preparations.

Another important duty for the CMO is to be an acting member of the crisis management group. Guidelines on how to deal with a serious or fatal injury must be drawn up together with the event coordinator and other members of the management group.

It is important that there are two separate medical services—one dedicated to athletes and one for the general public. It is imperative that the two services are completely separate and independent in order to guarantee maximum efficiency for both parts.

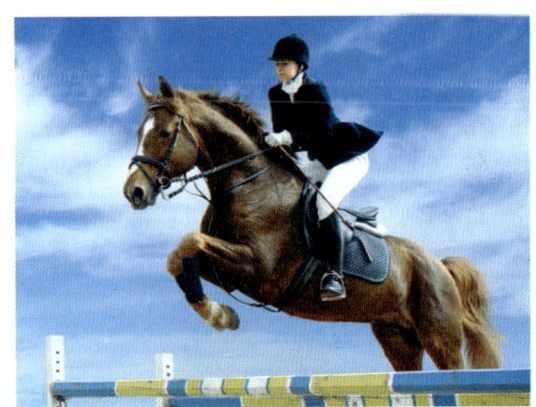

Radio and Communication Control at All Course Locations

In order to be able to offer medical intervention, it is essential that radio signals reach all areas of the course. Radio also allows medical staff to be prepared for when horses are approaching.

Cross-country events consist of courses with variable distances and with up to 30 to 40 jumps over solid obstacles and fences, hence the greater number of accidents occurring in this discipline; in many cases, there is no visibility between one jump and the next, though there is a fence judge at each jump to ensure regulation compliance.

It is, therefore, necessary for the medical staff to have their own exclusive medical channel dedicated exclusively to medical assistance (not veterinarian) that foresees the following:

1) Central post (preferably near to the control center) which receives information from all fence judges regarding the ongoing situation of the event.

2) In the case of an accident in which medical assistance is required, it will be the control center coordinator who will give the order for the doctor and paramedic equipped with resuscitation equipment and emergency medication of the concerned sector to intervene by car, with the help of the head of the sector who knows very well the displacement of the fences; in this way, the doctor can give assistance in a few minutes; in the case of a serious problem, the ambulance, which is strategically placed in the sector, is called.

3) If the ambulance is required to take the injured party to the hospital, its position must be replaced by a reserve ambulance.

Attendance of Qualified Personnel (For Rapid and Effective Intervention)

Medical personnel and paramedics must be expert and competent in dealing with the initial intervention of serious cases.

Communication of the state of health of the injured party must be communicated to the control center together with the decision to hospitalize or not, choosing not necessarily the nearest hospital but that which is specialized in dealing with the injury sustained.

Availability of Adequate Equipment

Adequate equipment includes an ambulance equipped with instruments and pharmaceuticals, an experienced crew (driver, medical and paramedic personnel), and a medic with his or her own vehicle.

The ambulance should be a designated four-wheel-drive vehicle conforming to current regulations for the recovery and transportation of injured and seriously ill patients; it must contain resuscitation equipment, emergency medication, and immobilization and transportation equipment.

Resuscitation Equipment

- Oxygen with tubing and mask
- Self-inflating bag/valve/mask with reservoir bag
- Masks for adult and children
- Powered suction with Yankauer attachment
- Oropharyngeal and nasopharyngeal airways
- Laryngoscope, blades, spare bulbs, and batteries
- Tracheal tubes, connectors, introducers/bougie
- Lubricant, adhesive tape, or securing bandage
- Syringes, various sizes
- Emergency chest drain kit
- Intravenous cannulae, 14- to 20-gauge, and syringe needles
- Crystalloids for infusion and intravenous sets for rapid fluid infusion
- Defibrillator
- Sphygmomanometer

Emergency Medication

- Adrenaline
- Antihistamine dextrose
- Atropine
- Diazepam
- Entonox
- Furosemide
- Hydrocortisone
- Lignocaine
- Metoclopramide
- Nonopiate analgesic
- Salbutamol
- Sterile water for injection

Immobilization and Transportation

- Rigid cervical collars

- Scoop stretcher and/or long board and/or lifting frame

- Splints to include: traction splint, securing straps, and bandages

14.11 GYMNASTICS EVENTS

Contributed by Michel Léglise, MD, Vice President, Fédération Internationale de Gymnastique (FIG), President, FIG Medical Commission, Coordinator, IOC Medical Commission Working Group "Sports, Children, and Adolescents," Paris, France; and Michel Binder, MD, Sports Pediatrician, FIG Medical Commission, Paris, France

Gymnastics comprises a number of competitive disciplines grouped under the umbrella of the Fédération International de Gymnastique (FIG). As these disciplines require relatively similar skills and make similar physical demands, injuries tend to be common to most facets of the sport. Factors that expose the gymnasts to injury are

- Acrobatic sequences

- Balance positions

- Extreme joint loading

- Dismounting, landing, or exit

- Choreographic and artistic elements

Furthermore, gymnasts in all disciplines are mostly adolescents and have thus not reached full development. Therefore, all of the acute injuries in the different disciplines as described in this chapter are of particular concern when affecting the growth plates due to their possible long-term implications.

Factors that trigger disorders and injuries in other sports are also present in gymnastics (neglectful physical, technical, and psychological preparation; lack of general hygiene; insufficient diet; etc.). In gymnastics, all disciplines place exceedingly rigorous technical demands on the athlete but those requiring extreme precision are particularly demanding. The technical requirements of particular exercises (as defined by the rules and points scoring code) obviously play an important part in the onset of specific conditions. Mental factors also exert considerable influence in potentially dangerous exercises. Further, each discipline has its own physical requirements and specific mechanical constraints, of which the physician must be aware in order to understand and prevent acute and chronic lesions. In injury prevention, good quality gymnastics equipment such as apparatus, mats and floors is also essential.

Despite the fact that acrobatic elements are becoming increasingly more spectacular and sensational with rotations, etc., the number of injuries seems relatively low. Injury frequency statistics based on insurance company accident reports show that artistic gymnastics ranks between sixth and ninth position among the major sports. Gymnastics, however, generate a large variety of chronic peripheral and spinal joint disorders—lesions that are exaggerated when they affect the growth plates, particularly in girls. Chronic lesions may become acutely exacerbated and vice versa.

In general, the treatment of acute medical conditions in gymnastics does not differ from other sports. Accidents can also happen to coaches, notably when they approach the horizontal bar/uneven bars or during a tumbling sequence, the most common accident being a complete or partial rupture of the brachial biceps tendon.

Men's Artistic Gymnastics

This discipline comprises six apparatus with different biomechanical constraints requiring dynamic and static effort, flexibility, momentum, strength, speed of execution, and rhythm to varying degrees, often choreographed to music.

Chronic lesions in men's artistic gymnasts occur most frequently at the

- Lumbar spine: Preexisting lumbago often intensifies in cases of isthmus lysis and spondylolisthesis (predisposing apparatus: floor and vault, drop landings from the horizontal bar)

- Shoulder: When exercising at the rings or, less frequently, at the horizontal bar; labrum lesions predominate, but also proximal long head of the biceps tendonitis and acromioclavicular joint pathology occur

- Wrist: Chronic pain (pommel horse), scaphoid pathology, stress fractures

- Hand: Previously gymnast's hands and wrists were dry, callous, often cracked with deep and bleeding dermal lesions, and often infected, but due to modern protective measures—in particular with the horizontal bar and parallel bars—these conditions are now rare

- Knee: Chronic lateral collateral ligament sprain (floor, vault)

- Ankle: Chronic sprain (floor, vault)

Floor Exercises: Gymnasts are expected to use the entire floor area for their routine (12 m × 12 m). Routines mainly consist of series of acrobatic elements on the diagonal covering as much floor area as possible. Tumbling runs, flips, and a combination of the two alternate with shows of balance, flexibility (splits, etc.), and strength (handstand position from scale position, etc.). Acute lesions in competition commonly affect the

- Knee (cruciate ligaments, collateral ligaments, meniscal lesions)
- Ankle (lateral ligaments, dislocation of the ankle, dislocation of the peroneal tendon)
- Achilles tendon (rupture)
- Cervical spine (much less common)

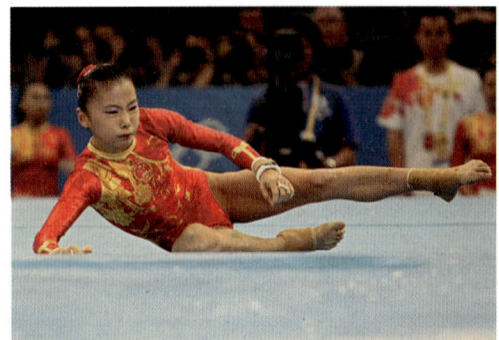

He Kexin, 2008 Beijing Olympic Summer Games. (Photo courtesy of Dr. Leglise.)

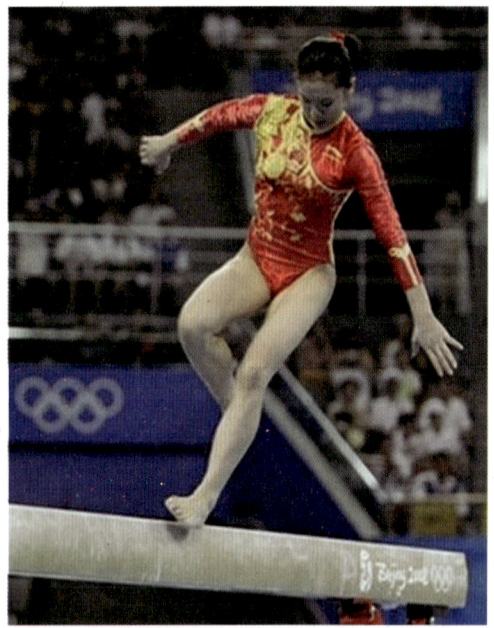

Cheng Fei, 2008 Beijing Olympic Summer Games. (Photo courtesy of Dr. Leglise.)

Pommel Horse: The entire exercise is performed on the wrists and hands as they make their way over the full length of the horse and back, pressing and pivoting on the two pommels. The gymnast performs rhythmic, straight, closed-leg circular movements interrupted only by scissor elements (pendulous swings with spread legs). The routine ends with a handstand dismount. Acute injuries in competition are very rare and almost exclusively cause acute wrist pain or sprains.

Rings: This is the apparatus that requires most muscular strength; the exercise combines rapid, dynamic swinging moves with static strength and control elements (cross, Maltese cross scale position, etc.) and also a number of handstand elements. Routines end with an acrobatic dismount.

Acute lesions mainly affect the shoulder with labrum, infraspinatus and supraspinatus muscle injuries, joint sprain, and acromioclavicular dislocation being the commonest. A poorly executed dismount may cause a sprain to the ankle or knee, and, in rare cases, cervical injury.

Vault: After a 25 m approach to develop the necessary power and a flic flac, the gymnast takes off from the springboard to the table in preflight (first vault), briefly touching the table with his hands prior to executing an acrobatic element in flight (second vault), then landing on a mat in the same axis (exit). Vaults differ widely and feature saltos and twists in midair. Acute injuries during the first vault usually affect the thorax and cervical spine, while landing injuries involve the knees, ankles (inferior tibiofibular joint sprains, dislocations, heel bone pathology) and the cervical spine. Other, more severe injuries can occur in uncontrolled dismounts or when a gymnast falls off the landing mat or from the podium to the floor.

Parallel Bars: Gymnasts perform acrobatic and swinging elements with changes in direction, smoothly and dynamically executed both over and under the bars in longitudinal and lateral positions and featuring elements of strength and balance, and handstands. Routines end with an acrobatic landing.

In competition, injuries include

- Sprains and dislocations of the fingers
- Sprains of the elbows and wrists
- Skin erosions on the inner part of the arm from rubbing on the bars if arms have not been properly protected
- Occasional ankle or knee sprains due to uncontrolled falls

Horizontal Bar: Routines are composed of giant forward and backward swings with changes in direction, in-bar skills with pirouettes, kips, release moves with acrobatic elements, saltos, twists, and combinations. Exercises end with acrobatic, stuck landings from a height of roughly five meters. In competition, injuries primarily occur during falls due to failure to regrasp the bar or due to inaccurate dismount landings (knee, ankle dislocation or sprain, cervical spine injury) or due to direct falls from the bar (head and thorax).

Women's Artistic Gymnastics

This discipline includes four apparatus with an assortment of biomechanical constraints that require varying degrees of dynamic and static effort, flexibility, balance, rhythm, and a certain level of choreographic creativity. Gymnasts may compete on one, two, three, or all four apparatus, depending on competition formats.

Chronic conditions in women's artistic gymnastics are often compounded by the fact that gymnasts have not always completed their osteoarticular growth, notably the

- Lumbosacral spine (lumbago, especially if there is preexisting lysis or listhesis, frequently osteochondrosis)

- Ankle, foot, knee, hip (osteochondrosis)

- Wrist, elbow (osteochondrosis)

- Pelvis (tearing of the iliac and ischial tuberosity due to overstretching)

Acute injuries include bruising of the vertebral spine when rolling on the beam and bruising of the anterior superior iliac spine due to repeated blows to the pelvis by the uneven bars.

Vault: When approaching the table, a poorly executed backward salto at entry (first vault) may result in a direct impact on the front of the table, with potential trauma to the cervical or thoracic spine being of particular concern; after pushing off with the hands (second vault) the main acrobatic sequence (in the case of forward or backward salto with or without sagittal rotation) may on landing result in injury of the ankles (sprain, dislocation, fracture), the knees (cruciate ligaments, meniscus, lateral ligaments), the feet (plantar aponeurosis, calcaneus fractures) and, again, of the cervical spine. Trauma injuries are worsened if vaults are unbalanced and gymnasts fall outside of the zone protected by the landing mat. Certain joint injuries may affect the growth plates of adolescent gymnasts (fracture and epiphyseal dislocation).

Uneven Bars: The upper bar usually is 2.2 m high and the distance between bars may vary. The gymnast executes giant forward and backward swings, release and regrasp moves, changes in direction, and acrobatic sequences on or between the bars. Routines end with an acrobatic dismount. Acute injuries due to falls in competition, be they in front, behind, or in between the bars often result from a loss of balance during the exercise or at the time of release. Poorly executed dismounts may cause ankle (sprain, dislocation), knee (sprain), and, less frequently, elbow (sprain, dislocation) and cervical spine injuries. Direct hits on the bars may result in hematomas.

Balance Beam: Gymnasts perform their exercise on beams that are 5 m long and 10 cm wide. Choreographed routines include alternating leaps (saltos, turns) and balance sequences. Acute injuries in competition due to acrobatic sequences on the beam may result in falls or direct blows on the beam with subsequent hematomas and muscular or osseous contusions, notably of the tibia, pelvic, and adductor muscles (fall astride the beam). Acrobatic mounts and dismounts may result in trauma to the lower limbs and the cervical spine.

Floor Exercises: Women's exercises differ from those of men in that they are accompanied by music: A gymnast performs an artistic sequence of acrobatic and balance movements lasting one and a half minutes on a 12 × 12 m floor; acrobatics and choreography form the basis of these floor exercises.

The most frequent injuries are in the lower limbs (lateral ligaments of the knees and ankles, Achilles tendon, including partial or total ruptures and, less frequently, the elbow (dislocation) and the cervical spine. An acute avulsion of the ischial tuberosity in adolescents is rare; this lesion results from repeated overstretching and affects the ischial crural region.

Acrobatic Gymnastics

In acrobatic gymnastics, there are no apparatus, just a series of collective and individual acrobatic elements, combined with choreographic sequences. There are five different types of events: men's pairs, women's pairs, mixed pairs, groups (women), and groups of four partners (men).

Acrobatics include base (the gymnast who carries or supports the others), top and flyer positions. A 2½-minute routine includes static elements (static pyramids, strength, balance), dynamic elements (vault, salto, dynamic pyramids, etc.), combined exercises and numerous displays of balance.

The type of acute and chronic conditions that affect these gymnasts depends on which position they have and the different physical demands placed upon them. Flyers are more prone to acute injuries, whereas base gymnasts are more susceptible to chronic disorders.

Chronic conditions are usually to be found in the lumbar spine (lumbago, lumbocrural sciatica). Also seen are tendinopathies of the wrist and elbow. In competition, injuries result primarily from the acrobatic elements and from falls of the tops and flyers, some of whom reach great heights (e.g., the fourth gymnast at the top of the pyramid); these include knee sprains, dislocations of the ankle, sprains to the forefoot, heel bone pathology, and, in some cases, trauma to the cervical spine. For the base gymnast, muscular lesions in the upper limbs and acute lumbago are frequent.

Tumbling

Tumbling is practiced on an extremely soft 25-m long dynamic track. The gymnast performs eight acrobatic elements without change in rhythm; only hands and feet are allowed to make contact with the track. An exercise closes with an exit on the landing mat.

The most frequent injuries involve

- Complete or partial ruptures of the Achilles tendon due to overstretching

- Microtears in the Achilles tendon leading to chronic tendonitis

- Partial tearing of the posterior leg muscles including gastrocnemius (also known as tennis leg)

- The knee, wrist and lumbar spine

As the track is rather narrow, a gymnast may lose balance and accidentally leave the track, resulting in a variety of osteoarticular injuries, particularly of the lower limbs (sprain, dislocation of the ankle) and the feet (heel bone pathology, rupture of the plantar aponeurosis, sprain to the forefoot). A poorly executed exit on the mat may cause lower limb joint injuries or, less frequently, injuries to the cervical spine.

Aerobics

An exercise lasts about two minutes and is really an anaerobic activity. It requires dynamic and static strength, jumps and leaps, and displays of balance and flexibility; rhythm and choreographic elements are also evaluated by the judges.

Typically, injuries cause wrist pain and swelling, often without a precise diagnosis, and, less frequently, elbow conditions (epicondylitis, epitrochleitis) and lumbago.

Acute osteoarticular and muscular lesions are rare; they primarily include wrist sprains and, in the case of adolescents, fractures of the growth plate. Ankle sprains and muscular injury are also seen in the lower limbs.

Aerobic gymnastics requires intensive cardiovascular training, and in cases where a gymnast is insufficiently prepared, or where an underlying cardiac disease has been overlooked, cardiac symptoms of varying degree may appear—from a feeling of general discomfort to full-blown cardiac emergencies. Careful preparticipation examinations may identify certain predisposing conditions and initiate further assessment to be able to either correct the condition or recommend appropriate restrictions for participation in sports.

Trampoline Gymnastics

Individual gymnasts or pairs (synchronized trampoline) perform on a 4 × 2 m piece of fabric fitted into a 5 × 3 m frame by steel springs. Ten different acrobatic elements are performed, after each rebound. The most frequent chronic pathologies involve the lumbosacral spine (lumbago, sciatica), the ankles and knees (chronic sprains). Falls in trampoline gymnastics may occur and may on occasion lead to severe injuries: A large majority of acute injuries could be avoided if better technical control is applied and if more progressive learning processes are enforced. The deceptive ease of the rebound phase on the trampoline sometimes causes beginners to take thoughtless risks without having a sufficient technical base. Exiting the fabric or landing on the frame supporting the fabric generates a variety of osteoarticular injuries, notably to the ankle and foot (sprain, fracture). Sometimes, athletes can fall to the ground and suffer various injuries, mainly to the ankles and legs. Stuck or hyperlordosis landing may bring on episodes of acute lumbago.

The most feared accident in trampoline is a fall with landing on the head in cervical hyperflexion or, more rarely still, in cervical hyperextension. This may lead to fractures or dislocations of the cervical spine and may have serious neurologic consequences. Performing first aid on the trampoline and evacuating an injured gymnast is problematic, especially with injuries to the spine. The fabric is unstable, and it would be wise to use a rigid surface or long board that could be slid under the gymnast or placed under the fabric from underneath the trampoline.

Rhythmic Gymnastics

This is a discipline for individuals or for groups of five gymnasts. Gymnasts use a different apparatus for each exercise (two for certain group exercises). These are rope, hoop, clubs, ribbon, and ball. A gymnast handles an apparatus primarily with her bare hands, but also with her feet and body. She performs fast and varied movements during throws (leaps, rolls on floor, etc.). In certain static positions, the peripheral and/or the spinal joints are loaded through their full range of motion. Choreography is highly important in this discipline. Chronic pathologies are rather frequent. They primarily cause lumbago, lumbosciatic syndrome, or may affect the pelvis (avulsion or chronic inflammation of the anterosuperior iliac spine and of the ischial tuberosity, especially in growing young girls), ankles (chronic sprains), and feet (chronic sprains and fatigue fractures). Accidents in competition are very rare. Injuries affect the ankles, knees (sprains), posterior leg muscles, and in some cases the feet (fall of the clubs may cause a fracture to the toe or, on rare occasions, injuries of the plantar aponeurosis).

14.12 TENNIS

Contributed by Babette M. Pluim (Netherlands), Miguel Crespo (Spain), Nicky Dunn (UK), Brian Hainline (USA), Stuart Miller (UK), Dave Miley (Ireland), Bernard Montalvan (France), Ann Quinn (Australia), Per Renström (Sweden), Kathleen A. Stroia (USA), Karl Weber (Germany), and Tim Wood (Australia), who are all members of the ITF Medical Committee

The Tournament Physician

An event physician is responsible for player medical services and the supervision of the medical team during a tournament, and is in tennis referred to as the "tournament physician." Presence of a tournament physician during all hours of play is mandatory for qualifying and main draw matches at Grand Slams and the Olympic Games, main draw Davis Cup and Fed Cup matches, ATP international series, and all WTA Tier I–V tour events. At smaller events, such as Challenger tournaments, Satellite tournaments, and the ITF Futures, the rules require a doctor to be on-call. Rules of National Federations regarding national championships and other events vary. The tournament physician is generally assisted by one or more (sports) physiotherapists and/or certified athletic trainers (called sports medicine therapists by the ATP, and primary health care provider by the WTA), depending on the size and needs of the event. There may be massage therapists as well. A well-prepared tournament physician will be in local contact with consulting specialists and access to a facility for performing diagnostic studies (e.g., x-rays, diagnostic ultrasound, MRIs and bone scans). Further, the tournament physician is aware of nearby pharmacies and their addresses, phone numbers and business hours for prescription medications. Most often, the background of the tournament physician is primary care sports medicine or orthopedic surgery.

The tournament physician must function as a generalist physician to detect and treat a variety of illnesses and injuries and provide or coordinate the care of players during the event. The tournament physician should have a working knowledge of tennis-specific injuries and medical conditions encountered in sports in general. It is recommended that he or she is trained and certified in CPR. The tournament physician must be aware of which players have a serious illness or have special medical needs, to allow the physician to be prepared to manage any emergencies.

Court-side assessment and triage and managing of routine injuries on court are generally not the task of the tournament physician but of the sports medicine therapist/primary health care provider. The sports medicine therapist/primary health care provider may call the tournament physician for assistance in the evaluation and/or treatment.

The tournament physician is responsible for developing and implementing an organizational plan for the sports medical team to handle medical emergencies, including the safe and expeditious evacuation of an injured player. This also includes contact with the closest hospital emergency room before the tournament begins. The tournament should have an emergency plan in place, whereby the tournament physician should have a working knowledge of evacuation procedures for emergencies, including fire, bomb warnings, and catastrophic illnesses.

The tournament physician may be requested to have certain medications—including special medications for players with certain medical illnesses or needs—crutches, and intravenous fluids available at the tournament.

It is recommended that the tournament physician write a report at the end of the week, summarizing the main issues and including recommendations to the tournament director for the next year.

Medical Rules

Several of the rules of the ITF, ATP, WTA Tour and/or National Federation pertain to medical conditions (e.g., the Medical Time-Out Rule, the Extreme Weather Conditions Rule, and the Tennis Anti-Doping Programme). The tournament physician should have working knowledge of the medical rules in tennis that are applicable to the event. It is recommended that the tournament physician checks the current status of the rules prior to an event by consulting the relevant rulebook or discussing those rules with an official.

The Medical Time-out Rule: The rule books of the Grand Slams, ITF, ATP, and WTA Tour all contain a paragraph regarding medical conditions for which a player may request a medical time-out. Generally, if a player develops a medical condition during the match or warm-up, or believes that medical diagnosis and treatment are required for a medical condition, he or she may request through the chair umpire to see the sports medicine therapist/primary health care provider. The sports medicine therapist/primary health care provider may call the tournament physician for assistance in the evaluation and/or treatment. The sports medicine therapist/primary health care provider or tournament physician may determine (authorization is done by the chair umpire) a one-time, three-minute medical time-out to treat the injured or ill player for that condition.

The time-out begins after the completion of the evaluation and diagnosis of the medical condition by the sports medicine therapist/primary health care provider or tournament physician.

Treatable medical conditions can be either acute or nonacute. An acute medical condition is the sudden development of a medical illness or musculoskeletal injury during the warm-up or the match that requires immediate medical attention. A nonacute medical condition is a medical illness or musculoskeletal injury that develops or is aggravated during the warm-up or the match and requires medical attention at the changeover or set break.

Players may not receive treatment for the following: any medical condition that cannot be treated appropriately or that will not be improved by available medical treatment within the time allowed; any medical condition that has not developed or has not been aggravated during the warm-up or the match; general player fatigue; or any medical condition requiring injections, intravenous infusions, or oxygen, except for diabetes, for which prior medical certification has been obtained, and for which subcutaneous injections of insulin may be administered.

During a match, if there is an emergency medical condition and the player involved is unable to make a request for a sports medicine therapist/primary health care provider, the chair umpire shall immediately call for the sports medicine therapist/primary health care provider and tournament physician to assist the player.

Either before or during a match, if a player is considered unable physically to compete, the sports medicine therapist/primary health care provider and/or tournament physician should inform the supervisor and recommend that the player is ruled unable to compete in the match to be played, or retired from the match in progress.

Extreme Weather Conditions Rule: To protect players from heat illness, the WTA Tour and ITF Juniors, Wheelchair, and Seniors have implemented a rule that pertains to play under conditions of high heat stress. The extreme weather condition rule is invoked when the heat stress meets or exceeds a WBGT of 28°C, or an apparent temperature of 32°C, following which a 10-minute break will be allowed between the second and third sets. There may also be a delay in the starting time of the matches scheduled for play that day. The referee has the discretion to suspend play if the conditions are considered too extreme.

The Medical Bag: The tournament physician should always carry a medical bag. The organization of the bag is important to ensure easy access for the physician as well as for anyone sent by the physician to retrieve an item for him or her. The bag should be arranged with different compartments, so the contents will fit in an organized manner. The bag should offer enough room to store all the required items and still be manageable when carrying it through airports or at tournament sites. The contents may vary slightly, depending on local conditions of the country where the tournament or event is being held.

The following equipment should be readily available on-site: resuscitation equipment, automatic external defibrillator (Grand Slams, ATP, and WTA events), ventilation mask, infusion set, and limb immobilization.

Essential Medications: This list of medications (Table 14.2) below will allow a physician to readily treat the majority of medical conditions and ailments. The list does include medications for emergency situations (heart attack, asthma, anaphylactic shock). The tournament physician should establish a pharmacy contact near the tournament site, including address, phone number, and hours open for business, which will be used for prescription medications.

The Tennis Anti-Doping Programme: Tournament physicians must be aware of substances and methods that are on the current WADA Prohibited List. To allow the administration/use of such substances or methods for valid therapeutic purposes (e.g., corticosteroids, adrenaline, bronchodilators, and diuretics), players will normally have been granted a TUE in advance of the tournament. If necessary, however, the tournament physician may submit an application for a TUE on behalf of a player during an event. In case of a medical emergency (e.g., severe asthma attack, anaphylactic shock), or exceptional circumstances, the TUE application may be submitted following administration of the substance in question. If the circumstances are not an emergency or an exception, a TUE would not be granted retroactively, in which case the player would participate entirely at his or her own risk.

Common Injuries and Medical Conditions in Tennis:

- Sliding/tripping/falls on the court: Ankle sprains; muscle strains (mainly posterior calves and thigh); abrasions on hands, elbows, and knees

- Ball in the eye/racket impact/foreign object in the eye: Injury of the eyelid, corneal erosion, conjunctivitis

- Knee rotation/valgus injury/overuse: Meniscal tear, MCL/ACL injury, patellar tendinopathy, patellofemoral pain

- Serving: Abdominal muscle strain, low-back pain, sprain of the ulnocarpal ligament of the elbow, medial epicondylitis, shoulder impingement, rotator cuff tendinopathy/partial tear

- Forehands: Medial epicondylitis, tendinopathy/rupture of the extensor carpi ulnaris tendon

- Backhands: Tennis elbow (lateral epicondylitis), injury of the nondominant extensor carpi ulnaris tendon, ankle sprains

- Volleys: Subluxating extensor carpi ulnaris tendon, TFCC lesions

- Heat problems: Cramps, heat syncope, heat exhaustion, and heat stroke

- Skin: Blisters, tennis toe, ingrown toenail

- Hip: Bursitis, labral tears, piriformis syndrome

- Digestive: Traveller's diarrhea, viral gastroenteritis, food poisoning. heartburn

- Neurologic: Exercise-induced headache, tension headache, migraine

- Respiratory problems: Hay fever, viral upper respiratory tract problem, (exercise-)induced asthma

- Cardiac problems: Tachycardia, heart attack, sudden exercise-related cardiac death, myocarditis

- Diabetes (hypoglycemia)

- Anemia

- Burnout

- Heat problems: Sunburn, cramps, heat syncope (vasovagal collapse), heat exhaustion, heat stroke

- Injuries in juniors: Sever's/Osgood–Schlatter/Sinding–Larsen–Johannsson diseases, osteochondritis dissecans (ankle, elbow, knee), spondylolysis/ spondylolisthesis, Panner's disease, Little Leaguer's elbow/shoulder

Summary

The tournament physician in tennis is responsible for player medical services and the supervision of the medical team during a tournament and is assisted by a sports medicine therapist/primary health care provider. The tournament physician functions as a

TABLE 14.2	**Contents of the Medical Bag**

Oral	Nonsteroidal anti-inflammatory drugs (NSAIDs): for treatment of pain and inflammation associated with musculoskeletal conditions
	Muscle relaxers: for musculoskeletal pain and stiffness associated with muscle spasm
	Analgesics: for treatment of mild to moderate pain, for example, paracetamol/acetaminophen
	Antibiotics: for common infections, for example, amoxycillin, azithromycin, erythromycin, flucloxacillin, doxycycline
	Antihistamines: for allergic reactions, for example, loratadine
	Antidyspeptics (antacids): for example, hydrotalcite, magnesium oxide.
	Antidiarrheals: for example, loperamide, bismuth subsalicylate
	Antiemetics: for example, metoclopramide; for motion sickness, for example, cyclizine, meclizine
	Cough suppressants: for symptomatic treatment of cough
	Decongestant/expectorant: for URTI, for example, acetylcysteine
	Migraine preparation: for example, sumatriptan
	Secretion inhibitors: for gastroesophageal reflux and gastric ulcers, for example, ranitidine, omeprazole
	Sleeping tablets: jet lag or long intercontinental flights, for example, temazepam.
Nasal/inhaler	Bronchodilator: for treatment of bronchoconstriction secondary to intrinsic asthma, exercise-induced asthma, infection, or allergy, for example, salbutamol[a]
	Nasal decongestant spray: for acute symptomatic relief of nasal congestion, for example, oxymetazoline, livocab
	Nitrolingual spray: for treatment of angina pectoris
Topical	Antibiotic ointment: for superficial skin infection.
	Antiviral cream: for treatment of cold sores, for example, acyclovir, penciclovir
	Corticosteroid cream: for noninfectious skin rashes
	Antifungal cream: for fungal skin infections, for example, miconazole
	Eye drops (neutral): for irritated eyes, for example, Visine
	Antibiotic eye drops or creams
	Eardrops: for earache
Injectable	Adrenaline[a]: for treatment of anaphylactic shock or life-threatening coronary syndromes
	Atropine: for treatment of bradyrhythmia
	Corticosteroid[a]: for soft-tissue and intra-articular injections in inflammatory conditions and for anaphylactic shock
	Anaesthetic: for use with or without corticosteroid for soft-tissue and intra-articular injections.
	Bronchodilator: for severe asthma—for example, terbutaline
	Diclofenac: for colic pain (kidney stone)
	Intravenous fluids: for intravenous infusion[a] for the treatment of severe dehydration or when oral hydration is not possible
	Diuretics[a]: for treatment of asthma cardiale
	Glucose and/or GlucaGen: for severe hypoglycemia in diabetics

[a]Medications or methods with an asterisk are on the WADA list of prohibited substances and methods.

generalist physician to detect and treat a variety of illnesses and injuries, and to provide or coordinate the care of players during the event. Court-side assessment and triage and managing of routine injuries on court are generally not the task of the tournament physician, but of the sports medicine therapist/ primary health care provider. The tournament physician should have working knowledge of the medical rules in tennis that are applicable to the event. Finally, the tournament physician should always carry a medical bag with essential medications and equipment and should have working knowledge of evacuation procedures for emergencies.

14.13 SOCCER DOCTOR

Contributed by Derek McCormack, Team Doctor, Glasgow Celtic FC, Scotland

As a doctor covering a soccer event, preparation is essential. During the game, your focus should change from spectator to professional. This may seem obvious, but it is remarkably easy to slip into fan mode and follow the flow of the game rather than watching for injuries and tracking players for hints of difficulties. The relationship you have with players and management should be empathetic but somewhat detached. Medical coverage at a soccer event will range from a small local amateur match to elite professional level, but I hope the following advice will be pertinent to most.

Match Preparation

Venue: Check the availability of first aiders and paramedics should assistance be required for a player on the field of play. Make sure you know where the nearest accident and emergency unit is. I program my car's satellite navigation system with this information prior to the game. For larger games, discuss with the security division to enable you to park your car as close as possible to the ground and in a position to enable a rapid exit. I always take my car to away games if at all possible. Should a player be injured during a game and require hospital assessment then I can take the player myself and the team bus can leave as scheduled.

This ability is also useful in the event of doping testing. Unfortunately, it may mean missing the start of the celebrations after a cup win.

If you have responsibility for first aiders/ paramedics, ensure you are aware of their competence level and their specific remit. I would advise practicing common requirements such as immobilizing a player, transfer of a spinal injury, and even simple transfer of an injured player off the pitch. I have witnessed first aiders at the front of a stretcher move in the opposite direction to those at the rear. Take charge when on the pitch and give clear, definitive commands.

Clothing: Be aware of changing weather conditions. Being hypothermic makes suturing more difficult. Likewise, the doctor going down with sunstroke presents the wrong image. Make sure your footwear is appropriate for running onto the pitch. I recall once running onto an icy pitch wearing normal footwear, slipping, and injuring my coccyx, then performing the standard "I haven't injured myself" funny walk.

Make sure the contents in your pockets are secure. Zip or Velcro closure is ideal. Make sure you have an adequate number of pockets.

Air Flights: Airport security may not allow medication, especially injectables, for hand luggage. If you have a player who has a condition such as IDDM or is a high anaphylactic risk, ensure you have named authorization from a hospital specialist to carry medication on board. Remember that insulin and other emergency fluids will be ineffective if they have been stored in the hold, so these must be taken onboard as hand luggage.

Select which medications you are likely to require during a flight and keep this in your hand luggage. Divide the remaining medication in both the team hamper and check-in luggage (especially if transfer flights are required), so that if one piece of luggage is lost or delayed, a backup is available.

Away Trips: If possible, arrange for an extra room to be made available in the event of a player presenting with symptoms of an infectious disease so he can be isolated.

Send menu requirements to the hotel in advance.

Medical Issues

Medical Insurance Coverage: Make sure you check with your medical defense to ensure you are covered for the level of player you are providing care for. Be especially careful to inform your medical defense union when you are traveling abroad.

Medical Confidentiality: Don't forget that footballers are patients. Members of the media will attempt to entice you to divulge information; don't fall for their subtle seductions. It is very easy to regard the sporting environment as being different from a consulting room, but the reality is this is your clinical workstation and the usual rules apply. History taking and examination should parallel those in the consultation room, albeit adapted to the sporting arena.

Player Medical History: Ensure you are aware of the medical problems players have, medications they use and allergics they have. For confidentiality reasons this information should be collated by you.

Medical Records: It is all too easy to forget to record information when you get involved in a game and you are in a sporting environment; however, remember your role as a doctor means you must keep *clear*, concise, *contemporaneous* notes. I would suggest you take a notepad and record relevant information on this for transfer as soon as possible to the medical record database.

Equipment

Gloves: Use universal protection at all times. I wear plastic gloves at all times as attempting to put gloves on in an acute situation can take up valuable time, and they will inevitably burst, the more important the occasion. In cold conditions, I would recommend wearing windproof and waterproof gloves that are insulated and one size larger than you normally require so they will fit on top of the plastic gloves and can be easily removed without catching on the underlying gloves.

Ensure players wear shin guards, and adjust footwear according to conditions. Make sure players have several pairs of football boots they can use. I have known players who have a favorite pair of boots that eventually wear out. New boots are then used with resultant blisters.

Have players assessed for orthotics if they appear to have poor mechanical alignment, and have players assessed for biomechanical issues if they have recurrent injuries. Renew footwear on a regular basis to maintain shock absorption and control mechanism.

Medication: Medication and equipment will be tailored to a degree by circumstances.

Suggested medication:

- Antacid
- Antiemetic (e.g., Buccastem)
- Antihistamines
- Aspirin
- Benzylpenicillin injection (plus water for injection)
- Co-Amoxiclav
- Dioralyte
- Erythromycin
- Flucloxacillin
- GlucoGel
- GTN
- Hydrocortisone
- Hydrocortisone cream
- Lamisil
- Loperamide
- Metronidazole
- NSAID oral and IM
- Paracetamol
- Penicillin V
- Prefilled adrenaline, IV
- Proton pump inhibitor
- Rectal diazepam
- Salbutamol (remember TUE)
- Strepsils

Suggested eye medication:

- Amethocaine eyedrops
- Chloramphenicol eye ointment
- Cotton buds
- Diclofenac eyedrops
- Fluorescein eyedrops
- Opticrom eyedrops
- Consider oxygen and Entonox (ensure you know how to connect and use)

A useful tip to protect an injured eye from compression is the bottom of a polystyrene cup.

Check stock requirements and expiry dates on a regular basis. When ordering from the pharmacy, ask for medication with as long an expiry date as possible—many pharmacists will dispense medication which is soon to expire.

Remember to document batch number and expiry date in the medical records when administered.

Medical Equipment

- Swabs
- Gloves
- Sterile water
- Clinical waste bag
- Sharps box
- Scissors
- Alcohol gel for hand cleaning
- Tape—I prefer Transpore, as it is very easy to tear into whatever size you wish
- Thick tape
- Dressings
- Blister pads—I would recommend Compeed. If there is room in the boot, two thin cotton socks (avoid nylon and wool) with a layer of Vaseline between the socks is useful. If prominent areas on the foot are liable to blister, a thin layer of Vaseline on the skin may be all that is required. Lacing boots at a slight angle is also a useful tip to avoid blisters by reducing in-shoe movement.
- Compression bandages
- Nasal tampons for epistaxis—but ensure you know how to use them
- Steri-Strips
- Glue
- Splints
- Disposable suture kit—for air travel, remember to put these in the hold. I forgot once and took them in my hand luggage and, of course, they were confiscated by airport security
- Sutures—cross section for face, mouth, limbs
- Tourniquet
- Venflons
- Syringes
- Needles
- Local anaesthetic—lignocaine—remember, take care if using adrenaline mix on distal structures such as toes
- Insect repellent
- Sunblock (even in Scotland!), minimum SPF of 15
- Sphygmomanometer
- Airway—use airways you feel confident with

- Resus mask
- Defibrillator
- Nebulizer
- Cervical collar—one adjustable will be easier than a set; whichever you use, make sure you are up to speed with usage, such as sizing
- Opthalmoscope/otoscope
- Stethoscope
- Thermometer
- The availability of a walking boot and crutches can be very useful
- Preprinted head injury advice cards are useful

You may wish to consider strapping materials. It would be most worthwhile if you could learn basic ankle strapping. For this, I would recommend underwrap be applied before an elastic adhesive bandage. Cohesive elastic bandage has the advantage that no underwrap is required, but I prefer adhesive. Zinc oxide tape can be used for reinforcement. Bandage scissors or tape cutters are helpful for removal, especially in an acute situation.

Match Day

Referees: Never argue with referees, but do not be intimidated or pressurized to remove a player off the pitch unless you are certain it is safe for the player to do so. I have been in a position where a senior referee demanded an injured player be removed immediately, but the player had a leg fracture and removing him without adequate splintage could have exacerbated his condition.

In the event of what looks like a serious injury or medical problem, do not wait for the referee to signal to you, but do try to ensure you are correct about the serious nature of the incident.

Communication: If you are working with a physiotherapist, ensure you have a system of hand signs if the physiotherapist treats a player on the pitch and also to signal the coaches if a player requires to be substituted. I have tried various radio systems but have yet to find one that is effective. I now enter the field of play with the physiotherapist unless it is obviously a minor problem.

Return-to-play of Injured Player: On-field assessment can be complicated by noise, time constraints, and the determination of some injured players to continue no matter what. When adrenaline is pumping, a player also has a much higher pain threshold than normal, which can mask the severity of some injuries. I would suggest you develop a rapid method of observation, palpation, active and passive movements, resisted tests, and finishing with functional tests. In the case of knees, perform ligament stability tests before the player stands up. With ankle injuries, the player may have a strapping on along with boot and sock. Rule out a fracture and ligament injury prior to functional tests of jogging and hopping. Do not be overrushed by coaches to return the player. Make sure there is no active bleeding and you are convinced of the safety of not only the injured player but also others when the player returns to the field of play. Be especially cautious when dealing with head injuries and be aware of associated neck trauma.

Hydration and Nutrition: Adequate hydration and a varied diet are very important to optimize a player's fitness. Well-chosen foods will help players train harder, reduce risk of illness and injury, and optimize performance. A good hydration strategy is an essential part of every player's preparation. Cramps are often linked to dehydration. Dehydration, by as little as 2% of body mass, can reduce concentration, reaction time, coordination, muscle strength, and endurance performance. A simple way for a player to monitor his hydration levels is using a urine chart. Be sure players begin exercise in a hydrated state. Drinking water or sports drinks during and after both training and games is important, especially when sweat loss is high.

Hot Conditions: Monitor hydration, especially in hot and humid environments. Encourage management to arrange training sessions during the cooler part of the day.

Pre- and postexercise weight measurements are often not practical. Players still use thirst as a subjective guide to hydration. By this stage, the player is already dehydrated.

During games, have fluids at the dugout so they can be provided to players during breaks in play such as injuries or substitutions. Be ready to respond rapidly in relation to this as often little time is available.

Cold water is absorbed more rapidly, but avoid ice cold water.

Sunblock protects against skin cancer and sunburn. Sunburn has a negative impact upon thermoregulation.

Cold Conditions: Ensure substitutes warm up on a regular basis and wear warm layers of clothing while sitting on the bench. Players who are substituted should immediately return to the dressing room for a shower rather than sitting and watching the game in cold, wet clothing.

Other Issues

Female Players: If you have responsibility for female players (I used to be the doctor for the Scottish Ladies' International Team), add sanitary pads to the list of medical equipment.

Liaise with obstetric specialists and adjust activities as appropriate during pregnancy. Playing soccer risks abdominal trauma, but most players are keen to continue with training, and it is important to keep them involved as part of the group if at all possible. Swimming, low-impact aerobics and static cycling are potential appropriate activities.

Monitor for the female triad. Remember that amenorrhea may not be exercise induced. Other causes include pregnancy, endocrine and genetic disorders, and polycystic ovary syndrome.

Contact Lenses: Check which players have contact lenses. Keep spare lenses nearby ensuring they are labeled for player and which eye.

Injuries: Most matches will produce only minor injuries, but major events do occur. I have experienced a rather dramatic ankle fracture/dislocation where the player's foot began to turn black due to the circulation being compromised, and have dealt with a cardiac emergency in the coaching staff. It is also worth bearing in mind that players suffer the same medical problems as the general population.

There is a natural tendency to focus on musculoskeletal causes in a soccer player, but I have been caught out with pain presenting with classical symptoms of calf strain being a DVT in a player who had a blood dyscrasia and hamstring symptoms proving to be early herpes zoster. Also, never forget referred pain.

Sudden cardiac death is rare in soccer, but it does occur. An increasing number of associations are recommending testing for HOCM and other cardiac disorders. All our players have a physical examination and blood tests, complete a questionnaire, and have an ECG and echocardiogram performed. Of course, this is not practical for all, but it maybe worthwhile discussing with a cardiologist what he or she would recommend in your area.

Have ice available for strains, sprains, and contusions. It is easiest to prepare plastic bags with melting ice beforehand and keep these in a vacuum container. Melting ice is much safer for direct contact and can readily be contoured around a joint.

Supplements/Banned Substances: Be wary of advising soccer players about supplements. An increasing number are requesting these. Many are ineffective, and the risk of contamination with banned substances is high.

Remember to ensure medications do not contain prohibited substances. An excellent online drug information database to check for banned ingredients is http://www.didglobal.com.

14.14 RUGBY UNION

Contributed by MG Molloy, Professor, University College Cork, Medical Officer, International Rugby Board (IRB); and Eanna Falvey, University College Cork and Cork University Hospital, Ireland

Introduction

William Webb Ellis is credited with first picking up the football and running with it at Rugby School in 1823. Men, women, boys, and girls play rugby worldwide. More than three million people aged from 6 to 60 regularly participate in the playing of the game, and the Rugby World Cup is now the second largest global international team competition. While the vast majority of rugby players are amateur, since 1998, professional rugby has been played by the world's elite.

The potential for serious and catastrophic injury in rugby, *though rare*, means a need for familiarity with airway management, cervical spine immobilization, and advanced life support measures is essential for any EP covering this sport. The specifics of acute management of these issues are addressed in depth in their respective chapters in this document. This chapter aims to familiarize an EP, however unfamiliar with the game of rugby union, with various unique features of play. We highlight the injuries that may be encountered, when and where they may be seen, and, most importantly, how best to identify them early and safely.

Rugby Injury Rates

Injury rates vary greatly according to the age, gender, and level of experience of those playing.

The incidence of injury increases as the standard of competition increases. An IRB study of the 2007 Rugby World Cup in France, found that

- The knee was the most commonly injured structure during both matches and training, followed by the posterior thigh and shoulder (matches) and the posterior thigh (training). Knee ligament and posterior thigh muscle injuries also caused the greatest loss of time for players for both match and training injuries.

- The tackle was the activity/event responsible for the highest incidence of injury; a higher proportion of tackle injuries were the result of being tackled rather than from tackling.

Phases of Play

Several unique phases of play are seen in rugby. These situations generate potential for injury with which the attending physician should be familiar.

The Scrum: A scrum is formed in the field of play when eight players from each team, bound together in three rows for each team, close up with their opponents so that the heads of the front rows are interlocked. This creates a tunnel into which a scrum half throws the ball so that these front-row players can compete for possession by hooking the ball with their feet.

Injury mechanism: The compressive forces generated by a "pack" (the eight forwards) is somewhat less than the force individual players may exert. It can nevertheless exceed 0.8 metric tons in international rugby, a considerable force on front-row players' necks. Seventy percent of the force is generated by the first (38%) and second rows (42%). The majority of injuries in the scrum occur at engagement either by "collapse" or "popping." In all circumstances, the players' positions in the scrum, either around their teammates or binding to the opposition, means the cervical spine is unprotected at the time of collapse.

Injuries seen: Injuries to the shoulder, soft-tissue injury to the neck, and superficial injuries to the head and face predominate. Catastrophic injury to the cervical spine and serious lumbar spine injury are rare, but the team physician must be prepared for them.

The Lineout: The purpose of the lineout is to restart play, quickly, safely, and fairly, after the ball has gone into touch, with a throw-in between two lines of players. The receiver is the player in position to catch the ball when lineout players pass or knock the ball back from the lineout. Any player may be the receiver, but each team may have only one receiver at a lineout.

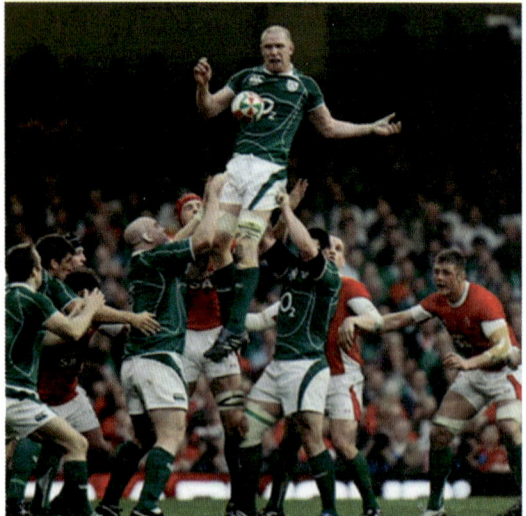

Lineout. (Photo courtesy of Dr. Molloy.)

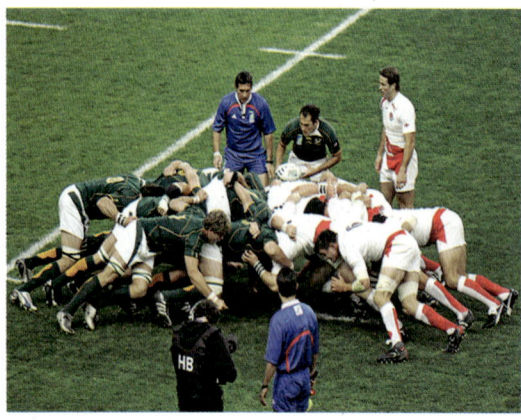

Scrum. (Photo courtesy of Dr. Molloy.)

Injury mechanism: This usually results from a fall, particularly from a height. Contact may also occur between players competing for the ball.

Injuries seen: Fall from a height onto the lower limb means injury to the knee and ankle can occur. Where the player loses balance, shoulder, neck or head injury may occur.

Important points: Injury resulting from a fall from the lineout may not be immediately obvious.

The Tackle: A tackle occurs when the ball carrier is held by one or more opponents and is brought to the ground.

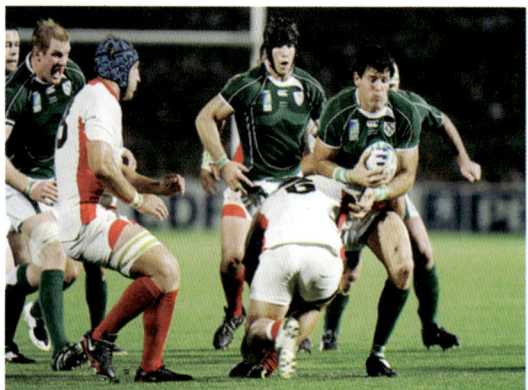

Tackle. (Photo courtesy of Dr. Molloy.)

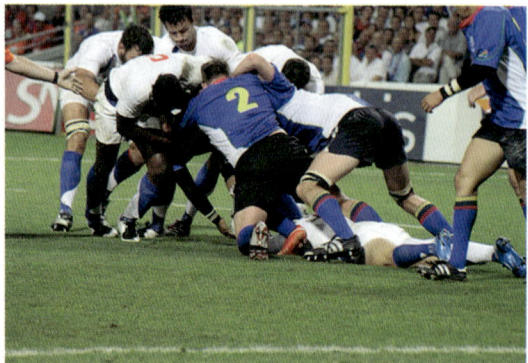

Ruck. (Photo courtesy of Dr. Molloy.)

Injuries seen: The injury profile in the tackle differs between the tackler and ball carrier. Using the shoulder and arms to tackle a ball carrier means head and neck injury may occur. While superficial injury predominates, contact between the head or neck and the lower limb or trunk of the ball carrier means significant injury such as concussion, facial fracture, shoulder injury, or cervical spine injury may be seen. Impact from a second player means the ball carrier may be at risk of knee, shoulder, or chest injury in addition to those seen in the tackler. Knee injuries are common in the tackle, as are dead legs after the game,

The Ruck: A ruck is a phase of play where one or more players from each team, who are on their feet, in physical contact, close around the ball on the ground. Players are rucking when they are in a ruck and using their feet to try to win or keep possession of the ball, without being guilty of foul play.

Injury mechanism: The ruck signifies an end to open play; as such it may be a focal point on which many players will converge. Players traveling at speed to join less mobile ruck means that significant energy exchange occurs. The additional use of feet to "clear" the ruck of opponents who have fallen to the wrong side is also a potential cause of injury.

Injuries seen: Injury to the head, face, and shoulder may occur due collision. Rucking injury may mean superficial injury to the chest and back. Inadvertent treading on fallen colleagues may lead to crush injury to extremities. If an opposition player falls to ground in an offside position (on the incorrect side of the ball), he may be moved by players' feet. Overzealous clearance is often termed "raking" and sometimes results in superficial injury to the trunk, upper limbs, and lower limbs.

The Maul A maul occurs when a player carrying the ball is held by one or more opponents, and one or more of the ball carrier's teammates bind on the ball carrier. A maul, therefore, consists of at least three players—the ball carrier and one player from each team—all on their feet. All the players involved must be caught in or bound to the maul and must be on their feet and moving toward a goal line.

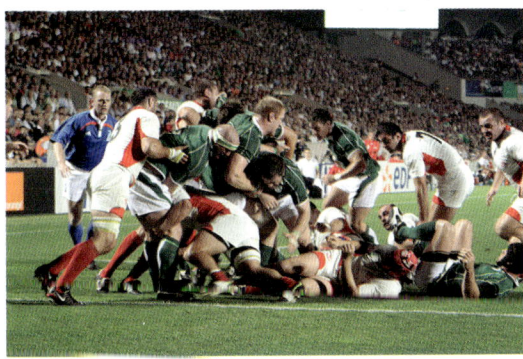

Maul. (Photo courtesy of Dr. Molloy.)

Injury mechanism: As the maul lacks the structure of a scrum, the same compressive forces are not exerted. Nonetheless, most of the forwards will engage in a maul situation, and when a mobile, or "rolling," maul ensues, significant speeds may be produced. Players losing their foot may be trodden upon, and collapse of the maul means a number of players will fall on each other. Injuries seen are very similar to those in the ruck.

A standard rugby game is of 80 minutes' duration, with two 40-minute halves. Team physicians are allowed on to the pitch at any time if they deem an injury has occurred. It is worthwhile briefly discussing this with match officials prior to the game.

Blood substitutions: These are permitted to afford team doctors the time necessary to properly attend to lacerations or abrasions. The player is substituted with an appropriate teammate while repairs are made, and the player is allowed to reenter play once blood flow has stopped and all blood has been cleaned from the injured party's clothes and person.

Emergency coverage at the game (covered elsewhere): If the sports physician does not feel competent in acute emergency airway management, then provisions should be made for access to emergency medical services.

14.15 CROSS-COUNTRY AND ALPINE SKIING EVENTS

Contributed by David McDonagh

The marathon event, cross-country skiing, downhill skiing, and mountain bike events all pose difficult challenges for rescue personnel. Most modern cross-country skiing arenas consist of laps of up to 5 to15 km, making them much easier to cover than the more classical events, which can be up to 50 km and more in open terrain. Usually tracks are prepared by snow scooters, thus allowing the EP access to all parts of the track. If available, it is advisable to have a scooter at the main medical station and two scooters spaced at approximately 3 km apart out on the track. Another option is to place a scooter at the sharp downhill swing (there is always at least one), where athletes tend to fall. Having mentioned all this, cross-country athlete injuries are extremely rare, but I have treated athletes with cervical facet joint fractures.

Downhill skiing is quite another matter. The athlete can slide out of the track and into woods, deep snow, even buildings and sheds. Getting to the athlete with skis and a sled requires great skiing competence, so the EP must be an experienced skier. Due to the high velocities achieved by downhill skiers, crashes may lead to head and neck injuries, thorax and abdominal injuries, as well as pelvic and extremity fractures.

On-site treatment is often extremely difficult due to slope incline, ice, deep snow, etc.

Obviously, treatment starts with emergency ABC, which means one has to be kitted with a "ventilation and circulation" backpack or belt system.

Fracture and luxation reductions are particularly difficult if the patient is on an icy surface; similarly, in deep snow, such activities can be quite taxing. Immobilizing the patient is the next task, followed by transfer to a transportation sled—this can be exhausting if a heavy athlete (downhill skiers can be a chunky lot) has to be moved over a distance in deep snow, particularly when spinal immobilization is a priority. Alternatively, helicopter transfer may be adjudged necessary, so continuous reanimation and spinal/limb immobilization may become a priority. Helicopters cannot always be relied upon due to weather conditions—fog, dark, wind, etc.—and one must also move the patient away from trees to ensure winch access. Not all rescue helicopters have winches. So even with a helicopter rescue, some form of patient movement is necessary.

Gross dislocations must be reduced before placing the athlete in the sled, due to several reasons, the most obvious being that the athlete cannot fit into the sled with a gross deformity. If distal pulses are absent, the onsite reduction must be attempted.

Then comes the task of pulling the sled by skis or by ropes down to the medical area. The best and most experienced skiers are needed for this task.

If the athlete has to be ventilated during descent, then transfer by sled must be limited and a helicopter should be used if available.

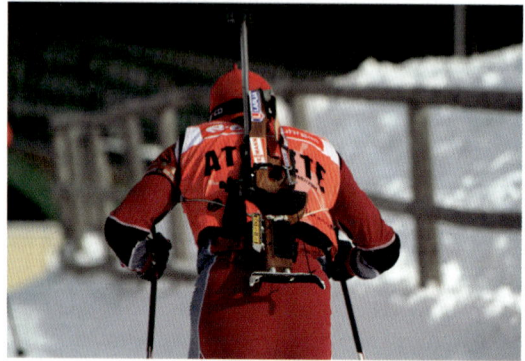

Ole Einar Bjørndalen.

14.16 TRIATHLON EVENTS

Contributed by Doug Hiller, CMO for Triathlon, Athens 2004 Summer Olympic Games and Beijing 2008 Summer Olympic Games, and has completed three Ironman Kona races, Hawaii, United States

A Brief History

Triathlon is a race consisting of consecutive swimming, bicycling, and running. The first race was held in 1974, and since then a huge variety of distances, courses, and rules have evolved internationally. The IF for the sport of triathlon is the International Triathlon Union (ITU), which was formed in 1989 under the leadership of Les McDonald and the representatives of 40 nations. The first Olympic triathlon competition was in Sydney in 2000, at which time, the woman's race helped open the Olympic Games. The sport continues in its prominent position on the Olympic program.

This chapter concerns medical care for "Olympic distance" races: 1.5-km open water swim, 40-km bike, and 10-km run.

Race-day Medical Care

Race-day medical care in this chapter is based upon our ITU experience at 20 World Championships. The worst problems the ITU medical committee has seen over the past 20 years have been the result of organizers and medical teams who underestimated the potential for disaster at World Championships, thereby almost creating impossible medical situations. Fortunately, there have always been adequate backup resources available on race day, but these problems could have been preempted.

Therefore, ITU guidelines are predicated not on what will "probably" happen with the athletes and race conditions but are based upon worst-case scenarios. While typically 1% to 2% of athletes may be seen in the medical tent under benign conditions, we have seen up to 15% of competitors on race days in very hot environments, for example. With 2,000 competitors, this provides the medical team with the opportunity to assess and provide care for up to one athlete per minute for five hours. This can be a daunting task.

Successful medical care is dependent upon many things: No race is safe without the complete commitment of the race organizing committee and race director, and no physician should agree to participate in race-day care without complete commitment from each of these entities.

The Medical Team

All medical team members should be clearly identified with scrub or other shirts.

Race medical director: This should be a well-respected physician who is experienced in the treatment of mass events, has good connections in the local medical community, and has the necessary time and energy to invest in the project. The race medical director (RMD) is recruited by the local organizing committee/race director, and should be brought onboard at least 6 months and hopefully a year in advance of the race.

Typically in well-established races, the new RMD is chosen by the previous RMD with the race director's blessing. The best races have long-standing, if ever-changing, medical teams who show up year to year with multiple physicians, nurses, and technicians who can fill in for each other in any role needed.

The RMD has overall responsibility for organization and race-day care, but should not try to be all things to all people at all times: Delegation of authority and responsibility without relinquishing oversight is critical.

Medical Team Members: These people should be recruited 6 months in advance if possible, and organizational meetings should be held as necessary, typically once 6 months in advance then again at least monthly until the race day. The medical team will staff the medical tent(s), and there should be roving medical teams available to care for injuries in situations where the patient cannot be easily brought to a medical area.

It is recommended that there be one physician per 200 athletes, and one nurse or paramedical person per 100 athletes. It is important to have experienced IV starters available in the medical tent if IV fluids are provided.

There should be about one "spotter" per 100 athletes (i.e., experienced people to stand at the finish line to immediately identify people who require medical attention or evaluation). Typically, this role will be filled by physicians, nurses, athletic trainers, or other race-experienced medical personnel. These people should stay out of the way of finishers and media except as absolutely necessary to help athletes.

There should be a security team of several experienced people to direct traffic around the medical tents and to gently assure the privacy of the medical area: This is most often a problem with intrusive press members, but family and friends, sponsors, and managers also must be appropriately reassured and directed.

Massage therapists should have a separate area, but it is helpful to have a number of massage therapists available in or around the medical tent.

The Medical Tent

The Function of the Medical Tent: The medical tent is not an emergency room nor is it an intensive care unit. It is a place to evaluate athletes (and sometimes spectators), to immediately stabilize and transport people with serious problems, and to treat relatively minor medical problems.

The size of the tent is a function of the number of contestants and the worst-case weather scenario. ITU recommends beds/cots/tables for 5% of competitors, which would indicate a tent of at least 10 × 12 m for 1,000 competitors. Each contestant cot area requires about two square meters, and there needs to be room in the tent for communication desks, supplies, heaters or cooling tubs, etc.

The main medical tent should be located as close as possible to the finish line. This is obviously of great importance to the athletes and medical team, but there is great pressure from the sponsors and media to occupy a large area around the finish line. If necessary, it may be helpful to remind the race director that it is bad press to have athletes collapse at the finish line, and then be shown throughout a tortuous parade to the distant medical area. It is, therefore, in everyone's best interest to situate the medical area as close as possible to the finish area. If the primary medical tent is not within a few steps of the finish line, there should be some wheeled transport immediately available—this can be modified golf carts, wheeled stretchers, etc. Wheelchairs are of minimal assistance with a dehydrated, hypotensive athlete. All medical tents should be designed to provide adequate privacy. There should be restrooms or portable restrooms available by the medical tents.

Secondary Medical Tents: It is not unusual to have the swim finish at some distance from the finish line itself. In this case, there should be a tent and medical team at the swim finish, prepared for evaluation, emergency transport, emergency care of near drowning, contusions, ocular abrasions, lacerations of the feet, stings by marine organisms, if any, and other mass swim-type injuries and maladies. For cool- or cold-water swims, adequate preparations for hypothermia should be made, and, of course, there should be established communication between this area, the main medical tent, and RMD and the race officials.

Similarly, if the bike finish is different from the run finish, a tent, medical teams, supplies, and communications should be provided.

In each medical tent, there should be a large, well-marked map of the course with the swim, bike and run legs clearly marked, and numbers to call as necessary.

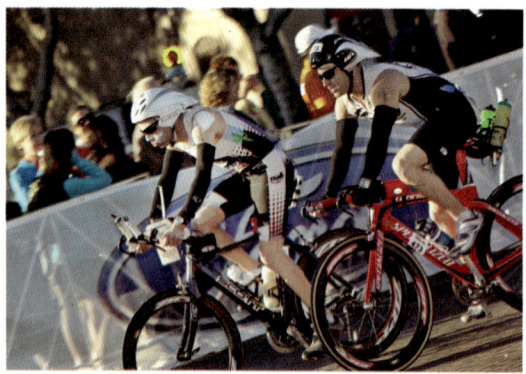

Communication: A formal communication system must be established for the medical team, and between the medical team and ambulance dispatch, ERs and the race organization. Typically, this is done with a dedicated radio system provided by the race organization, although some races use cell phones. A cell phone can be difficult in a noisy environment.

It is essential to have communication that blankets the race course. This is the responsibility of the race director/organizing committee. It is especially important to have designated people available at potentially dangerous corners on the bike course.

There should be an explicit method established to communicate athletes' identities and race numbers to the race organization, and an explicit and published way for families to find out where the athletes are and to communicate with them. This is especially important for athletes who are transported to hospitals: The information should be available from the race organization and from the medical area.

Medical Records: A medical record form should be created and used for every patient: It should include name, race number, age, vital signs, lab work, if any, treatment details, outcome and disposition. The Triathlon Canada Medical Committee has recommended that there be a medical form on the back of the athlete's race number that includes past medical history, medications, allergies, physician name, and phone number of a person to contact in emergencies. Other races require this information for race registration, computerize it, and have it available in the medical tent.

Prerace Medical Screening: It is the responsibility of each athlete to determine his or her fitness to participate in the race. Athletes with significant risks are responsible for communicating specific information to the race organization and RMD.

Race-day Medical Problems

Race course, environmental conditions, race length, age, physical conditioning, experience, and underlying medical conditions each have significant effects on what we see in the medical tent.

The Swim: The RMD has little or no control over what happens in the water but inherits the problems that do occur. Potential problems range from serious facial and other contusions to corneal abrasions, rib fractures, hypothermia, marine life contact, lacerations, water ingestion or aspiration, panic, nausea, confusion, dizziness, and even chest pain, which may represent myocardial infarction. Some swim exits unavoidably contribute to lacerations about the feet. The decision as to whether the athlete is to continue is both a matter of medical recommendation and the rules of the particular race as they relate to withdrawal.

The Bike: Accidents are unfortunately not uncommon on the bicycle leg of triathlons: These usually are limited to abrasions, but deep lacerations and fractures of the wrist, clavicle, humerus, and even femur are encountered occasionally. Closed head injury is rare but can occur. Every competitor in every race must be required to wear an appropriate helmet or be disqualified from the race.

The Run: Triathletes begin the run portion of the race tired and frequently not in fluid balance. Problems encountered during the run can run the gamut, including exhaustion, nausea, vomiting, muscle cramping, severe headache, and clinical dehydration (or, more rarely, overhydration). Heat injury or hypothermia may present, depending upon environmental conditions. Hyponatremia, with or without overhydration, may occur, especially in longer races.

Postrace: Athletes who have performed at a high level up to the finish line, as well as athletes who have walked the course to the finish line, frequently collapse at or shortly after finishing. This is a variable phenomenon that is related both to physiological as well as psychological causes. To keep the athlete ambulating, albeit with assistance, is helpful. Having a triage physician and/or nurse at the finish line and at the medical tent entrance is important, and many athletes do well in a monitored rest area without any medical intervention.

Athletes who do require evaluation and/or treatment in the medical tent should be identified, a medical record begun, and the race officials notified that the athlete is in the medical area.

Ambulances

There should be a minimum of two available, and ITU recommends 4 per 1,000 athletes. These should be fully equipped for CPR and trauma, and be able to communicate not only with the ER but with the medical tent. There must be a meeting with the drivers to explain the race course, to identify access points on the course, and to insure that the ambulances do not run counter to bike or run traffic in places where it would be dangerous to the athletes.

Local Hospitals

The local hospitals and their ERs should be informed well in advance that the race is occurring and that they may be seeing certain kinds of problems. It is advisable for the RMD to speak with the ER medical directors prior to the race. An excellent scenario is to have the local hospital(s) sponsor the medical tent, providing medical personnel and supplies for the race.

Medical Supplies

Supplies needed will be dictated by the race course, weather, and other factors.

- Medical tent: There should be room in the tent for the number of cots available (see below), as well as seats for athletes who do not need to lie

down, and for medical personnel, communications personnel, and supplies.

- There should be enough cots available for 5% of the competitors: In very hot environments, this could be 10% to 15%. These are recommendations only (see index).

Training Injuries

Typical injuries sustained during training are those expected of endurance swimmers, bicyclists, and runners. Overuse injuries are rampant and range from tendonitis to stress fractures. Traumatic injuries commonly seen from cycling include acromioclavicular separation, wrist fractures, shoulder injuries, and, rarely, long bone fractures and head injuries.

The editor extends his thanks to Andy Hunt for assistance in writing this chapter.

For a list of recommended equipment, see Appendix, page 524.

14.17 SKATING SPORTS

Contributed by Julia Alleyne, Canadian Skating Team, University of Toronto, Canada; Victor Lun, Associate Professor, University of Calgary and Canadian National Bobsleigh, Skeleton, Luge, and Long Track Speed Skating Teams; and Jim Thorpe, Canadian Men's Olympic Ice Hockey Team and Calgary Flames Hockey Club

Competitive ice sports generally included men's and women's hockey, figure skating, synchronized skating, as well as long and short track speed skating. As a rule, the severity of the injuries and complexities of the emergency situation increase with the number of skaters on the ice; the force of contact with the ice, boards, or other athletes; and any unnecessary delay in removing the athlete from the cold surface. Each sport has unique equipment rules, procedural rules and technical skills that increase risk of injury. In ice hockey and figure skating, the ice venue is bordered by wooden hockey boards in most competitions with no padding. In speed skating events, padding is used. Access to the ice is usually limited to two gates and thus medical personnel often have to walk across the ice surface to attend an injured athlete. Ambulance access to the venue is also limited and often shared with the Zamboni ice maker access. Air quality can be a problem in the arena and is related to poor ventilation systems or gas-fueled Zamboni ice makers versus electrical ones.

Through good planning and a thorough understanding of the sports, many emergencies can be predicted and even prevented. For those situations that do occur, we aim to handle them quickly and safely evacuate the athlete from the ice surface.

Figure Skating

Figure skating is divided into four Olympic disciplines (men's and women's singles, ice dance, and pairs) with differences related to technical components and rules that often affect risk of injury. Men's and women's singles skating is considered low risk since one skater is on the ice surface during competition and a maximum of six are on the ice together during warm-up or practice. The skaters jump and spin in a choreographed pattern and there are rules of etiquette to reduce the risk of collision. Ice dance is a moderate risk and performed in couples where lifts are permitted, but not above the shoulders, and fast choreography is executed with little space between the couple's blades. Pairs skating is high risk, as the couple skates with mandatory above-head lifts, partner throws, and side-by-side jumps and spins with elevated legs. All dance and pairs practices and warm-ups have 8 to 10 skaters on the ice surface at once. Synchronized skating is a team figure skating competition with 16 skaters on the ice at one time performing line splices, rotating wheels, and transitional pattern movements. This is high risk for collisions. The majority of skaters incur overuse type of injuries from training affecting their lower extremities, shoulders and spines. However, if they enter the competitive rink in an injured state, they may be putting not just themselves at risk for increased injury but also their partner, and often medical clearance is not granted as the skater is not able to provide a safe and stable lift, spin or throw technique.

Speed Skating

Speed skating is divided into long track and short track disciplines. In long track speed skating (also called Speed Skating in Europe), athletes race in pairs, skating counterclockwise on two lanes of a 400-m oval track. At the 2010 Olympics both men and women will have five individual distances as well as a team pursuit event.

In contrast to long track speed skating, short track speed skating (also called short track skating in Europe) has a mass start with four to eight skaters all starting at the same time. The race takes place on a 111.12-m oval track within a hockey rink. At the 2010 Olympics, men and women skated four distances and each had a relay event.

The main concerns in long track speed skating are falls and collisions at high velocity, particularly in the sprint racing distances (500 m and 1,000 m). The risk and severity of injury is further magnified by the long and sharp blades of the speed skates that are worn and the lack of protective body wear. Although long track speed skaters have a lower incidence of falling compared to short track speed skating, they can achieve speeds in excess of 60 km per hour. Falls most often occur as the skaters negotiate the turns at the ends of the oval track. If a skater falls on the inside lane, there is also potential for a collision with the skater on the outside lane. In short track speed skating, there is greater potential for falling, as the smaller track and tight corners can make it difficult for the athlete to maintain control. As there are also more skaters on the ice, there is also a greater chance for collisions with multiple skaters. However, short track speed skaters do wear helmets and gloves, and their body suits are constructed from cut-proof material like Kevlar.

To reduce the incidence and severity of injury in the event of a fall, the Olympic and most other high-performance long and short tracks are surrounded by free-standing, covered, open-cell foam padding. The foam padding is covered with a vinyl-like covering for durability and protection from ice and water. The foam pads are linked together with Velcro flaps and seat belt–like strapping in a way to completely enclose the skating track. There may also be some anchoring at the base of the pads to reduce their motion when a skater crashes into them. However, there are no boards or other structure supporting the pads from behind. The weight and shape of the foam pads usually prevent the athlete from sliding under or flying over these pads. In short track speed skating, there are often two layers of padding and the pads are taller compared to those used in the long track speed skating.

Ice Hockey

Ice hockey can be divided into men's hockey and women's hockey. There can also be a division with regard to the rules played, being that of the North American rules or that of the International Ice Hockey Federation (IIHF) rules, which the Olympics follow. Men's hockey tends to be a faster game with more body contact as the athletes are bigger in size in general than the women, and men's game allows body checking, while the women's game does not. The women's game has limited contact. In the men's game, facial protection and mouth guards are optional, whereas in the women's game, full facial protection is mandatory and mouth guards are usually worn. In the IIHF rules, men born after 1977 must wear the half visor, but mouth guards are not mandatory, only recommended. There is, however, pressure to make mouth guards and possibly neck guards mandatory within the next few years. Because the women's game has limited contact, full face mask, mouth guards, and generally smaller athletes with less speed, there tends to be fewer major injuries, concussions, lacerations, and spine injuries. However, the game is still fairly ballistic, with stops, starts, and rapid changes in direction. There can still be incidental collisions at speed, and there are the associated issues with strained groins and related shoulder and knee injuries. In comparing the North American and international game, the international game is generally safer with fewer injuries. The reasons for this are partly in the dimensions of the ice, where international ice is 200 ft × 100 ft and North American ice is 200 × 85 ft. The extra 15 ft of width makes for much more room on the ice, and thereby less board play and more room to get away from open ice hits. Also there is almost no fighting in international play because of the immediate game ejections as well as possible suspension from subsequent matches. International rules also play a no-touch icing whistle, which makes for fewer collisions with fore-checking forwards coming down on defenseman at speed near the end boards. Both games now play a no–center line rule, which takes away the old two-line pass, and this lets the athletes spread out more, so there is less contact. The international game also places more emphasis on speed and skill and less emphasis on physical intimidation.

Inherent with all types of hockey is the issue that it is a high-speed, multidirectional sport with 12 players in the field of play using hockey sticks that can propel hockey pucks at speeds in excess of 100 mph. The borders of the field of play are hockey boards with a rim of dasher about 3 in. wide topped by a fairly heavy and not very movable Plexiglas. This, combined with sharp hockey skates that are sharpened daily, can make for a risky environment. Because of this, emergency action plans that are clear and rehearsed are mandatory. Physicians are generally required to be within 50 ft of the ice surface. Trainers qualified in first responder training are usually on the bench, and first onto the ice surface when an athlete is injured. Spine boards, AEDs, major wound kits, airway kits, and first aid supplies are usually very near the players' bench. There are also emergency dental kits, as well, for any major dental trauma. Also, there are special eye kits for any significant eye trauma. At Olympic, NHL, and most professional hockey venues, there is usually an ambulance unit with qualified staff in the building near the Zamboni entrance.

To reduce the risk of catastrophic injury, there has been a push to increase players' respect for each other and their ability to continue their careers. This includes "RESPECT" or "STOP" signs on the back of players' jerseys, as well as implementation of rules to decrease the number of head blows and hits from behind that are occurring in hockey. This is especially true in the officiating of international matches.

Understanding Sport Equipment

Skates consist of a boot and blade. The blades are slightly different for each sport. In figure skating, the skates have an inside and outside edge and a set of toe picks at the front, which are used strategically to initiate movements. The blades are fastened to the boot by screws, and if these loosen, then injuries can happen quickly and so the rinkside physician should have the appropriate tools on hand. The boot is tightened by a set of laces, and, again, this can be a hazard if they come loose; this is reason to interrupt the competition to correct the lacing. Helmets are not worn in figure skating but are in speed skating and ice hockey. In ice hockey, injuries can be caused by blows from the hockey sticks or pucks.

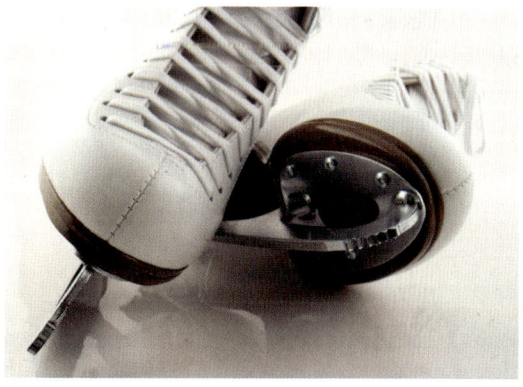

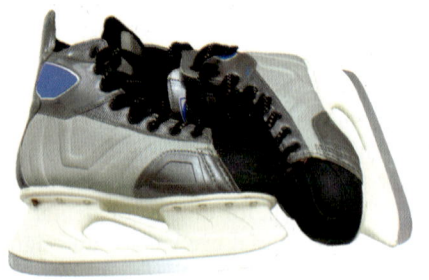

Common Injuries on Ice

Most emergency injuries are a result of a fall, contact with the boards or another skater or the ice, laceration with the skate blade, or stick injuries in ice hockey. Emergencies injuries in skating may include

- Lacerations to the face, neck, groin, legs
- Head injury and concussion
- Spinal trauma
- Fractures
- Facial trauma
- Hyperventilation and respiratory compromise
- Chest and abdominal contusions from stick injuries
- Ice burns
- Cardiac arrest

Medical Equipment

Laceration supplies are essential for skating coverage, but in addition to pressure bandages and suture kits, skin glues, abrasion sprays, and cushioned blister bandages are commonly used. Splinting devices for upper and lower extremity are essential, as is a full neck collar for immobilization off the ice. A wheeled roller stretcher with straps is best for evaluation. Each venue should have oxygen, an automated defibrillator, airways, spinal board and Ventolin inhalers. All medical personnel should have ice grips for the soles of their shoes, warm gloves, and layered clothing.

Emergency Care on Ice

Prior to each competitive event, it is recommended that a mock off-ice evacuation be practiced with full equipment and timing. It is recommended that at least three medical personnel be on duty with the ice dance, pairs and synchronized skating events; however a successful evacuation will often take four people to assist. The ice captain provides the communication support for the transport and additional services to be arranged. The medical team should have communication radios for detailed medical commands.

After an incident has occurred on the ice, the ice has to be inspected and usually flooded to ensure that there are no obstructions, blood, or even tiny contaminants on the ice surface that could cause further falls or injury.

Rink-side Rules for Return-to-play

All types of figure skating have a standard 2-minute rule where the skater can request medical attention or the medical personnel can assess an injured or ill skater to make a decision about return to play. If the assessment requires more time then the skater should be assisted from the ice for complete evaluation in the medical room.

Rules for return to play in hockey are important for player safety. These athletes are known to be proud of their toughness and may try to get back when it is not quite safe to do so. With regard to musculoskeletal trauma, it is generally said that the injured joint must have full pain-free range of motion and at least 85% to 90% of strength compared to the uninjured paired limb. With regard to lacerations, the laceration must be closed and covered and all bloodstained garments or jerseys must be changed over. In regards to concussion, the current consensus is that if a player has sustained a head trauma or a suspected concussion, he is removed from that particular contest and reassessed daily. He is not returned to play until he has gone through a graduated exercise program that is outlined in the recent Zürich "Consensus Statement on Concussion" document. At no time should a person still suffering postconcussion symptoms be returned to play. Also players should not be returned to play if suffering an illness that includes a fever greater than 38.5°C.

14.18 MOTOR SPORTS EVENTS

Contributed by Nils Kaehler, Norwegian Motorsports Federation, Trondheim, Norway; and Vlad Haralambie, Romanian Motorsports Federation, Gavrielescu, Bucharest

Motor sports are growing in popularity and are supported by millions of fans around the world. The sports include several disciplines, from the exclusive world of Formula 1 racing to swamp drag racing, from offshore boat races to motorcycle trials, from hill climbs to endurance rallies. But despite all the thrills and excitement, there are spills and danger involved. Motor racing is a potentially dangerous sport. It is an inherently risky activity. Regardless of efforts made by organizing bodies and engineers to enhance safety, and despite safety improvement in both equipment and tracks, motor sports will never be totally safe. Regrettably, fatal accidents do occur. Working as an EP at a motor sports event is extremely exciting but also a tremendous challenge. A well-organized medical team is therefore absolutely necessary. Fear the worst.

The following thoughts are supposed to give you some ideas about planning and structuring your job as the medical officer. For a more comprehensive and specific information I refer you to your national updated "medical code."

The first thing an EP should ensure before accepting the task is that he or she has sufficient emergency medical diagnostic and treatment skills. You may need them. You should also check that

- Medical staff are sufficiently trained and experienced to take action independently and immediately in case of an accident

- You and your staff have the necessary equipment

- Your equipment is suited to the event environment (cold temperature, high temperature, water/land, high risk of burn injuries/inhalation injuries, etc.)

- You and your staff have proper clothing

- You know the people you are going to work with (paramedics, track marshals, rescue workers, race control, security, etc.) and how to contact them (radio communication, are they visible, signals, etc.)

- You have access to ambulance or helicopter transport. Where are they located?

- You walked or drove around the track. Know your track. How do you access the various parts of the track?

- You and your helpers are positioned at suitable locations around the circuit so as to provide rapid intervention and evacuation if necessary

- You are recognizable as the race doctor/event physician and the other track workers know how to contact you

- You have local/track information about previous races (black spots), drivers, or vehicles that may concern you

- You have adequate information about the drivers' physical and mental health—is it acceptable to participate in the race?

- That athlete health information is available

Furthermore, a continuous flow of relevant information between the medical officer and the race control staff is of highest importance. If the EP is not positioned at the same location as the race control, then effective communication routes are essential. The medical officer should preferably attend all event management committee meetings and be informed about organizational changes.

The last but probably most important thing a medical officer should never forget is to prevent personal damage and injury. Never go to the accident site and initiate treatment without ensuring that your own safety is assured. You cannot help people if you yourself are injured—ensure that the accident site is safe and secured before entering.

What to Expect

In most cases, the medical officer will probably be confronted with minor injuries such as bruises, burns, and sprains. However, as these are high-velocity/high-energy sports, there is the potential of life-threatening and even fatal injuries.

The medical officer should therefore always be prepared for the worst.

- Facial and cerebral injuries

- Neck and spinal lesions

- Thorax injuries (lung contusion, rib fractures, pneumothorax, foreign body injuries)

- Pelvic injuries (contusion, fractures, bleeding, abdominal organ injury)

- Burns (various grades; be aware of dehydration)

- Lacerations (often simple; be aware of nerve and vascular damage)

- Extremity injuries (fractures/dislocations; check peripheral pulse and sensibility)

These injuries are addressed later in this manual.

However the following skills are obligatory (ABCDE):

- Airway maintenance with cervical spine protection

- Breathing and ventilation

- Circulation with hemorrhage control

- Disability: Neurologic status

- Exposure/environmental control: Undress the patient to examine for injuries, but avoid hypo-/hyperthermia (usually off the race track)

It is expected that a medical officer is familiar with these skills and has the necessary equipment to carry out this basic treatment. To avoid cooperation problems with other paramedics, and possible other doctors, the leader of the *trauma team* should be predefined (i.e., before the race). Other physicians should be informed of this. This can be a potential area of conflict. It is best to have a meeting with other physicians before the race to avoid this type of situation.

Lack of teamwork during rescue can have fatal consequences. We recommend that all medical staff should be familiar with the same trauma system and would recommend ATLS/FIMS and regular refresher courses in addition to regular team training exercises.

It is also important to instruct the medical team and other track staff (track marshals) what not to do in case of an accident:

- Do not try to raise a driver onto his or her feet until you are sure that there is no fracture (risk of further soft tissue damage) or spinal injury (risk of exacerbating a spinal injury).

- If the driver lifts himself or herself out of the car or stands up after a motorbike accident, and does not wish to continue the race, accompany him or her out of the track firmly.

- Do not try to solve all problems in situ; stabilize the athlete as best you can and evacuate the athlete from the track as soon as possible.

- Do not expect the race to be stopped (races can be stopped if the pilot or the vehicle remains on the track or in a dangerous position); if necessary, get track staff to protect the injured athlete with straw bales until you have completed your clinical evaluation and treatment.

If the athletes are available for consultation, then a medical control should be carried out 24 hours after a crash—particularly if there has been an injury to the head, lung, liver, or spleen—to endeavor to detect the presence of insidious hemorrhage or hematoma. Measure pulse and blood pressure, make a neurologic evaluation, palpate the abdomen, and auscultate the lungs. If it is not possible to evaluate the athlete 24 hours after a crash, then inform him or her of the need to complete a medical check within 24 hours.

Do not forget to mention in the pilot's health book any loss of consciousness and your opinion regarding quarantine.

If there is a briefing session with the drivers before the race, it is important to participate at this briefing and to instruct drivers in what they should and should not do in the event of an accident.

14.19 BOXING—AN INTRODUCTION TO RINGSIDE MEDICINE

Contributed by Abdelhamid Khadri, Vice President, AIBA Medical Committee, Rafat, Morocco; and David McDonagh, Secretary, AIBA Medical Commission, Trondheim, Norway

Boxing is one of the world's oldest sports, and evidence of its existence was found in Egypt as early as 3000 BC. The sport has continuously evolved and was first accepted as an Olympic sport in 688 BC at the 23rd Olympiad in Olympia, where Onomastos of Smyrna became the first Olympic champion. More than 2,600 years later, boxing remains on the Olympic Games program. The first boxing competition at the Olympic Games of modern times was at the St Louis (United States) Olympic Games in 1904 with bouts in seven weight divisions.

The word "amateur" is no longer used and the sport now includes women who perform at the highest level. A new competition form, the World Series of Boxing (WSB), has been introduced, where boxers fight for seven 3-minute rounds, without helmets—so the sport is midway between Olympic style and professional boxing. There are 12 teams around the world, and the boxers are paid. WSB boxers are allowed to participate in the Olympic Games. The sport is run by the International Boxing Association, AIBA.

Olympic-style boxing is now composed of 10 weight classes for men and for women, men's bouts consisting of three 3-minute rounds, while women box four 2-minute rounds. As women's boxing is new to the Olympics, there will be 10 weight classes for men and three classes for women at the London Games. In the WSB, there are only five weight classes.

Boxing is unique in many ways, particularly due to the emphasis on safety. Amateur boxing has always, unfairly, been associated with professional boxing, which is a far more dangerous sport. In an AIBA tournament, all boxers are checked medically every day to exclude injuries that may expose them to further injury. Athletes who are hurt in the ring have an obligatory medical check after an event. At AIBA events, there are at least two AIBA physicians as well as local organizers' physician staff present. AIBA physicians are approved ringside physicians and must complete both a course and an exam, as well as have years of boxing experience.

Referees receive constant drilling on safety issues and are also regularly reevaluated. If a referee allows a boxer to continue when a bout should have been stopped, he or she will be demoted. A referee can stop a bout at anytime and is encouraged to do so if another boxer is being overpowered or is in danger of being injured. Similarly, the AIBA physician can also stop a bout at any time by notifying the competition jury.

If a referee stops a bout due to a boxer being unable to continue or defend himself after one or a series of head blows, the referee declares an RSCH (referee stops contest due to head injury). The same decision is reached when the boxer has three eight counts in the same round or four eight counts in the whole bout. A boxer who is knocked down and who cannot stand up after a 10-second count, with or without a loss of consciousness, is declared to have suffered a knockout (KO).

Any RSCH or KO carries an automatic suspension period from all forms of sparring and boxing—this obligatory rest period is for 30 days for a single occurrence.

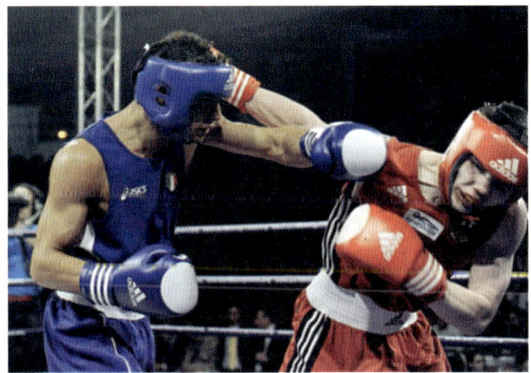

A second KO or RCSH within a 3-month period mandates a 180-day suspension, whereas a third decision within a 1-year period results in a 360-day suspension. When a boxer finishes a suspension period, a mandatory neurologic evaluation must be conducted before resumption of boxing activity is allowed.

Injuries in Olympic-style boxing, both short-term and long-term, are now rare. As opposed to professional boxing, Olympic-style boxing is seldom blighted by major head injuries, with injuries more likely to be seen in rugby, American football, diving, and equestrian sports. As with all high-energy sports, ringside physicians must be able to diagnose and treat concussion, cerebral contusions, and cerebral bleeding. Ringside physicians must be updated in head injury diagnostic and treatment modalities.

Boxers are susceptible to nasal injuries, facial cuts and hand conditions. The most frequent injury is a nosebleed as a result of numerous blows to the boxer's face. Nosebleeds are rarely caused by nasal fractures, but the ringside physician must identify a fracture if one is present. Similarly, the presence of a septal hematoma must be examined for and excluded. Untreated septal hematomas may lead to cartilaginous collapse, as seen with the saddle-nose deformity, so rapid referral for incision is recommended. Most nosebleeds are venous bleeds from the anterior nose, but on occasion there may be arterial bleeds or posterior venous bleeds. If the nosebleed is arterial in origin, the bout should be stopped, pressure should be applied to the bleeding site, and the boxer should be referred to an ENT specialist. Posterior bleeds will bleed into the back of the mouth despite anterior packing of the nose. The boxer must cease boxing and be referred to an ENT unit. In most cases, bleeding is mild and benign and the boxer can continue the bout.

Facial cuts are more frequent in professional boxing than in Olympic-style boxing mainly because of the head guard. Superficial and peripheral cuts are not usually severe and boxers may continue to box. Deep cuts are another matter, particularly in the infraorbital/supraorbital areas, the eyelids, the lachrymal ducts, the nose and the lips. Boxers with deep cuts in these areas should not continue, due to the potential risk of damaging underlying nerves. Cuts to the lips and nose can worsen and should be stopped if there is the likelihood of cosmetic damage.

Classically, the boxer is exposed to hand injuries due to repetitive microtrauma to the hand or by a strong blow when the opponent's head or elbow meets the boxer's hand.

In such cases, one often finds that the injured boxer has used poor-quality hand bandages or gloves. Boxers who do not firmly close their fists inside the gloves are more exposed to hand injury. Fractures of the scaphoid bone are, by far, the most common of all carpal bone fractures in boxers. Fractures of the proximal one-third of the scaphoid have a high risk of nonunion, pseudoarthrosis, and bone avascular necrosis. Correct and early diagnosis is important to help prevent these complications.

Boxer's fracture—fracture of the head of the fifth metacarpal bone—can on occasion be treated conservatively, but if there is rotational deformity, angulation, or displacement, then surgical fixation may be required.

The most common and most significant ligamentous injury of the wrist is that of the scapholunate ligament. Failure to diagnose and treat this condition may lead to instability of the scaphoid and lunate bones and thus cause long-term dysfunction.

Surgery is usually not required for boxers with distal extensor tendon injury of the finger—mallet finger or drop finger—but flexor tendon injuries of the finger require surgical intervention.

Mandibular fractures, particularly condylar fractures, are occasionally seen.

Referral for OPG or CT scan examinations are recommended.

CHAPTER 15

Muscle and Joint Injuries

Contributed by Emin Ergen, Professor, Ankara University, Turkey; Chair, International Archery Federation Medical Committe

Reviewer: Walter R. Frontera, Professor and Dean, University of San Juan and Past President of FIMS, Puerto Rico; and Konstantinos Natsis, Professor, Aristotle University of Thessaloniki, Thessaloniki, Greece

15.1 MUSCLE INJURIES

Skeletal muscle makes up 40% to 45% of total body weight. Muscle injuries are common both in competitive and recreational physical activities. These injuries may also lead to complications like myositis ossificans and muscle hernia. Delayed onset muscle soreness (DOMS) is another frequently occurring muscle problem associated with strenuous exertions.

There are two main causes of muscle injuries:

- Direct trauma (contusions): Traumatic injury to muscle due to direct force may produce superficial or deep muscle contusions in contact sports. Myositis ossificans is a complication following direct (or sometimes indirect) trauma and a permanent loss of function may occur. Contusions (and some tears) may also be subdivided into intermuscular and intramuscular hematomas.

- Indirect trauma: Muscle activation results in force production within the muscle. Eccentric muscle actions generate higher levels of force or tension within the muscle compared to concentric actions, thus making the muscle more susceptible to rupture or tear. Injuries can often be seen at the myotendinous junction. In younger individuals, the weakest point in the muscle-tendon-bone complex is the apophysis. Factors that may contribute to muscle strain injury include inadequate flexibility, inadequate strength or endurance, dyssynergistic muscle contraction, insufficient warm-up, or inadequate rehabilitation from previous injury. Indirect traumas may also lead to inter- or intramuscular hematoma.

Classification of Muscle Injuries

Muscle injuries can be complete or partial. Muscle strain commonly occurs in the lower extremities but may also occur in the upper extremities depending on the sport.

Commonly injured muscles include

- Biceps femoris
- Rectus femoris
- Semitendinosus
- Adductors
- Vastus medialis
- Soleus

Degrees of Injury

First degree—mild injury:

- Tear of only a few muscle fibers
- Mild swelling, pain, and disability
- Characterized by the patient's ability to produce strong, but painful, muscle contraction

Second degree—moderate injury:

- Disruption of a moderate number of fibers
- Moderate amount of pain, swelling and disability
- Partial loss of strength

- Characterized by the patient's weak and painful attempts at muscle contraction

Third degree—severe injury:

- Complete rupture of muscle–tendon unit
- More easily detected by physical examination
- Complete loss of function
- Characterized by the patient's extremely weak but painless attempts at muscle contraction
- May require surgical repair

Hematomas

A muscle strain or blow usually causes a hematoma. The localization of hematoma is important in chosing the type of treatment and in making return to sport activity decisions. Intermuscular hematomas are localized near the large intermuscular septa or muscle fascial sheaths. Their location facilitates early dispersal of the extravasated blood with the help of gravity, which minimizes the inflammation response and the potential scarring, allowing early resolution.

Intramuscular hematomas are localized within muscles and usually take longer to recover compared to intermuscular lesions. The hemorrhage tends to be more confined, the mass is often palpable, and the inflammatory response is greater. The myositis ossificans risk is higher in intramuscular hematomas. There is also the danger of developing a compartment syndrome after intramuscular hematoma in some locations. Due to severe pain and limited function, restoration of the joint range of motion (ROM) and subsequent muscle function is relatively slower. In some rare cases, surgical repair or open drainage of a large intramuscular hematoma is indicated. In the latter situation, diagnosis depends on noting the tenseness of the swelling as well as the diminishing peripheral pulses, sensation and function. When these signs

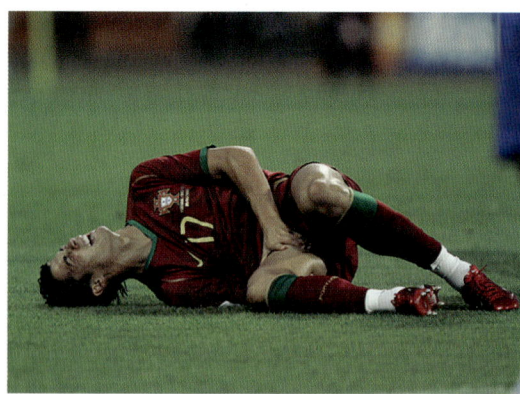

FIGURE 15.1. Ronaldo, Portugal.

are present, early surgical intervention, with release of the fascia and aspiration of the clot, is necessary.

Diagnosis of Muscle Injuries

History and Complaints: Pain is the major complaint after a muscle injury. Generally, a sharp or stabbing pain is felt at the moment of injury and reproduced by contracting the muscles involved. In the resting position, the pain is not very severe. Pain can inhibit muscle contraction. In total ruptures, the muscle is unable to contract and therefore no movement is produced.

Inspection: Only after about 24 to 48 hours, bruising and discoloration may be seen, often below the site of injury. If the hematoma is large enough, swelling may be noted (Fig. 15.2).

Palpation: There is often localized tenderness and swelling over the damaged area. A slight defect may be palpable in partial ruptures, whereas there is a significant gap in total ruptures.

Laboratory: Laboratory tests are not routinely used for the diagnosis of muscle injuries.

TABLE 15.1	Clinical Findings—Muscle Injuries				
Degree	**Pain**	**Swelling and Bruising**	**Structural Defect**	**Loss of ROM**	**Loss of Function**
First (mild)	+	Minimal	0	Minimal	Minimal
Second (moderate)	++	Moderate	±	Significant	Significant
Third (severe)	+++	Extensive	+	Severe	Complete

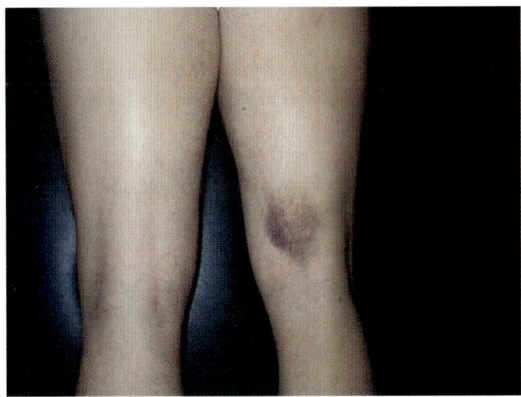

FIGURE 15.2. Ecchymosis after a hamstring strain.

Imaging: Ultrasound (Fig. 15.3) and magnetic resonance imaging (MRI) are superior to plain radiography and have become the techniques of choice for imaging muscles, tendons and ligaments over the last decades. Because the majority of muscle injuries are self-limiting and the cost of MRIs is rather high, specific indications for the use of MRI in patients suspected of having muscle tears should be taken into account. MRI findings in muscle strains depend on whether the rupture is complete or partial. In the acute partial tear, blood and edema may infiltrate between the muscle bundles, especially in the region of the myotendinous junction. Blood and edema may also collect between the fascial planes. A mass may be detected at the site of the injury in acute cases. In the chronic phase, a defect is detected at the site of the rupture. Complete tears show total disruption of the muscle; muscle retraction, blood, and edema within the lesion and surrounding fascial planes can also be seen. Blood degrades in time, resulting in changed signal characteristics. Intramuscular hematomas and hemorrhages are often encountered on MRI examinations without a clear history

of trauma. Typically, an intramuscular hematoma resorbs spontaneously over a period of 6 to 8 weeks. Careful palpation during the first 3 weeks after injury and magnetic resonance imaging investigation performed during the first 6 weeks after injury provide valuable information that can be used to predict the time to return to preinjury level of performance.

Treatment of Muscle Injuries

PRICES is the general approach after an acute strain or contusion followed by progressive symptom-guided rehabilitation.

- **P**rotection: The area should be protected from further injury.
- **R**est will help the regeneration process.
- **I**ce: Application of cold will reduce bleeding and control edema.
- **C**ompression: Pressure application helps reduce bleeding and controls swelling, together with cold.
- **E**levation: Elevating the extremity will also be helpful.
- **S**upport: The area or extremity should be supported to diminish further trauma risk.

Other physical modalities may be started within 24 to 36 hours by the physician and physiotherapist. Oral anti-inflammatory medications: Nonsteroidal anti-inflammatory drugs (NSAIDs) are commonly used in treatment of musculoskeletal sport injuries. Their use is based on physicians' experience rather than objective scientific studies. When choosing an NSAID, knowledge of potential side effects should be taken into consideration (e.g., renal and gastrointestinal complications). NSAIDs are not recommended during later phases due their reported inhibitory effect on tissue healing. Myorelaxants and analgesics can be prescribed if there is severe pain and muscle spasm. Corticosteroid injection to the injured area is not indicated due to the risk of scar tissue formation, increased rupture potential, and the greater risk of bacterial infection.

Physical Modalities: Cold during the initial phase and heat, ultrasound, iontophoresis and electrical muscle stimulation at different points during the progression of healing are commonly employed physical modalities.

Therapeutic Exercises: Therapeutic exercises are very important but are the most commonly

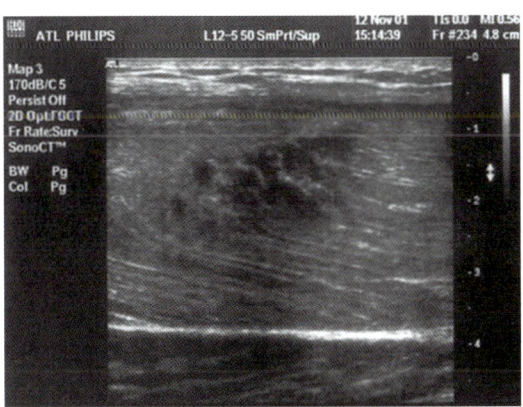

FIGURE 15.3. Intramuscular hematoma, ultrasonic image.

underutilized means of treating and rehabilitating musculoskeletal sport injuries. These exercises are not only important to correct the deficits (weakness, reduced joint ROM, loss of endurance) resulting from injury but also to prevent a recurrence of injury.

Rehabilitation should be aimed at restoration of muscle strength, flexibility, and endurance to preinjury levels. High-speed motion, with rapid development of peak torque and sudden deceleration, has to be introduced with caution and certainly not until full ROM has been restored. Active muscle exercises should adhere to specific principles and should be introduced in the following order:

- Static exercises without load
- Static exercises with load
- Limited dynamic muscle training with exercises within active ROM to the pain threshold
- Dynamic exercises with increasing load
- Proprioceptive training
- Protected load-bearing activities
- Sport-specific exercises

In the case of hamstring injuries, there is limited evidence to suggest that the rate of recovery can be increased with an increased frequency of flexibility (stretching) exercises. Consideration should be given to the lumbar spine, sacroiliac and pelvic alignment, and to postural control mechanisms when managing hamstring injuries.

Other Treatment Options: Proliferative therapy, local administration of autologous conditioned serum (ACS), herbal substances, hyperbaric oxygen therapy, and gene therapy are some other treatment modalities used on muscle injuries, although the evidence supporting them is not strong.

For information on return-to-sport activity, see Chapter 73.

15.2 JOINT INJURIES

Joint ligament injuries (sprains) are common injuries. Due to the complex structure of joints, associated injuries to neighboring tissues—such as capsule, bone, cartilage, tendons, and muscles—are frequently underdiagnosed, and the rehabilitation of ligamentous injuries is often inadequate leading to a high rate of recurrence.

Clinical Perspective

Joints are vulnerable regions and generally injured at their weakest point. For example, inversion injuries to the ankle are far more common than eversion injuries, due to the relative instability of the lateral aspect of the joint and weakness of the lateral ligaments compared to the medial ligament. Medial ligament sprains usually take longer to rehabilitate. This also applies to the knee joint where the medial collateral ligament is weaker than the lateral collateral ligament.

The most important part of the assessment of ligamentous injuries is the determination of the degree of instability present in the joint. This will determine the management of the injury. A well-planned rehabilitation program is required to ensure return to sport with full functional capacity and to avoid recurrence of the injury.

Occasionally, other structures (e.g., bone, cartilage) are damaged in addition to the ligaments. If these additional injuries are not diagnosed and treated properly, prolonged pain and disability may result.

Diagnosis of Joint Ligament Injuries

History: The mechanism of injury is an important clue in making a diagnosis. An inversion ankle sprain suggests lateral ligament damage, an eversion injury suggests medial ligament damage, and valgus stress to the knee may suggest a medial collateral lesion. The presence of a compressive force suggests the possibility of an osteochondral injury.

At the time of the injury, the athlete may have heard a noise or snap. This may be significant in an acute knee injury but may not have diagnostic significance in ankle injuries.

The location of pain will often indicate which ligaments have been injured. Most joint injuries are accompanied by swelling. The site of the swelling may provide an indication of the location of the pathology. The degree of swelling is usually, but not always, a reliable indication of severity.

The degree of disability, both immediately following the injury and subsequently, is an important indicator of the severity of the injury. The initial management with the PRICES regimen and the duration of restricted weight bearing after the injury should all be noted.

Physical Examination: Examination of the joint requires an assessment of the degree of instability present and the grading of the ligamentous injury. Examination should also detect losses in ROM, muscle strength, and proprioception.

Imaging: Standard radiographs including anteroposterior views, lateral views, and at least one oblique view should be performed after sprains in situations where instability is present and/or if bony tenderness is present to exclude associated fractures.

IMPORTANT NOTE: An osteochondral fracture may not be apparent on initial radiographs. If significant pain and disability persist despite appropriate treatment 4 to 6 weeks after an apparent sprain, a referral to a specialist sports physician or orthopedic surgeon is indicated. A radioisotope bone scan may be necessary to exclude an osteochondral fracture.

Treatment of Ligament Injuries

The initial management of ligament sprains follows the same principles, independent of the degree of injury.

Initial Management: The initial management of ligament injuries requires the PRICES regimen. This is probably the single most important approach in treatment, particularly with grade I and grade II injuries. Many of the problems resulting from sprains are due to the presence of excess blood and edema in and around the joint. This limits the ROM of the joint and can act as an irritant, causing excessive synovial reaction. In addition to PRICES, it is important for the injured athlete to avoid factors that will increase blood flow and swelling (e.g., hot showers, heat rubs, alcohol, excessive weight bearing).

Control of Pain and Swelling: Pain and swelling can be controlled with the use of electrotherapeutic modalities (e.g., TENS, interferential). Analgesic agents may be prescribed. Gentle, soft-tissue therapy and mobilization after the first 48 hours also may help to reduce pain. By reducing pain and swelling, muscle inhibition around the joint is minimized, enabling ROM exercises to be performed. Physicians have a tendency to prescribe NSAIDs in cases of joint injuries/ligament sprains, although evidence of their efficacy is not convincing. However, it may be appropriate to start NSAIDs medication after an injury and continue for about 4 to 5 days in order to reduce the risk of developing synovitis.

Restoration of the Full Range of Motion: Non–weight bearing on crutches for the first 24 hours is advised, but partial weight bearing in normal heel–toe gait after lower extremity problems should then be encouraged. The damaged joint may be protected with strapping or bracing. This will allow partial and ultimately full weight bearing without danger of aggravating the injury. As soon as pain allows, active ROM exercises (e.g., stationary cycling) can be started.

Regaining Muscle Strength: Strengthening exercises should be initiated as early as possible, if pain allows. Active exercises should be performed initially with gradually increasing resistance. Weight-bearing activities should be carefully commenced after structural tissue healing.

Reeducation of Proprioception: Proprioception is often lost or severely reduced following joint injuries. Proprioceptive exercises can be incorporated early in the ankle rehabilitation program and should be gradually increased from balancing on one leg to the use of the rocker board or minitrampoline and finally to more functional activities while balancing.

Functional Exercises: During the later phases of rehabilitation, functional exercises (e.g., jumping, hopping, twisting, figure-of-eight running) should be performed when the injured athlete is pain-free, has full ROM, and has sufficient muscle strength and proprioception.

Treatment of Grade III Injuries

Treatment of grade III injuries requires initial conservative management, but also surgery in some cases, for example, lateral ligament of the knee. If the patient shows good progress and is able to return to full sporting activity with the aid of external supports, surgery may not be indicated for most ligaments. If, however, despite a proper conservative approach, the patient continues to complain of recurrent episodes of instability or persistent pain, then surgical intervention is recommended. Following surgery, it is very important to implement an intensive rehabilitation program to restore full joint ROM, strength, and proprioception.

In some cases, even if the rehabilitation has been adequate, the symptoms may persist. In this case, it is necessary to take into account the presence of other pathology. Symptoms of intra-articular pathology include clicking, locking, and joint swelling. Examination may reveal effusion, bony tenderness, or swelling. The joint should be reassessed for evidence of chronic ligamentous instability.

Recommended Reading

Askling CM, Tengvar M, Saartok T, Thorstensson A. Acute first-time hamstring strains during high-speed running: a longitudinal study including clinical and magnetic resonance imaging findings. *Am J Sports Med* 2007;35(2):197–206.

Khan K, Bruker P. Ankle acute injuries. In: Fahy TD, ed. *Encyclopedia of Sports Medicine and Science.* http://www.sportsci.org/encyc/index.html. Published March 7, 1998. Accessed March 31, 2011.

Malone TR, Garrett WE, Zachazewski JE. Muscle: deformation, injury, repair. In: Zachazewski JE, Magee DJ, Quillen WS, eds. *Athletic Injuries and Rehabilitation.* Philadelphia, PA: Saunders; 1996.

Mason DL, Dickens VA, Vail A. Rehabilitation for hamstring injuries. *Cochrane Database Syst Rev* 2007;1:CD004575. doi: 10.1002/14651858.CD004575.pub2.

Peterson L, Renström P. *Sports Injuries: Their Prevention and Treatment.* 3rd ed. London, UK: Martin Dunitz; 2001.

Reid D. *Sports Injury Assessment and Rehabilitation.* New York, NY: Churchill Livingstone, Inc.; 1992.

Walsh M, Mellion MB. Injury prevention, diagnosis and treatment. In: Mellion MB, Walsh M, Shelton GL, eds. *Musculoskeletal Injuries in Sport.* 1997:361–370.

CHAPTER 16

Corticosteroid Injections

Contributed by David McDonagh, Deputy CMO, Lillehammer 1994 Olympic Winter Games

Reviewer: Richard Budgett, IOC Medical Committee and CMO, London 2012 Olympic Summer Games

If an athlete presents with acute severe joint or tendon pain, one must always endeavor to make a correct diagnosis take appropriate radiological examinations, exclude infection or the possibility of referred pain, and attempt conservative treatment before suggesting corticosteroid injections. If the cause of pain is recent trauma, then remember that a painkilling injection may mask substantial injury; many physicians believe this to be both ethically and clinically dubious practice. Athletes are often looking for a "quick-fix," that is, relief of symptoms, rather than receiving curative treatment. Corticosteroid injections can be effective in reducing inflammation but posttraumatic inflammation is an essential part of the healing process. If the cause of the pain is unknown, then a corticosteroid injection should not be administered.

16.1 CHOICE OF CORTICOSTEROID AGENT AND DOSE

Studies suggest that more water soluble preparations are better suited for acute inflammatory conditions, whereas less water-soluble preparations are more suited to chronic inflammatory conditions. Studies have demonstrated that the more water-soluble the corticosteroid, the shorter is the duration of action. There are variations in patient response, but most patients have symptomatic relief for 1 to 3 weeks, and the less water-soluble corticosteroids seem to have a longer effect. So why don't we use less water-soluble preparations in all cases? The answer of course is that there seem to be more complications associated with corticosteroids that stay longer in the body.

Therefore, for the EP who primarily treats acute conditions, water-soluble agents (e.g., hydrocortisone) would seem to be the most practical agents if the need for an injection arises. For chronic conditions, methylprednisolone and triamcinolone are often used, and appear to have beneficial effect compared to other preparations. The dose to be injected varies dependent on the lesion—obviously, less of the agent is used for a tennis elbow (epicondylitis) than with an intra-articular knee condition.

16.2 INJECTION TECHNIQUE AND PRINCIPLES

The objective for any injection procedure is to insert the needle into the correct site without injuring any structures and causing a minimum of pain to the athlete. Similarly, it is essential to avoid the introduction of infectious agents into the body. A sterile injection technique should be utilized and gloves should be worn. I often mark the desired entry site using a sterile pen. The skin should be cleaned with alcohol or chlorhexidine (with or without iodine) and allowed to dry completely. The needle is then inserted and advanced to the desired area. Tendons should not be injected, but if one pierces a tendon by mistake, there will be significant resistance on injecting. If one injects into peritendinous tissue, a bursa, or joint space, there is usually no significant resistance—if there is, you are doing something wrong.

There are many injection techniques and various entry portals for different joints and peritendinous sites; however, it goes beyond the scope of this manual to go into great detail on this issue. An increasing number of practitioners use guided injection (employing ultrasound). Having received a corticosteroid injection, athletes should limit loading the affected joint or tendon for 3 to 7 days to avoid steroid flares and the danger of muscle/tendon ruptures.

16.3 CONTRAINDICATIONS

Contraindications to corticosteroid injection are many:

- Local infection in the inflammatory site
- Systemic infection or major organ infection (e.g., pneumonia, nephritis)
- Significant skin breakdown at the proposed injection site
- Known hypersensitivity to the proposed injection substance
- The presence of a joint prosthesis
- Local bone or osteochondral fracture
- Severe joint destruction (e.g., Charcot joint)
- Unstable diabetes—corticosteroid injections can cause blood sugar elevations

16.4 COMPLICATIONS

If one uses an aseptic (or sterile) technique and one carefully places the needle in the correct position (ideally confirmed by imaging) without damaging structures, then corticosteroid injections are usually of minimal risk to the patient. There is slightly higher risk of complication with soft tissue injections due to the possibility of damaging tendons and the effect of corticosteroids on healthy tissue.

Reported side effects of corticosteroid injection therapy include

- Systemic effects
- Skin and pigment changes
- Fat atrophy
- Muscle wasting
- Tendon rupture—injections directly into a tendon
- Septic arthritis—fortunately rare
- Nerve and blood vessel damage
- Postinjection symptoms
- Anaphylaxis
- Steroid arthropathy
- Blood sugar elevations
- Steroid flare—which is usually a self-limiting, painful inflammation that lasts for 1 to 2 days and believed to be caused by the leucocyte phagocytosis of corticosteroid crystals.

Informed consent should be obtained with a discussion of the risks and benefits and recorded in the patient/athlete medical file. There is still no universal agreement regarding the maximum number of injections and time interval between these injections. Some physicians recommend a 3-month interval between injections, and most at least 1 month. Many recommend a maximum of three injections per inflammation site; some recommend one injection only. There are not enough scientific data available to clarify these issues.

Joint and tendon pain are common clinical complaints, and a combination of precise history taking, physical examination, laboratory testing, and imaging may be needed to determine the underlying cause of pain. Once the diagnosis is established, conservative measures are generally employed and offer most patients symptomatic relief.

CHAPTER 17

Wounds

Contributed by David McDonagh, Secretary AIBA Medical Commission

Reviewer: Angela D. Smith, Clinical Associate Professor of Orthopaedic Surgery, University of Pennsylvania; Attending Faculty, The Sports Medicine and Performance Children's Hospital, Philadelphia; Chair, Education Commission, FIMS 2002–2005; Past President, ACSM

17.1 WOUND CLASSIFICATION

A wound is the term given to tissue damage caused by mechanical force. When evaluating wounds, one must consider

- The nature of the wound (bruise, abrasion, burn, laceration, combination, etc.)
- The wound dimensions—length, width, depth (superficial, partial, full thickness), etc.
- The anatomical position of the wound and relation to fixed anatomical landmarks (supraclavicular, midclavicular line, distance from the umbilicus, etc.)
- Underlying or nearby structures
- Time since injury
- Clean or contaminated wound

A good case history and/or injury observation is important in order to allow one to evaluate if a wound is clean or if it has been contaminated. Wounds can then be classified as

- Clean
- Clean-contaminated: a wound involving normal but colonized tissue
- Contaminated: a wound containing foreign or infected material
- Infected: a wound with pus present

This an important classification, as clean wounds should be closed immediately; clean-contaminated can usually be close; whereas contaminated and infected wounds should be left open, treated with oral antibiotics and left to heal by secondary intention.

When clean and clean-contaminated wounds are more than 6 to 8 hours old (opinions vary on this time factor), many recommend that the wound be cleaned, left open, and then closed by delayed primary closure after 48 hours. Prophylactic peroral antibiotics are often used with delayed closure.

17.2 WOUND HYGIENE

Today, saline solution and tap water are the most commonly used wound-cleansing agents. The aim of wound cleaning is to remove foreign bodies and dead tissue and also to maintain the healing environment. For the EP, simple cleansing is usually adequate and further wound debridement usually takes place somewhere else. Remember that exudates in acute wounds contain essential nutrients that benefit healing. Be careful using ice packs on swollen and lacerated wounds—the best temperature for wound healing is body temperature. Macrophages do not function properly at lowered temperatures.

Tap Water or Saline?

Sandy Thompson, Manchester Royal Infirmary, has reviewed 397 papers on this topic (see http://www.bestbets.org) and found that "Tap water is a safe and effective solution for cleaning recent wounds requiring closure and is the treatment of choice." While this may be true in most western countries, we know that tap water quality varies around the world. I would support the above statement with the addendum "if the tap water is of good quality."

Wound debridement is sometimes necessary, but be careful when removing full-thickness tissue. This is usually not necessary, unless the tissue is obviously devitalized, has little or no attachment to surrounding tissue, or is extremely contaminated; it is often best left alone.

17.3 LACERATIONS

Cuts can occur in all sports. For the EP, the following situations may be addressed:

- Does the athlete have to leave the field of play (FoP)?
- Can the cut be treated with tape, strips, and wound glue, or is immediate suturing required?
- Is the wound clean enough to close?
- Is the wound superficial or deep and is there a ligament, muscle, capsule, nerve, blood vessel, or bone injury as well?
- Can the athlete return to play (RTP)?

Usually, if the athlete has a cut, then he or she should leave the FoP for wound inspection.

First, evaluate the wound: Is there arterial bleeding? Serious arterial bleedings usually occur in the femoral triangle, popliteal fossa, axilla, or neck but are rare in sport. However, in some sports (e.g., ice skating, short-track skating, ice hockey), there is a danger of deep lacerations and the potential for large artery damage due to deep cuts from sharp skating blades.

Here, compression is the answer. Suturing large artery lacerations in the field is nigh impossible and one risks worsening the injury. Compression with a sterile glove and a thin compress is the only viable option. Do not use too many bandages, as this only reduces the amount of pressure that can be applied and soaks up more blood.

Ensuring circulation by giving intravenous fluid is essential. If you are the only medical person present, then get assistance from another player or coach and get him or her to compress the bleeding artery at the site of the cut. Then put in at least one, preferably two, IV cannulas, hang up two infusion bags with saline or plasma expanders (if you have them), check that the airways are free (insert a tongue depressor if necessary), give oxygen via a mask, and then change positions with your assistant. Get someone nearby to ring the helicopter or ambulance; let him or her hold the phone while you speak to the emergency central, informing them of the seriousness of the injury and keeping your hand compressing the wound at all times. Ask for immediate helicopter or ambulance assistance. Be prepared for a rapid clinical deterioration. If the ambulance does not have a competent physician or paramedic on board, then I would advise the event physician to travel with the patient to the hospital in these exceptional circumstances. If the sports event has to be stopped because the event physician has left the arena, then so be it. A life is more important than a game.

Minor arterial bleeds are much less dramatic, but blood loss can be significant if ignored. Once again, compression is the key. Observe the patient throughout the period of treatment. If you choose to ligate the small artery with a suture, then do this in the medical room. Remove the patient from the field of play, clean the wound thoroughly, seriously consider giving the patient a tetanus vaccine (check your national guidelines here), and suture, if you are competent and if the situation demands it. If you do not feel competent enough to suture the wound, transfer the athlete to a hospital or suitable clinic, compressing until there is hemostasis. One may then apply an elasticized stretch bandage to compress the wound.

Major venous bleeds are rare in the thigh—again, you need to have a deep gash. The leg veins are more exposed but again serious bleeds from cuts are rare. Compression is often enough to give adequate hemostasis. Suture if necessary. Again, wound hygiene and an antitetanus booster vaccine should be considered.

If the wound is over the knee joint or ankle joint, then inspect the wound for muscle and ligament injury (look for ruptures of the patellar ligament, in particular, as there is little fat protection); check muscle and ligament function distal to the wound. If intact function, evaluate the wound for bleeding; if none, then close the wound after thorough cleaning. Again, apply an elasticized stretch bandage to compress the wound afterwards.

Never close the wound if you suspect or are unsure of a muscle, ligament, major nerve, or capsule injury. If in doubt, cover the wound with a wet saline bandage and transfer the patient to a hospital for further evaluation.

Scalp wounds can cause profuse venous bleeding (see Head Injuries, Chapter 27).

Arterial bleeds require compression and possibly suturing, so the athlete should thus leave the

FoP and receive treatment in the medical room. Glue and tape seldom work with arterial bleeds as the wound usually swells up and the tape loosens. The bleeding also affects the tape's adhesiveness. Give local anesthetics, clean the wound, and inspect the wound for other damage. If no structural damage is apparent, close the wound with sutures (ligation of small arterial bleeds may be necessary). Apply a compression bandage and evaluate the athlete's ability to return to play. As a rule, athletes can return to play (depending on the sport) if there is no fracture, head injury, organ contusion, or muscle/ligament or joint injury.

Venous bleeds, if superficial, can usually be treated with tape and glue. Clean the wound and assess wound depth and associated structural damage. If none, close the wound with tape and glue. As a general rule, if there is no bleeding, tape and glue are effective. If there is bleeding, suturing is usually necessary.

I usually apply tape at a 90-degree angle to the wound and use the glue to adhere the tape to the skin. Some physicians put glue into the wound and then apply tape. I only use this technique in extreme circumstances as wound glue gives a burning sensation, may cause pigmentation of wounds, is in itself a foreign body, and makes strip removal difficult.

I usually leave some space in between the tape strips because then you can follow the line of the cut. If you place the tape strips immediately beside each other, then the skin may buckle, so allow some space in between for better visual control.

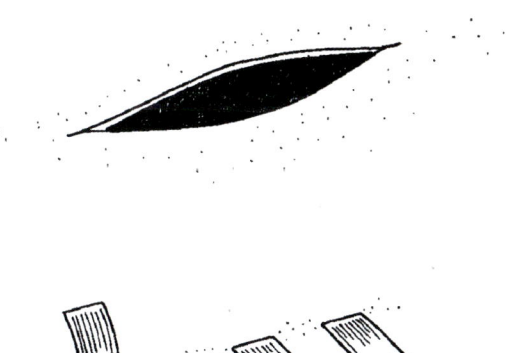

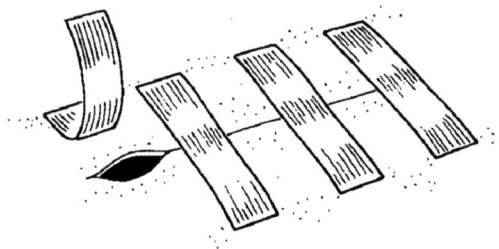

FIGURE 17.1. Taping of wounds.

Cover the wound with a thin dressing and then apply an elasticized stretch bandage to compress the wound. Do not use too thick a dressing, as this will just soak up more blood and reduce the compression effect.

Remove devitalized skin flaps (epidermal) as these often become necrotic. If the skin flap includes dermis, then it usually survives, so removal is not recommended unless circulation is definitely compromised.

Consider the use of antibiotics and vaccines (as discussed below).

17.4 TETANUS VACCINES

Tetanus is acquired when a wound is infected with the spores of the bacterium *Clostridium tetani*. Unfortunately, the spores are to be found all over the world and can affect people of all ages. Tetanus can be prevented through immunization, but there is no standard practice worldwide for the issuing of vaccines (World Health Organization Position Paper, May 19, 2006—"The exact timing of the booster doses should be flexible to take account of the most appropriate health service contacts in different countries"). In the same paper, the WHO recommend a total of six vaccinations; basic vaccination programs should include three doses of DTP in infancy, followed by a TT-containing booster at school-entry age (4 to 7 years), in adolescence (12 to 15 years), and in early adulthood stating, "Three DTP doses in infancy will give 3 to 5 years' protection, a further dose or booster (e.g., in early childhood) will provide protection into adolescence, and 1 or 2 more booster(s) will induce immunity well through adulthood—a duration of 20 to 30 years has been suggested."

There is still a lot of confusion and varying practices around the world regarding the need for further vaccination in patients with open wounds. WHO states, "Passive immunization using tetanus antitoxin, preferably of human origin, is essential for treatment and occasionally also for prophylaxis (e.g., in cases of dirty wounds in incompletely immunized people)." This poses the following diagnostic challenges:

- Is a wound clean or contaminated?

- What is the patient's vaccination status—unknown, no vaccination, incomplete vaccination, fully vaccinated?

TABLE 17.1	Clean Wounds		
Vaccination Status	**Time Since Last Vaccine**		**Recommended Vaccine**
Fully vaccinated	<10 y since last booster		None necessary
Fully vaccinated	>10 y since last booster		Vaccine booster
Received only one vaccine			Vaccine ×2 with at least 6 month interval
Received two vaccines with correct interval <12 mo	<12 mo		None
No vaccine			Full vaccination
Unknown status			Full vaccination

In Norway, we use the regime as shown in Figures 17.1 and 17.2:

It is beyond the scope of this manual to address all the national guidelines for tetanus vaccination. Contact your national health authority for local routines. Here are some English language Web sites:

- WHO: http://www.who.int/immunization/wer8120tetanus_May06_position_paper.pdf

- USA: http://wwwn.cdc.gov/travel/yellow-BookCh4-Tetanus.aspx

- UK: http://www.dh.gov.uk/en/Publichealth/Healthprotection/Immunisation/Greenbook/DH_4097254

- Canada: http://www.phac-aspc.gc.ca/im/is-cv/index-eng.php

Clean Wound versus Contaminated Wound

A wound that looks dirty, that is, covered with oil or soot, is not necessarily an infected wound. A contaminated wound is a wound that has been exposed, or has been potentially exposed, to bacteria or toxins or substances that can potentially contain bacteria or other harmful microbes.

So a cut in a squash court or at a badminton game is unlikely to be contaminated, unless caused by a punch, tooth mark, or contact with another player (organic origin). In ice hockey or boxing, cuts are often caused by opponents, so while the environment is relatively clean, the human factor may cause contamination. The risk of tetanus contamination is greater at outdoor events. Where animals wander, the risk of tetanus infection is present.

TABLE 17.2	Contaminated Wounds		
Vaccination Status	**Time Since Last Vaccine**		**Recommended Vaccine**
Fully vaccinated (3 or 4 doses at correct interval)	<5 y since last booster		None necessary
Fully vaccinated	>5 y since last booster		Vaccine booster
Received only one vaccine			HTIg + vaccine (at least 2 with 6 mo in between)
Received two vaccines with correct interval	<12 mo		None
Received two vaccines with correct interval	<5 y		Vaccine booster
Received two vaccines with correct interval	>5 y		HTIg + vaccine booster
No vaccine			HTIg + full vaccination
Unknown status			HTIg + full vaccination

Clinical Findings

The incubation period of tetanus usually varies between 3 and 21 days (median, 7 days; range, 0 to 60 days), so the event physician is not likely to see the characteristic features of the disease:

- Trismus—early spasms of the facial muscles (trismus or "lock-jaw" and "risus sardonicus")

- Followed by spasm of the back muscles (opisthotonos)

- Sudden, generalized tonic seizures (tetanospasms)

- Spasm of the glottis, which may cause sudden death

Diagnosis is based on clinical findings and not on laboratory results. For an event physician, tetanus prevention is important. One must first differentiate between contaminated and clean wounds as this affects vaccination treatment. Wound care is important and wounds should be cleansed and kept clean; earth or organic material must be removed as soon as possible and foreign bodies removed. In vaccinated patients, if you decide to give a tetanus vaccine, you should usually think about giving antibiotics as well, due to the risk of bacterial contamination from earth. In the unlikely event of encountering a patient with acute onset tetanus, prompt admission to hospital and treatment with antitetanus immunoglobulins and appropriate antibiotics may prevent tetanus progression, but is unlikely to influence established pathology.

17.5 BURNS AND ABRASIONS

Burns

First- and second-degree burns and abrasions are not uncommon on asphalt, cement, and artificial surfaces (cycling, road races, tennis, field hockey, winter sliding sports, etc.) so one should be prepared to offer elementary wound care.

Clean the wound with sterile water/saline. Hand injuries can be placed in a bowl of sterile water. Remove foreign bodies, stones, grass, etc. Creams and bandages: White Vaseline gives good sore protection and prevents bandages sticking to the wound. Vaseline grid bandages are also very useful. (Some people prefer silver sulphadiazine, though care must be used in case of bright sunlight—silver can give skin discoloration when exposed to sunlight. Beware also sulpha reactions/allergies; there is little evidence to show that the use of silver sulphadiazine reduces bacterial wound infections or sepsis in patients with burns.) Finally, cover the wound with a nonabsorbent bandage. Recommend the changing of bandages the next day.

Blisters can be emptied on the second day and dead skin removed using small scissors. Leave 2 to 3 mm of skin at the sore's edge. For athletes wishing to continue their sport, a Duoderm, Comfeel, or Angel Skin pad can be applied. Make sure the pad covers the whole of the sore and at least 10 mm of healthy skin. Based on the current available evidence, blisters should wherever possible be left intact to reduce the risk of infection, but if anatomical position necessitates intervention for functional purposes, aspiration appears to result in less pain than deroofing.

Remember to check tendon function with finger burns.

Third-degree burns are unusual in most sports, but can occur. Treatment is as above, but as most surgical centers recommend skin transplantation, a referral to the local burn/surgical unit may be advised. Prophylactic antibiotics are recommended in some centers as infection increases the depth of tissue damage. It is not absolutely vital that surgery takes place immediately, so an athlete may wait a couple of days, and thus travel home before receiving a surgical evaluation.

Abrasions

For asphalt burns, scrubbing the wound may be necessary. (This is painful. Dripping local anesthetic onto the wound may help; anesthetic creams tend to have a slow onset.) I often use a sterile surgical hand-and-nail scrub brush and try to remove all discoloration from the skin. This prevents infection and discoloration of scars. Remove devitalized skin flaps (epidermal), as these often become necrotic. If the skin flap includes dermis, then it usually survives, so removal is not recommended unless circulation is definitely compromised.

Artificial Grass Burns

While artificial grass surfaces have several advantages, they also have some potential drawbacks. Obviously, there is a risk of abrasions/burns caused by sliding over these synthetic fibers, but increased

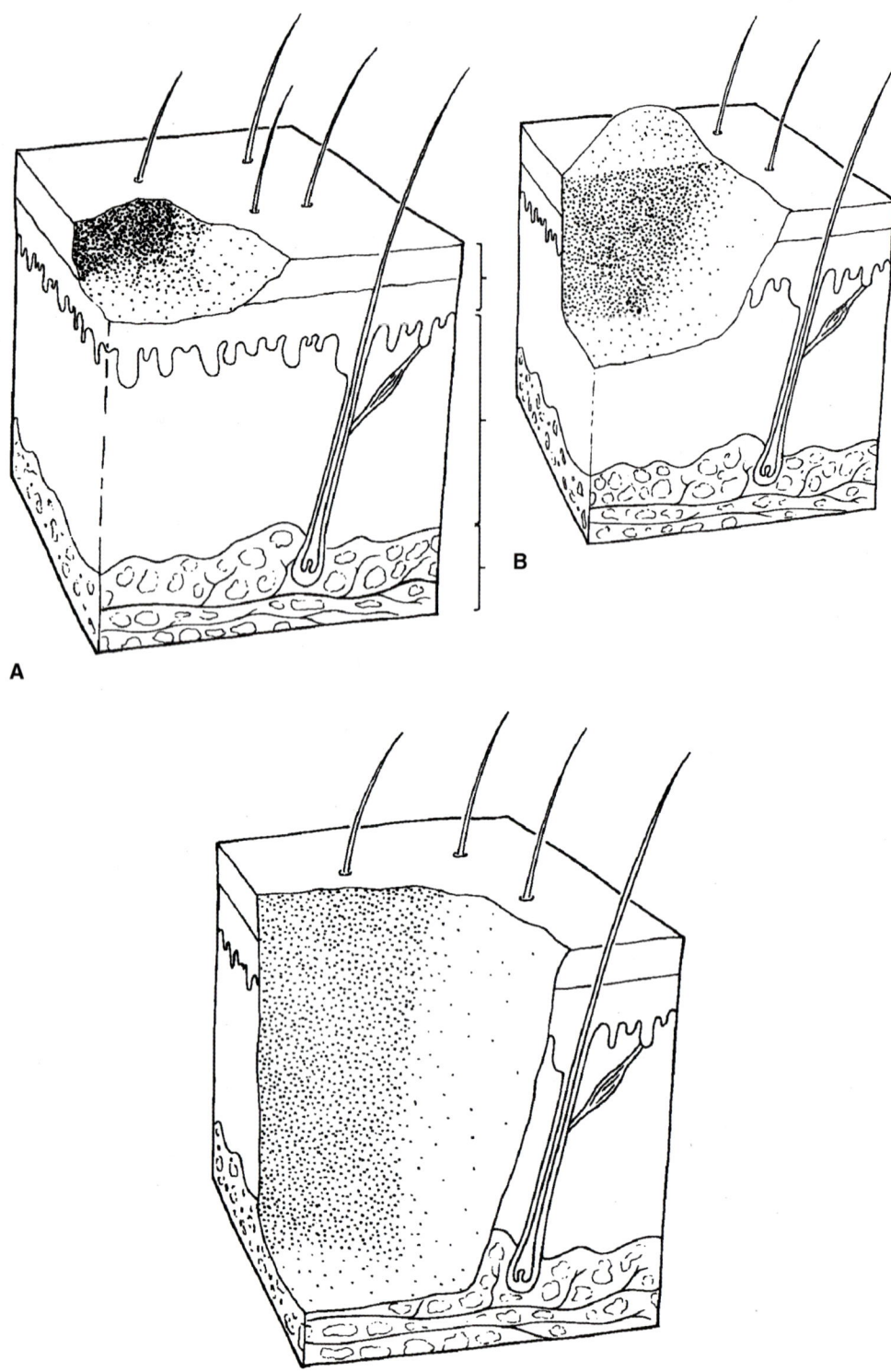

FIGURE 17.2.　Burns. A: First-degree burn; B: Second-degree burn; C: Third-degree burn.

rates of MRSA infections have also been reported in these wounds. Similarly, artificial surfaces seem to absorb heat more than natural surfaces, so there is a possibility of heat-related illness when athletes have to perform for longer periods of time in the heat.

17.6 FRICTION BLISTERS

These develop in areas of constant friction, most typically on the feet or hands. Moisture contributes to their development. There have been some conflicting studies about the use of antiperspirants to prevent friction blisters. If blisters are painful, a small incision to allow drainage, but leaving the roof intact, may help during competition. There may be predisposing inflammatory conditions such as allergic or contact dermatitis, urticaria, or exercise-induced angioedema. Blister prevention can be achieved by keeping the feet dry, choosing correctly fitting shoes, using a thick pair of socks, removing foreign bodies from the shoe, etc., but they can still occur despite these preventative procedures. Blisters can be treated as burn injuries, above, and by using sterile hydrocolloid bandages.

17.7 BRUISES AND CONTUSIONS

There are several scales for classifying bruises, but they remain rather esoteric and obviously open for individual interpretation by the physician.

As an example, here is the Bruise Harm Score.

Use of Topical NSAID Creams: According to Whitefield et al. in 2002, topical 5% ibuprofen is as effective as oral ibuprofen in the treatment of superficial soft-tissue injuries.

TABLE 17.3	Bruise Harm Score	
Harm Score	**Severity Level**	**Notes**
0	Light bruise	No damage
1	Less than moderate bruise	Little damage
2	Moderate bruise	Some damage
3	Serious bruise	Dangerous
4	Extremely serious bruise	Dangerous

17.8 FROSTBITE

When exposed to subzero temperatures, blood vessels close to the skin start to vasoconstrict. While vasoconstriction may help in preserving the body's core temperature, it will inevitably lead to lead to ischemia, tissue hypoxia, and damage. Exposed tissue may also freeze over, thus further damaging tissue. This combination of hypoxia and freezing causes an inflammation, which is probably prostaglandin mediated.

There are several ways of classifying frostbite from that similar to burns classification (with first, second, third, and fourth degrees) to Liebl (superficial and deep) to Cauchy et al., who developed a classification based on recovery, need for surgery, etc.

Frostbite is not, and should not be, common in organized sport. This is due to the fact that the development of frostbite is dependent of a number of factors: temperature, exposure time, and clothing protection. As far as organized sports are concerned, we are basically talking about long-distance skiing events, but some incidents have occurred in other sports where poorly clad or shod athletes have been exposed to the cold over time. FIS, the International Ski Federation, has developed guidelines to prevent cold-induced injuries. The following rules apply for Telemark skiing:

- At temperatures down to minus 15°C— obligatory warm shelter in the area

- Between minus 15°C and minus 20°C—at any point on the course, there must be a warm shelter available

Recommendations regarding cold weather protection must be given to competitors and to competition officials. Medical personnel must check competitors for frostbite, particularly in the face. Having a warm tent for the competitors at the start area is recommended. Warm clothing must be available in the arrival area. At temperatures below minus 22°C in a major portion of the course, all competitions must be delayed or cancelled.

Strong wind worsens the effect of cold. A useful wind chill factor converter is available from Environment Canada Wind Chill Calculations at http://www.msc.ec.gc.ca/education/windchill/WindChill_Calculator_e.cfm

Frostbite in organized skiing events should not occur; however, it may be seen in mass participation events, with brave but inexperienced athletes (often decent skiers from warmer countries) who are inadequately prepared or dressed for colder climates.

There are several types of clothing accessories that may be useful in prevention (e.g., extrathermal/windproof socks, gloves, balaclavas and neck-warmers, underwear and vests). Creams and lotions may reduce the skin exposure to cold air, though they are by nature sticky and messy and not often used by top athletes. Ski glasses or goggles may prevent both dryness of the eyes and snow blindness.

Clinically, frostbite presents with an initial burning sensation, followed by a feeling of numbness, and then finally (often but not always) intense pain. When the pain becomes more intense, the skin begins to discolor: red, then blue, then black. Clear or purple-colored blisters may occur. The affected area is cold to touch and looks necrotic. The disappearance of pain is not a good sign as this usually indicates nerve destruction. In the intermediary phase, before necrosis begins, palpation often reveals that the surrounding skin and subcutaneous tissues are stiff and immovable (frozen).

Treatment

- Get the patient to a warm area and keep him or her there until he or she has been adequately rewarmed.

- Immerse the affected body part in clean, warm water (104°F [39°C]) for approximately 30 minutes until normal skin coloration has returned. The final part of this process may be painful, but the patient must persevere. Hot water may be needed to be added to keep the temperature even. Avoid using water that is too hot.

- Do not scrub dry the skin; dry by placing absorbent towel on the skin, and then remove without irritating the skin.

- Do not puncture any grade 2 blisters initially.

- All wound care must be conducted in as sterile an environment as possible to prevent infection.

- Cover sores with Vaseline bandages or with Flamazine cream against the skin.

- Rest the injured body part.

- Check tetanus status.

- Ensure that the athlete leaves the sports arena in a warmed vehicle and leaves for a warm

environment. Refreezing of tissue has a bad prognosis. The Lapps of northern Europe (the Sami people) have by experience learned that it is better to keep walking to a final warm shelter and then start the rewarming process, than to temporarily rewarm frozen toes and then reexpose them to more cold.

- Most experts now agree that the old "trick" of rubbing the injured area with snow is not a good idea.

- Oral and/or topical NSAIDs may help prevent further prostaglandin activity.

- Hyperbaric oxygen therapy may be useful in advanced cases.

- Conclusion: Get the injured area into a warm environment, keep it warm there, and treat as a burn injury.

- The prognosis for frostbite injuries depends on the extent of injury and whether or not complications, such as infections, occur.

Nonfreezing cold injuries can also occur when conditions are cold and wet:

Chilblains: Red, swollen, tender, painful, warm skin patches, often with hyperesthesia, "pins and needles," or numbness. Unless there are underlying microangiopathies or neuropathies, these conditions recover spontaneously when the athlete receives sufficient warmth.

Trench Foot: Develops when the skin of the foot is exposed to *both* cold and moisture for 12 hours or more (but more often for days or weeks,

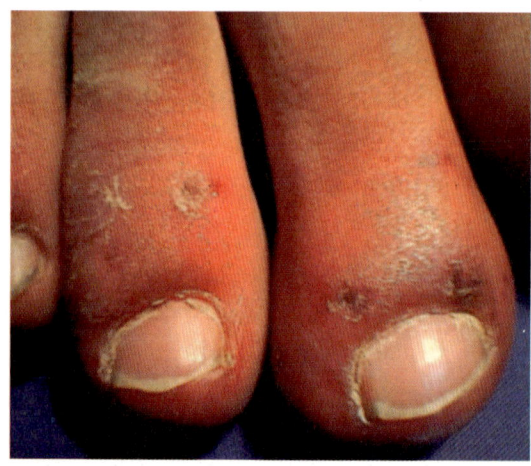

FIGURE 17.3. Chilblains.

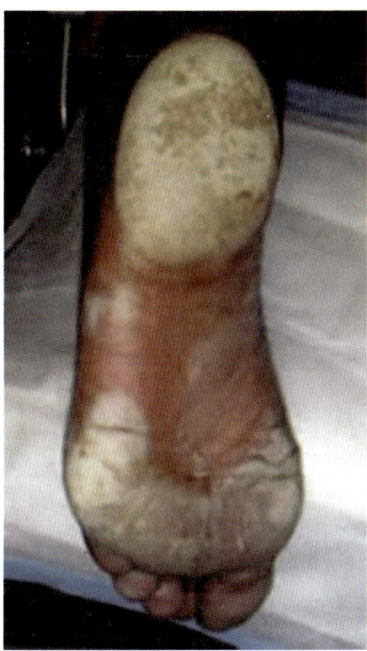

FIGURE 17.4. Trench foot.

as seen in polar or military expeditions of yore). This combination of cold and moisture weakens the skin, causing small skin tears, small ulcers, and infection. Initially, trench foot may present with "pins and needles" or numbness or pain. The skin looks like skin looks when it immersed in water for longer periods. With continued exposure, the feet may swell and become red, then bluish, then black. Treatment of mild cases is conservative and requires the athlete to desist activity until the lesions heal. The athlete will need to discuss shoe/ boot type and training procedures with his or her coach.

17.9 BITES AND STINGS

Though uncommon in sport, bite wounds do occur, either from humans, animals, insects, reptiles, or other creatures. The clinical findings in a bite wound depend on its source. Clinical findings with human or dog bites are usually not very dramatic; however, when infections do occur, findings may present as early as 24 hours after a bite, though Malinowski stated that signs of moderate infection develop first after 2½ days. Symptoms from spider or venomous reptile bites may be severe and appear shortly after the bite.

- General wound considerations (see Sections 17.6 and 17.8, above)
- Specific infection risks and the need for prophylactic antibiotics: dog/cat bites—*Pasteurella*; Humans—*Staphylococcus aureus*
- Wound location: a bite on the hand is potentially more serious than a bite on the leg
- Potential complications: systemic complications
- Anaphylactic reactions
- Wound symptoms

Human Bites

Bites by humans do occur and can be intentional (Hello, Mr. Tyson) or accidental, classically when a wound has been caused by another athlete's teeth puncturing the skin of the hand.

These wounds are seldom large and the main concern is that of infection after a puncture wound. It is rare to have structural damage to muscles, nerves, capsules, etc. as human teeth are not that sharp. The commonest site of injury is over the dorsal surface of the MCP joints. The human mouth is reckoned to contain more than a hundred different types of microorganisms including *Staphylococcus aureus*, various streptococci, enterobacteria, proteus, etc. It is important to prevent or appropriately treat infections. Approximately 10% to 15% of human bite wounds become infected (Marr et al., 1994). Athletes, particularly the fighting variety, often wait until infection is established before contacting an EP by which time there are usually several competing bacteria active in the wound. As most of these injuries occur on the hands, and hand wounds have a higher infection rate than similar wounds, the event physician must be alert, even if the wound looks simple and clean.

The commonest organisms isolated from human bites are *Eikenella corrodens,* alpha-hemolytic streptococci, anaerobic bacteria, beta-lactamase producing bacteria including *Staphylococcus aureus* and *Bacteroids*, and seem to confirm that bite infections are caused by oral rather than skin bacteria.

There is also the possibility of viral transmission with hepatitis B and C, though this risk is considered low. If the likelihood of the "biter" being infected with hepatitis B or C is low, then a hepatitis B vaccine program may be recommended while informing the athlete of the low level of transmission risk. Herpes simplex virus (HSV) as well as syphilis, tuberculosis, actinomycosis, tetanus, and HIV infections can be transmitted through human bites, though the likelihood is considered rare.

Human bite wounds usually present in two ways:

Clenched-fist injury: These are the most common variety and occur when a clenched fist comes into contact (i.e., hits) with another individual's teeth, causing a usually small wound, usually less than 10 mm in length. The wound usually occurs on the dorsal aspect of the third metacarpophalangeal (MCP) joint of the dominant hand. As well as skin injuries, capsule injuries, extensor tendon lacerations, and even fractures may occur. Once they have established a base in the finger, bacteria may spread along the extensor tendons and cause purulent infections, even abscesses. These infections can present several centimeters away from the initial bite. Such wound infections require hospitalization with intravenous antibiotics and, not unusually, open surgery.

Occlusive bites: Occlusive bites occur when teeth penetrate the skin, often at two locations (e.g., on the dorsal and palmar aspects of the hand). Regrettably, bites are not unknown, but seriously frowned upon, in boxing and rugby. Once again, bites to the hand, but also ear and nose, must be given greater attention, and the use of prophylactic antibiotics for these locations is advised. As these wounds often develop polymicrobial colonizations, with both aerobic and anaerobic as well as beta-lactamase–producing species, dicloxacillin is often an effective antibiotic. Bites to the hand have a high risk of infection due to the risk of teeth penetrating tendon sheaths or the closed midpalmar space. Wounds must be examined carefully, including specific nerve and tendon function tests. If you suspect damage to major nerves or tendons, then athletes should be referred to a hand surgeon. Open wounds that require suturing should probably be referred to a hand surgeon.

Dog Bites

The likelihood of being bitten by a dog in sport is not very great; however, stray mutts do appear on football pitches and sometimes players kick out at these in an effort to remove the canine intruders from the playing field. This sometimes provokes a retaliatory bite, usually in the legs or arms. In adult athletes, this is rarely a dangerous issue, unless the dog has rabies or some other disease, but it can be serious in younger children, particularly if the face is attacked.

The commonest injuries are

- Puncture wounds
- Lacerations, with or without deeper soft-tissue injuries
- Infections due to *Pasteurella multiocida* (usually penicillin sensitive) or *Staphylococcus intermedius*
- *Capnocytophaga canimorus*—usually only dangerous to elderly, sick patients, particularly homeless alcoholics

Treatment

Treatment is pretty straightforward: wound cleansing, suturing of skin if necessary. If damaged deep soft tissue, then a referral to a specialist unit is recommended due to the risk of infection. Cover with a wound dressing and give a tetanus booster.

To Suture or Not to Suture? A lot has been written about this subject, but little research has been carried out. Microbiologists state that wounds should be left open due to the risk of infection, but as trauma physicians, we cannot allow all our patients to walk around with gaping wounds. Most physicians now agree that most wounds should be closed with primary suture, but that wounds to the hand and face should be referred to a specialist. Garbutt reviewed 74 papers and concludes, "Bite wounds to the hand should be left open. Nonpuncture wounds (lacerations, etc.) elsewhere may be safely treated by primary closure after thorough cleaning."

Prophylactic Antibiotics? Again, this is not a very well-documented area, and further research needs to be conducted. The most commonly quoted article is from Cummings et al.[5] One hundred patients with no sign of infection were given prophylactic antibiotics: eighty-four avoided infection, nine returned with infected wounds. In the control group, 16 had infected wounds. The conclusion was that 7 infected wounds per 100 bites could be avoided if prophylactic antibiotics were administered. Herren[6] reviewed 120 papers and concluded that "the use of oral antibiotics for all types of dog bite wounds reduces the risk of infection by nearly half. A prescribing policy that limits antibiotics to higher risk wounds may be effective."

Which Antibiotic? Again, there are many variations, but in Europe, the drug of choice is penicillin for dog and cat bites, and dicloxacillin for humans.

Swabs: There is not much point in taking a wound swab immediately after an injury. Most microbiologists recommend a wait of at least 6 to 8 hours until there is adequate colonization.

Rabies: The danger is always present after a dog bite. Rabies is prevalent in all the continents, with a few exceptions, usually island or peripheral states. If a dog bite occurs in an region with known rabies, then patients should be referred to a specialist unit, a combination of rabies vaccine and human rabies immune globulin is recommended. If an athlete is partially vaccinated, then two booster doses are recommended. Intensive wound irrigation is of vital importance. Follow local guidelines here. For an overview, the Centre for Disease Control and Prevention (http://www.cdc.gov/) gives a good overview, as always.

Cat Bites

Cat bites should not be expected at a sporting event, although an athlete may turn up with a bite. *Pasteurella* and *Staphylococcus aureus* are not unusual pathogens. Fresh wounds should be washed carefully, a tetanus booster should be given and the wound dressed. Iqbal has reviewed 56 papers (and concludes, "Antibiotic prophylaxis should be given to all cat bite wounds unless a superficial wound is present. Most importantly, oral antibiotics should be given when presented with a puncture wound or low extremity wound. This area requires further large scale RCTs as previous studies involved small groups of patients."

Snake Bites

An event physician may be required to treat athletes who have been bitten by snakes, though this is an unlikely scenario. Snake bites are rare in most countries: approximately 10 bites per 100,000 population in the United States and 15 per 100,000 in Australia, with only 2 to 4 deaths per annum in both countries (even though the population of the United States is far greater than Australia). Sri Lanka, on the other hand, is known for having a very high rate of snakebites and deaths, though it is not easy to find precise data. India has between 15,000 to 20,000 deaths annually due to snake bites, mainly in Tamil Nadu, Kerala, Rajasthan, and West Bengal. Even though there are several hundred species of venomous snakes, only about 250 species can give fatal bites—not a very consoling thought.

Venomous snakes are classified in two groups:

a) Elapids—cobras, kraits, mambas, Australian copperheads, sea snakes, and coral snakes

b) Viperids—vipers, rattlesnakes, copperheads/cottonmouths, adders, and bushmasters

A third group, colubrids, contain some species that are venomous. Colubrids include boomslangs, tree snakes, vine snakes, and mangrove snakes, some of which are venomous.

Venom is injected into a body through the snake's fangs and may be

■ Cytotoxic or dermatotoxic: causing necrosis of skin, fat, fascia, and muscle

■ Neurotoxic: causing a neuromuscular blockade that may lead to cardiac or respiratory failure

■ Hemotoxic: causing embolisms and coagulopathies

It is important to get as accurate a history as possible. Allergic patients may have exaggerated responses to nonlethal envenomations. The history should include details of the snake itself if possible, such as color, size, rings, patterns, and special features. In many countries, people try to capture the snake to assist identification. Knowledge of local snake species is vital to allow early antiserum treatment, if appropriate. The actual time that the bite incident occurred is important to estimate and also the time involved from the bite to the onset of symptoms—pain and pain intensity, paresthesia, swelling. Often, the more intense the pain, the more toxic the envenomation. There may be systemic symptoms such as nausea and vomiting, diarrhea, chest or abdominal pain, dyspnea, and dysphagia.

Clinically, one must examine the bite site and check the vital signs. When examining the bite wound, look for signs of dermatotoxic venom—local tissue destruction, edema, or lymphadenitis. There may be local or distant angioedema. Check the patient for neurotoxicity—cardiac or respiratory distress. Look for signs of hemorrhage or embolisms. Check the vital signs. Is the patient drowsy or confused? Gauge the level of consciousness.

For the EP, the goal must be to get the patient to a hospital as soon as possible.

Ring an ambulance and get the patient to lie down. Establish an intravenous line as soon as possible. Make sure the airways are patent and give oxygen if necessary. Apply a splint to the injured extremity. No other first-aid techniques have any documented effect (i.e., suction, etc.).

Antivenom may be effective; however, this may not be readily available and it is difficult to know which species-specific (monovalent) antivenom to administer. Antivenom for cobras, mambas, and taipans are available in India, the United States, South Africa, and Australia. However, some polyvalent serums are available.

One of the world's leading authorities on snake bites, Dr. Ian Simpson, of the WHO's Snakebite Treatment Group in South Asia, has developed the "Do it RIGHT" concept for snakebite treatment:

- **R**—Reassure the patient. Seventy percent of snakebites come from nonvenomous species. In half of the remaining 30%, venom is not injected, and these are called "dry bites." The victim is usually not at risk. (Is this why traditional treatments appear to work?)

- **I**—Immobilize the affected limb in the same way as a fracture. Do not tie tight bandages; simply stop the limb from moving, as movement helps venom spread.

- **GH**—Get to Hospital fast. If the patient has been envenomed, then antivenom can be administered. Studies from West Bengal show that victims who do not survive are those that come late to the hospital.

Prophylactic Antibiotics after Nonvenomous Snake Bites: Terry reviewed 67 papers and concludes, "Prophylactic antibiotics are not indicated in the routine management of patients with snakebites from nonvenomous snakes if no necrosis is present."

Fish, Jellyfish, and Other Aquatic Nasties

Jellyfish: Swimmers can on occasion come in contact with jellyfish tentacles that contain venom. Some jellyfish release venom that causes a mild burning sensation, while others release powerful life-threatening toxins (the most deadly jellyfish are to be found in the Indian Ocean and around Australia). There are several hundred types of jellyfish.

Symptoms include a whole panorama of local symptoms, from mild stinging pain, itching, erythema, and a blistering rash; to nausea, vomiting, diarrhea, lymphadenopathy, intense pain, paresthesia, and muscle spasms; to severe reactions, with dyspnea, chest pain, coma, and death. Some stings can cause death in minutes (e.g., box jellyfish).

Many old-hands swear by vinegar baths, where one covers the stung area or attached tentacle with vinegar for 15 to 30 minutes—this is believed to hinder the nematocysts from releasing their toxins. Alternatively, rinse in sea water or alcohol. Fresh water is believed by some to aid nematocysts' toxin release; others believe that fresh water can be used. There are different attitudes to the use of ice. Remove tentacles with a forceps. Do not use pressure bandages.

Eye lesions should be rinsed with saline. Obviously, vinegar must not be dripped into the eyes. Stings in the mouth can be treated with gargling diluted vinegar (three parts water to one part vinegar).

In the event of a serious sting or anaphylactic reaction, the event physician must be versed in reanimation techniques and in the treatment of shock. Before an event, the event physician should consult the event organizers about the presence of jellyfish and other aquatic organisms. Event organizers are usually aware of these problems and try to avoid hosting events in infested areas.

Sea Urchins: Swimmers may pierce their skin with sea urchin pedicles. These usually break off, leaving bony foreign bodies in the skin. These spikes may be coated in toxin and thus cause local inflammation. As foreign bodies, they may also predispose to infection. Toxic symptoms include local pain, burning, and dye discoloration from the spines. Spines should be removed using a forceps. If these are deep sitting, then athletes may have to be referred for surgical removal. Hot water is reputably useful in minimizing the toxin effect, though this is poorly documented in literature.

Stingrays: Stingrays are large, bottom-dwelling fish that can be stepped upon by divers. Contact with stingrays is not common in sport and fatalities are rare. These fish have a venomous spine at the base of their tail. This venom causes local vasoconstriction that may lead to poor wound healing, tissue necrosis, and infection. The spine may remain in the skin and needs to be removed. Clinically, findings are similar to other aquatic stings with local pain, erythema, and swelling, but systemic symptoms may present due to the effect of the toxin—nausea, vomiting, headaches, cramps, dyspnea and even cardiac arrhythmias. Once again, treatment requires wound lavage with salt water and foreign body removal.

Shark Attacks: I have no experience or knowledge of shark attacks and could not find an author willing to write a small chapter. The incidence of shark attacks is relatively low, and South Africa seems to be unusually exposed to these attacks. For more information on this topic, I refer to the International Shark Attack File (http://www.flmnh.ufl.edu/fish/Sharks/Statistics/2002attacksummary.htm).

Mycobacterium marinum: This is a rare condition that can affect open-water swimmers. If the swimmer has a cut or skin lesion, this can be infected by the mycobacteria, causing a painful papule, nodule, or ulcer at the injury site. The infection can cause lymphadenitis, lymphadenopathy, fever, and, rarely, even systemic infections. Clarithromycin may be effective, but I would refer patients to a specialist as these lesions may take months to resolve.

Insect Bites

As this is primarily a sports manual, I will not go into great detail about the array of nasty little bugs that inhabit our planet. I will focus on the commoner types of insect bites and hope my colleagues in far-off lands excuse my exclusion of what may be more common insects in their countries.

- Wasps and bees
- Mosquitoes
- Flies
- Fleas
- Ticks
- Spiders

Wasps and Bees: Bee and wasp stings are usually just uncomfortable, but some unfortunate individuals may receive multiple stings and become quite ill. Stings in the mouth or to the tongue may cause swelling and impair respiration. In the United States, approximately 40 deaths are reported each year from insect venom anaphylaxis, most, but not all, having had a previous wasp or bee allergic reaction. Most allergic reactions occur within an hour of being stung. According to Pumphrey, most sting-induced anaphylactic reactions come within 10 to 20 minutes of exposure.

For a normal sting reaction, oral antihistamines and topical hydrocortisone creams are usually effective, but soreness lasts for a few days. A one-off high dose of oral prednisolone can have a dramatically positive effect, but this is not allowed in sport, unless a TUE has been applied. Ice packs and cold water cloths can alleviate symptoms. The stinger should be removed. Prophylactic antibiotics are not indicated. If bacterial skin infections at the sting site do occur, they should be treated accordingly. (For anaphylactic reactions see Chapter 23.)

Mosquitoes: Mosquitoes are irritating, annoying creatures that bite both at day and night. Normally, bites are just itchy and uncomfortable but can on occasion become infected. The infecting bacteria vary, depending on what part of the world you are in, but the usual causal agents are streptococci (superficial, erythema, warm) or staphylococci (deep, sores, pus, crusts). For a normal bite reaction, oral antihistamines and topical hydrocortisone creams are usually effective, but itching may disturb an athlete's sleep. Hot showers make things worse. There are many topical agents around the world with purportive anti-itching effect; some help a little and some not at all. Some bites occur on exceptionally sensitive areas such as the eyelids or genitals and athletes have been forced from competition due to noninfected mosquito bites.

Mosquitoes are also bearers of several serious microorganisms that may cause a multitude of debilitating illnesses such as

- Malaria (South and Central America, Africa, Asia)
- Dengue fever (tropical North, South, and Central America; Africa; Asia; and Australia)
- Yellow fever (South and Central America, Africa)
- Elephantiasis (Tropics)
- Japanese encephalitis (East and South East Asia)
- Leishmaniasis (Afghanistan, Algeria, Bangladesh, Brazil, India, Iran, Iraq, Nepal, Peru, Saudi Arabia, Sudan, and Syria)
- Viral meningitis and encephalitis, among others

Ticks: Ticks are small arachnid parasites that live on the blood of mammals, birds, and reptiles. They are often found in tall grass and low bushes or shrubs and attach themselves to their victims, both humans and animals, by biting onto their victims who brush against these bushes. Athletes may encounter tick bites in golf or in terrain sports. Ticks bite through the skin and will stay there until they choose to drop off or they are physically removed. They can be very difficult to remove, but it is important for the physician to remove all parts of the tick. According to the Norwegian Institute of Health, there is a greater risk of infection if the tick is allowed to remain on the skin for more than 24 hours.

Remove the tick by using tweezers (special tick-removing forceps have been designed). Try to hold the forceps around the creature's neck, and then pluck straight out. Some people twist the tweezers 90 degrees while plucking. Try to remove all parts of the head and mouth as remains often cause infection (not necessarily the tick-borne infections). Try to avoid pulling the tick by the body, as this just causes it to burst and makes removal of the mouth and head more difficult.

Tick-borne illnesses are caused by infection with a variety of pathogens, including bacteria (e.g., *Rickettsia*), viruses, and protozoa. Ticks can transmit one or several varieties of these pathogenic agents. The list of potential diseases is long and includes, among others, Lyme disease, tick-borne relapsing fever, Rocky Mountain spotted fever, babesiosis, ehrlichiosis, tick paralysis, and Tularemia.

Tick-borne encephalitis (TBE) is caused by a viral infection and is to be found from France to Eastern Russia, in northeastern China, in northern Japan, and from Scandinavia to Italy, Greece, and the Crimea in the south. Acute cases can present with a variety of neurological symptoms and findings including, obviously, encephalitis. Some patients have symptoms within a day of being bitten, but most patients need up to 7 days before they develop symptoms. The disease can lead to long-term neurological sequelae or even death. Traditionally, the TBE virus has been divided into two subtypes, and they appear to cause slightly different clinical presentations, though the eastern variant (Russia, Asia) is believed to be the more virulent. Vaccinations do appear to be effective, and there are several products on the market.

The EP is unlikely to encounter acute cases and even less likely to diagnose such difficult condi-

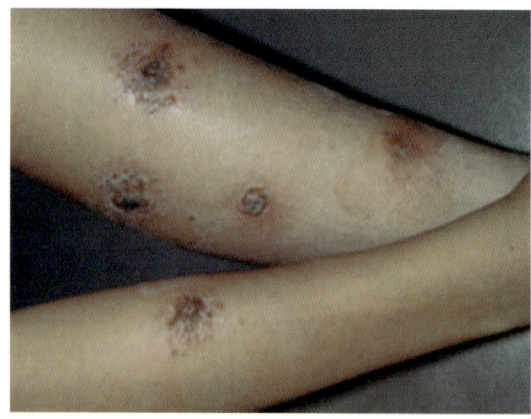

FIGURE17.6. Flea bites.

tions during a short sporting event, but will be expected to be able to remove a tick and treat primary skin infections. The EP should be aware of local protocols for the treatment of bites.

An athlete may present with an erythema be administered migrans rash a week or two after a bite. These are classical bull's-eye lesions with a central reddish lesion, surrounded by a pale ring, surrounded by another reddish ring. The patient may feel tired and ill, and have a fever, headache, and/or arthralgia. Early oral antibiotics are usually effective. Choice of antibiotic will vary from place to place, but penicillin, erythromycin, or doxycycline can be used.

Should prophylactic antibiotics be administered after tick bites? There is no real consensus on this topic, but the general opinion is that antibiotics are only necessary if there is a known risk of *Borrelia burgdorferi* in an area.

Various antibiotics are effective for different diseases in different countries, so follow these recommendations.

Tsetse Flies: These flies are known to breed along rivers in sub-Saharan Africa. They feed exclusively on blood. They can transmit trypanosomiasis and nagana.

Sand Flies/Fleas: These small flies are found in sandy areas and can go by other names, such as sand gnats, jiggers, etc. Sand fleas (*Tunga penetrans*), as the name implies, can burrow into the skin and have to be literally scraped or cut out using a needle or a scalpel. Be careful not to rupture the flea's body, as rupturing the female's egg sac may increase the risk of infection. Local know-how suggests the cleaning of wounds with

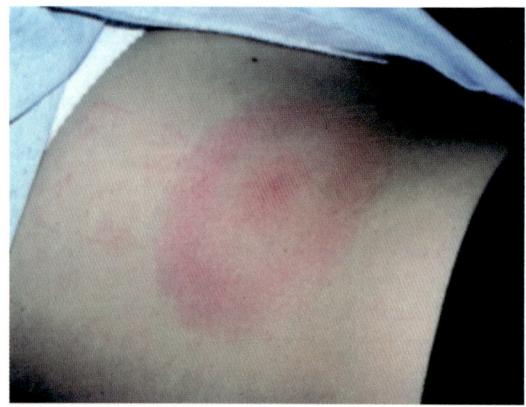

FIGURE 17.5. Erythema migrans.

antiseptic swabs, preferably alcohol, and covering the wound with an iodine solution and small plaster. Sand fleas are to be found in the tropics and subtropics in Central and South America, the West Indies, Asia, and Africa. Some strains are vectors for severe illnesses such as leishmaniasis. Wearing sandals in known infected areas can help in preventing flea bites. According to the CDC, over 90% of new cutaneous leishmaniasis cases (approximately 1.35 million new cases yearly) occur in Afghanistan, Algeria, Brazil, Iran, Iraq, Peru, Saudi Arabia, and Syria. Over 90% of new visceral leishmaniasis cases (450,000 cases) occur in India, Bangladesh, Nepal, Sudan, and Brazil.

Flea Bites: Flea bites can occur when fleas are transferred from animals (contact with dogs and cats; cats lying on a bed) or birds (nests near an air vent). Bites are commonest around the waist or on the legs. They cause itching (which can be intense if the patient is allergic), which may in turn result in rashes that may become infected. They can also act as vectors for *Yersinia pestis*, endemic typhus, and other conditions.

Antihistamine tablets or topical hydrocortisone creams may be effective against itching; however, the only way to get rid of these nasties is to remove the animals that are carrying them and to use insecticides and other debugging techniques in the residence.

Spiders: Spiders do not usually bite humans, and even if they do, they seldom cause problems. Nearly all spiders can produce venom. Spiders may creep into football boots or kit bags, and athletes in Australia, South Africa, the United States, etc. have been known to have been bitten by an array of these nasty little critters. However, only few species possess dangerous neurotoxic venoms, while others can bite and inject venom that causes skin and connective tissue necrosis.

Spiders that produce neurotoxins include

- Widow spiders (United States), button spiders (southern Africa)
- Sydney funnel-web spiders, redback spiders (Australia)
- Mouse spiders
- Brazilian wandering spiders

Spiders that produce dermatonecrotic venom:

- Recluse spiders (United States)

- Six-eyed sand spiders (Southern Africa)
- White-tailed spiders, house spider, brown spider (Australia)
- Black widow spider bites may produce mild or severe symptoms, varying from local pain at the site of the bite to severe muscle cramps, muscle weakness, tremor, intense abdominal or chest muscle pain, nausea, vomiting, dizziness, and dyspnea. These bites are seldom fatal in healthy athletes, though patients can be extremely ill, requiring hospitalization, narcotic analgesia, and a specific antitoxin (antivenin). Black widows are found in large parts of the United States and parts of Canada

Dermatonecrotic spiders are believed to possess sphingomyelinase D, which is a highly toxic agent that can cause major tissue destruction in skin, fat, fascia, muscle. For those of us not used to seeing severe spider bites, the effects are not dissimilar to those found with aggressive group A streptococcal necrotizing dermatitis and fasciitis. Some spiders are supposedly more venomous than others including the Chilean recluse spider and the six-eyed sand spiders of Southern Africa.

Bites by these spiders can produce lesions that are local and minor or severe dermatonecrotic lesions that may lead to death.

My advice to the EP here is to ensure that one is aware of local venomous arachnoids and to be familiar with diagnostic and treatment modalities.

Tarantulas are big, hairy spiders that can be found in southern Europe (Spain, Portugal, Italy, Turkey, and Cyprus); North, Central, and South America; Africa; and Asia. Though large, hairy, and scary, they are not now believed to possess deadly venom; however, anaphylactic reactions to bites can occur.

Good Advice in Avoiding Bites

- Close the windows at night time—at least keep the windows closed when the lights are on
- Use a mosquito net
- There are various forms of mosquito repellents—some work and some do not
- Wear sandals or shoes in the tropics
- In known poison spider country, shake and empty your shoes before putting them on
- Avoid walking in high grass in known snake areas

- Do not wear shorts when playing golf in tick-infested areas

- Avoid patting strange animals

- Never try to separate two fighting dogs

Recommended Readings

Auerbach PS. *Wilderness Medicine.*

CDC. Parasites: leishmaniasis. http://www.cdc.gov/ncidod/dpd/parasites/leishmania/default.htm. Accessed March 31, 2011.

Cummins et al. Antibiotics to prevent infection in patients with dog bite wounds: a meta-analysis of randomized trials. *Ann Emerg Med* 1994.

Dire DJ, Welsh AP. A comparison of wound irrigation solutions used in the emergency department. *Ann Emerg Med.* 1990;19(6):704–708.

Iqbal, (Manchester Royal Infirmary, 2005) has reviewed 56 papers (Best Bets: submitted but not checked).

Journal of Wound Care Fernandez.

Katrina Herren, Manchester Royal Infirmary, on BestBETS.

Mitnovetski, 2004; Elenbaas,1984; Dire, 1991.

Pumphrey. *Clin Exp Allergy* 2000.

Revis, 2008, University of Florida College of Medicine gives an excellent overview of this topic at http://www.emedicine.com/med/topic1033.htm

Terry, Manchester Royal Infirmary, 2002 has reviewed 67 papers (BestBets).

World Health Organization. Tetanus vaccine: WHO position paper. *Weekly Epidemiol Rec.* 2006;81(20):198–208.

CHAPTER 18

Fractures and Dislocations

Contributed by David McDonagh, Chair, FIBT Medical Committee

Reviewer: Angela D. Smith, Clinical Associate Professor of Orthopaedic Surgery, University of Pennsylvania; Attending Faculty, The Sports Medicine and Performance Children's Hospital, Philadelphia; Chair, Education Commission, FIMS 2002–2005; Past President, ACSM

18.1 OPEN FRACTURES

Classification

An open fracture can be defined as a broken bone that is in communication through the skin with the environment. The amount of communication can vary from a small puncture wound in the skin to a large avulsion of soft tissue that leaves the bone exposed. The diagnosis is usually obvious but may be missed, especially if the puncture wound is very small.

The most-used classification system was developed by Gustilo and Anderson. This system grades open fractures combined with wound size and soft-tissue injury and correlates the likelihood of infection and amputation (Table 18.1).

Examination

Limb examination should consist of a detailed examination of the vascularity of the limb, including limb color, warmth and perfusion, palpable pulses, capillary return (normal <3 seconds), and transcutaneous oxygenation and pulse wave forms using pulse oximetry. A detailed neurologic examination should document the sensory and motor function.

The skin over the fracture should be carefully examined. Any break in the skin at the level of the fracture should be considered indicative of a possible open fracture. Remember that wounds away from the fracture can communicate with the fracture. Periarticular open fractures almost always contaminate the associated joints.

Signs of crush injury should be sought if indicated by the mechanism of injury (e.g., horse falls on jocket). These injuries may exhibit few external signs.

Management

- The treatment of open fractures should be considered as an emergency. Adequate fluid/blood replacement, analgesia, splinting, antibiotics, and tetanus prophylaxis are required before surgical treatment.

- Initially, irrigate with saline, cover with a sterile, moist dressing, and ideally then keep the wound covered until surgery in order to reduce the risk of infection.

- The aims of management are to prevent infection, ensure healing of the fracture, and promote the restoration of function.

- Associated injuries may be severe and also require urgent treatment.

Drugs

- Intravenous antibiotics should be started immediately (e.g., cefuroxime or alternative antibiotic in line with local guidelines). First-generation cephalosporins (gram-positive coverage) such as cephalothin (1 to 2 g every 6–8h) suffice for Gustilo–Anderson type I fractures. An aminoglycoside (gram-negative coverage), such as gentamycin (120 mg every 12h; 240 mg/d), is added for types II and III injuries.

| TABLE 18.1 | Gustilo–Anderson Classification of Open Fractures | | | |

Type	Wound Description	Other Criteria	Infection Rate	Amputation Rate
I	<1 cm (puncture wound)		0%	2%
II	1–10 cm		0%	2%–7%
IIIA	>10 cm, coverage available	Segmental fractures, farm injuries, injury occurring in a highly contaminated environment	7%	2.5%
		High-velocity gunshot injuries		
IIIB	10 cm, requiring soft-tissue coverage procedure	Periosteal stripping	10%–50%	5.6%
IIIC		With vascular injury requiring repair	25%–50%;	25%

Additionally, metronidazole (500 mg every 12h) or penicillin (1.2 g every 6h) can be added for coverage against anaerobes. Tetanus prophylaxis should be instituted. Antibiotics are generally continued for 72 hours following wound closure.

Complications

- Patients with open fractures are at risk of acute wound infection and osteomyelitis. Infection can result in nonunion of the fracture, chronic osteomyelitis, and possibly result in the need for amputation.

- There is also a risk of tetanus infection.

- Infection rates vary but remain as high as 20% in severe cases. This risk depends on the degree of associated soft-tissue injury and the initial management of the patient. Infections may be caused by bacteria that contaminate the wound at the time of injury or by hospital-acquired pathogens.

- Complications other than infection and failure of skeletal fixation and nonunion of fracture will depend on the location and extent of soft-tissue damage.

- Both neurovascular injury and compartment syndrome can occur.

18.2 CLOSED FRACTURE CLASSIFICATION WITH SOFT-TISSUE INJURIES

The Tscherne and Oestern is a widely accepted classification system for soft-tissue injuries in closed fractures.

- Grade 0, simple fracture configuration, with little or no soft-tissue injury (e.g., indirect violence as with torsional injury to the tibia in downhill skiers).

- Grade 1, mild to moderately severe fracture configuration. Superficial skin abrasion. Mild to moderate soft-tissue damage due to bone fragment pressure (e.g., fracture with lateral dislocation of the distal tibia and fibula ankle with medial skin pressure).

- Grade 2, moderately severe fracture configuration. Deep contaminated abrasion with local skin and muscle damage (includes compartment syndrome). The injury is caused by direct trauma (e.g., motorbike crash).

- Grade 3, severe or comminuted fracture configuration. Extensive contusion or crushing of skin or subcutaneous tissue. There may be avulsion of skin. There is destruction of muscle. This type includes decompensated compartment syndrome and a major arterial injury (e.g., crush injury with closed fracture).

Using this classification system for closed fractures helps one to be aware of the potentially serious complications of closed injuries (Table 18.2).

TABLE 18.2	Tscherne and Oestern Classification of Soft-tissue Injuries		
Grade	Soft-tissue Injury (Superficial)	Soft-tissue Injury (Deep)	Compartments
0	Absent or negligible	Absent or negligible	Soft and/or normal
1	Superficial abrasion	Contusion from within	Soft and/or normal
2	Deep contaminated abrasion	Significant contusion	Impending compartment syndrome
3	Crushed skin, subcutaneous avulsions	Crushed devitalized muscle	Compartment syndrome

18.3 FRACTURES—IMMOBILIZATION

The treatment of gross fracture dislocations is always difficult. Many physicians avoid reducing fractures due to a lack of experience or for fear of worsening the situation. Several aspects must be considered before reducing a fracture: distance to a hospital, ETA of ambulance/helicopter, the patient's hemodynamic situation, local procedures, the availability of and need for anesthesia, etc.

In my opinion, gross fracture distortions should be reduced as soon as possible for several reasons.

- Transport—it is extremely difficult to transport a patient with a 40-degree laterally displaced femur fracture. How do you place the patient on the stretcher/gurney? How do you support the unreduced limb during transport? Have you tried to airlift a patient in this position? Have you seen the inside of smaller rescue helicopters?

- Gross fracture deformities almost always have concomitant vascular and nerve injuries. Reduction of the fracture will often (but not always) alleviate the vessel and nerve injury somewhat.

- The longer the dislocation lasts, the greater the risk of ischemia and hypoxia to the damaged area.

So which reduction criteria should be considered when faced with a fracture/dislocation?

- Gross fracture dislocation and reduced/absent distal arterial pulses

- Worsening of swelling in a closed fracture with gross dislocation

- Continuous bleeding from an open fracture with gross dislocation despite arterial compression

- Gross fracture dislocation and falling blood pressure (hemorrhagic shock?)

I would strongly advise event physicians to consult with their local surgical units and request written guidelines for this specific form of care.

18.4 LUXATIONS, DISLOCATIONS

There are several matters to be considered here:

- Are anesthetics required?

- Does the athlete need a radiological examination before reduction is attempted?

- Does the athlete need a radiological examination after reduction?

- May the athlete return to play without a radiological examination?

- Should the athlete be sent immediately to a hospital or can he or she wait until after the event? Many athletes want to see the event to its conclusion even if they cannot participate themselves.

In certain situations, *luxations can be reduced immediately without anesthetic.*

- Finger DIP and PIP joint subluxations and luxations (Fig. 18.1). Immediate manual reduction is necessary and recommended. Afterwards, use tape to stabilize the finger to the neighboring finger (preferably a longer finger). Athlete consent should also be present before the reduction procedure. After reduction, palpate the bones for fracture signs. Apply ice to prevent swelling. Return to play—maybe, depending on the exclusion of a fracture, the level of pain, the range of motion, the sport, and the risk of exacerbation. Hospitalization—not necessary. Radiological examination is recommended.

- Toe DIP and PIP joints—as above

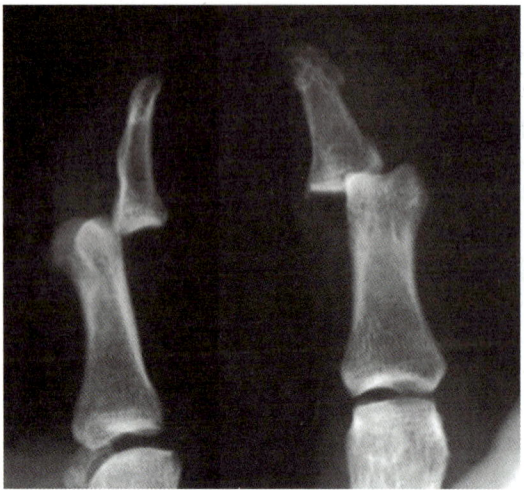

FIGURE 18.1.

- Mild grade 1 to 2 acromioclavicular joint subluxations (no manual reduction necessary). Use only tape to reduce the subluxation. After reduction, palpate the bones for fracture signs. Apply ice to prevent swelling. Return to play—maybe, depending on the exclusion of a fracture, the level of pain, the range of motion, the sport, and the risk of exacerbation. Immediate hospitalization—not necessary; the patient can wait. Radiological examination is recommended.

- Glenohumeral luxations. In some cases, an immediate reduction is possible without anesthetic (particularly if there is a history of previous luxation). Response time must be quick, and diagnosis must be confident and correct. Athlete consent should also be present: "Can I try, Jimmy? It will be painful but quick." After reduction, palpate the bones for fracture signs. Apply ICE principles and tape the shoulder to give support and prevent swelling. Return to play—no. Immediate hospitalization—not necessary; if there is no fracture, the patient can wait until after the event. Radiological examination is recommended.

- Patella luxation. As with glenohumeral dislocations above, immediate reduction can be considered with patient consent. After reduction, palpate the bones for fracture signs. Apply ICE principles and tape the patella to give support and prevent swelling. Return to play—doubtful. Immediate hospitalization—not necessary; the patient can wait. Radiological examination is recommended.

Luxations that Should Be Reduced as Soon as Possible with Anesthetic

- Most glenohumeral dislocations
- Elbow joint
- Hip joint
- Some patella dislocations
- Ankle joint

Recommended Reading:

Gustilo RB, Anderson JT. Prevention of infection in the treatment of one thousand and twenty-five open fractures of long bones: retrospective and prospective analyses [abstract]. *J Bone Joint Surg Am.* 1976;58(4):453–458.

Gustilo RB, Mendoza RM, Williams DN. Problems in the management of type III (severe) open fractures: a new classification of type III open fractures [abstract]. *J Trauma.* 1984;24(8):742–746.

Tscherne H, Oestern HJ. Pathophysiology and classification of soft tissue injuries associated with fractures. In: Tscherne H, Gotzen L, eds. *Fractures with Soft Tissue Injuries.* Berlin, Germany: Springer Verlag; 1984:1–9.

CHAPTER 19

Bursitis

Contributed by David McDonagh, Chair, FIBT Medical Committee

Reviewer: Richard Budgett, CMO, IOC Medical Committee, London 2012 Olympic Summer Games

There are a myriad of bursae in the body, and at times it is difficult to differentiate between a bursitis of traumatic or infective origin or a combination of both (Fig. 19.1). Here is a handy rule of thumb for the pathogenesis of the various bursal inflammations seen by an EP:

- Olecranon—usually traumatic but often infected

- Subacromial—always traumatic, often history of previous injury, often microtrauma

- Trochanter—often referred from the back or the hip

- Prepatellar—usually traumatic but occasionally infected

- Infrapatellar—usually traumatic but occasionally infected

- Runner's knee—usually due to overuse injury

- Jogger's knee—usually due to overuse injury

19.1 OLECRANON BURSITIS

This bursitis is usually caused by irritation (friction) or by a mild trauma to the point of the elbow. Swelling can come rather quickly and has a tendency to increase after a few days, thus stretching the covering skin and thereby increasing the risk of bacterial infection. If there is a skin puncture or penetrating wound, then that risk is further increased. It is important to consider the potential presence of these bacterial agents when choosing medication therapy, antibiotics, or NSAIDS. The possible presence of an infection should also rule out steroid injection treatment.

Treatment

If the athlete presents with a 1-day-old swelling, then I usually prescribe NSAIDS and a tight compressing bandage. I also inform the athlete of the risk of infection occurring within some days and of the need for a new appointment. The temptation to aspirate the bursa should be resisted, particularly if an infection is present as swellings often return and one risks introducing bacteria into these periarticular structures. I usually wait until the swellings are fairly large—strawberry size, approaching 4 cm—before aspirating. Unaspirated lesions can take many months before they resolve. Protective elbow pads can be worn during sporting activity.

19.2 SUBACROMIAL BURSITIS

This painful phenomenon is almost always associated with some form of supraspinatus pathology and leads to impingement symptoms and is almost always associated with previous trauma or microtrauma. See Chapter 51

19.3 TROCHANTER BURSITIS

This condition can be a primary condition, but is often secondary to pathological processes in the back or in the hip. Trochanter bursitis can cause discomfort at rest leading to sleeping difficulties. It is often challenging to investigate the underlying cause of the lesion (if there is one) and medication is often required by the athlete.

Clinical findings: Palpation of tenderness over the trochanter. The actual site of tenderness may

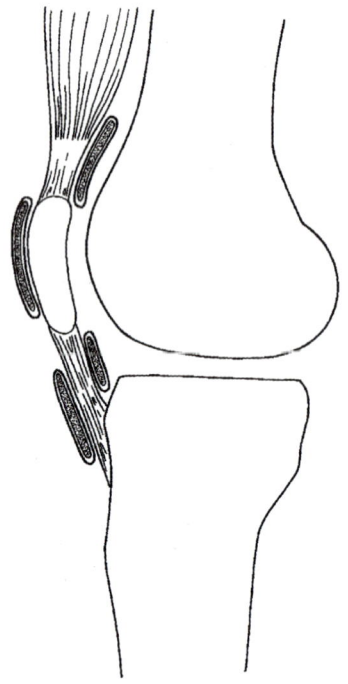

FIGURE 19.1. Bursa of the knee.

vary somewhat from slightly in front of, on top of, or slightly posterior to the trochanter. The more posterior the discomfort, the more one approaches the piriformis and sciatic area, so one may have to reconsider one's diagnosis with posterior trochanter lesions.

Treatment: RICE principles and NSAIDs may be attempted but do not always help. The athlete may benefit from sleeping on a softer bed or putting a pillow under the trochanter. Hydrocortisone combined with lignocaine injections can be effective and may give symptomatic relief. There is a relatively small risk of complication in this area but one should endeavor to diagnose and treat any underlying conditions, if any.

19.4 JOGGER'S KNEE—DISTAL ILIOTIBIAL BAND SYNDROME

Jogger's knee is characterized by pain or aching on the lateral aspect of the knee where the iliotibial band lies over the lateral femoral condyle and down to its attachment on the proximal tibia. Symptoms are usually more pronounced during or after a run. Repetitive knee flexion and extension causes irritation as

the iliotibial band rubs over the lateral femoral condyle. Contributing factors are genu varum, subtalar joint pronation, anisomelia, and running on an uneven surface where one leg is constantly higher than the other, for example, running up a hill at an angle. When presented with an acute situation, it is difficult to recommend treatment that will definitely remove discomfort in the short term. Treatment is more about correction of the contributing factors and reducing tightness in the iliotibial band. Gentle massage may help, as may gentle stretching exercises, a decrease in training, correction of training errors, a shortening of the stride, or the use of insoles or shoes that limit pronation. NSAIDS in the acute phase may or may not help. Icing may have some limited effect. For chronic or prolonged acute conditions, corticosteroid injections behind the band may have some effect, though in the initial acute phase, this may be a contentious form of treatment. When insoles are required then there is usually a period of adaptation before improvement.

19.5 PREPATELLAR BURSITIS

Usually caused by repetitive local friction, the "Washerwoman's" knee arises over the front of the patella. The bursa may swell considerably and cause pain on knee flexion, during activity, but also at rest if very swollen. As with other bursitis, it is usually reddish in color, warm, and tender. The amount of fluctuation depends on the amount of fluid in the bursa. The condition is not very common in sport, although sometimes wrestlers may be bothered, as well as athletes who receive direct blows or falls on the knee, such as footballers, basketball players, motorbike riders. It is more commonly seen in the workforce in tilers, plumbers, roofers, etc. Prepatellar bursitis is sometimes seen with an underlying rheumatoid arthritis or gout. If there is bone tenderness after trauma then x-rays should be taken to exclude a patella fracture.

Treatment is again based on the PRICES principles: Protect; Rest (until the bursitis has gone); Ice (for 20 minutes several times daily); Compression (gentle compression may help); Elevation; Support (with kneepads). Medication: NSAIDS may give relief. Antibiotics are indicated if there are signs of infection. I rarely, if ever, needle aspirate these bursae and have not been placed in the position where an athlete needed to have it done before a competition. Think twice before aspirating if the athlete is participating outdoors. Steroid injections can be effective but should be conducted in a sterile environment by an experienced practitioner.

19.6 POSTERIOR HEEL BURSITIS

This condition is usually caused by the prolonged use of tight or ill-fitting boots or shoes and can occur in prolonged walking or skiing sports, as well as in ice skating. Treatment is based on icing, NSAIDS, padding, and shoe wear adaptation.

CHAPTER 20

Injuries and Illnesses that Require Treatment on the Field of Play

Contributed by David McDonagh, Secretary, AIBA Medical Commission

Irrespective of how much time has passed since the time of injury, trauma care must start as soon as the patient arrives under your care. By doing so, an EP save lives, prevent complications and disability, and save careers.

Obviously, the most basic task for an EP is to provide emergency lifesaving treatment and hopefully prevent death by trauma or acute illness. Here are some basic emergency care principles:

- Examine, diagnose, and treat life-threatening complications of trauma as soon as the patient comes under your care.

- Use the simplest treatment possible to stabilize the patient's condition.

- Perform a complete, thorough examination of the patient to ensure that no other injuries are missed.

- Constantly reassess the patient for response to treatment, if the patient's condition deteriorates, reassess the patient.

- Start definitive treatment only after the patient is stable.

- When definitive treatment is not available locally, transfer the patient to another center.

Trauma deaths occur in three time periods:

- *Immediate deaths*: Patients who do not reach the hospital alive die from overwhelming injuries, including rupture of the heart or pulmonary artery, overwhelming hemorrhage, or massive destruction of brain or other neural tissue.

- *Early deaths*: Patients who arrive alive at the hospital need immediate resuscitation to survive. Many deaths in the early time period are preventable with appropriate early diagnosis and treatment of severe life-threatening injuries such as pneumothorax, flail chest, and abdominal hemorrhage.

- *Late deaths*: Late deaths occur as a result of infection and multiple organ failure.

Appropriate initial care can prevent late complications and death.

The successful management of severe trauma is dependent on the following six steps:

- Triage

- Primary survey + resuscitation

- Secondary survey

- Stabilization

- Transfer

- Definitive care

Start resuscitation at the same time as making the primary survey.

- Do not start the secondary survey until you have completed the primary survey.

- Do not start definitive treatment until the secondary survey is complete.

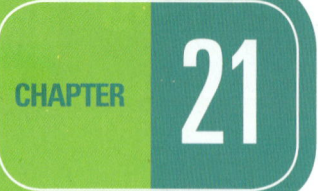
Airways, Oxygenation, and Ventilation

Contributed by Johan Arnt Hegvik, Anesthetics Department; and David McDonagh, Emergency Department, St. Olavs University Hospital, Trondheim, Norway

Reviewer: Ian Cohen, Sports Physician, Assistant Professor, University of Toronto, Canada

21.1 AIRWAY MAINTENANCE (WITH CERVICAL SPINE PROTECTION)

As we all know, the A in ABC (or CAB after 2010) has now been expanded to include cervical spine protection as the technique used in repositioning the head and neck to the neutral anatomical (inline) position also facilitates in opening the airway. To stabilize the neck takes usually only a few seconds longer so, in most situations, one can stabilize the neck before proceeding to airway management. In the event of this not being possible, airway management should be prioritized over cervical immobilization.

- Firstly, the airway must be inspected for patency. To do this, you must perform a chin lift or jaw thrust, always supporting the head and neck to protect the spinal cord.

- Having inspected the airway, remove any foreign bodies. These may include vomitus, mouth guards, dental implants, teeth, etc.

- Insert an oropharyngeal or nasopharyngeal airway.

- Initiate high-concentration oxygen therapy with equipment that allows maximum oxygen concentration.

- Ensure that the patient is ventilating adequately. If not, assisted ventilation may be necessary—either by mouth-to-mouth (MTM) or by bag and mask. If a pneumothorax is present, this should be decompressed. An open pneumothorax should be bandaged in such a way as to avoid the buildup of pressure under the bandage (and thus potentially cause a tension pneumothorax). Bandages can be taped on three sides, leaving the fourth side untaped.

- Apply a cervical collar.

21.2 WHEN TO INTUBATE

Indication: Intubation should be considered when inadequate oxygenation or ventilation is not corrected by mask or nasal ventilation with oxygen.

Signs of inadequate oxygenation include

- Observed cyanosis

- Lowered oxygen saturation measured on a pulse oximeter indicating inadequate oxygenation

- Abnormal respiratory rate (<12 or more than 20 respirations per minute)

- Auscultation revealing reduced or absent breath sounds

Inadequate ventilation can occur if there is

- A nonpatent airway, (swollen, inflamed, or injured airway)

- Inadequate chest wall expansion

- Asymmetrical chest wall expansion (flail chest, pneumothorax, tension pneumothorax, hemothorax)

- A foreign body in the airways

- Airway damage (e.g., oropharyngeal bleeding, fracture of the larynx)

- Chest wall damage (rib fractures)

- Diaphragmatic damage (penetrating injury)

- Pneumothorax or tension pneumothorax
- Spinal cord injury with reduced intercostal and diaphragmatic muscle function
- Cerebral injury with abnormal respiration patterns

Intubation Contraindications

None, if there is serious and increasing hypoxemia.

In cases of severe airway trauma or obstruction, safe intubation may not be possible. Emergency cricothyroidotomy is indicated in such cases. Extreme care is also needed when intubating a patient with an existing or potential spinal injury.

Preparation

Do you have to intubate?

- Probably, if there is increasing and life-threatening hypoxemia or hypercapnia
- If ventilation and oxygenation via bag and mask are not improving the patient's condition
- If there is severe airway trauma or obstruction, then emergency cricothyroidotomy may be a better option

Equipment

- An experienced assistant—plan what to do and how
- Pulse oximeter—to observe a fall in O_2 saturation
- End-tidal CO_2 detector device—to be connected immediately after intubation, to ensure that the tube is in the trachea and not the esophagus, later, to correct the ventilation (frequency or tidal volume)
- Suction unit—test before use
- Tongue depressor–C—choose the right size
- Mask and bag connected to an oxygen source—test before use
- Laryngoscope—choose correct blade and check both bulb and battery before you start
- Tracheal tube with cuff—choose the correct size and test before use (7.0 mm can be used on most adults; for children, a quick rule of thumb is to measure the circumference of the child's fifth fingertip or nostril and use a similar-dimensioned tube)
- Syringe to inflate the tracheal tube cuff

- Introducer and a sterile lubricant—install the lubricated introducer into the tracheal tube before you start
- Magill forceps
- Oxygen source
- Precut tape to secure the tracheal tube after intubation

Backup

- Laryngeal mask
- Emergency cricothyroidotomy set

21.3 OXYGEN ADMINISTRATION AND VENTILATION

Oxygen should be delivered at a rate of 10 to 15 L/min. If using a facial mask, it is important that the mask sits snugly on the patient. A pulse oximeter is extremely useful in monitoring the level of oxygen saturation. A value of 95% or more would imply that there is adequate oxygenation. Values of 94% or less would imply that the patient is not receiving enough oxygen. Incorrect values can occur in anemic or severely hypothermic patients.

Remember, oxygen is explosive, so beware when taking oxygen tanks into areas where there is a fire or a risk of explosion.

Mask Ventilation

Place a correctly sized facemask over the patient's mouth and nose. Remember the adage: "Left hand, mask; right hand, bag." The patient should be in the sniffing position (unless spinal injury dictates otherwise). Using the left hand, apply the jaw thrust: Lift the mandible anteriorly to open the airway using your fourth and fifth fingers, whilst using the thumb and index finger to hold the mask in place. Compress the bag with the right hand. The chest should expand with each breath. If chest expansion is not optimal, try repositioning the mask and try again. If this does not help, try inserting an oral tongue suppressor.

Direct Laryngoscopy

If mask ventilation is not giving adequate oxygenation or ventilation, recheck the airway and apply suction. Place the patient in the sniffing position. Ensure that all materials are assembled and close at hand. If there is time and if the patient is awake, then try to anesthetize the mucosa by dripping Xylocaine 2%, from a syringe into the oropharynx. Now, there are two main options:

- The first is to insert the orotracheal tube without any more medications or light sedation. As soon as the tube is in the trachea, the patient should receive a strong sedative, analgesia, and a muscle relaxant.

- The second is to give the analgesia, sedative, and muscle relaxant (in this order), then wait until the patient is fully relaxed and insert the tube.

In both situations, we have to be prepared to handle hypotension.

Hold the laryngoscope in the left hand. Open the patient's mouth with the right hand and insert the blade, being careful not to break a tooth. Pass the blade to the right of the tongue and advance the blade into the hypopharynx, pushing the tongue to the left. Lift the laryngoscope upward and forward, without changing the angle of the blade, to expose the vocal cords.

Insert the orotracheal tube between the vocal cords and advance the tube 2 cm further into the trachea. If the patient is not sleeping well, he or she must receive further sedation/analgesia. If the tracheal tube is correctly placed in the trachea, the patient can be given a long-acting muscle relaxant as well.

Inflate the cuff, connect the oxygen device, and give the patient some breaths. Connect the end-tidal CO_2 detector device to ensure that the tube is in the trachea/airway and not in the esophagus. Listen over both lungs as well as over the epigastrium to ensure that the tube is in the trachea and not in one of the bronchi or in the esophagus. Ensure that the end-tidal CO_2 device demonstrates the presence of CO_2 (you now know that the tube is in the airway).

Secure the placement of the tube with precut tape. Watch for desaturation and hypotension and be prepared to treat these conditions.

21.4 EMERGENCY CRICOTHYROIDOTOMY

In the event of a mask ventilation failing to give adequate ventilation and where endotracheal intubation is not possible (due to airway obstruction or damage), emergency cricothyroidotomy will have to be performed. There are two techniques available, the standard surgical (optimal) approach and the percutaneous dilation method. The operator should use the technique with which he or she is more experienced. Be aware, performing a cricothyroidotomy on a patient with a thyroid or cricoid cartilage, or laryngeal fracture injury may worsen the injury.

Surgical Cricothyroidotomy

- Gently hyperextend the neck taking care not to damage the spine.

- Identify the space/groove between the cricoid and thyroid cartilages.

- Clean and infiltrate this area with local anesthetic.

- Make a vertical incision 1.5 cm long and dissect down to the membrane between the cricoid and thyroid cartilages (Fig. 21.1).

- Cut through this membrane and rotate the blade 90 degrees and insert a curved artery forceps.

- Remove the blade and open the forceps, thus widening the space between the cricoid and thyroid cartilages.

- Pass a 4- to 6-mm endotracheal tube into the trachea (if the space is very small, a nasogastric tube can be used).

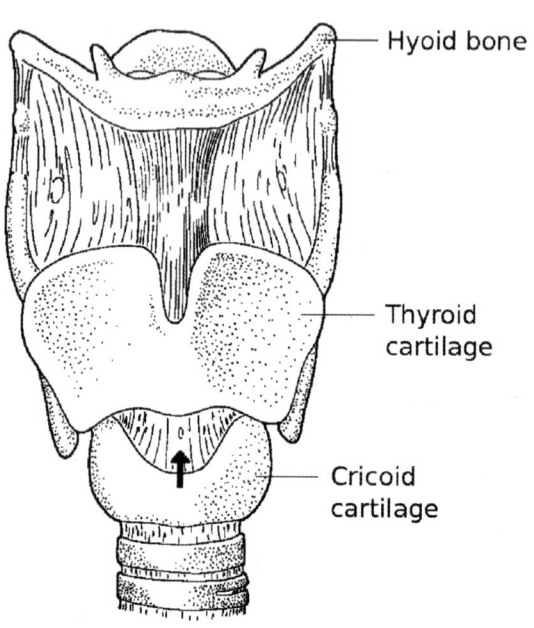

Hyoid bone

Thyroid cartilage

Cricoid cartilage

FIGURE 21.1. Bony anatomy of the cricothyroid region.

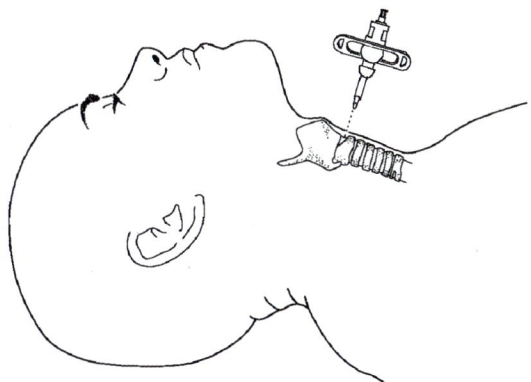

FIGURE 21.2. Insertion site for needle cricothyroidotomy.

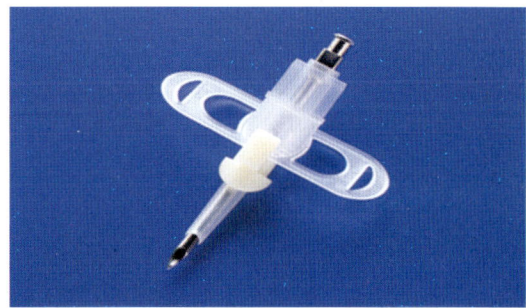

FIGURE 21.4. Trocar with needle.

- Palpate the space between the cricoid and thyroid cartilages (Fig. 21.1).

- Stabilize the larynx and trachea with one hand.

- With the other hand, insert the cricothyroid needle with trocar into this space, penetrating the cricothyroid membrane (Figs. 21.2, 21.3, and 21.4).

- Once in the trachea, with the syringe attached, aspirate air from the trachea.

- Once air is aspirated, push the needle and trocar approximately 1 cm further into the trachea.

- Remove the inner needle, leaving the trocar in place.

- Secure the trocar with tape to avoid movement— avoid bending or kinking the trocar.

- Attach an oxygen delivery tube to the hub of the trocar, being careful not to displace the trocar.

Needle Cricothyroidotomy

Both forms of cricothyroidotomy may allow for emergency oxygenation of the lungs, which may or may not be adequate. The amount of oxygen that can be given through the needle trocar is obviously less than the amount that can be given through an endotracheal tube. Patients need to be urgently transferred to hospital. Marked rises in $PaCO_2$ may occur due to inadequate exhalation of CO_2.

A computer-based simulation is available on the Ethernet—look up the National Capital Area Medical Simulation Center, Cricothyroidotomy.

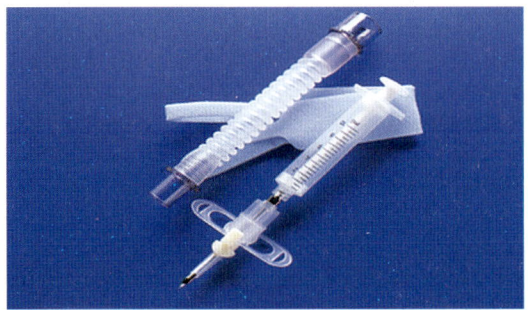

FIGURE 21.3. Trocar with needle, syringe and oxygen delivery tube.

CHAPTER 22

CPR—Practical Issues and Updates

Contributed by Gary Mak, Consultant Cardiologist, Hong Kong Sports Institute, Hong Kong

Reviewers: Fabio Pigozzi, Professor, University of Rome "Foro Italico," and President, FIMS, Rome, Italy; and Johan-Arnt Hegvik, NTNU, Trondheim, Norway

Note from the book editor, David McDonagh:
When describing CPR guidelines, one must always refer to up-to-date best practice–based principles. These are usually supplied by the American Heart Association or the European Resuscitation Council and are under constant review and development. New guidelines are produced regularly and one should be aware of changes. Hopefully, all national guidelines should be based on these best practice principles. As an EP, you should follow your own national guidelines and hope that these are updated to accepted international standards.

The chapter below describes the accepted guidelines for 2010.

I am aware of the fact that AEDs are expensive and not readily available in all parts of the world. Another question altogether is if a state with limited resources should invest such large sums in AEDs when other issues may be more pressing. Fortunately, I am not a politician. My advice here is that if at all possible ensure that AEDs are present at a sporting event. If impossible, for whatever reason, then you must have a procedure in place that compensates, however inadequately, for this lack of accepted equipment and, not least, have trained staff adequately to perform optimal resuscitation based on the circumstances. It is one thing to have inadequate equipment; it is something completely different to be inadequately trained in your local procedures. Staff must be trained to supply optimal treatment for athletes, coaches, staff, guests, and spectators.

If you do not have an AED, then you should open the mouth, remove foreign bodies, and supply CPR (30 compressions then two breaths) with cardiac massage at a rate of a minimum of 100 compressions per minute, at a depth of a minimum of 5 cm

(2 in.) until a defibrillator is available, be that in the ambulance, medical room, or hospital.

Nontraumatic sporting cardiac arrests are usually cardiovascular in origin. Sudden cardiac arrest (SCA) in athletes is fortunately uncommon but still potentially catastrophic. SCA is usually associated with congenital or structural abnormalities in younger athletes (<35 years), whereas coronary artery disease is a more common cause in those 35 years and above.

Ventricular fibrillation (VF) is the most common arrhythmia found in victims of nontraumatic SCA in athletes. Resuscitation is most successful if defibrillation is performed as soon as possible and within 5 minutes after collapse; however, successful resuscitation is less likely once the rhythm deteriorates into asystole. As successful resuscitation is dependent on early CPR and defibrillation, all sporting venues should consider having defibrillators and trained staff present at sporting events.

22.1 DEFIBRILLATION PLUS CPR: A CRITICAL COMBINATION

Treatment of VF-induced SCA requires early CPR and shock delivery with a defibrillator. High-quality bystander CPR can double or triple survival rates from cardiac arrest. CPR should be provided until an automated external defibrillator (AED) or manual defibrillator is available. Recent guidelines (American Heart Association, http://www.americanheart.org/; or European Resuscitation Council, http://www.erc.edu/) recommend integrated CPR and AED use.

The ILCOR "Chain of Survival" is attached below (Fig. 22.1). All EPs, coaches and trainers

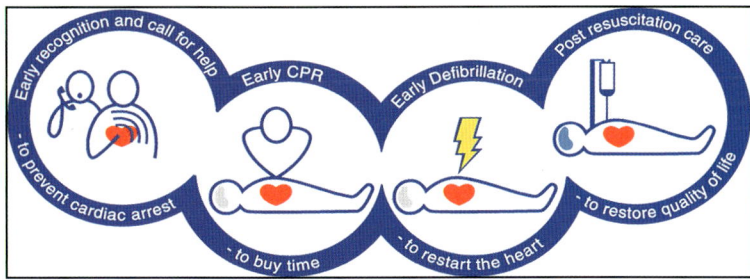

FIGURE 22.1.   ILCOR Chain of Survival, 2010.

should be trained to provide effective CPR and defibrillation with AEDs.

22.2 2010 GUIDELINES UPDATES

Both the American Heart Association Guidelines for Cardiopulmonary Resuscitation and Emergency Cardiovascular Care and the European Resuscitation Council Guidelines for Resuscitation focused on the improved delivery of lifesaving CPR. The simplified adult BLS algorithm (Fig. 22.2) and the algorithm for adult BLS healthcare providers (Fig. 22.3) can be seen. For updates, please visit the American Heart Association's Web site at http://www.americanheart.org/, or the European Resuscitation Council's Web site at http://www.erc.edu/.

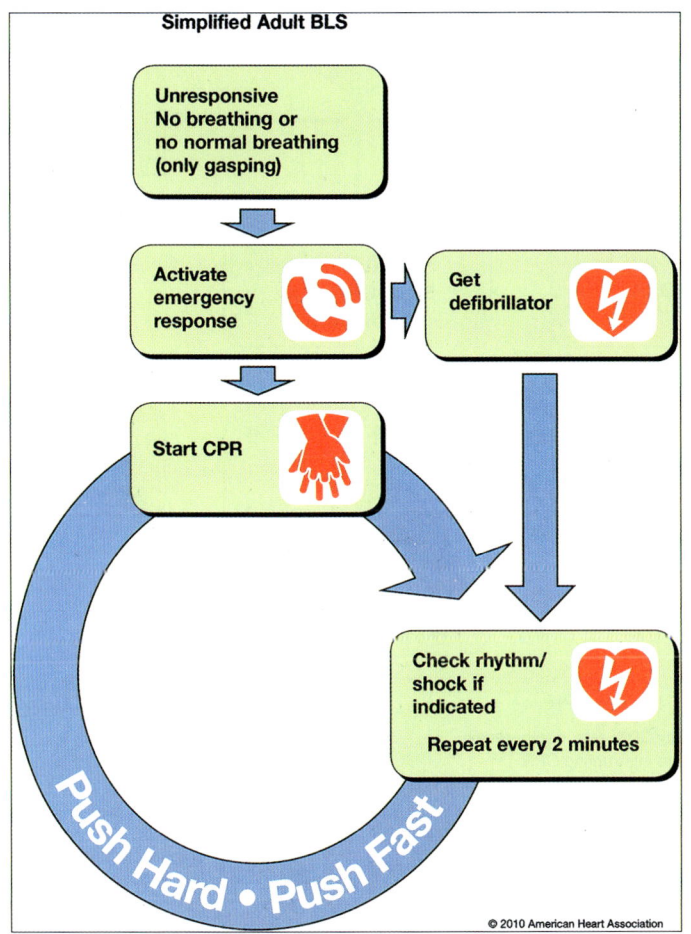

FIGURE 22.2.   Simplified adult BLS algorithm.

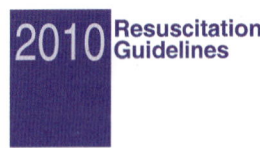

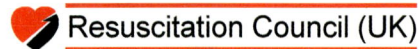

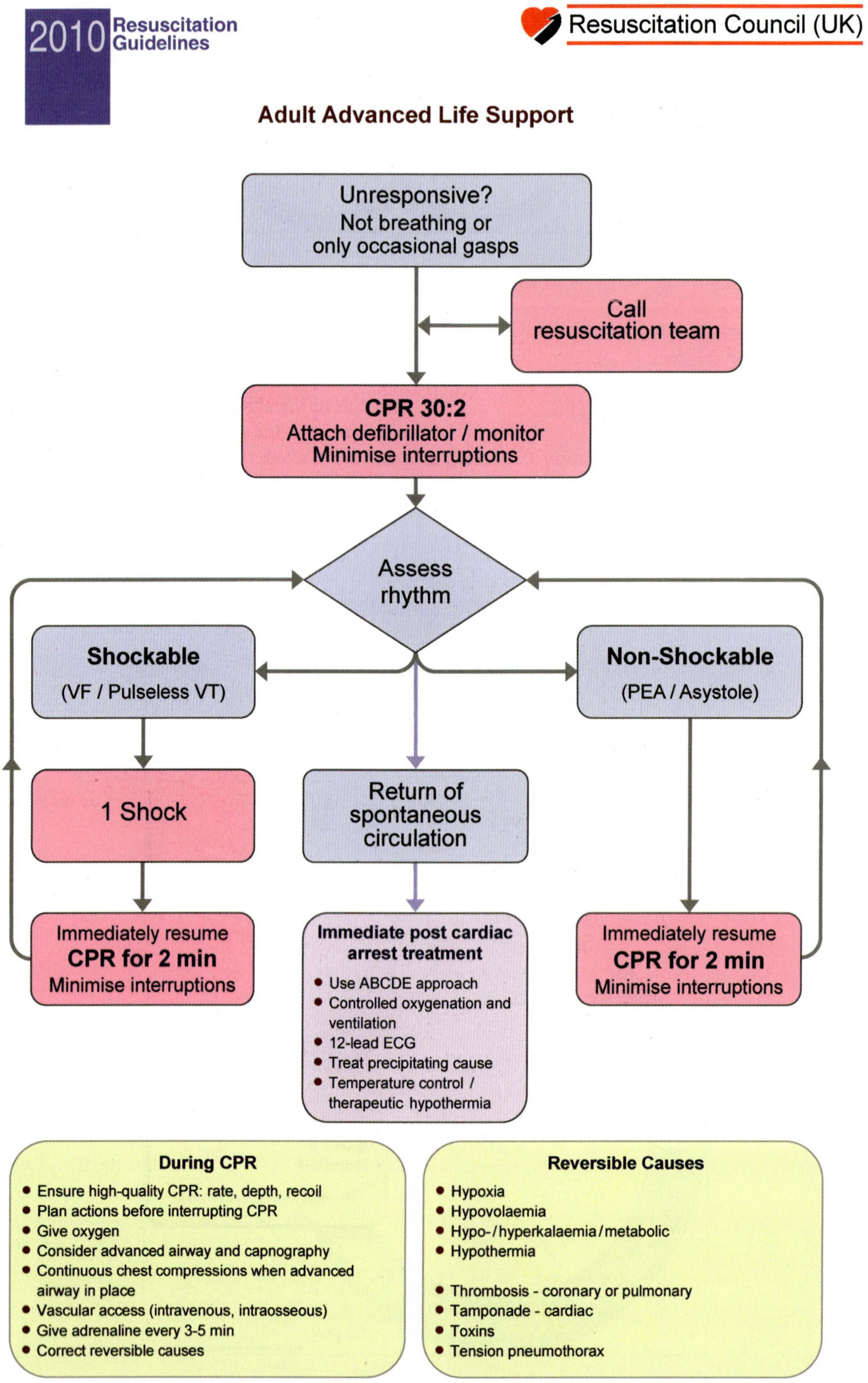
2010 Resuscitation Guidelines
Resuscitation Council (UK)
Adult Advanced Life Support
Unresponsive?
Not breathing or
only occasional gasps
Call
resuscitation team
CPR 30:2
Attach defibrillator / monitor
Minimise interruptions
Assess
rhythm
Shockable
(VF / Pulseless VT)
Non-Shockable
(PEA / Asystole)
1 Shock
Return of
spontaneous
circulation
Immediately resume
CPR for 2 min
Minimise interruptions
Immediate post cardiac
arrest treatment
• Use ABCDE approach
• Controlled oxygenation and ventilation
• 12-lead ECG
• Treat precipitating cause
• Temperature control / therapeutic hypothermia
Immediately resume
CPR for 2 min
Minimise interruptions
During CPR
• Ensure high-quality CPR: rate, depth, recoil
• Plan actions before interrupting CPR
• Give oxygen
• Consider advanced airway and capnography
• Continuous chest compressions when advanced airway in place
• Vascular access (intravenous, intraosseous)
• Give adrenaline every 3-5 min
• Correct reversible causes
Reversible Causes
• Hypoxia
• Hypovolaemia
• Hypo-/hyperkalaemia/metabolic
• Hypothermia
• Thrombosis - coronary or pulmonary
• Tamponade - cardiac
• Toxins
• Tension pneumothorax

FIGURE 22.3. ALS algorithm.

1. Immediate delivery of effective chest compressions

   Immediate recognition of cardiac arrest is essential. If a patient is unresponsive or there are absent or "gasping" breaths, immediately apply rhythmic compression pressure over the lower half of the sternum, thus increasing intrathoracic pressure and directly compressing the heart to create blood flow. Blood flow generated by chest compressions may deliver a small but critical amount of oxygen and substrate to the brain and myocardium. "Look, Listen, and Feel" have been removed from the BLA algorithm.

The key elements of effective CPR are:

- Do not waste time whilst performing the primary survey. Use <10 seconds to ascertain the presence or absence of normal breathing.

- If the patient has an open airway and is unresponsive, or if there is absent or occasional gasping breathing, initiate CPR.

  It may be difficult to accurately determine the presence or absence of adequate or normal breathing in unresponsive victims. This may be because the airway is not open or because the patient has only occasional gasps (which are not necessarily adequate ventilation). The EP should treat the victim who has occasional gasps as if he or she is not breathing. This means initiating adult basic life support/automated external defibrillation (ADBS/AED).

- The 2010 AHA Guidelines for CPR and ECC also deemphasize the pulse check as a mechanism to identify cardiac arrest. Healthcare providers may have difficulty in finding a pulse and this activity may use up valuable time. There is no evidence, however, that checking for breathing, coughing, or movement is superior for detection of circulation. To avoid delays in chest compressions, the event physician should take no more than 10 seconds to check for a pulse; and if this is not found, start chest compressions.

- Push hard and push fast at a rate of at least 100 compressions per minute with adequate depth (at least 5 cm—2 in.).

- Allow full chest recoil with equal compression and relaxation times.

- Minimize interruptions in chest compressions to 10 seconds or less (e.g., for shocks).

- Change the person compressing every 2 minutes or after five cycles of 30:2.

2. A universal 30:2 compression-to-ventilation ratio for all victims to provide longer periods of uninterrupted chest compressions

3. A sequence change to chest compressions rather than rescue breaths is recommended (CAB rather than ABC)

4. 1-second rescue breaths with sufficient volume to achieve visible chest rise and to avoid hyperventilation

5. When AED is available, the rescuer should give one shock followed by immediate CPR for VF cardiac arrest (no "stacked" shocks). As the rhythm analysis by current AEDs after each shock typically results in substantial interruptions of chest compressions, rescuers should not check the rhythm or pulse immediately after shock delivery. There is a continued deemphasis on pulse check. They should immediately resume CPR, beginning with chest compressions, and should check the rhythm after five cycles (or about 2 minutes) of CPR.

6. Current guidelines extended the use of AEDs for children aged 1 year or older.

New Recommendation: Hands-only CPR

The outcome of chest compressions without ventilation is significantly better than no CPR for adult cardiac arrest. Studies of adults with cardiac arrest treated by lay rescuers have shown similar survival rates among victims receiving hands-only CPR versus conventional CPR with rescue breaths. Animal studies and extrapolation from clinical evidence suggest that rescue breathing is not essential during the first 5 minutes of adult CPR for VF SCA. If the airway is open, occasional gasps and passive chest recoil may provide some air exchange. In addition, a low minute ventilation may be all that is necessary to maintain a normal ventilation–perfusion ratio during CPR.[1] At some stage, supplementary oxygen with assisted ventilation is necessary; however, the precise length of time is not known at this time.

These new guidelines were supported by both the ERC and the UK Resuscitation Council with the goal of increasing the rate of bystander CPR.

Simple barrier devices, such as pocket masks, increase the public acceptability of mouth-to-mouth (MTM) ventilation. MTM ventilation is preferred to nose-to-mouth ventilation. These devices are quite cheap and portable.

Lay Rescuer AED Programs

AEDs are sophisticated, reliable computerized devices that use voice and visual prompts to guide lay rescuers and health care providers to safely defibrillate VF SCA. Since 1995, the AHA has recommended the development of lay rescuer AED programs. As the improvement in survival rates in AED programs is affected by the time to CPR and to defibrillation, sites that deploy AEDs should establish a response plan, train likely responders in CPR and AED usage, maintain equipment, and coordinate with local EMS units. (See Fig. 22.2 for lay rescuer BLS algorithm.)

An event physician who has regular contact with a particular team or arena should develop a local AED program to prepare for this type of emergency.

Induced Hypothermia

About 60% of cardiac arrest survivors regain consciousness; of these, one-third experience irreversible cognitive disabilities due to anoxic brain injury. Mild hypothermia is thought to suppress many of the chemical reactions associated with reperfusion injury. Despite these potential advantages, hypothermia can also produce adverse effects, including arrhythmias, infection, and coagulopathy.

Induced hypothermia (cooling within minutes to hours after return of spontaneous circulation [ROSC]) has been shown, in two randomized clinical trials, to improve outcome in adults who remained comatose after initial resuscitation from out-of-hospital VF cardiac arrest. Recent reports from other centers have reproduced similar results.

The 2003 ILCOR Advisory Statement on Therapeutic Hypothermia after Cardiac Arrest, recommends initiating cooling to a target core temperature of 32°C to 34°C within 6 hours in selected unconscious adult patients with return of spontaneous circulation after out-of-hospital VF cardiac arrest.

According to ERC, inducing hypothermia is "safe and effective even if there is lack of experience (in performing induced hypothermia)."

In the field, when there is an ROSC and the survivor remained unconscious, one should start with simple external cooling methods. These techniques include the use of cooling blankets; application of ice packs (partially filled with water) or even chilled soft drink cans to the groin, axillae, and neck, using a protective cotton or flannel sheet barrier to minimize frostbite injury; use of wet towels and fanning; and use of a cooling helmet. If there is expected delay before retrieval, one should also start chilling using an intravenous crystalloid solution at 4°C and infuse at a rate of 30 mL/kg of body weight over 30 minutes. This has been showed to reduce core temperature significantly and does not cause pulmonary edema.

Core body temperature (e.g., rectal temperature) should be monitored and maintained in the range of 32°C to 34°C. Excessive cooling below 32°C is likely to *increase* the incidence of complications such as arrhythmias, infection, and coagulopathy.

The development of shivering during cooling leads often to core warming and will increase overall oxygen consumption. In experienced hands, shivering may be prevented by an anesthesiologist by using a neuromuscular blocker (e.g., pancuronium, 0.1 mg/kg every 2 hours for a total of 32 hours) and sedation (e.g., midazolam, 0.125 mg/kg of body weight per hour, and fentanyl, 0.002 mg/kg/h).

22.3 CONCLUSION

To rescue SCA victims, the need for "effective" CPR—push hard, push fast (100 compressions per minute—followed by two rescue breaths); allow complete chest recoil; and minimize interruptions in chest compressions—is essential. Whenever defibrillation is attempted, rescuers must coordinate proper CPR with defibrillation to minimize interruptions in chest compressions (no longer than 10 seconds) and to ensure immediate resumption of chest compressions after shock delivery. Compression-only CPR is recommended to untrained or unwilling laypersons. For unconscious survivors with return of spontaneous circulation, early induction of hypothermia would help to improve outcome. Well-planned and organized lay rescuer AED programs are essential for a successful resuscitation of the unfortunate athlete.

Remember, there may be other reversible conditions present, which, if detected and treated, will have a dramatic effect on patient survival—the 4Hs and 4Ts are

- Hypoxia, hypovolemia, hypokalemia/hyperkalemia/metabolic conditions, hypothermia

- Thrombosis, tamponade (cardiac), toxins, tension pneumothorax

Recommended Reading

www.erc.edu European Resuscitation Council. Guidelines developed by Europeans and have been written with European practice in mind

http://circ.ahajournals.org/cgi/content/full/122/18_suppl_3/S685 - B121#B121

Bernd W Böttiger et al. Number needed to treat = six: therapeutic hypothermia following cardiac arrest—an effective and cheap approach to save lives. *Crit Care.* 2007;11:162.

Feld JM, Hazinski MF, Sayre MR, et al. 2010 American Heart Association guidelines for cardiopulmonary resuscitation and emergency cardiovascular care science. *Circulation.* 2010;122(18)(suppl 3):S640–S933.

International Liaison Committee on Resuscitation. Consensus on science and treatment recommendations. *Resuscitation.* 2005;67(2–3):181–314.

Nolan JP, Morley PT, Vanden Hoek TL, et al. Therapeutic hypothermia after cardiac arrest: an Advisory Statement by the Advanced Life Support Task Force of the International Liaison Committee on Resuscitation. *Circulation.* 2003;108:118–121.

Sayre MR, Berg RA, Cave DM, Page RL, Potts J, White RD. Hands-only (compression-only) cardiopulmonary resuscitation: a call to action for bystander response to adults who experience out-of-hospital sudden cardiac arrest: a science advisory for the public from the American Heart Association Emergency Cardiovascular Care Committee. *Circulation.* 2008;117;2162–2167.

CHAPTER 23

Acute Anaphylactic Reactions

Contributed by David McDonagh, Secretary, AIBA Medical Commission

Reviewer: Sven Erik Gisvold, Professor of Anesthetics, St. Olavs University Hospital, NTNU, Trondheim, Norway

Anaphylaxis is characterized by the rapid development of life-threatening airway, breathing, and/or circulation problems usually associated with skin and mucosal changes. The European Academy of Allergology and Clinical Immunology Nomenclature Committee defines *anaphylaxis* as "a severe, life-threatening, generalized or systemic hypersensitivity reaction." The American College of Allergy, Asthma and Immunology Epidemiology of Anaphylaxis Working Group has concluded that the overall yearly frequency of episodes is a minimum of 30 cases per 100,000 persons.

Anaphylaxis can be triggered by a wide variety of substances, most commonly food (nuts, milk, fish, crustaceans, fruit), drugs (antibiotics, NSAIDS, aspirin, anesthetic drugs), and venoms (wasps, bees), and as many as 9% of sufferers may be exposed to recurrent anaphylactic reactions.

According to Pumphrey (*Clin Exp Allergy* 2000), fatal anaphylaxis can occur within minutes (usually intravenous medication), 10 to 15 minutes (insect stings), and after 30 to 35 minutes with food reactions, causing respiratory arrest.

23.1 CLINICAL FINDINGS

Always suspect anaphylaxis if an athlete who is exposed to a trigger becomes suddenly ill with rapidly progressing skin changes (flushing, urticaria, angioedema) and life-threatening airway, breathing, and/or circulation problems. The diagnosis can be supported by a positive history of recent allergen exposure.

- The patient: Is often anxious, feels and looks unwell

- May have neurological symptoms due to cerebral ischemia or anoxia (e.g., confusion, agitation, and loss of consciousness)

- Can also have vomiting and abdominal pain

- May react after several minutes—the speed of symptom debut often depending on the trigger

- May develop skin changes, often the first feature, present in over 80% of anaphylactic reactions

  - Skin changes may be subtle or dramatic and may involve mucosa, skin, or both
  - And may be erythematous—a patchy, or generalized, red rash
  - Or may be urticarial (pale, pink or red), with different shapes and sizes, can appear anywhere on the body, and are usually itchy
  - May have angioedema with swelling of deeper tissues, such as the eyelids, lips, and occasionally the mouth and throat.

  To make the diagnosis of anaphylaxis the patient may have one/any of the above.

- And one of the following three presentations: **Airways, respiratory, or circulatory**

  - Airway Findings—Swelling in the mouth and pharynx
    - Airway swelling with edema of the pharynx/larynx or tongue
    - Breathing or swallowing difficulty
    - Hoarseness
    - Stridor—a high-pitched inspiratory noise caused by upper airway obstruction

- Respiratory Findings (Lower Respiratory Tract)
  - Acute asthma-like findings—wheezing, prolonged expiration
  - Dyspnea and increased respiratory rate
  - Exhausted, tired patient
  - Confusion (cerebral hypoxia)
  - Cyanosis
  - Asthmatic findings
  - Respiratory arrest
  - Anaphylaxis can present with purely acute asthma findings without skin or circulatory features (is often triggered by food allergy)
- Circulatory Findings
  - Pale, clammy, dizzy, collapsed
  - Tachycardia initially, bradycardia in advanced stage
  - Hypotension
  - Decreased level of or loss of consciousness
  - Myocardial ischemia and angina (even if normal coronary arteries)
  - Cardiac arrest due to direct myocardial depression, vasodilation, and capillary fluid loss
  - Circulatory collapse may occasionally be the only finding in anaphylaxis, without other respiratory or cutaneous signs

Remember:

- Skin or mucosal changes alone are not a sign of an anaphylactic reaction
- Skin and mucosal changes can be subtle or absent in up to 20% of reactions

23.2 DIFFERENTIAL DIAGNOSIS

- Severe asthma—most often in children
- Septic shock—hypotension and a petechial or purpuric rash
- Vasovagal episode
- Panic attack—particularly those who have had a previous anaphylactic reaction
- Idiopathic (nonallergic) urticaria or angioedema

23.3 TREATMENT

- Early recognition of main problem—airway, breathing, circulation (ABCDE)
- An early call for help
- Clear the airways
- CPR if necessary

- Highest available oxygen concentration with mask and reservoir
- IV line and fluid immediately if hypotensive, pre-shock, or in shock—administer rapid IV fluid (20 mL/kg in a child or 500 to 1,000 mL in an adult): Use Ringer's lactate or acetate solution; sometimes large amounts of fluids are necessary due to excessive capillary leakage and vasodilation
- Medication—adrenalin.
  - Adrenalin is the drug of choice in all serious situations.
    - Intramuscular adrenalin: 1 mg/mL (0.1%)
    - Adults: 0.3 to 0.5 mg, depending on how serious the condition is
    - Children: 0.015 to 0.03 mL/kg or 0.15 to 0.3 mg for every 10 kg of body weight, depending again on the seriousness of the condition.
    - Give IM unless experienced with IV adrenalin.
    - Occasionally large amounts of adrenalin may be needed.
    - If IV access is established, dilute adrenalin to 0.1 mg per mL (9 mL saline + 1 mL adrenaline) and titrate IV 0.1 mg (= 1 mL of the diluted solution) as needed according to vital signs.
    - Infiltration adrenalin—if anaphylactic reaction is due to an insect bite or injection, infiltrate the site with 0.2 mL adrenalin 1 mg/mL.
- Other medications:
  - *If the patient has had a respiratory failure, follow the appropriate adrenalin treatment above and, once the patient's condition is more stabile, add*
    - Antihistamines, both H1—dexlorfeniramine 10 mg, IM, and—H2—ranitidine, 50 mg dissolved in 20 mL, slowly IV
    - Hydrocortisone 100 mg, IV over 30 seconds
  - If convulsions, IV or rectal diazepam: adults, 10 to 20 mg; children, 0.5 to 1 mg/kg
- Remove trigger if easily accessible and easily removed
- Depending on the seriousness of the situation, lie the patient on his or her back and elevate the legs if hypotensive
- Breathing but unconscious patients should be placed in the recovery position
- Some patients with milder airway and respiratory problems may wish to sit to facilitate breathing
- If the patient feels faint, do not sit or stand him or her up, as it is reported that this may instigate cardiac arrest

CHAPTER 24

Emergency Medications for Emergency Conditions

Contributed by David McDonagh, Chairman, FIBT Medical Committee

Reviewer: Sven Erik Gisvold, Professor or Anesthetics, St. Olavs University Hospital, Trondheim, Norway

Certain medications are an absolute necessity in an emergency bag. To be able to treat an acute asthmatic attack, a myocardial infarction, or an anaphylactic shock, as well as oxygen, you will need

- Adrenalin 1 mg/mL (0.1%), injectable
- Morphine 5 mg/mL, injectable
- Diazepam 5 mg/mL, injectable, or 10 mg, rectal suppository
- Glyceryl nitrate 0.25, sublingual tablets
- Hydrocortisone 100 mg, injectable
- Prednisolone 20 mg, tablets
- Salbutamol 5 mg per puff, pressure dose inhaler
- Ipratroprium 0.5 mg per puff, pressure dose inhaler
- Nebulizer
- Antiemetic
- Antihistamine tablets
- Dexclorfeniramine 10 mg/mL, injectable
- Ranitidine 50 mg, tablets, 30 seconds

Below, I have listed a series of treatment modalities for serious medical conditions. Routines and practices vary from country to country. Please check that these recommendations are in line with your national guidelines. The guidelines given below are based on those used in Norway and are based on the European Resuscitation Guidelines 2010 (http://www.erc.edu).

24.1 ACUTE LIFE-THREATENING OR SEVERE ASTHMATIC ATTACK

Diagnosis of a severe asthmatic attack in adults:

- Hunched forward
- Agitated or drowsy
- Exhausted, confused, or coma
- Wheeze is loud or absent
- Respiratory rate of 25 or more
- Heart rate of 110 or more
- Inability to complete sentences—talks only with a few words
- If you have the ability to measure PEF, the peak flow between 33% and 50% of best or predicted

The condition may deteriorate and patients may develop:

- $SpO_2 < 92\%$
- Silent chest
- Cyanosis
- Poor respiratory effort
- Bradycardia or hypotension
- Confusion or coma
- Peak flow <33% of expected or best
- Remember, anaphylaxis can present with asthma symptoms and findings only

Treatment (GINA Guidelines)

- Oxygen—enough to raise O_2 sat to 94% to 98%

- Beta-2 agonists—salbutamol 5 mg, preferably via a nebulizer and pressure dose inhaler

- Hydrocortisone, 100 mg IV over 30 seconds (alternatively IM, but with slower onset)
  - Or prednisolone—40 to 50 mg per os
  - If the situation is obviously very severe, adrenalin should be given as described under treatment of anaphylactic reactions

- Short-acting bronchodilator—ipratropium 0.5 mg, preferably via nebulizer and pressure dose inhaler; if you do not have a nebulizer, then inhale two to four puffs every 20 minutes; for a milder attack, two to four puffs every 3 to 4 hours

24.2 ACUTE CORONARY SYNDROMES

- Oxygen—Give supplementary oxygen (4 to 8 L/min) to all patients with arterial oxygen saturation <90% and/or pulmonary congestion.

- Oxygen should be given generously to all patients with suspected coronary syndrome/chest pain, not only those with desaturation and/or congestion. The goal is 94% to 98% O_2 sat

- Glyceryl nitrate is an effective treatment for ischemic chest pain. Glyceryl trinitrate may be considered if the systolic blood pressure is >90 mm Hg and the patient has ongoing ischemic chest pain. Glyceryl trinitrate can be useful in the treatment of acute pulmonary congestion. Glycerol trinitrate is *not* recommended with hypotension (systolic blood pressure ≤90 mm Hg), particularly if combined with bradycardia, nor in patients with inferior infarction and suspected right ventricular involvement. Use of nitrates under these circumstances may cause decrease in blood pressure and cardiac output.
  - If indicated, use either
    - Sublingual, 0.25 to 0.5 mg, repeat after 5 minutes if no effect
    - Mouth spray, 0.4 mg, repeat after 5 minutes if no effect
    - Isosorbide dinitrate tablet, 2.5 to 5 mg
- Morphine—analgesic of choice for nitrate-refractory pain; it may also benefit patients with pulmonary congestion. Give morphine in initial doses of 3 to 5 mg IV and repeat every few minutes until the patient is pain-free.

- Antiemetic—nausea is common during an infarction and also as a side effect of morphine

- Acetylsalicylic acid—several large, randomized controlled trials indicate decreased mortality when acetylsalicylic acid (ASA), 75 mg, 300 mg, or 325 mg, is given to patients in the hospital with ACS. Some studies suggest reduced mortality if ASA is given earlier. ASA should be given as soon as possible to all patients with suspected acute coronary syndromes unless the patient has a known ASA allergy. The initial dose of ASA to be chewed is 160 to 325 mg. Soluble IV ASA may be as effective.

24.3 ACUTE ANAPHYLACTIC REACTION

- Oxygen—usually atleast 10 L/min
- Intramuscular adrenalin 1 mg/mL (0.1%)
  - Adults: 0.3 to 0.5 mL, depending on how serious the condition is
  - Children: 0.015 to 0.03 mL/kg or 0.15 to 0.3 mL for every 10 kg of body weight, depending again on the seriousness of the condition

- Infiltration adrenalin—if due to insect bite or injection, infiltrate the site with 0.2 mL adrenalin 1 mg/mL

- IV Ringer's lactate, acetate, or NaCl

- *If respiratory failure as well, administer adrenalin first and once the patient is under control:*

- Antihistamines, both H1—dexclorfeniramine 10 mg, IM; and
  - H2—ranitidine, 50 mg dissolved in 20 mL, slowly IV
  - Hydrocortisone 100 mg, IV over 30 seconds
  - *If convulsions*:
  - IV or rectal diazepam: adults, 10 to 20 mg; children, 0.5 to 1 mg/kg

24.4 ACUTE EPILEPTIC ATTACK

Most seizures are self-limiting and treatment is supportive as described above. However, if the tonic–clonic phase of the seizure lasts longer than 5 minutes or if there are repeated seizures, then more active treatment is required. This will require urgent transfer to hospital.

Convulsions may hinder normal ventilation and these patients are often hypoxic and cyanotic during attacks.

Always check the airway first. Ensure the patency of the airway and then administer oxygen if available.

Without IV access:

- Rectal diazepam 10 to 20 mg, repeated after 15 minutes if needed, or

- Buccal midazolam 10 mg (not available in all countries)

With IV access:

- Diazepam IV 5 mg initially may be repeated with 2.5- to 5-mg increments

- Consider IV glucose (50 mL of 50% solution).

24.5 PREHOSPITAL ANALGESIA

The EP should be able to administer adequate pain relief in the prehospital setting.

Analgesics should be administered if the athlete is in pain and especially if there is considerable transport time. In general, analgesia should be avoided if the athlete has had a head injury; strong analgesia may result in a change in the athlete's level of consciousness and thus mask cerebral deterioration. Analgesics can be administered by several different routes:

- Intravenous—quickest, most effective route to achieve pain relief, though many EPs choose not to establish IV access for various reasons

- Intramuscular—easy, effective, but slower onset than with IV administration

- Oral—should be avoided if the patient is vomiting or likely to require general anesthesia

- Inhalation—may be effective but beware of contraindications

- Rectal—effective but often impracticable due to the sporting setting

NSAIDs (Nonsteroid Anti-inflammatory Drugs)

Early oral administration is useful for the alleviation of pain and swelling, particularly in acute joint injuries when used in combination with ice, compression and elevation. All oral agents should be avoided if there is a likelihood that the athlete will require surgery as most anesthetists prefer the patients to have fasted for 6 hours or more. NSAIDs in the prehospital setting should be avoided if there is a history of peptic ulcer disease, renal dysfunction, allergy, or asthma.

Morphine

Intravenous morphine is a highly effective drug, often producing an analgesic effect within a few minutes, and the effect may last for hours, having a half-life of 2 to 4 hours. Dosage varies, but most adults respond to 5 mg given slowly IV. On occasion (e.g., with shoulder dislocations or leg fractures), higher doses of up to 15 mg may be required. Nausea and vomiting are not uncommon complications, so antiemetics are often administered simultaneously. There is a danger of respiratory depression, so avoid use in head injuries. If the patient is hypotensive, the administration of morphine may exacerbate the situation, so beware.

Nalaxone is an effective opiate antagonist and particularly useful with respiratory depression—40 μg up to 2 mg is recommended.

Nitrous Oxide/Oxygen Inhalation Agents

In certain countries, portable tanks containing 50% nitrous oxide and 50% oxygen are used for rapid analgesia. The patient should be fully conscious and have normal respiration. The effect is short acting and may have to be repeated during transport. As the nitrous oxide gas diffuses rapidly into air-filled spaces, its use is contraindicated with head injuries, pneumothoraces, explosion injuries, abdominal perforations, otitis media, and diving/decompression disorders.

Recommended Reading

1. European Resuscitation Council Guidelines for Resuscitation 2010. *Resuscitation 81.* Elsevier, 2010:1219–1276.

CHAPTER 25

Emergency Intravenous Therapy

Contributed by David McDonagh, Chairman, FIBT Medical Committee

Reviewer: Sven Erik Gisvold, Professor of Anesthetics, NTNU, St.Olavs University Hospital, Trondheim, Norway

In certain emergency conditions, such as shock or intravascular volume depletion due to diarrhea or heat stroke, the event physician may be obliged to administer intravenous fluids. *Note*: The EP should also be aware of the restrictions on intravenous fluid use in the WADA list (http://www.wada-ama.org/en/prohibitedlist.ch2).

If the intravascular volume is reduced, either by hemorrhage or by dehydration, the body attempts to compensate by inducing vasoconstriction and by initiating fluid migration from the extravascular compartment to the vascular system. This compensatory system does have limits and cannot cope with major blood loss, particularly if this loss is rapid. When hemorrhage occurs, oxygen-transferring red blood cells will be lost. The body attempts to compensate by increasing cardiac output—pumping faster and thus delivering more blood—and by increasing oxygen extraction from the blood. If the blood volume is increased by giving intravenous fluids, even if they do not carry oxygen, adequate oxygen delivery to the body tissues can be maintained with mild to moderate blood loss for a period of time. If, however, there is a severe hemorrhage and hemoglobin levels fall to 7 g/dL, blood must also be given.

- Crystalloid solutions: These are usually isotonic and include Ringer's lactate and 0.9% saline; they are commonly used and are purported to be equally effective. Many physicians prefer to use Ringer's lactate with hemorrhagic shock, but recommend 0.9% saline for hemorrhagic shock combined with brain injury. Hypertonic solutions will pull extravascular water into the vascular system and can thus be considered to be plasma expanders; they may have short-term volume benefits but can cause other problems later. These are used on occasions where there is a combination of head injury (with cerebral edema) and significant blood loss. If one suspects cerebral pathology (e.g., injury or edema due to high altitude), saline 0.9% is preferable to Ringer's lactate, as saline contains more sodium (154 mmol/L contra 130 mmol/L). This helps raise osmolality and can potentially draw more fluid out of the edematous brain.

- Colloid solutions are also plasma expanders and are primarily used to restore the circulating volume in hypovolemic patients. Combinations of colloids and hypertonic crystalloid solutions are also used. Colloid solutions are effective volume expanders but may interfere with coagulation, particularly when large volumes are administered, and may also cause acute renal failure in predisposed patients. The inexperienced physician should probably refrain from using these solutions.

- Blood is usually given as packed red blood cells and should be cross-matched before transfusion; however, in urgent situations, type-O Rh-negative blood can be administered.

  - *Note.* I have never seen blood units at a sports event. I would strongly recommend not having blood units available in this prehospital environment, for several reasons:
    - They are *not* necessary—this is sport we are talking about, not war.
    - Blood should be given in hospitals.
    - Serious transfusion complications can occur (hemolytic anemia, lung injury, infections, etc.).

- Finally, you will probably be suspected of organizing some form of doping activity.
- Rate of fluid administration, remembering that overly rapid infusion may lead to pulmonary edema:

■ Shock: Adults can be given 1 L of crystalloid solution as quickly as possible, but beware patients with cardiogenic shock who do not need large volumes of fluid. Children can be given crystalloid solutions at a rate of 20 mL/kg body weight.

■ Hemorrhagic shock: Adults can be administered colloids at a rate of 5 to 10 mL/kg body weight. I would recommend not administering colloids to children. If there is internal bleeding, rapid transfusion may worsen the situation. If you do not have colloids, establish an IV line and administer other IV fluid slowly and carefully. If the patient is awake and has a pulse and a systolic pressure of at least 80, then continue with slow IV.

■ Fluid depletion: For patients with symptomatic dehydration that is not due to hemorrhaging (e.g., heat), adults will need between 1 and 3 L of Ringer's lactate/acetate. Give an initial 1 L IV bolus over a 30-minute period. If dehydration is symptomatic, the patient usually needs several liters of fluid, so continue giving up to 3 L at a rate of 500 mL/h. For children with symptomatic dehydration, a bolus of approximately 30 mL/kg of body weight is often given over a 30-minute period.

Recommended Reading

1. European Resuscitation Council Guidelines for Resuscitation 2010. *Resuscitation 81*. Elsevier, 2010:1219–1276.

CHAPTER 26

The Unconscious Athlete

Contributed by David McDonagh, Secretary, AIBA Medical Commission

Reviewer: Sven Erik Gisvold, Professor of Anesthetics, St. Olavs University Hospital, NTNU, Trondheim, Norway

It is difficult to assess an unconscious patient due the lack of diagnostic facilities at a sports event and the necessary urgency to transfer the patient to a hospital as soon as possible. A delay in transporting the patient to a hospital where more efficient diagnostic and therapeutic services are available may have fatal consequences. In a sporting environment, it is natural to assume that cerebral trauma is the cause of the loss of consciousness, but this may be an incorrect and potentially dangerous assumption. Unconsciousness is defined as loss of awareness of the environment and it has previously been classified as

- Obtundation—slow and inappropriate response to a continuous verbal stimuli

- Stupor—no response to verbal stimulus, requires vigorous and repeated noxious stimuli before responding

- Coma—does not respond to verbal or noxious stimuli and is thus unarousable and unresponsive

As we all know, a variety of conditions can cause the patient to collapse into unconsciousness—be they sudden cardiovascular episodes (e.g., sudden cardiac death, subarachnoid hemorrhage), neurologic disorders (e.g., epilepsy, head injury, spinal cord lesion), metabolic disorders (e.g., diabetes), etc. The duties of the event physician are thus to make a rapid triage, request ambulance/helicopter support, and stabilize the patient by initiating ABCDE while endeavoring to gain a medical history from onlookers, coaches, friends, family, etc.

Causes

The variety of causes is legion and can include

- Head injury/concussion, cerebrovascular accident, cranial fracture

- Epileptic attack

- Meningitis, encephalitis

- Asphyxia

- Syncope, fatigue

- Body temperature disorders—hypothermia, hyperthermia

- Cardiac arrest

- Hemorrhage

- Hypoglycemia, hyperglycemia

- Drug overdose

- Poisoning or intoxication (fume inhalation, etc.)

History

History from relatives, friends, or witnesses:

- What happened? Did anyone see the athlete collapse? Head injury?

- Onset of coma (abrupt, gradual)

- Recent injury—for example, head injury, concussion

- Recent complaints (headache, nausea, focal weakness, vertigo)

- Previous medical illness (diabetes, uremia, heart disease)

- Medication/drugs (medicinal, recreational)

History taking should be as extensive as possible given the limitation of time and the time required to examine and treat the patient. An accurate description of events leading up to the patient's collapse may provide valuable information as will a previous history of diabetes, epilepsy, medications, etc. Sudden coma is commonly the result of a vascular lesion. A history of systemic illness (e.g., diabetes, liver diseases) may point to a metabolic cause. Assess the accident scene—this may provide some information on the injury mechanism or precipitating factors. Look for patient identification, bracelets, neck pendants, or wallet cards containing medical information.

General Physical Examination

- When approaching an unconscious/potentially lifeless patient, always start with a brief ABC procedure: airway, breathing, and circulation.

- Assess: Check the level of consciousness by talking to the patient or checking for a pain reaction and then see if the patient breathes voluntarily. Is the patient cyanotic? Then check for a radial or carotid pulse, but don't waste time.

- Respiratory rate: normal between 12 and 20/min

- Respiratory pattern

- Cyanosis

- Oxygen saturation

- Pulse

- Blood pressure: Check blood pressure. Normal pressure is a good sign; raised blood pressure or pressure that is increasing may indicate raised intracranial pressure. Low blood pressure in an unconscious athlete may indicate advanced severe head injury or that the athlete may be in a preshock condition due to hypovolemia, anaphylaxis, hypoglycemia, etc.

- Evidence of trauma

- Thorax: clavicles, sternum, ribs, wound, asymmetrical respiration

- Abdomen: rigidity and guarding, pulsating masses, bruising, pelvis fractures

- Head: cranial deformity, scalp wounds, ears (CSF or blood), jaw, bitten tongue

- Limbs: fracture, deformity, distal pulses, color, capillary refill

- Back: wounds, deformities

- Evidence of acute or chronic systemic illness

- Nuchal rigidity (examine with care in case of cervical spinal injury)

Neurologic Examination

- Level of consciousness

- Level of intellectual function: concentration, memory, orientation

- Respiratory pattern

- Pupillary size and pattern

- Eyes and eye movements

- Motor function

- Coordination

Level of Consciousness

It is important for the EP to determine the patient's level of consciousness both in regard to defining the level of care required and also due to the need to define a baseline neurologic status. Altered levels of consciousness are an important clinical finding and may be the only indicator of major cerebral injury. An initial evaluation should be followed by regular reevaluations as deterioration may occur. One should look for such signs as confusion, aggressivity or passivity, drowsiness, difficulty in staying awake, difficulty in awakening the athlete—shouting, shaking, pain stimulus—slurring of speech, slow mental functioning, difficulty with counting or solving problems, poor memory, intoxicated appearance, etc. The Glasgow Coma Scale is a commonly used tool in the prehospital environment (see below). If the patient is unconscious, has deteriorating consciousness, or is moving between an unconscious and partially conscious state, then urgent intervention is required and rapid transfer to a hospital is essential (if head injury is the suspected cause, then refer to a hospital with a neurologic unit). If the patient regains consciousness, try to evaluate the extent of preincident and postincident amnesia, as well as his or her level of intellectual function.

Level of Intellectual Function

Patients may remain conscious but still have serious cerebral lesions. It is important to examine for amnesia, concentration ability (count from 79 down to 70. What is your telephone number?

Repeat backwards, i.e., last number first.), memory (quiz about recent events you would expect the athlete to know about, e.g., Maddocks questions; give him or her a word and request this word after 4 to 5 minutes), and orientation (Where are you? How did you get here? What time is it?). In 1995, D. L. Maddocks developed the first qualitative assessment of a player's mental state and recommended removal from the field should any of the answers be incorrect:

- What field are we at?
- Who are we playing?
- Who is your opponent at present?
- What half/quarter are we in?
- How far into the period are we?
- Who scored last?
- Who did we play last week?
- Did we win last week?

Respiratory Pattern

The rate and depth of respiration are important to evaluate—there may be hyperventilation, hypoventilation, Cheyne-Stokes respiration, or ataxic respiration. The respiratory centers are found in the brainstem medulla and damage to this area may cause abnormal breathing patterns. Injury to the upper brainstem may cause Cheyne-Stokes respiration, whereas injury to the lower brainstem may cause central neurogenic respiration with shallow and rapid respiration—a most serious form of dysfunction.

Pupillary Size and Reaction

Pupils should be equal and react to light (ipsilateral and consensual—PEARL). If serious pathology is present, then you may find a normal-sized but unreactive pupil or a fixed, dilated pupil. Bilateral dilatation often indicates severe brain damage. Examine the pupils early and often, as unequal pupils and unequal reflexes are important signs of serious brain injury. The inequality may disappear later and thus mask an important sign of deterioration. If normal, photophobia may be present, which may indicate a cerebral lesion. Attempts have been made to categorize the various phases of pupillary reactions—initially, the pupils may constrict, become unreactive to light, and then dilate and remain dilated.

Eye Inspection and Eye Movements

The presence of binocular hematomas may indicate the presence of a facial/cranial fracture. Due to time constraints, papilloedema is not often looked for and even then is rarely found immediately after trauma, even though its presence may indicate raised intracranial pressure. Eye movements are difficult to evaluate in an unconscious patient. If one eye is sunken, there may be an orbital fracture present. Similarly, exophthalmos may also indicate a major fracture. Doll's eye movement—indicating brainstem dysfunction—should not be tested for due to the possibility of concomitant spinal injury. Nystagmus and diplopia may be present.

Motor Function

This is elicited by applying peripheral noxious stimuli (e.g., pinching of limbs, pinprick tests) to elicit (a) an appropriate response—brushing away the source of stimulus—or (b) an inappropriate response—indicating decerebrate or decorticate rigidity.

The motor response is also useful in localizing the level of a spinal injury. A paralyzed limb will show no response. Decerebrate rigidity indicates brainstem damage and, if bilateral, is usually associated with a very poor prognosis. Complete flaccidity with no response to stimuli usually indicates severe CNS depression due to intoxification (drug overdose).

A detailed neurologic examination may also reveal the presence of a cranial nerve injury (changes in smell, hearing, taste, speech, smiling, eye movement, shoulder shrugging) or raised intracranial pressure (papilloedema).

Coordination

If you have excluded a spinal injury and the patient is able to stand and has normal vital signs and mental status, then some elementary coordination and balance tests can be carried out: finger–nose test (with eyes closed and open), Romberg test, etc.

Treatment

In general, management of the comatose patient depends on the cause. However, while the patient is undergoing evaluation, it is essential to maintain adequate cerebral oxygenation and to establish an intravenous line for volume control and prompt medication if necessary, for example, intravenous glucose/insulin, antibiotic, high-dose steroid, anticonvulsants.

The evaluation and treatment of the unconscious patient is difficult and resource consuming. For the EP, the main task is to stabilize the patient, if possible, correct correctable conditions, and get the patient to a hospital as quickly as possible. When the patient has left the scene, try to gather more information about the injury or event.

■ Place the patient in the recovery position

■ Clear the mouth and pharynx; suction, if indicated

■ Establish and maintain an airway—insert an oral airway

■ If unconscious or severely impaired consciousness (no cough reflex), use a laryngeal mask airway or a laryngeal tube intubation, then pass an orogastric or nasogastric tube

■ Intubation should be attempted *only* if the patient appears lifeless and does not have pharyngeal reflexes. In all other situations, tracheal intubation is a specialist task that involves the use of anesthetic drugs

■ If intubation is impossible, perform cricothyroidotomy or tracheostomy

■ If consciousness is not so deeply impaired, a tracheal tube may be rejected by the patient

■ Consider cervical spinal precautions

■ Determine the presence of spontaneous respirations and pulse

■ Support respiratory and circulatory functions

■ Assess for sources of external bleeding

■ Manage any life-threatening conditions when identified

■ Reassess vital signs at regular intervals (5 to 15 minutes) or when necessary

■ Initiate transport to the nearest appropriate treatment facility; contact them, giving an update on the patient's status

■ Monitor and treat the patient en route

26.1 GLASGOW COMA SCALE

This scoring system is used the world over for classifying head injuries. It is useful for several reasons: Its universality allows physicians to communicate, so that if an event physician warns the hospital that a patient with a GCS score of 10 is on his way to the hospital, the receiving team has a pretty good idea of what to expect. The GCS is also useful for relatively quick triage and can be very helpful when large numbers of injured patients are involved. On the negative side, the scale is not very subtle and scores may vary depending on the physician. The scale does not accommodate subtle changes in consciousness very well and a patient can go from being relatively stable to being very ill despite small changes in GCS scores. The scale was also designed to be used in patients 1 hour or more after trauma; it was not designed for acute, on-the-spot evaluation of head injuries. So in the immediate posttrauma state, a patient may have a more normal GCS score even if he or she has a serious injury. But all in all, it is a useful tool. The scoring system is based on measuring three bodily functions:

■ Eye response

■ Motor response

■ Verbal response

And then summating the score to define the level of head injury.

■ Severe head injury: GCS score of 8 or less

■ Moderate head injury: GCS score of 9 to 12

■ Mild head injury: GCS score of 13 to 14

■ Minimal head injury: GCS score of 15

Patients scoring 3 or 4 have an 85% chance of dying or remaining vegetative, while scores greater than 11 indicate only a 5% to 10% likelihood of death or vegetative state and 85% chance of moderate disability or good recovery (Table 26.1).

26.2 PEDIATRIC GLASGOW COMA SCALE

As children are children and not fully developed, the GCS can be difficult to analyze. Now, while it is not normal to have infants at a sports event, the event physician may attend events where children are present. The Simpson and Reilly pediatric GCS may be of assistance (Table 26.2).

Adjustment to Age

■ During the first 6 months: The best verbal response is normally a cry, though some infants make vocal responses during this period: Normal verbal score expected is 2. The best motor response is usually flexion: Normal motor score expected is 3. Normal aggregate score is 9.

TABLE 26.1 Glasgow Coma Scale

Eye Opening (E)		Best Motor Response (M)	
Spontaneous	4	Obeys	6
To loud voice	3	Localizes	5
To pain	2	Withdraws (flexion)	4
Nil	1	Abnormal flexion posturing	3
		Extension posturing	2
		Nil	1
Sum:		*Sum:*	
Verbal Response (V)			
Oriented	5		
Confused, disoriented	4		
Inappropriate words	3		
Incomprehensible sounds	2		
Nil	1		
Sum:		**TOTAL**	

TABLE 26.2 Pediatric Glasgow Coma Scale

Eye Opening (E)		Best Motor Response (M)	
Spontaneous	4	Obeys command	5
To loud voice	3	Localizes pain	4
To pain	2	Withdraws (flexion to pain)	3
Nil	1	Extension to pain	2
		Nil	1
Sum:		*Sum:*	
Verbal Response (V)			
Oriented	5		
Words	4		
Vocal sounds	3		
Cries	2		
Nil	1		
Sum:		**TOTAL**	

- 6 to 12 months: The normal infant makes noises: Normal verbal score expected is 3. The infant will usually locate pain but not obey commands: Normal motor score expected is 4. Normal aggregate score is 11.

- 12 months to 2 years: Recognizable words are expected: Normal verbal score expected is 4. The child will usually locate pain but not obey commands: Normal motor score expected is 4. Normal aggregate score is 12.

- 2 to 5 years: Recognizable words are expected: Normal verbal score expected is 4. The child will usually obey commands: Normal motor score expected is 5. Normal aggregate score is 13.

- After 5 years: Orientation is defined as awareness of being in a hospital: Normal verbal score expected is 5. Normal aggregate score is 14.

Recommended Reading

http://www.pubmedcentral.nih.gov/articlerender.fcgi?tool=pmcentrez&artid=1462953

Consensus statement on Concussion in Sport—the 3rd International Conference on Concussion in Sport held in Zurich. *South African Journal of Sports Medicine.* McCrory, 2009;21(2):1015–5163.

Cantu R, ed. *Neurologic Athletic Head and Spinal Injuries.* Saunders Company, W. B.

CHAPTER 27

Severe Head Injuries and Cranial Fractures

Contributed by Nils Ericsson, Neurosurgeon, Accident and Emergency Department, Trondheim, Norway

Reviewer: Tomm Müller, Department of Neurosurgery, St. Olavs Hospital, Trondheim, Norway

Head injuries are common in sports; US data suggest an annual incidence of 300,000. According to the Head Injury Severity Scale (HISS) (Fig. 27.1), most of these sports-related head injuries may be classified as mild or minimal, in sports medicine, typically referred to as "concussion" or "mild traumatic brain injury (mTBI)." Chapters 29 and 30 discuss the whole issue of sports concussion and the difficult diagnostic and return-to-play decisions faced by the EP.

The immediate symptoms of mild and severe head injury may not differ significantly and it is also important to remember that an initially mild head injury may deteriorate into a more severe injury. The EP must always be prepared for a medical emergency. In this context, the importance of continuous observation and recording the level of consciousness is crucial. The commonest way to evaluate the development of a head injury is by using the universally accepted Glasgow Coma Scale, which is based on measuring three bodily functions: eye response, motor response, and verbal response, and then summating the score (Table 27.1).

27.1 TRAUMATIC BRAIN INJURY (TBI)

The brain may be damaged when exposed to torsional or direct forces. There are several injury mechanisms often caused by acceleration or deceleration of the brain tissue—at the point of impact (coup) or at its opposite pole (contrecoup) or diffusely, often affecting the frontal and temporal lobes. Structural damage may occur with torsion or shearing forces causing tears of axons in white matter, so-called diffuse axonal injury (DAI). These small lesions are typically found in the brainstem, the corpus callosum, and supratentorial white

matter tracts and are clinically associated with long-term coma. Damaged blood vessels leak, causing contusions and intracerebral or subarachnoid hemorrhages (Fig. 27.1). Tears may also occur in the extracerebral, epidural, or subdural vessels, thus causing acute epidural or subdural hematomas.

The brain has a high metabolic demand and is dependent on a constant supply of oxygenated blood. The intracranial space is a rigid cavity of fixed volume with nonelastic walls and rigid meninges and brain tissue. There is not a lot of room for expansion. The integrity of the brain is highly vulnerable to alterations in blood flow and changes in intracranial volume. TBI may cause disruption of cerebral blood flow, regionally or globally. The resulting cerebral ischemia causes a cerebral edema that may lead to raised intracranial pressure (ICP). The presence of a traumatic intracranial hemorrhage or hematoma will further increase the ICP and thus worsen the situation and may eventually result in a herniation of brain tissue between the compartments or through the foramen magnum.

27.2 EXAMINATION OF AN ATHLETE WITH HEAD INJURY

The EP has limited diagnostic capabilities and hence his/her main task is to identify a serious head injury, to initiate correct management and to evacuate the patient to a neurosurgical unit (see Chapter 26). Recognition of a serious head injury begins with observation of the incident. The EP should if possible be watching the event at the field side or on a TV screen at the facility. This allows one to evaluate the trauma mechanism and may indicate other injuries, the presence of seizures, etc. A medical

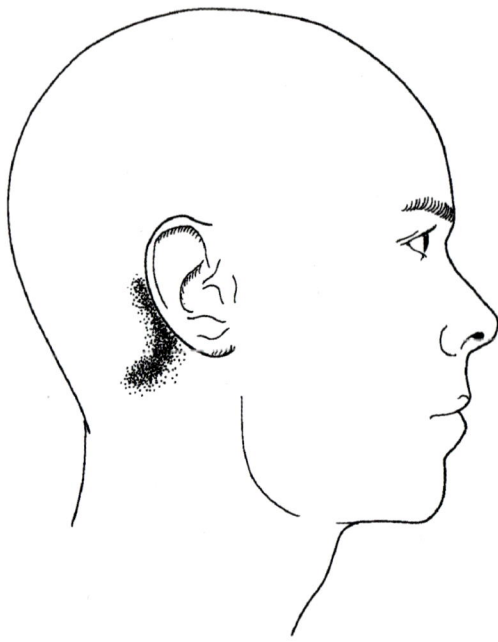

FIGURE 27.1. Battle's sign, or mastoid ecchymosis, indicates a posterior basilar fracture, but its absence does not exclude a fracture.

history should be taken from trainers, spectators, etc., whilst the initial triage is being carried out or even after the patient has been sent to hospital. Important information can then be forwarded to the hospital.

History

- Time of accident
- Cause of accident, injury mechanism
- Loss of consciousness—description by patient and/or observers
- Observed seizures or vomiting
- Nausea, headache, paresthesia, weakness
- Visual defects
- Symptoms indicative of injury to other organs
- Previous illnesses, medications, family history of stroke, SAH, bleeding, alcohol, drugs, etc.

Clinical Examination

- Vital signs
  - Pulse, blood pressure, respiration
- Local inspection of the scalp and scull
  - Cuts and bruises
  - There may be a depressed fracture area in the skull, so look for indentations; beware when palpating a fractured skull—you may make things worse by pressing fracture segments further into the brain
  - CSF leakage to the ears, mouth, nose; sweet taste of sugar in CSF

TABLE 27.1	Glasgow Coma Scale		
Eye Opening (E)		**Best Motor Response (M)**	
Spontaneous	4	Obeys	6
To loud voice	3	Localizes	5
To pain	2	Withdraws (flexion)	4
Nil	1	Abnormal flexion posturing	3
		Extension posturing	2
		Nil	1
Sum:		*Sum:*	
Verbal Response (V)			
Oriented	5		
Confused, disoriented	4		
Inappropriate words	3		
Incomprehensible sounds	2		
Nil	1		
Sum:		**TOTAL**	

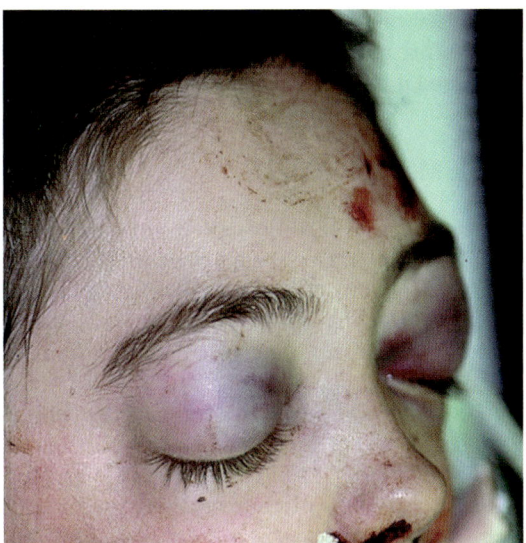

FIGURE 27.2. Raccoon eyes, also called binocular hematoma, indicate a frontal basilar fracture. (Reprinted from Fleisher GR, Ludwig S, Baskin *MN. Atlas of Pediatric Emergency Medicine.* Philadelphia, PA: Lippincott Williams & Wilkins; 2004.)

- • A bleeding nose may indicate a basal fracture; a bleeding ear almost always does
- • Battle's sign—takes time to develop and is often absent in the early injury phase
- • Binocular hematomas—note white corneas, often associated with basilar fractures; may also take time to develop
- • Otoscopy—blood behind an intact drum; this may indicate a basal fracture
- ■ Short neurologic exam
  - • Level of consciousness
  - • Motor function
  - • Pupillary size and reaction to light

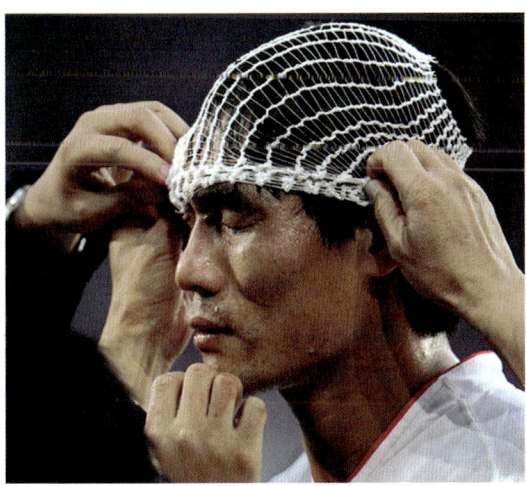

FIGURE 27.3. Jin Cheu. (Courtesy FIFA.)

27.3 MANAGEMENT AND TREATMENT

As for all medical emergencies, the patient with a serious head injury must be stabilized according to general emergency principles. Pulse and breathing must be evaluated as soon as possible and this examination should take no more than 10 seconds. If the athlete has absent or occasional gasping respiration, sweep the mouth for a mouth guard or gum shield and initiate chest compressions immediately. An athlete who has absent or gasping breathing should be treated as a sudden cardiac arrest (with cervical caution). The current American Heart Association 2010 Guidelines support this statement.

This excellent body of researchers also states that no studies had evaluated the routine use of the finger sweep to clear an airway. Despite this, I would recommend the use of the finger sweep, as the gum shield is the most likely cause of foreign body airway obstruction in sport (along with chewing gum). However, the finger sweep must be performed carefully as reports have also documented harm to the victim.

Hypotension and/or hypoxia dramatically increase mortality in patients with severe head injury. Always suspect a cervical injury in the head-injured athlete and apply a cervical collar and use a spinal board/vacuum mattress or both, if possible. The following check list may be helpful in an emergency situation:

- ■ Check pulse (carotid) and breathing (normal or abnormal/gasping)
- ■ Check level of consciousness
- ■ Finger sweep to remove mouth guard
- ■ If pulseless or abnormal/gasping breathing, treat as SCA—initiate chest compressions, consider defibrillation (see Chapter 26).
- ■ Insert oral airways and administer oxygen
  - • If pulse present but breathing is compromised, give rescue breaths every 5 to 6 seconds and be prepared for cardiac arrest
  - • If pulse present with normal breathing but reduced level of consciousness, give oxygen (10 to 15 L)
- ■ Establish IV lines; normotension is the goal
- ■ Stop scalp bleeding and cover cranial wounds
- ■ Apply semirigid cervical collar in the absence of a fixed neck fracture dislocation
- ■ Use a spinal board or vacuum mattress or a combination of both

- Never remove penetrating intracranial foreign bodies—bleeding will worsen
- Elevate the upper body, always protecting the cervical spine

Transport

- The patient should lie in a supine position with the head elevated
- The patient should not lie on a wound or fracture site
- Continuous neurologic evaluation—use a check list
- Continuous respiratory and circulatory evaluation
- Ensure correct cervical and spinal immobilization
- Ensure careful lifting and movement of the patient

Contact with Hospital

Inform the hospital of the patient's status and expected time of arrival, so that the trauma team is prepared. In case of patient deterioration, recontact the hospital and inform them of these changes.

27.4 SCALP LACERATIONS AND BLEEDING

Scalp wounds may on occasion bleed profusely and must be stopped. Simple suturing is usually adequate but may not be possible on the field of play. Venous bleeding can usually be stopped by applying digital compression adjacent to the wound. Bleeding that does not stop may be arterial in origin and may be due to a cranial fracture. Due to this risk, digital compression should not be excessive as there is a risk of pressing fractured bone further

into the cranium. If necessary, cover the wound and apply a turban bandage. Occasionally, IV fluid may be needed if blood loss is significant.

27.5 SMELLING SALTS

Smelling salts are a combination of ammonium carbonate salt (a white crystalline structure) and water. The combination of these two substances causes the release of ammonia gas (NH_3), which, when placed under an athlete's nose, causes irritation of the nasal, buccal, and pharyngeal mucus membranes, triggering an inhalation reflex. Addressing the question, "Are smelling salts likely to work for sport-related mild head injury?" Prof. Paul McCrory in the *British Journal of Sports Medicine* in 2006 states,

> It is unlikely that the induced inhalational reflex has a significant therapeutic effect over and above the natural history of the condition. Increasing the respiratory rate alone certainly has no beneficial pathophysiological effect on the nature or underlying cause of concussive injury. Whether the salts increase alertness or improve reaction times or have other positive cognitive benefits remains to be proven scientifically.

Following on this, McCrory concludes, "In modern sports medicine, however, when used correctly, smelling salts are unlikely to have significant benefit or cause significant adverse effects in sport-related head injury."

Recommended Reading

http://www.pubmedcentral.nih.gov/articlerender.fcgi?tool=pmcentrez&artid=1462953

Consensus statement on Concussion in Sport—the 3rd International Conference on Concussion in Sport held in Zurich. *South African Journal of Sports Medicine*. McCrory, 2009;21(2):1015–5163.

Cantu R, ed. *Neurologic Athletic Head and Spinal Injuries*. Saunders Company, W. B.

CHAPTER 28

Syncope

Contributed by David McDonagh, Secretary, AIBA Medical Commission

Reviewer: Sven Erik Gisvold, Professor of Anesthetics, St. Olavs University Hospital, NTNU, Trondheim, Norway

Unfortunately, athletes can faint. It is always difficult to differentiate between a "faint" and a serious disorder. Syncope may be caused by the same conditions that cause unconsciousness, some of which are life threatening, but most episodes are more gentle affairs. The problem for the EP is at least twofold.

Is there any serious underlying pathology? If not, can and when can the athlete return to play? Difficult questions, with no easy answers.

Obviously, if the patient has a history of benign syncope, then a return-to-play decision is easier. Similarly, if the sport is relatively safe with little inherent danger, it is easier to allow an earlier return-to-play. But what about boxing, rugby, American football, and downhill skiing?

How do you know that this syncope was not in fact a "second impact" head injury? Patients with fulminant cerebral edema can collapse after insignificant blows to the head. Before allowing an athlete to return immediately to play, consider some of the potential syncopal causes: cardiac ischemia or arrhythmia; vascular disease, hemorrhage, or hypovolemia; neurologic abnormality including subarachnoid hemorrhage, meningitis, epilepsy; hypoglycemia or other metabolic abnormality; heat-related illness and dehydration

Obviously the patient's condition during the episode, the length of the episode, and the patient's recovery after the episode all influence one's decision. Syncopal patients have usually regained consciousness by the time the EP or emergency medical staff have arrived. Obtain as thorough a history as possible, but beware, athletes and coaches will try to belittle the seriousness of the event and will almost always want to continue activity.

However, considering all the potentially serious causes of a syncopal episode, one should definitely err on the side of safety. Healthy athletes do not usually "just faint."

Treatment

- Position the patient on his or her back being careful to protect the cervical spine.

- Be prepared to turn the patient onto his or her side at the first sign of vomiting or choking.

- Elevate the lower limbs, unless other injuries suggest otherwise. (If he or she has other injuries, then other causes of unconsciousness should be considered.)

- Check vital signs.

- Be prepared to treat respiratory and cardiac arrest, having suction, oxygen, infusion sets, even defibrillators ready or nearby.

- Assess the patient thoroughly and try to find the underlying cause of the episode—easier said than done.

- If syncope persists, then there is probably a more serious condition present.

- Check the airway for patency.

- Administer high-concentration oxygen and assist ventilation, if necessary.

- Assess the need for an IV infusion. Consider the need for glucose, diazepam.

- Maintain the patient in the recovery position until and during transport.

- If the patient recovers, he or she should rest for a while before standing up, walking, etc.

- Reevaluate the patient after some minutes.

- Retake a medical history and evaluate the need for further investigation before even thinking about a return-to-play.

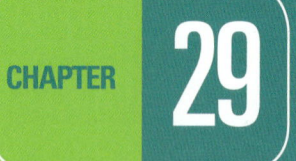

CHAPTER 29

Zurich Consensus Statement on Concussion in Sport

The 3rd International Conference on Concussion in Sport held in Zurich, November 2008

McCrory P, Meeuwisse W, Johnston K, Dvorak J, Aubry M, Molloy M, and Cantu R

PREAMBLE

This paper is a revision and update of the recommendations developed following the 1st (Vienna) and 2nd (Prague) International Symposia on Concussion in Sport (1,2). The Zurich Consensus statement is designed to build on the principles outlined in the original Vienna and Prague documents and to develop further conceptual understanding of this problem using a formal consensus-based approach. A detailed description of the consensus process is outlined at the end of this document under the "background" section (see Section 11). This document is developed for use by physicians, therapists, certified athletic trainers, health professionals, coaches and other people involved in the care of injured athletes, whether at the recreational, elite or professional level.

While agreement exists pertaining to principal messages conveyed within this document, the authors acknowledge that the science of concussion is evolving and therefore management and return-to-play decisions remain in the realm of clinical judgment on an individualized basis. Readers are encouraged to copy and distribute freely the Zurich Consensus document and/or the Sports Concussion Assessment Tool (SCAT2) card and neither is subject to any copyright restriction. The authors request, however that the document and/or the SCAT2 card be distributed in their full and complete format.

The following focus questions formed the foundation for the Zurich concussion consensus statement:

Acute Simple Concussion

- Which symptom scale, which sideline assessment tool is best for diagnosis and/or follow up?
- How extensive should the cognitive assessment be in elite athletes?
- How extensive should clinical and neuropsychological (NP) testing be at nonelite level?
- Who should do/interpret the cognitive assessment?
- Is there a gender difference in concussion incidence and outcomes?

Return-to-play (RTP) Issues

- Is provocative exercise testing useful in guiding RTP?
- What is the best RTP strategy for elite athletes?
- What is the best RTP strategy for nonelite athletes?
- Is protective equipment (e.g., mouthguards and helmets) useful in reducing concussion incidence and/or severity?

Complex Concussion and Long-term Issues

- Is the Simple versus Complex classification a valid and useful differentiation?

- Are there specific patient populations at risk of long-term problems?

- Is there a role for additional tests (e.g., structural and/or functional MR Imaging, balance testing, biomarkers)?

- Should athletes with persistent symptoms be screened for depression/anxiety?

Pediatric Concussion

- Which symptoms scale is appropriate for this age group?

- Which tests are useful and how often should baseline testing be performed in this age group?

- What is the most appropriate RTP guideline for elite and nonelite child and adolescent athlete?

Future Directions

- What is the best method of knowledge transfer and education

- Is there evidence that new and novel injury prevention strategies work (e.g., changes to rules of the game, fair play strategies etc)?

The Zurich document additionally examines the management issues raised in the previous Prague and Vienna documents and applies the consensus questions to these areas.

SPECIFIC RESEARCH QUESTIONS AND CONSENSUS DISCUSSION

29.1 Concussion

1 Definition of Concussion

Panel discussion regarding the definition of concussion and its separation from mild traumatic brain injury (mTBI) was held. Although there was acknowledgement that the terms refer to different injury constructs and should not be used interchangeably, it was not felt that the panel would define mTBI for the purpose of this document. There was unanimous agreement however that concussion is defined as follows:

Concussion is defined as a complex pathophysiological process affecting the brain, induced by traumatic biomechanical forces. Several common features that incorporate clinical, pathologic and biomechanical injury constructs that may be utilized in defining the nature of a concussive head injury include:

1. *Concussion may be caused either by a direct blow to the head, face, neck or elsewhere on the body with an "impulsive" force transmitted to the head.*

2. *Concussion typically results in the rapid onset of short-lived impairment of neurologic function that resolves spontaneously.*

3. *Concussion may result in neuropathological changes but the acute clinical symptoms largely reflect a functional disturbance rather than a structural injury.*

4. *Concussion results in a graded set of clinical symptoms that may or may not involve loss of consciousness. Resolution of the clinical and cognitive symptoms typically follows a sequential course however it is important to note that in a small percentage of cases however, postconcussive symptoms may be prolonged.*

5. *No abnormality on standard structural neuroimaging studies is seen in concussion.*

2 Classification of Concussion

There was unanimous agreement to abandon the simple vs. complex terminology that had been proposed in the Prague agreement statement as the panel felt that the terminology itself did not fully describe the entities. The panel however unanimously retained the concept that the majority (80%–90%) of concussions resolve in a short (7–10 day) period, although the recovery time frame may be longer in children and adolescents (2).

29.2 Concussion Evaluation

1 Symptoms and Signs of Acute Concussion

The panel agreed that the diagnosis of acute concussion usually involves the assessment of a range of domains including clinical symptoms, physical signs, behavior, balance, sleep and cognition. Furthermore, a detailed concussion history is an important part of the evaluation both in the injured athlete and when conducting a preparticipation examination. The detailed clinical assessment of concussion is outlined in the *SCAT2* form, which is an appendix to this document. The suspected diagnosis of concussion can include one or more of the following clinical domains:

(a) Symptoms—somatic (e.g., headache), cognitive (e.g., feeling like in a fog) and/or emotional symptoms (e.g., lability)

(b) Physical signs (e.g., loss of consciousness, amnesia)

(c) Behavioral changes (e.g., irritability)

(d) Cognitive impairment (e.g., slowed reaction times)

(e) Sleep disturbance (e.g., drowsiness)

If any one or more of these components is present, a concussion should be suspected and the appropriate management strategy instituted.

2 On-field or Sideline Evaluation of Acute Concussion

When a player shows **ANY** features of a concussion:

(a) The player should be medically evaluated onsite using standard emergency management principles and particular attention should be given to excluding a cervical spine injury.

(b) The appropriate disposition of the player must be determined by the treating healthcare provider in a timely manner. If no healthcare provider is available, the player should be safely removed from practice or play and urgent referral to a physician arranged.

(c) Once the first aid issues are addressed, then an assessment of the concussive injury should be made using the SCAT2 or other similar tool.

(d) The player should not be left alone following the injury and serial monitoring for deterioration is essential over the initial few hours following injury.

(e) A player with diagnosed concussion should not be allowed to return to play on the day of injury. Occasionally in adult athletes, there may be return to play on the same day as the injury (see Section 4.2). It was unanimously agreed that sufficient time for assessment and adequate facilities should be provided for the appropriate medical assessment both on and off the field for all injured athletes. In some sports this may require rule change to allow an off-field medical assessment to occur without affecting the flow of the game or unduly penalizing the injured player's team.

Sideline evaluation of cognitive function is an essential component in the assessment of this injury. Brief neuropsychological test batteries that assess attention and memory function have been shown to be practical and effective.

Such tests include the Maddocks questions (3,4) and the Standardized Assessment of Concussion (SAC) (5–7). It is worth noting that standard orientation questions (e.g., time, place, person) have been shown to be unreliable in the sporting situation when compared with memory assessment (4,8). It is recognized, however, that abbreviated testing paradigms are designed for rapid concussion screening on the sidelines and are not meant to replace comprehensive neuropsychological testing

which is sensitive to detect subtle deficits that may exist beyond the acute episode; nor should they be used as a stand-alone tool for the ongoing management of sports concussions.

It should also be recognized that the appearance of symptoms might be delayed several hours following a concussive episode.

3 Evaluation in Emergency Room or Office by Medical Personnel

An athlete with concussion may be evaluated in the emergency room or doctor's office as a point of first contact following injury or may have been referred from another care provider. In addition to the points outlined above, the key features of this exam should encompass:

(a) A medical assessment including a comprehensive history and detailed neurological examination including a thorough assessment of mental status, cognitive functioning and gait and balance.

(b) A determination of the clinical status of the patient including whether there has been improvement or deterioration since the time of injury. This may involve seeking additional information from parents, coaches, teammates and eyewitness to the injury.

(c) A determination of the need for emergent neuroimaging in order to exclude a more severe brain injury involving a structural abnormality

In large part, these points above are included in the SCAT2 assessment, which forms part of the Zurich consensus statement.

29.3 Concussion Investigations

A range of additional investigations may be utilized to assist in the diagnosis and/or exclusion of injury. These include:

1 Neuroimaging

It was recognized by the panelists that conventional structural neuroimaging is normal in concussive injury. Given that caveat, the following suggestions are made: Brain CT (or where available MR brain scan) contributes little to concussion evaluation but should be employed whenever suspicion of an intracerebral structural lesion exists. Examples of such situations may include prolonged disturbance of conscious state, focal neurological deficit or worsening symptoms.

Newer structural MRI modalities including gradient echo, perfusion and diffusion imaging have greater sensitivity for structural abnormalities. However, the lack of published studies as well as absent preinjury neuroimaging data limits the usefulness of this approach in clinical management at the present time. In addition, the predictive value of various MR abnormalities that may be incidentally discovered is not established at the present time.

Other imaging modalities such as fMRI demonstrate activation patterns that correlate with symptom severity and recovery in concussion (9–13). Whilst not part of routine assessment at the present time, they nevertheless provide additional insight to pathophysiological mechanisms. Alternative imaging technologies (e.g., positron emission tomography, diffusion tensor imaging, magnetic resonance spectroscopy, functional connectivity), while demonstrating some compelling findings, are still at early stages of development and cannot be recommended other than in a research setting.

2 Objective Balance Assessment

Published studies, using both sophisticated force plate technology, as well as those using less sophisticated clinical balance tests (e.g., Balance Error Scoring System (BESS)), have identified postural stability deficits lasting approximately 72 hours following sport-related concussion. It appears that postural stability testing provides a useful tool for objectively assessing the motor domain of neurologic functioning, and should be considered a reliable and valid addition to the assessment of athletes suffering from concussion, particularly where symptoms or signs indicate a balance component (14–20).

3 Neuropsychological Assessment

The application of neuropsychological (NP) testing in concussion has been shown to be of clinical value and continues to contribute significant information in concussion evaluation (21–26). Although in most case cognitive recovery largely overlaps with the time course of symptom recovery, it has been demonstrated that cognitive recovery may occasionally precede or more commonly follow clinical symptom resolution suggesting that the assessment of cognitive function should be an important component in any return-to-play protocol (27,28). It must be emphasized however, that NP assessment should not be the sole basis of management decisions rather it should be seen as an aid to the clinical decision making process in conjunction with a range of clinical domains and investigational results.

Neuropsychologists are in the best position to interpret NP tests by virtue of their background and training. However, there may be situations where neuropsychologists are not available and other medical professionals may perform or interpret NP screening tests. The ultimate return-to-play decision should remain a medical one in which a multidisciplinary approach, when possible, has been taken. In the absence of NP and other (e.g., formal balance assessment) testing, a more conservative return-to-play approach may be appropriate.

In the majority of cases, NP testing will be used to assist return-to-play decisions and will not be done until patient is symptom free (29,30). There may be situations (e.g., child and adolescent athletes) where testing may be performed early whilst the patient is still symptomatic to assist in determining management. This will normally be best determined in consultation with a trained neuropsychologist (31,32).

4 Genetic Testing

The significance of Apo lipoprotein (Apo) E4, ApoE promotor gene, Tau polymerase and other genetic markers in the management of sports concussion risk or injury outcome is unclear at this time (33,34). Evidence from human and animal studies in more severe traumatic brain injury demonstrate induction of a variety of genetic and cytokine factors such as: insulin-like growth factor-1 (IGF-1), IGF binding protein-2, Fibroblast growth factor, Cu-Zn superoxide dismutase, superoxide dismutase-1 (SOD-1), nerve growth factor, glial fibrillary acidic protein (GFAP) and S-100. Whether such factors are affected in sporting concussion is not known at this stage (35–42).

5 Experimental Concussion Assessment Modalities

Different electrophysiological recording techniques (e.g., evoked response potential (ERP), cortical magnetic stimulation and electroencephalography) have demonstrated reproducible abnormalities in the postconcussive state; however, not all studies reliably differentiated concussed athletes from controls (43–49). The clinical significance of these changes remains to be established.

In addition, biochemical serum and cerebral spinal fluid markers of brain injury (including S-100, neuron specific enolase (NSE), myelin basic protein (MBP), GFAP, tau etc) have been proposed as means by which cellular damage may be detected if present (50–56). There is currently insufficient evidence, however, to justify the routine use of these biomarkers clinically.

29.4 Concussion Management

The cornerstone of concussion management is physical and cognitive rest until symptoms resolve and then a graded program of exertion prior to medical clearance and return to play. The recovery and outcome of this injury may be modified by a number of factors that may require more sophisticated management strategies. These are outlined in the section on modifiers below. As described above, the majority of injuries will recover spontaneously over several days. In these situations, it is expected that an athlete will proceed progressively through a stepwise return-to-play strategy (57). During this period of recovery while symptomatic following an injury, it is important to emphasize to the athlete that physical AND cognitive rest is required. Activities that require concentration and attention (e.g., scholastic work, videogames, text messaging etc) may exacerbate symptoms and possibly delay recovery. In such cases, apart from limiting relevant physical and cognitive activities (and other risk-taking opportunities for reinjury) while symptomatic, no further intervention is required during the period of recovery and the athlete typically resumes sport without further problem.

1 Graduated Return-to-play Protocol

Return-to-play protocol following a concussion follows a stepwise process as outlined in Table 29.1.

With this stepwise progression, the athlete should continue to proceed to the next level if asymptomatic at the current level. Generally each step should take 24 hours so that an athlete would take approximately one week to proceed through the full rehabilitation protocol once they are asymptomatic at rest and with provocative exercise. If any postconcussion symptoms occur while in the stepwise program then the patient should drop back to the previous asymptomatic level and try to progress again after a further 24-hour period of rest has passed.

2 Same Day RTP

With adult athletes, in some settings, where there are team physicians experienced in concussion management and sufficient resources (e.g., access to neuropsychologists, consultants, neuroimaging, etc.) as well as access to immediate (i.e., sideline) neurocognitive assessment, return-to-play management may be more rapid. The RTP strategy must still follow the same basic management principles namely, full clinical and cognitive recovery before consideration of return to play. This approach is supported by published guidelines, such as the American Academy of Neurology, US Team Physician Consensus Statement, and US National Athletic Trainers Association Position Statement (58–60). This issue was extensively discussed by the consensus panelists and it was acknowledged that there is evidence that some professional American football players are able to RTP more quickly, with even same day RTP supported by NFL studies

TABLE 29.1 **Graduated Return-to-play Protocol**

Rehabilitation Stage	Functional Exercise at Each Stage of Rehabilitation	Objective of Each Stage
1. No activity.	Complete physical and cognitive rest.	Recovery.
2. Light aerobic exercise.	Walking, swimming or stationary cycling keeping intensity <70% MPHR. No resistance training.	Increase HR.
3. Sport-specific exercise.	Skating drills in ice hockey, running drills in soccer. No head impact activities.	Add movement.
4. Noncontact training drills.	Progression to more complex training drills (e.g., passing drills in football and ice hockey. May start progressive resistance training).	Exercise, coordination, and cognitive load.
5. Full contact practice.	Following medical clearance participate in normal training activities.	Restore confidence and assess functional skills by coaching staff.
6. Return to play.	Normal game play.	

without a risk of recurrence or sequelae (61). There is data, however, demonstrating that at the collegiate and high school level, athletes allowed to RTP on the same day may demonstrate NP deficits postinjury that may not be evident on the sidelines and are more likely to have delayed onset of symptoms (62–68). It should be emphasized however, the young (<18) elite athlete should be treated more conservatively even though the resources may be the same as an older professional athlete (see Section 6.1).

3 Psychological Management and Mental Health Issues

In addition, psychological approaches may have potential application in this injury, particularly with the modifiers listed below (69,70). Care givers are also encouraged to evaluate the concussed athlete for affective symptoms such as depression as these symptoms may be common in concussed athletes (57).

4 The Role of Pharmacological Therapy

Pharmacological therapy in sports concussion may be applied in two distinct situations. The first of these situations is the management of specific prolonged symptoms (e.g., sleep disturbance, anxiety, etc.). The second situation is where drug therapy is used to modify the underlying pathophysiology of the condition with the aim of shortening the duration of the concussion symptoms (71). In broad terms, this approach to management should be only considered by clinicians experienced in concussion management.

An important consideration in RTP is that concussed athletes should not only be symptom free but also should not be taking any pharmacological agents/medications that may mask or modify the symptoms of concussion.

Where antidepressant therapy may be commenced during the management of a concussion, the decision to return to play while still on such medication must be considered carefully by the treating clinician.

5 The Role of Preparticipation Concussion Evaluation

Recognizing the importance of a concussion history, and appreciating the fact that many athletes will not recognize all the concussions they may have suffered in the past, a detailed concussion history is of value (72–75). Such a history may preidentify athletes that fit into a high risk category and provides an opportunity for the healthcare provider to educate the athlete in regard to the significance of concussive injury. A structured concussion history should include specific questions as to previous symptoms of a concussion; not just the perceived number of past concussions. It is also worth noting that dependence upon the recall of concussive injuries by teammates or coaches has been demonstrated to be unreliable (72). The clinical history should also include information about all previous head, face or cervical spine injuries as these may also have clinical relevance. It is worth emphasizing that in the setting of maxillofacial and cervical spine injuries, coexistent concussive injuries may be missed unless specifically assessed. Questions pertaining to disproportionate impact versus symptom severity matching may alert the clinician to a progressively increasing vulnerability to injury. As part of the clinical history it is advised that details regarding protective equipment employed at time of injury be sought, both for recent and remote injuries. The benefit a comprehensive preparticipation concussion evaluation allows for modification and optimization of protective behavior and an opportunity for education.

29.5 Modifying Factors in Concussion Management

The consensus panel agreed that a range of 'modifying' factors may influence the investigation and management of concussion and in some cases, may predict the potential for prolonged or persistent symptoms. These modifiers would also be important to consider in a detailed concussion history and are outlined in Table 29.2.

In this setting, there may be additional management considerations beyond simple RTP advice. There may be a more important role for additional investigations including: formal NP testing, balance assessment, and neuroimaging. It is envisioned that athletes with such modifying features would be managed in a multidisciplinary manner coordinated by a physician with specific expertise in the management of concussive injury.

The role of female gender as a possible modifier in the management of concussion was discussed at length by the panel. There was not unanimous agreement that the current published research evidence is conclusive that this should be included as a modifying factor although it was accepted that gender may be a risk factor for injury and/or influence injury severity (76–78).

1 The Significance of Loss of Consciousness (LOC)

In the overall management of moderate to severe traumatic brain injury, duration of LOC is an

TABLE 29.2	Concussion Modifiers
Factors	**Modifier**
Symptoms	Number
	Duration (> 10 days)
	Severity
Signs	Prolonged LOC (> 1 minute), Amnesia
Sequelae	Concussive convulsions
Temporal	Frequency—repeated concussions over time
	Timing —injuries close together in time
	"Recency" —recent concussion or TBI
Threshold	Repeated concussions occurring with progressively less impact force or slower recovery after each successive concussion.
Age	Child and adolescent (< 18 years old)
Co and Premorbidities	Migraine, depression or other mental health disorders, attention deficit hyperactivity disorder (ADHD), learning disabilities (LD), sleep disorders
Medication	Psychoactive drugs, anticoagulants
Behavior	Dangerous style of play
port	High risk activity, contact and collision sport, high sporting level

acknowledged predictor of outcome (79). Whilst published findings in concussion describe LOC associated with specific early cognitive deficits it has not been noted as a measure of injury severity (80,81). Consensus discussion determined that prolonged (>1-minute duration) LOC would be considered as a factor that may modify management.

2 The Significance of Amnesia and other symptoms

There is renewed interest in the role of posttraumatic amnesia and its role as a surrogate measure of injury severity (67,82,83). Published evidence suggests that the nature, burden and duration of the clinical postconcussive symptoms may be more important than the presence or duration of amnesia alone (80,84,85). Further it must be noted that retrograde amnesia varies with the time of measurement postinjury and hence is poorly reflective of injury severity (86,87).

3 Motor and Convulsive Phenomena

A variety of immediate motor phenomena (e.g., tonic posturing) or convulsive movements may accompany a concussion. Although dramatic, these clinical features are generally benign and require no specific management beyond the standard treatment of the underlying concussive injury (88,89).

4 Depression

Mental health issues (such as depression) have been reported as a long-term consequence of traumatic brain injury including sports related concussion. Neuroimaging studies using fMRI suggest that a depressed mood following concussion may reflect an underlying pathophysiological abnormality consistent with a limbic-frontal model of depression (52,90–100).

29.6 Special Populations

1 The Child and Adolescent Athlete

There was unanimous agreement by the panel that the evaluation and management recommendations contained herein could be applied to children and adolescents down to the age of 10 years. Below that age children report different concussion symptoms different from adults and would require age appropriate symptom checklists as a component of assessment. An additional consideration in assessing the child or adolescent athlete with a concussion is that in the clinical evaluation by the healthcare professional there may be the need to include both patient and parent input as well as teacher and school input when appropriate (101–107).

The decision to use NP testing is broadly the same as the adult assessment paradigm. However, timing of testing may differ in order to assist planning in school and home management (and may be performed while the patient is still symptomatic). If cognitive testing is performed then it must be developmentally sensitive until late teen years due to the ongoing cognitive maturation that occurs during this period which, in turn, makes the utility of comparison to either the person's own baseline performance or to population norms limited (20). In this age group it is more important to consider the use of trained neuropsychologists to interpret assessment data, particularly in children with learning disorders and/or ADHD who may need more sophisticated assessment strategies (31,32,101).

The panel strongly endorsed the view that children should not be returned to practice or play until clinically completely symptom free, which may require a longer time frame than for adults. In addition, the concept of 'cognitive rest' was highlighted with special reference to a child's need to limit exertion with activities of daily living and to limit scholastic and other cognitive stressors (e.g., text messaging, videogames etc) while symptomatic. School attendance and activities may also need to be modified to avoid provocation of symptoms. Because of the different physiological response & longer recovery after concussion and specific risks (e.g., diffuse cerebral swelling) related to head impact during childhood and adolescence, a more conservative return-to-play approach is recommended. It is appropriate to extend the amount of time of asymptomatic rest and/or the length of the graded exertion in children and adolescents. It is not appropriate for a child or adolescent athlete with concussion to RTP on the same day as the injury regardless of the level of athletic performance. Concussion modifiers apply even more to this population than adults and may mandate more cautious RTP advice.

2 Elite Versus Nonelite Athletes

The panel unanimously agreed that all athletes regardless of level of participation should be managed using the same treatment and return-to-play paradigm. A more useful construct was agreed whereby the available resources and expertise in concussion evaluation were of more importance in determining management than a separation between elite and nonelite athlete management.

Although formal baseline NP screening may be beyond the resources of many sports or individuals, it is recommended that in all organized high risk sports consideration be given to having this cognitive evaluation regardless of the age or level of performance.

3 Chronic Traumatic Brain Injury

Epidemiological studies have suggested an association between repeated sports concussions during a career and late life cognitive impairment. Similarly, case reports have noted anecdotal cases where neuropathological evidence of chronic traumatic encephalopathy was observed in retired football players (108–112). Panel discussion was held and no consensus was reached on the significance of such observations at this stage. Clinicians need to be mindful of the potential for long-term problems in the management of all athletes.

29.7 Injury Prevention

1 Protective Equipment—Mouthguards and Helmets

There is no good clinical evidence that currently available protective equipment will prevent concussion although mouthguards have a definite role in preventing dental and orofacial injury. Biomechanical studies have shown a reduction in impact forces to the brain with the use of head gear and helmets, but these findings have not been translated to show a reduction in concussion incidence. For skiing and snowboarding there are a number of studies to suggest that helmets provide protection against head and facial injury and hence should be recommended for participants in alpine sports (113–116). In specific sports such as cycling, motor and equestrian sports, protective helmets may prevent other forms of head injury (e.g., skull fracture) that are related to falling on hard road surfaces and these may be an important injury prevention issue for those sports (116–128).

2 Rule Change

Consideration of rule changes to reduce the head injury incidence or severity may be appropriate where a clear-cut mechanism is implicated in a particular sport. An example of this is in football (soccer) where research studies demonstrated that upper limb to head contact in heading contests accounted for approximately 50% of concussions (129). As noted earlier, rule changes also may be needed in some sports to allow an effective off-field medical assessment to occur without compromising the athlete's welfare, affecting the flow of the game or unduly penalizing the player's team. It is important to note that rule enforcement may be a critical aspect of modifying injury risk in these settings and referees play an important role in this regard.

3 Risk Compensation

An important consideration in the use of protective equipment is the concept of risk compensation (130). This is where the use of protective equipment results in behavioral change such as the adoption of more dangerous playing techniques, which can result in a paradoxical increase in injury rates. This may be a particular concern in child and adolescent athletes where head injury rates are often higher than in adult athletes (131–133).

4 Aggression Versus Violence in Sport

The competitive/aggressive nature of sport which makes it fun to play and watch should not be discouraged. However, sporting organizations should be encouraged to address violence that may increase concussion risk (134,135). Fair play and respect should be supported as key elements of sport.

29.8 Knowledge Transfer

As the ability to treat or reduce the effects of concussive injury after the event is minimal, education of athletes, colleagues and the general public is a mainstay of progress in this field. Athletes, referees, administrators, parents, coaches and health care providers must be educated regarding the detection of concussion, its clinical features, assessment techniques and principles of safe return to play.

Methods to improve education including web-based resources, educational videos and international outreach programs are important in delivering the message. In addition, concussion working groups plus the support and endorsement of enlightened sport groups such as Fédération Internationale de Football Association (FIFA), International Olympic Commission (IOC), International Rugby Board (IRB) and International Ice Hockey Federation (IIHF) who initiated this endeavor have enormous value and must be pursued vigorously. Fair play and respect for opponents are ethical values that should be encouraged in all sports and sporting associations. Similarly coaches, parents and managers play an important part in ensuring these values are implemented on the field of play (57,136–148).

29.9 Future Directions

The consensus panelists recognize that research is needed across a range of areas in order to answer some critical research questions. The key areas for research identified include:

- Validation of the SCAT2
- Gender effects on injury risk, severity and outcome
- Pediatric injury and management paradigms
- Virtual reality tools in the assessment of injury
- Rehabilitation strategies (e.g., exercise therapy)
- Novel Imaging modalities and their role in clinical assessment
- Concussion surveillance using consistent definitions and outcome measures
- Clinical assessment where no baseline assessment has been performed
- "Best-practice" neuropsychological testing
- Long term outcomes
- On-field injury severity predictors

29.10 Medical Legal Considerations

This consensus document reflects the current state of knowledge and will need to be modified according to the development of new knowledge. It provides an overview of issues that may be of importance to healthcare providers involved in the management of sports related concussion. It is not intended as a standard of care, and should not be interpreted as such. This document is only a guide, and is of a general nature, consistent with the reasonable practice of a healthcare professional. Individual treatment will depend on the facts and circumstances specific to each individual case. It is intended that this document will be formally reviewed and updated prior to 1 December 2012.

29.11 Statement on Background to Consensus Process

In November 2001, the 1st International Conference on Concussion in Sport was held in Vienna, Austria. This meeting was organized by the IIHF in partnership with FIFA and the Medical Commission of the IOC. As part of the resulting mandate for the future, the need for leadership and future updates were identified. The 2nd International Conference on Concussion in Sport was organized by the same group with the additional involvement of the IRB and was held in Prague, Czech Republic in November 2004. The original aims of the symposia were to provide recommendations for the improvement of safety and health of athletes who suffer concussive injuries in ice hockey, rugby, football (soccer) as well as other sports. To this end, a range of experts were invited to both meetings to address specific issues of epidemiology, basic and clinical science, injury grading systems, cognitive assessment, new research methods, protective equipment, management, prevention and long term outcome (1,2).

The 3rd International Conference on Concussion in Sport was held in Zurich, Switzerland on 29/30 October 2008 and was designed as a formal consensus meeting following the organizational guidelines set forth by the US National Institutes of Health. (Details of the consensus methodology can be obtained at: http://consensus.nih.gov/ABOUTCDP.htm)

The basic principles governing the conduct of a consensus development conference are summarized below:

1. A broad based nongovernment, nonadvocacy panel was assembled to give balanced, objective and knowledgeable attention to the topic. Panel members excluded anyone with scientific or commercial conflicts of interest and included researchers in clinical medicine, sports medicine, neuroscience, neuroimaging, athletic training and sports science.

2. These experts presented data in a public session, followed by inquiry and discussion. The panel then met in an executive session to prepare the consensus statement.

3. A number of specific questions were prepared and posed in advance to define the scope and guide the direction of the conference. The principle task of the panel was to elucidate responses to these questions. These questions are outlined below.

4. A systematic literature review was prepared and circulated in advance for use by the panel in addressing the conference questions.

5. The consensus statement is intended to serve as the scientific record of the conference.

6. The consensus statement will be widely disseminated to achieve maximum impact on both current health care practice and future medical research.

The panel chairperson (WM) did not identify with any advocacy position. The chairperson was responsible for directing the consensus session and guiding the panel's deliberations. Panelists were drawn from clinical practice, academic and research in the field of sports related concussion. They do not represent organizations per se but were selected for their expertise, experience and understanding of this field.

See Appendix pages 530–535 for Pocket Scat2 and Scat2 Forms.

Reference

See original document McCrory P, Meeuwisse W, Johnston K, et al. Consensus statement on Concussion in Sport—the 3rd International Conference on Concussion in Sport held in Zurich, November 2008. *J Sci Med Sport* 2009;12(3):340–351; *Phys Sportsmed* 37(2):141–159; *Pm R* 2009;1(5):406–420; *J Athl Train* 2009;44(4):434–448; *Clin J Sport Med* 2009;19(3):185–200. *J Clin Neurosci* 2009;16(6):755–763.

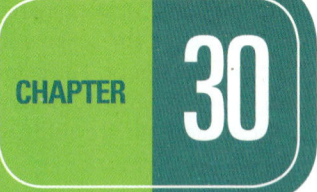

Sports Concussion—A Pragmatic Approach for Event Physicians

CHAPTER 30

Contributed by Jon Patricios, Sports Concussion South Africa, Johannesburg, South Africa

The most beautiful thing we can experience is the mysterious. It is the source of all true art and all science. He to whom this emotion is a stranger, who can no longer pause to wonder and stand rapt in awe, is as good as dead: his eyes are closed — Albert Einstein

Concussion is a trauma-induced change in mental state that may or may not involve loss of consciousness (LOC). The injury may manifest with any combination of physical, cognitive, emotional, and sleep-related symptom clusters including headache, dizziness, nausea, visual disturbances, amnesia, poor concentration, irritability, depressed affect, fatigue, and drowsiness.

Whereas previous definitions and classification systems emphasized LOC and amnesia as the primary manifestations of concussion, the revised definition since 2001 specifically acknowledges that this form of mild traumatic brain injury may present with a wide spectrum of symptoms. Previously, our definition of concussion was far simpler and management (apparently) easier; we now acknowledge that our previous understanding was invalid and our treatment inappropriate. Current models of understanding and management incorporate broader definitions and more thorough clinical evaluations and have introduced neuropsychologic testing. This appears to have widened the safety net around the concussed athlete, but protocols appear confusing and intimidating. As a result, the prospect of identifying and managing sports concussion from field side to return-to-play has perhaps become more daunting than ever, especially to clinicians who may not regularly face such clinical conundrums. This need not be so.

This chapter seeks to briefly review the historical evolution of concussion management, convey an understanding of the pathophysiology and potential immediate and long-term complications, and, most importantly, allow the event and team physician to develop a template for managing these injuries.

30.1 HISTORICAL REVIEW

Scientific research into many aspects of concussion has been impaired as much by differences in definition as by the ethical and practical issues involved in inducing and monitoring brain injury. From this has stemmed controversy regarding the ideal management of concussion in sport and a lack of objective data guiding return-to-play decisions, resulting in sports organizations relying on broad, subjective guidelines for head injury management and applying rigid, compulsory exclusion periods from sport depending on unvalidated grading systems of injury severity. The last 7 years have seen a more collated approach to head injury management in sports persons. Acknowledging that concussion is a potentially serious injury and that, as clinicians, we were found wanting with regards to a more objective assessment protocol, the first of a series of international collaborations took place in 2001.

This watershed occurred at the First International Conference on Concussion in Sport, Vienna (2001). During this conference, a comprehensive systematic approach to concussion was formulated for application in sport, which included computer-based neuropsychologic testing as an integral part of a comprehensive clinical concussion evaluation. Since then, consolidation of the Vienna guidelines has taken place at the Second International Conference in Prague (2004), and the National Athletic Trainers Association (United States, 2004) and the American College of Sports Medicine (2005) have published clinical management guidelines based on these consensus meetings. Most recently, in Zurich (October 2008), a review of scientific evidence in

TABLE 30.1	Symptoms of Concussions		
Physical	**Cognitive**	**Emotional**	**Sleep**
Headache	Poor concentration	Depression	Drowsiness
Photophobia	Problems remembering	Irritability	Insomnia
Dizziness	Feeling "foggy"	Mood swings	Sleeping more
Phonophobia	Feeling "slowed down"	Aggressiveness	Difficulty getting to sleep
Nausea			
Numbness/tingling			
Vomiting			
Fatigue			
Visual changes			
Balance problems			

the field was again presented, current protocols debated, and the Concussion in Sport Group again tasked with reviewing recommendations.

To summarize the findings and recommendations of all of these documents is beyond the scope of this chapter, but the most important common threads include the following:

- Concussion represents a serious neurologic injury that may present with a wide spectrum of symptoms and signs.

- Previous concussion assessment protocols were varied, subjective, and inconsistent.

- The emergence of computerized neuropsychological testing has both provided a useful diagnostic and monitoring tool and given impetus to concussion understanding and research but has limitations, especially when relied upon without clinical input.

- Serial clinical assessments both neurologic and cognitive remain the cornerstones of management.

- Certain sporting populations require a more specialized and conservative approach; these include pediatric participants (15 and under), those with a history of recurrent concussion, and those with neurologic and psychological comorbidity (e.g., depression, epilepsy, attention deficit disorder).

- Educating athletes, parents, coaches, and colleagues remains paramount to successful concussion programs.

The precise pathophysiology of concussion remains unclear. Research has shown that moderate to severe brain injury causes a complex cascade of neurochemical changes in the brain. The assumption is that similar changes occur in concussion. Immediately after biomechanical injury to the brain, abrupt, indiscriminant release of neurotransmitters and unchecked ionic fluxes occur. These ionic shifts lead to acute and subacute changes in cellular physiology. A "hypermetabolism" occurs in the setting of diminished cerebral blood flow, and the disparity between glucose supply and demand triggers a cellular energy crisis. The resulting energy crisis or "mismatch" may account for the symptoms and behavioral changes (Table 30.1) as well as being a likely mechanism for postconcussive vulnerability, making the brain less able to respond adequately to a second injury and potentially leading to longer lasting deficits.

30.2 THE POTENTIAL COMPLICATIONS OF CONCUSSION

Early Complications

Intracranial Space-occupying Lesions: Concussion may be, but is not usually, associated with damage to cerebral arteries and veins. Bleeding from these vessels may lead to epidural, subdural, or intracerebral hematomas. Signs of raised intracranial pressure have to be recognized immediately and treated surgically to decompress the brain.

This is a medical emergency and needs to be red-flagged by the event or team physician, and the player stabilized and removed to a hospital with brain imaging facilities and neurosurgical cover.

Dysautoregulation Syndrome

Diffuse cerebral swelling is a rare but well recognized complication of minor head injury and occurs mainly in children and teenagers. Second-impact syndrome was first reported to occur in American football players who died after relatively minor head injury. This injury may occur if a player returns to play prematurely following a previous head injury, hence the term "second impact." Brain edema and an increased vulnerability to injury during the biochemical "mismatch" described earlier may still be present from the previous blow. A second blow results in further swelling, followed by loss of the brain's ability to control blood inflow (autoregulation). Cerebral blood flow increases rapidly and brain pressure rises uncontrollably, leading to cardiorespiratory failure and possible death.

Impact Convulsions

Convulsions (seizures) in collision sports are not common but can appear as a dramatic event. They characteristically occur within 2 seconds of impact, but are not necessarily associated with structural brain damage. The good outcome with these episodes and the absence of long-term cognitive damage reflect the benign nature of these episodes, not necessarily warranting antiepileptic treatment and prolonged preclusion from contact sports.

30.3 MORE ENDURING COMPLICATIONS

Prolonged Postconcussion Syndrome

The clusters of symptoms manifesting after a concussive blow may persist for days to weeks. The consequences of symptoms such as headache, dizziness, memory loss, and fatigue are particularly significant in young people who may be in a learning environment, making decisions concerning rest from cognitive as well as physical stresses important.

Chronic Traumatic Encephalopathy

This condition reflects the cumulative effect of long-term exposure to repeated concussive and subconcussive blows. Certainly, there is growing concern that each episode of concussion may result in residual brain damage possibly associated with the cerebral deposition of abnormal Tau protein. This is most evident in the development of cognitive dysfunction in boxing, the degree of which is directly related to the number of bouts in a boxer's career. The cerebral damage that may occur is thought to be largely cortical and more subtle than the cerebellar and basal ganglia manifestations of dementia pugilistica. Cognitive deficits have also been documented in amateur, professional, and retired soccer players. Genetic factors, associated with the ApoE4 gene, may also increase the risk of developing chronic brain injury in sport. Future research will need to establish what severity of head injury causes summation and how long that residual effect may last. Thus, it would be responsible to want to document a player's cognitive function periodically and note whether any cognitive deficit is present.

The Risk of a Second Concussion

Players with a past history of concussion may be at increased risk of subsequent concussion. This, however, remains controversial, and it seems that certain players display a high-risk playing technique (tackling head-on) that places them at increased risk of concussion. The risk of concussion is a feature of any collision sport and is directly related to the amount of time spent actually playing the sport. Therefore, the chance of repeat concussion may reflect the level of exposure to injury risk.

The significance of these aspects for the event and team physician is the following:

- Red-flagging of potentially catastrophic injuries is a priority, and an efficient system for their management should be part of preevent planning.

- The acknowledgment of the risks of reexposure of the recently concussed athlete to a potential second blow must be acknowledged, and the player must not be allowed to return during the event.

- An understanding that the symptoms and signs of concussion may be diverse and vary in duration, necessitates referring the concussed player on, into a system capable of monitoring him or her and providing appropriate return-to-play guidance.

30.4 THE PRAGMATIC APPROACH

In order to crystallize the body of knowledge that has emerged over the last decade and practically apply the recommendations, the following steps need to be adhered to in the stepwise management of a concussed athlete:

- On-field—identify, stabilize, and remove the player

- Initial assessment—utilization of field side Sports Concussion Assessment Tool (SCAT)

- Formal clinical evaluation—emergency room/ consulting room

- Follow-up evaluation(s) (clinical +/− neuropsychological)

- Return-to-play—gradual reintroduction to contact and collision sport

In addition, it is essential to acknowledge that, at any stage in this process, an athlete may be red-flagged as having a potentially life-threatening head injury. This implies the need for an urgent brain CT or MRI scan and referral to a neurosurgeon (Fig. 30.1).

Signs of a potentially catastrophic injury that should be constantly monitored for include

- Headaches that worsen

- Severe neck pain

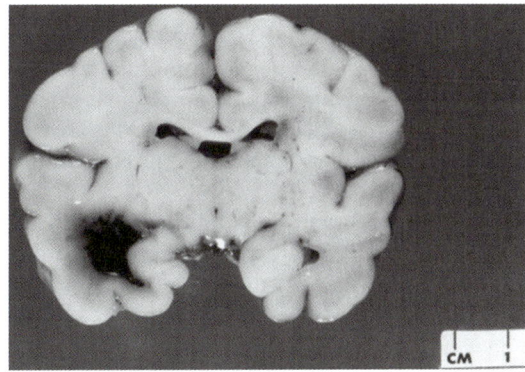

FIGURE 30.2. Postmortem specimen of intraventricular bleed.

- Looking very drowsy

- Being unable to recognize people or places

- Deteriorating consciousness

- Increasing confusion or irritability

- Unusual behavior change

- Repeated vomiting

- Slurred speech

- Focal neurologic signs

- Weakness/numbness in limbs

- Seizures

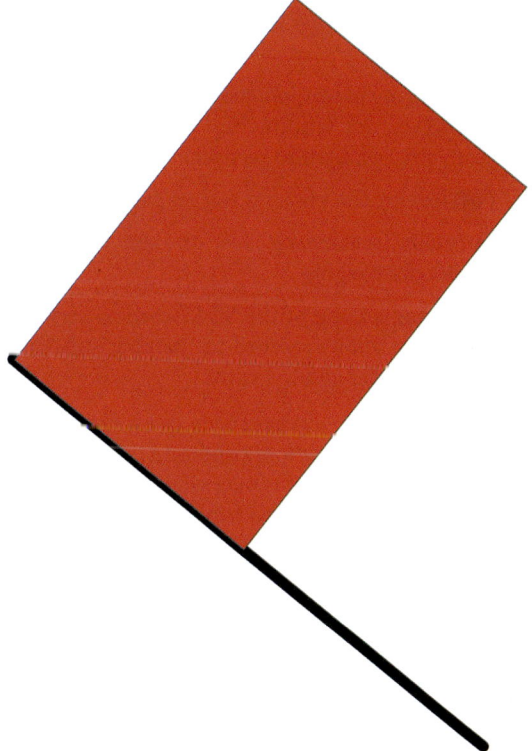

FIGURE 30.1.

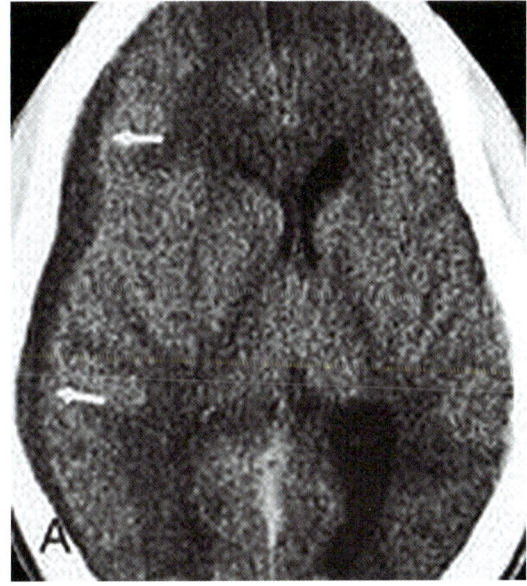

FIGURE 30.3. CT scan subdural hematoma. (Reprinted from Swischuk LE. *Emergency Imaging of the Acutely Ill or Injured Child.* 3rd ed. Philadelphia, PA: Lippincott Williams & Wilkins; 1994, with permission.)

On-field Management

This involves identifying the symptoms and signs of concussion, stabilizing the injured player particularly if an associated neck injury is in any way suspected, and removing the player from the field.

Asking appropriate questions that have been validated to demonstrate that brain function has been significantly enough affected to warrant removal from the field provides the first tool in concussion intervention. These eight questions described by D.L. Maddocks in 1995 serve as the first qualitative assessment of the player's mental state and indicate removal from the field should any of the answers be incorrect:

- What field are we at?
- Who are we playing?
- Who is your opponent at present?
- What half/quarter are we in?
- How far into the period are we?
- Who scored last?
- Who did we play last week?
- Did we win last week?

The typical signs of a concussed player on the field include confusion about on-field calls, being out of position, deterioration in play, or complaints of symptoms such as headache, nausea, dizziness, and blurred vision.

Should any of the symptoms and signs suggest a concussion, the player should be removed from the field. He or she should preferably be stretchered off and, if there is any suggestion of a neck injury, associated numbness, or paraesthesia, LOC, confusion, or seizures, the head and neck must be stabilized in a hard collar and head blocks as per neck injury protocol.

Field Side Assessment

This is the first opportunity to assess the player's neurologic status thoroughly and provides the first quantitative assessment of the injury, serving as the baseline measure of what should be a series of clinical evaluations before the player returns to play in the coming days or weeks.

This assessment should take place in a controlled environment sheltered from excessive light and noise stimulus and with restricted entry so that the clinician is able to work without interference of other players, coaches, spectators, and even family members. This will facilitate a more efficient and objective evaluation.

From the Prague conference in 2004 emerged a clinical tool that is specifically designed for field side concussion assessment. The Sports Concussion Assessment Tool or SCAT card has three purposes: education, red-flagging potentially catastrophic head injuries, and serving as the baseline clinical assessment. The original SCAT card (Fig. 30.4A) may be criticized for being a little cluttered with information, and is in the process of being revised following the Zurich meeting. There is no reason why the card cannot be customized for particular sporting codes as long as it contains the essential information that allows for education on the significance of concussion, red-flag criteria, a symptom scoring system and basic record of the clinical examination. Additional useful information may include emergency and follow-up contact numbers and concussion information Web sites. An example of a SCAT card modified for South African Rugby is given below (Fig. 30.4B).

The important tenet of clinical concussion evaluation is that the patient should be monitored serially to establish a trend in symptoms. Most cases of concussion will improve from soon after the time of injury and it is important to facilitate this by

- Keeping the player in a relatively quiet environment (i.e., not sending him or her back to the team environment to recover)
- Not leaving the player unaccompanied
- Formally reassessing his or her condition before discharging
- Providing a copy of the SCAT card to serve as a baseline clinical record for comparison with future assessments

Concussed players who have been assessed field side by a medical doctor, whose condition is improving, and have no red-flag signs may safely be discharged home in the care of a responsible adult.

Those who have been red-flagged, whose symptoms and signs are deteriorating or not improving or where no medical doctor is available, should be referred to an emergency department or doctor who should reassess the patient clinically, determine the need for brain imaging, and admit more neurologic observation if appropriate.

Pharos Sport Concussion Assessment Tool (SCAT)

The SCAT Card
(Sport Concussion Assessment Tool)
Athlete Information

What is a concussion? A concussion is a disturbance in the function of the brain caused by a direct or indirect force to the head. It results in a variety of symptoms (like those listed below) and may, or may not, involve memory problems or loss of consciousness.

Signs to watch for: RED FLAGS
GO TO HOSPITAL IMMEDIATELY
- Headache
- Very drowsy
- Can't recognise people and places
- Vomiting
- Confused
- Seizures
- Unsteady
- Slurred speech

How do you feel? You should score yourself on the following symptoms, based on how you feel now.

None = 0   Mild = 1   Moderate = 2   Severe = 3

PHYSICAL (9)					COGNITIVE (3)				
Headache	0	1	2	3	Feeling slowed down	0	1	2	3
Dizziness	0	1	2	3	Poor concentration	0	1	2	3
Nausea	0	1	2	3	Poor memory	0	1	2	3
Vomiting	0	1	2	3	**COGNITIVE TOTAL**				/9
Light Sensitivity	0	1	2	3	EMOTIONAL (4)				
Noise Sensitivity	0	1	2	3	Irritability	0	1	2	3
Visual changes	0	1	2	3	Sadness	0	1	2	3
Numbness / Tingling	0	1	2	3	More emotional than usual	0	1	2	3
Poor Balance	0	1	2	3	Nervousness	0	1	2	3
PHYSICAL TOTAL				/27	**EMOTIONAL TOTAL**				/12

SLEEP (4)				
Drowsiness	0	1	2	3
Sleeping less	0	1	2	3
Sleeping more	0	1	2	3
Trouble falling asleep	0	1	2	3
SLEEP TOTAL				/12

PHYSICAL + COGNITIVE + EMOTIONAL + SLEEP
= TOTAL SYMPTOM SCORE /60

Exertion:
Do these symptoms worsen with:
- Physical activity   Yes ☐ No ☐
- Cognitive activity   Yes ☐ No ☐

Overall Rating: How different is the person acting compared to his/her usual self? Normal 1 2 3 4 5 Very different

What should I do?
Any athlete suspected of having a concussion should be removed from play, and then seek medical evaluation.
Remember, it is better to be safe. **Consult your doctor after a suspected concussion.**

What can I expect?
Concussion typically results in the rapid onset of short-lived impairment that resolves spontaneously over time. You can expect that you will be told to rest until you are fully recovered (that means resting your body and your mind). Then, your doctor will likely advise that you go through a gradual increase in exercise over several days (or longer) before returning to sport.

www.sportsconcussion.co.za
Spineline: 0800 678678

A

The SCAT Card
(Sport Concussion Assessment Tool)
Medical Evaluation

Name: _____ Date: _____

Sport/Team: _____

1) SIGNS - Circle Yes or No
Was there loss of consciousness or unresponsiveness? Y N
Was there seizure or convulsive activity? Y N
Was there a balance problem / unsteadiness? Y N
Was there memory loss? Y N

2) MEMORY
Modified Maddocks questions (check correct)

At what venue are we?____; Which half is it?____; Who scored last?____

What team did we play last?____; Did we win last game?____

Which team are we playing? _____

3) SYMPTOM SCORE
Total number of positive symptoms (from opposite page) = _____

4) COGNITIVE ASSESSMENT

5 word recall		Immediate	Delayed
	Examples		(After concentration tasks)
Word 1_____	cat	____	____
Word 2_____	pen	____	____
Word 3_____	shoe	____	____
Word 4_____	book	____	____
Word 5_____	car	____	____

Months in reverse order:
Jun-May-Apr-Mar-Feb-Jan-Dec-Nov-Oct-Sep-Aug-Jul (circle incorrect)

Digits backwards (check correct)
5-2-8   3-9-1   _____
6-2-9-4   4-3-7-1   _____
8-3-2-7-9   1-4-9-3-6   _____
7-3-9-1-4-2   5-1-8-4-6-8   _____
Ask delayed 5-word recall now

Pulse _____ bpm
BP. _____ mmHg

5) NEUROLOGIC SCREENING

	Pass	Fail
PEARL	____	____
Light sensitivity	____	____
Eye motion	____	____
Balance test	____	____
Gait assessment	____	____
Any neurological abnormality	____	____

Any neurologic screening abnormality necessitates formal neurologic or hospital assessment

There should be approximately 24 hours (or longer) for each stage and the athlete should return to stage 1 if symptoms recur. Resistance training should only be added in the later stages. Medical clearance should be given by a doctor before return to play.

www.sportsconcussion.co.za
Spineline: 0800 678678

FIGURE 30.4.   **A:** Original SCAT card.

Instructions:

SCAT is for use by medical doctors, physiotherapists or athletic trainers. In order to optimise the information gathered from the card, it is strongly suggested that all athletes participating in contact sports complete a baseline evaluation prior to the beginning of their competitive season. This card is a suggested guide only for sports concussion and is not meant to assess more severe forms of brain injury. Please give a COPY of this card to the athlete for their information and to guide follow-up assessment.

Return To Play

Athletes should not be returned to play on the same day of injury. When returning athletes to play, they should follow a stepwise, symptom-limited program, with stages of progression. For example:
1. Rest until asymptomatic (physical and mental rest)
2. Light aerobic exercise (e.g. Stationary cycle)
3. Sport-specific exercise
4. Non-contact training drills (start light resistance training)
5. Full contact training after medical clearance
6. Return to competition (game play)

For More Information:

Johannesburg:
Dr Jon Patricios
Morningside Sports Medicine & CSMO
011-883 9000 / 011-442 8233
082-574 6918
e-mail: sportsconcussion@mweb.co.za

Cape Town
Dr Ryan Kohler
Western Province High Performance Centre
021-659 4524
082-784 5737
e-mail: ryank@yebo.co.za

www.sportsconcussion.co.za
Spineline: 0800 678678

B

Sports Concussion Assessment Tool (SCAT)

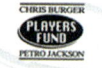 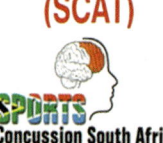 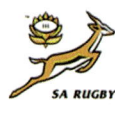

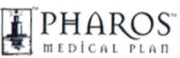 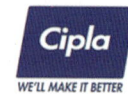

The SCAT Tool represents a standardized method of evaluating people after concussion in sport. This SCAT Tool has been modified as part of the Summary and Agreement Statement of the Third International Conference on Concussion in Sport, Zurich, 2008.

Post Concussion Symptoms

Ask the athlete to score themselves based on how they feel now. It is recognized that a low score may be normal for some athletes, but clinical judgment should be exercised to determine if the change in symptoms has occurred following the suspected concussion event.

It should be recognized that the reporting of symptoms may not be entirely reliable. This may be due to the effects of a concussion or because the athlete's passionate desire to return to competition outweighs their natural inclination to give an honest response.

If possible, ask someone who knows the athlete well about changes in affect, personality, behaviour etc.

Please see back page for further instructions
www.sportsconcussion.co.za
Spineline: 0800 678678

FIGURE 30.4. *(continued)* **B**: SCAT card modified for South African Rugby.

Whether discharging home or to hospital, emphasis must be paced on

- Appropriate behavior over the following 48 to 72 hours (Table 30.2)
- Monitoring for red-flag signs
- The importance of follow-up with a doctor (sports physician, neurologist, or neurosurgeon) familiar with modern concussion protocol
- Not exercising at all until cleared to do so by such a doctor

Formal Clinical Evaluation

A more structured assessment in the form of an emergency room evaluation or office consultation may be the first assessment postconcussion if the symptoms and signs were not acknowledged field side or, preferably, be a follow-up evaluation by a doctor well-versed in concussion management paradigms.

This setting allows for a more thorough history that includes an account of the mechanism of injury, LOC, anterograde and retrograde amnesia, a history of previous concussions and head

---

TABLE 30.2 **Patient Discharge Information for 48 Hours After Injury**

Patient Information—Important Reminders for the First 48 h

A normal x-ray, CT, or MRI scan *does NOT exclude concussion*.

You may be referred home after being assessed. In this case:

- Always make sure that you are in the presence of a responsible adult for 48 h.
- Record and monitor the symptoms of concussion including headache, nausea, dizziness, fatigue, sleep disturbances, memory lapses, mood swings, poor concentration, or any other feeling that concerns you.
- Complete rest and sleep will help recovery.

Do not

- Drive a motor vehicle or motorcycle if symptomatic.
- Consume alcohol
- Take excessive amounts of painkillers (follow the doctor's orders)
- Place yourself in an environment of loud noise and excessive light
- Study
- Work at the computer
- Exercise until reevaluation by a doctor

Contact your nearest emergency department immediately if

- Any of the symptoms deteriorate
- The headache becomes severe or does not respond to mild analgesics (e.g., paracetamol)
- You have a seizure (fit)
- You experience excessive irritability
- You experience visual disturbances
- You experience balance problems
- You or anyone else is concerned about your condition

Decisions regarding returning to sport will be made taking into consideration your individual circumstances including medical history, previous head injuries, and current symptoms.

You must receive clearance from a doctor before returning to sport.

and neck injuries, and associated comorbid factors such as other neurologic, psychological, and endocrinologic conditions that may impact on recovery.

The symptom score should again cover physical, cognitive, emotional, and sleep manifestations and be compared to earlier symptoms.

The controlled environment of the consultation room also lends itself to verbal screening of cognitive function via a short battery of tests such as immediate and delayed word recall, reverse digit recall, and reverse months of the year.

Assessment of balance is increasingly being recognized as a useful monitoring tool, especially where this may be compared to preinjury records. Either formal computerized test batteries or clinical evaluation using two-foot, one-leg, and tandem-stance assessments such as the Balance Error Scoring System (BESS) may provide further clinical insight. The BESS consists of three tests lasting 20 seconds each, performed on two different surfaces, firm and foam.

The athlete first stands with the feet narrowly together, the hands on the hips, and the eyes closed (double leg stance). The athlete holds this stance for 20 seconds while the number of balance errors (opening the eyes; hands coming off hips; a step, stumble, or fall; moving the hips more than 30 degrees; lifting the forefoot or heel; or remaining out of testing position for more than 5 seconds) are recorded.

The test is then repeated with a single-leg stance using the nondominant foot and a third time using a heel–toe stance with the nondominant foot in the rear (tandem stance).

All three tests are performed on a firm surface (grass, turf, court), and again on a piece of medium-density foam (a piece of foam can easily be carried in a travel trunk or equipment bag for road games).

The general medical examination should include blood pressure and pulse measurements, and an evaluation of associated injuries, especially neck and maxillofacial injuries.

Thereafter, a neurologic evaluation—including evaluation of all cranial nerves; pupil response; fundoscopy; and motor, sensory, and cerebellar function—should be performed.

An example of the clinical template that incorporates all of these assessment criteria is the Acute Concussion Evaluation (ACE) by Gioia and Collins (2006) available at http://www.cdc.gov/ncipc/tbi/ACE.pdf. Versions of this clinical evaluation (see Appendix), used to serially assess the athlete,

are likely to provide a further quantitative guide to recovery status and clinical trends.

Again, it should be emphasized that, at all times from field side through all office consultations, a high level of alertness for potential red-flag symptoms and signs should be maintained by the assessing clinician.

Neuropsychologic Evaluation

Since 2001, computerized neuropsychological test batteries have emerged as useful objective measures of alteration in brain function following a concussion, particularly where these can be compared to preinjury baseline scores for the same player. Postconcussion recovery rates vary between individuals. Some players may take days and others may take weeks to recover. Individual factors associated with each concussion injury are different and emerging evidence has suggested that genetic factors may be involved in both the response to head injury and recovery rates. There are dangers associated with universal mandatory exclusion criteria. It may be tempting to assume that a player has completely recovered from concussion as soon as an arbitrary time period has passed and that a medical assessment is not necessary, when in fact brain function, as measured by neuropsychological evaluation, is still abnormal. These test batteries help to provide an additional check particularly where players, under pressure to return to play, may mask symptoms.

A neuropsychological test is designed to assess the ability of the brain to process information (cognitive function). Traditional paper-and-pencil tests, such as the Digit Symbol Substitution Test, have been replaced by more practically applied computerized neuropsychological tests. Computer tests are quick and easy to administer, show fewer learning effects, and, more importantly, are able to detect very subtle changes in cognitive function by measuring response variability, a feature not found with the paper-and-pencil tests. Computerized tests are cost-effective and easily accessible to a large number of players. The tests are designed for medical doctors to administer, as the aim of the test is to determine whether cognitive dysfunction is present and not the reason for abnormal function.

Examples of computerized tests include Automated Neuropsychological Assessment Metrics (ANAM), CogState Sport, HeadMinders, and the Immediate Post-Concussion Assessment and Cognitive Testing (ImPACT). The test can be administered by team physicians and performed as part of a preseason evaluation forming a baseline neuropsychological assessment. The benefits are that the player returns to play cognitively as well as symptomatically recovered and has the ability to perform sports-specific skills optimally. Newer protocols suggest not testing the athlete whilst symptomatic as this may induce unnecessary cognitive stress, possibly increase the chances of a practice effect and not alter the immediate management of the player. Issues of cost and accessibility may prevent the use of computerized tests, and concussion management protocols should be able to be implemented without their use.

A neuropsychologist, as part of the multidisciplinary sports concussion team, should be consulted if cognitive function is severe and prolonged, in cases of recurrent concussion over a short period, in players who appear to suffer concussion with relatively minor impacts, where neurologic or psychological comorbidity exists (e.g., depression, attention deficit disorder, migraine sufferers), and in cases where a decision to stop a player partaking in contact or collision sport is to be considered. In these cases, the neuropsychologist will perform a more extensive battery of verbal, pencil-and-paper, and computerized tests to establish the cognitive implications of the injury.

Return to Play Protocol

The final phase of a safe, structured and supervised concussion rehabilitation protocol involves the progressive exposure of the recovering athlete to increasing degrees of exercise intensity whilst monitoring symptoms. This process should be preceded by both clinical and cognitive recovery. In other words, the player should be asymptomatic, have a normal neurologic examination, and have neuropsychological data (where utilized) that have returned to baseline or are comparable with age-appropriate norms. The end point is a return to match competition.

Return-to-play following concussion follows a stepwise process. No activity and complete rest until the player

- Is asymptomatic
- Has a normal neurologic and balance assessment
- Has neuropsychological test parameters that have returned to baseline preseason values or are comparable to age-appropriate norms

Exercise rehabilitation program:

- Light aerobic exercise (walking and stationary cycling)
- Sport-specific training (running drills, ball handling skills)
- Noncontact drills
- Full-contact practice
- Game play

An example of a return-to-play protocol is provided in Appendix. The player can proceed in a stepwise progression to the level above after 24 hours provided he or she is asymptomatic. This gradual reexposure to exercise serves as a final "stress test." If any postconcussion symptoms develop, the player should drop back to the previous asymptomatic level.

Support Network

The emphasis on a multidisciplinary approach to head injury management necessitates the need for a clinical support network able to manage the injured player from the time of injury to return-to-play. Essential for adequate cover at the event are

- Field side medical and paramedical personnel trained in concussion identification, head and neck stabilization, and removal of the head-injured player
- The equipment necessary to stabilize a head-injured player (hard collar, head block, spine board)
- A private room or medical facility appropriate for assessment of the player
- Field side ambulance
- On-call emergency room or casualty room
- On-call radiology center with CT and/or MRI facilities
- On-call radiologist and neurosurgeon
- For follow-up, contact should be established with
  - A sports physician or neurologist well-versed in sports concussion protocol
  - A neuropsychologist
  - Physiotherapists to help manage associated (especially neck) injuries

- Additional useful resources include
  - Field side SCAT cards
  - Pamphlets detailing the guidelines for the player and his or her family on discharge
  - Contact numbers of doctors and emergency rooms
  - Educational material and useful Web site information for the patient and family

30.5 CONCLUSION

Sports-related concussion management appears to have partially emerged from the somewhat nebulous and eclectic guidelines of the 20th century. The series of international consensus statements since 2001 appear to not only have consolidated expert opinion into a more unitary model but exponentially spurred research and interest in the field. The vast increase in concussion publications, seminars, and educational material may have led to a somewhat confusing management scenario for event and filed side clinicians. This review of current concepts in concussion management emphasizes a structured clinical protocol incorporating a thorough history, serial clinical assessments, and a graded return-to-play process. Where available, computerized neuropsychological testing is a useful adjunct and often the only objective representation of changes to the affected player's brain. Adopting international conventions in the management of players of all levels is in the best clinical interest of our players, will allow for a framework of practical research, and will help mitigate against the possible medicolegal consequences of poorly managed head injuries.

Recommended Reading

Aubry M, Cantu R, Dvorak J, et al. Summary and agreement statement of the First International Conference on Concussion in Sport, Vienna 2001. Recommendations for the improvement of safety and health of athletes who may suffer concussive injuries. *Br J Sports Med.* 2002;36:6–10.

Cantu RC. Second-impact syndrome. *Clin Sports Med.* 1998;17:37–44.

Collie A, Maruff P. Computerised neuropsychological testing. *Br J Sports Med.* 2003;37:2–32.

Collins MW, Iverson GL, Lovell MR, et al. On-field predictors of neuropsychological deficit following sport-related concussion. *Clin J Sports Med.* 2003;13(4):222.

Collins MW, Lovell MR, Iverson GL, et al. Cumulative effects of concussion in high school athletes. *Neurosurgery.* 2002;51:1175–1181.

Gioia G, Collins M. Acute Concussion Evaluation (ACE). Heads Up: Brain Injury In Sport Your Practice Tool Kit. Center for Disease Control, http://www.cdc.gov/ncipc/pub-res/tbi_toolkit/tbi/ACE, modified June 2007.

Giza GC, Houda DA. The neurometabolic cascade of concussion. *J Athl Train.* 2001;31(3):228–235.

Guskiewicz KM, Bruce SL, Cantu RC, et al. National Athletic Trainers position statement on the management of sports-related concussion. *J Athl Train.* 2004;39:278–295.

Herring SA, Bergfield JA, Boland A, et al. ACSM team physician consensus statement: concussion (mild traumatic brain injury) and the team physician. *Med Sci Sports Exerc.* 2006;2:395–399.

Maddocks D, Dicker G. An objective measure of recovery from concussion in Australian rules footballers. *Sport Health.* 1989;7:6–7.

Maddocks DL, Dicker GD, Saling MM. The assessment of orientation following concussion in athletes. *Clin J Sports Med.* 1995;5(1):32.

McCrory P, Johnston K, Meeuwisse W, et al. Summary and agreement statement of the 2nd International Conference on Concussion in Sport, Prague, 2004. *Br J Sports Med.* 2005.

CHAPTER 31

Acute Headache

Contributed by Bredo Knudtzen, Neurologist; Former Team Physician, Norwegian National Ice Hockey Team; Consultant, National Centre for Epilepsy, Norway

Reviewer: Prof. Lars Jacob Stovner, National Headache Centre, NTNU, Trondheim, Norway

An athlete who presents with an acute, new, severe headache is more likely to have a more serious underlying pathology than a patient with yearlong recurrent headache episodes. The event physician must especially consider the following conditions due to the seriousness:

- Subarachnoid hemorrhage (SAH)

- Epidural or subdural hematoma

- Meningitis

- Purulent sinusitis

At a sporting event, athletes may present to the event physician with acute headache. As usual, the event physician must think of the worst possible causal conditions and endeavor to exclude these first. A short but precise history is vital; ask the athlete the following questions:

- First-time episode (more dangerous?) or history of headaches?

- Pain intensity: mild, medium, or severe?

- Pain location: frontal/facial (sinusitis?), lower occipital (SAH?), band like (tension?)

- History of recent trauma? (epidural or subdural hematoma?)

- Fever? (meningitis, encephalitis, sinusitis, or SAH?)

31.1 ACUTE NONTRAUMATIC SUBARACHNOID HEMORRHAGES

These life-threatening hemorrhages may occur in the sporting environment. Usually, there is an underlying aneurysm or vascular malformation that may rupture either spontaneously or after a traumatic episode. As aneurysms take time to develop, these usually rupture later in life, whereas arteriovenous malformations (AVM) are congenital and are more likely to be the cause of SAH in younger athletes. Other rarer causes of hemorrhage include tumors and infection. Figures vary regarding the incidence of SAHs around the world but seem to be in the region of 8 cases per 100,000 person years (Linn et al., 1996).

If a major bleed occurs, then the patient may die within minutes. Other bleeds may be less severe and may be either due to the rupture of smaller aneurysms or due to a gradual leakage from an AVM. For these lesser bleeds, the main pathological consequence of a subarachnoid hemorrhage is local vasospasm, where a protective vasospasm may occur and lead to tissue ischemia and infarction. In-hospital treatment requires early surgical intervention to stop the bleeding (and treat other surgical complications such as hydrocephalus) and the administration of medications to reverse the vasospasm and increase cranial blood flow.

Therefore, in relation to an athlete with a SAH, the event physician has three fundamental tasks:

- Early suspicion and diagnosis

- Emergency treatment if necessary

- Immediate hospitalization

Early Suspicion and Diagnosis

Typically, patients present with a sudden, new, severe, and intense headache. The pain may intensify over several days (if the patient lives that long).

Intense pain, often described as "the worst pain in my life" is often accompanied by nausea and vomiting and many feel dizzy with disturbed balance. In one study, approximately 50% of patients who survived an SAH said that the onset of pain was instantaneous, 20% stated that pain developed over a 1- to 5-minute period, and the remaining 30% took even longer time to develop maximum pain. Apparently, the speed of onset cannot be relied on to identify all cases of SAH; however, those patients with classical sudden, intense headache should be investigated for the presence of a subarachnoid hemorrhage.

Loss of consciousness (LOC) occurs in about 50% of cases with spontaneous bleeding. Seizures may occur during or after this LOC.

On examination, there may be partial paralysis, loss of vision, photophobia, and dysphasia.

The classical finding of a stiff neck may be present, though the sensitivity of this test is disputed.

Spontaneous subarachnoid hemorrhages due to AVMs may be preceded by sentinel symptoms (headaches, nausea, blurred vision, vomiting, dizziness) in days leading up to the bleed. This headache is usually described as having a precise starting time, being constant (day and night without relief), and usually being progressive. So, if an athlete complains of extreme intense headache, a history of acute onset, and a new, constant headache combined with nausea or dizziness, alarm bells should ring. Many authors (Al Shahi et al., 1996) do not accept the existence of sentinel bleeds and believe the term should be abandoned[2]; however, if you encounter the above scenario, refer the patient to hospital, as CT scan, MRI, or spinal puncture is strongly recommended. Remember that noncontrast CT is not 100% sensitive, and negative CT scan does not always exclude an SAH.

MRI is more sensitive but not always immediately available.

SAH symptoms may be vague, but the presence of instantaneous, constant headache, without relapse, often worse for each day is not typical of tension or stress headaches. These symptoms may be present in cases of meningitis or encephalitis, but these cases too need referral to hospital.

Neck Stiffness (Nuchal Rigidity)

Passively flex the patient's neck and try to touch the patient's chest with his chin. If nuchal rigidity is present, then flexion may produce pain or muscle spasms that prevent the chin touching the chest (one must ensure that no cervical spine trauma is present).

Nuchal rigidity may indicate a life-threatening subarachnoid hemorrhage or meningitis. Unfortunately, studies indicate a poor diagnostic accuracy for this test in meningitis patients and the same assumption is made for its accuracy in diagnosing SAH.

Treatment: Stabilization is the primary goal, and in worse cases may involve intubation, ventilation, and the administration of supplemental oxygen or intravenous fluids. Should seizures occur, an anticonvulsant should be given, but be aware of oversedating trauma patients. If the headache is intense, pain killers may be administered intramuscularly.

Prognosis: The overall prospects for SAH are not good—approximately 10% to 15% of those who suffer an aneurysmal hemorrhage do not live long enough to get medical treatment, 20% to 40% die of complications, and approximately 12% of the survivors have permanent neurologic disability, such as partial paralysis, cognitive or speech difficulties, and vision problems. SAHs associated with traumatic brain injury have a poor prognosis with over half having being associated with death or severe disability.

31.2 ACUTE MENINGITIS

Various studies show that approximately 25% of adults with acute bacterial meningitis do not survive and that many survivors have to live with neurological sequelae. The longer one delays effective treatment, the worse the prognosis (Aronin et al., 1998).

This is one of those disorders where the event physician must think and act quickly. There are several treatment guidelines for acute meningitis available (e.g., the British Infection Society), but, as with SAH, the event physician has three fundamental tasks:

- Early suspicion and diagnosis
- Emergency treatment if necessary
- Immediate hospitalization

van de Beek et al., from the University of Amsterdam, conducted a nationwide study over a 4-year period in the Netherlands that included all adults with community-acquired acute bacterial meningitis. They found that the classic triad was present in only 44% of episodes:

- Fever
- Neck stiffness
- Changed mental status

However, they found that 95% of patients had at least two of the four symptoms:

- Headache
- Fever
- Neck stiffness
- Altered mental status

They concluded that the strongest risk factors for an unfavorable outcome were those where there was systemic compromise, a low level of consciousness, and infection with *Streptococcus pneumoniae*.

The take-home message here is that physicians must have a low threshold for referral when athletes present with acute headache, fever, nuchal rigidity, and altered mental status. In the early phase of illness, these are very difficult diagnoses to make when alone at a sports event without access to a laboratory and with little or no support around you. Unfortunately, the diagnosis may be a lot easier to make when the athlete is seriously ill, but by then it may be too late to prevent a catastrophic outcome.

Clinical findings may be minimal initially but if the patient has any of the following shock/ pre-shock findings, then a crisis is preimminent and urgent referral to a hospital—by helicopter if available and if faster—is advised.

- Poor peripheral perfusion, CRT > 4 seconds
- Falling systolic BP, particularly if under 90
- Respiratory rate under 8 or over 30
- Pulse rate under 40 or over 140
- Depressed conscious level (GCS < 12) or varying conscious levels (fall in GCS > 2)
- Focal neurology
- Seizures
- Bradycardia and hypertension
- Papilloedema
- Rash and particularly if rapidly progressive

Obviously ABC must be carried out and an intravenous line should be established.

The most common pathogens in acute bacterial meningitis are *S. pneumoniae* and *Neisseria meningitides*. For young patients with suspected meningococcal disease (they may have a rash and a meningococcal septicemia as well) the immediate use of intravenous/oral antibiotics (penicillin) followed by rapid admission to a hospital is considered by many to be correct treatment.

The problem with adult bacterial meningitis is that the causative agent is usually not a meningococcus. Sigurdardottir et al. in 1994, conducted a 20-year review of all acute adult bacterial meningitis in Iceland. They found a mean annual incidence of 3.8 per 100,000. The most common causative organisms were *N. meningitidis*, *S. pneumoniae*, *Listeria monocytogenes*, and *Haemophilus influenzae*. *N. meningitidis* caused 93% of the infections in the 16- to 20-year-old age group, but it caused only 25% of the infections in patients aged 45 years or older. A significant underlying illness or condition was present in 39% of the patients. They concluded that most cases were caused by pneumococci and *Listeria*.

In parts of the world, there is an increasing penicillin-resistance amongst pneumococci. There is also an issue of administering indiscriminate antibiotics that may or not have an effect and that may influence antimicrobial testing on arrival at the hospital. Some studies show that mortality rates have not been improved by preadmission antibiotics.

I can only recommend that you follow local guidelines on this issue.

However, there is no doubt that the earlier a patient arrives at a hospital (or arrives at a unit that has been alerted), the better are the chances of survival. This requires that the admitting physician is observant, lucky, has a low threshold for referral, organizes immediate admission to a hospital, and warns the hospital of the patient's imminent arrival.

Viral meningitis is commonest amongst children, but rare in healthy adults. Clinically, it is impossible to accurately differentiate between viral and bacterial causative agents. Enteroviruses are the most common cause at all ages. Most cases are self-limiting, although morbidity may be considerable. Herpes simplex virus may cause viral meningitis, so symptoms may recur.

All suspected cases of meningitis should be admitted to a hospital.

31.3 ACUTE ENCEPHALITIS

Acute encephalitis is a complex and severe inflammatory condition. The Event Physician is not likely to meet a case of acute encephalitis for the simple reason that an athlete will usually be too sick to turn up. The lesion may present with similar clinical findings as found in SAH and bacterial meningitis. However, the presentation is usually not as dramatic and the onset of symptoms is usually spread over some days, rather than an "out-of-the-blue" onset of SAH and acute bacterial meningitis. Symptoms may vary, depending on which part of the brain is most affected. Findings may include

- Fever
- Headache
- Photophobia
- Altered mental status with confusion, disorientation, irritability, anxiety
- Poor memory/memory loss
- Seizures
- Weakness or numbness of arm or leg

Acute encephalitis can be caused by a wide variety of conditions, viruses being the commonest causative agent. The list includes

- Viral infection: In Europe, herpes simplex virus is the commonest cause. Others include rash-causing viruses (e.g., mumps, measles, rubella); upper respiratory tract viruses (e.g., flu, enteroviruses); gut viruses (e.g., enteroviruses, echovirus); insect-borne viruses (e.g., Japanese encephalitis virus, West Nile virus); and tick-borne viruses (e.g., Central European tick-borne virus)
- Bacterial infections are rare (mycoplasma, meningococcal, pneumococcal, and listeria)
- Postinfectious autoimmune reactions and autoimmune reactions
- Fungi (e.g., histoplasma, cryptococcus, candida)
- Ingestion of toxic substances
- Parasites (e.g., malaria, toxoplasma)
- Drug reactions
- Underlying malignancy

Treatment: Once again, the symptoms are so similar to SAH and acute bacterial meningitis that admission to a hospital is the only option.

31.4 ACUTE MIGRAINE

The event physician is not often confronted with an acute first-time migraine attack. Having stated this, I have met scores of athletes with established migraine who suffer attacks before, during or after major sports events. As the diagnosis of migraine is complicated and time-consuming (diaries are often needed; neurological examinations, brain scans, and blood tests need to be taken; MIDAS disability scores may be needed; etc.), it is impossible for an EP to make a certain diagnosis on a first-time patient. I would recommend referral to a hospital of this first-time "migraine" headache as the headache may be due to some of the life-threatening disorders mentioned above (SAH, meningitis, etc.).

In patients with known migraine, the situation is different. Migraine patients are often well aware of the trigger factors that bring on an attack and recognize the accumulation of symptoms and headache characteristics. If the symptoms are typical and the patient can reassure the doctor (!) that he or she has experienced identical episodes before in similar situations, then it is reasonable to prescribe the migraine medication that the athlete is familiar with. Migraine athletes will probably only consult the EP if they have forgotten their migraine medication or if the medication does not work (beware). The fact that medication does not work may be due to the exceptional circumstances surrounding the athlete. At a major sports event, an athlete may be experiencing major stress and a lack of sleep due to all the excitement in the buildup to the event. The athlete may be surrounded by bright lights, media, and loudspeakers; a menstruation may be just around the corner; athletes in sports involving weight classes may not have eaten properly for several days. All of these factors may trigger a first-time migraine in a predisposed patient or they may trigger a more intense and atypical migraine attack in a patient with known migraine.

An acute migraine may present with intense headache, nausea, and altered mental status—the same symptoms that may be found with an SAH and with meningitis. The only course of action open to the event physician is to admit to a hospital patients with symptoms associated with SAH and meningitis. The classical migraine headache is moderate to severe, throbbing, unilateral, and worsened by movement. SAH and meningitis may also present with pain that may be unilateral (or expressed as being so by a patient in an altered mental status). In other words, the presence of unilateral headache does not guarantee the diagnosis of migraine.

If you decide that the headache warrants admission to a hospital, be prepared: This may not be a popular diagnostic conclusion for many athletes, particularly if it is on the morning of a major championship. Athletes may demand medication and say that they will seek medical attention after

TABLE 31.1	Clinical Findings in Migraine			
Nausea	Scalp Tenderness	Visual disturbances	Diarrhea	Seizure
Photophobia	Lightheadedness	Vertigo	Altered consciousness	
Phonophobia	Vomiting	Paresthesias	Syncope	

the event if symptoms have not improved. As physicians, we can only give advice; we cannot forcibly remove athletes from an event unless the rules of a particular sport or country allow us to do so. The final responsibility lies with the athlete, but the EP's advice must be based on sound clinical judgment and not on insecurity or the fear of legal reprimand. Remember that an unnecessary trip to a hospital may ruin an athlete's chances to win a gold medal; at the same time, if an athlete is cleared for competition and then dies on the sports field from an SAH, the EP will surely be held responsible and face investigation. These are not easy decisions; if in doubt, consult a specialist over the telephone. If you suspect SAH or meningitis, always admit the patient immediately.

Migraine is the second most common cause of headache, after tension headaches, affecting approximately 6% of men and 15% of women. Migraine attacks are episodic in nature and are often associated with a long list of symptoms (Table 31.1).

Attacks can be triggered by a variety of factors that are also common before, during, or after a sports event.

One of the gurus of modern migraine research, Dr. Neil Raskin, University of California, San Francisco, stated in 2006, "If the headaches are reliably caused by menstruation, hunger, lack of sleep, or physical exertion—among a number of other factors—they are likely the product of migraine." The causative factors mentioned here are commonly experienced by athletes at a sports event (Table 31.2).

Diagnosis: The International Headache Society issues guidelines on migraine diagnosis and treatment. They define migraine without aura as being a "Recurrent headache disorder manifesting in attacks lasting 4 to 72 hours. Typical characteristics of the headache are unilateral location, pulsating quality, moderate or severe intensity, aggravation by routine physical activity and association with nausea and/or photophobia and phonophobia."

Some of their diagnostic criteria are

A. At least five attacks fulfilling criteria B through D

B. Headache attacks lasting 4 to 72 hours (untreated or unsuccessfully treated)

C. Headache has at least two of the following characteristics:

1. Unilateral location

2. Pulsating quality

3. Moderate or severe pain intensity

4. Aggravation by or causing avoidance of routine physical activity (e.g., walking or climbing stairs)

D. During headache, at least one of the following:

1. Nausea and/or vomiting

2. Photophobia and phonophobia

E. Not attributed to another disorder

These guidelines are available on the web and can be found at http://ihs-classification.org/en/02_klassifikation/02_teil1/01.01.00_migraine.html.

TABLE 31.2	Factors That May Trigger a Migraine Attack		
Sunlight	Hunger	Stormy weather	Lack of sleep
Bright lights	Stress	Barometric pressure changes	Alcohol
Sounds	Physical exertion	Hormonal variations in the menstrual cycle	Chocolate

Treatment: There is an array of different medications available to physicians today. There is a large degree of individual variation regarding efficacy and response times.

There are three main groups:

- NSAIDS—usually more effective when taken early in a mild attack

- 5HT receptor agonists—include ergotamine and triptans

- Dopamine receptor antagonists—may enhance gastric absorption of the above medications, decrease nausea and vomiting, and help restore normal gastric motility

In general, in established migraine, medication should be administered as soon as possible after the onset of an attack. If symptoms have returned or are still present after 1 hour, a new increased dose may be taken. There are a multitude of factors to be considered when choosing the right medication, but I will just make a few pointers: Nasal sprays seem to work faster than oral preparations, though they seem to have less efficacy; monotherapy does not always work; triptans are reportedly only effective in migraine with aura after the aura is completed and administered when the headache commences; there is a role for nonpharmacological treatment (albeit anecdotal), particularly in the days before an event—avoid specific triggers, eat and sleep as well as possible, avoid computer games and iPods, go for a walk in the late evening, avoid excess caffeine, gentle massage may help (avoid the neck), yoga, meditation, etc.

31.5 TENSION-TYPE HEADACHE

Tension headache is usually described as a chronic condition characterized by a circular or bilateral, tight, pressing discomfort or pain. Athletes may develop symptoms in the buildup to a major event. Tension headaches have been previously defined as headaches that are not throbbing in nature and are not worsened by movement and that are without accompanying nausea, vomiting, photophobia, or phonophobia. However, this neat separation of tension headaches on the one hand and migraine on the other has recently been rebuked by the International Headache Society. Regrettably, it is not that easy. For more on this topic, I refer to the IHS website.

Treatment: Pain can usually be treated with mild analgesics.

31.6 POSTTRAUMATIC HEADACHE

Traumatic head injuries trigger a period of episodic or constant headache that can last for several months or even years. The patient often complains of associated dizziness, vertigo, and impaired memory. Patients find it difficult to work. Concentration may provoke headache or extreme tiredness. Loud music and TV viewing may exhaust the patient. Many patients avoid social gatherings. Neurological tests and CT/MRI studies are normal. Follow up CTs are recommended in case there is a chronic subdural hematoma present.

A similar clinical picture can be seen in athletes after an infectious mononucleosis, long-term mycoplasma infections, viral meningitis, Lamdia Giardiasis infections, flu-like illnesses, or parasitic infections. There is no convincing evidence that infectious mononucleosis predisposes to this condition, yet many young athletes in their late teens present with this clinical picture. Treatment is often empirical and, even though one is hesitant in initiating antidepressant treatment in young athletes, they do seem to work in some cases. These headaches may last for several years.

31.7 PRIMARY EXERTIONAL HEADACHE

This is obviously a condition that one must expect to find amongst athletes, although they are more common in patients over the age of 40. The headache occurs just after exercise (often associated with weight lifting, heading the ball in soccer, diving, aerobics, and jogging). Patients may also experience headache during sexual intercourse. Discomfort typically lasts for 15 to 20 minutes only, but may on occasion last a whole day. Exertional headaches are frequently found in migraine sufferers, but the vast majority of exertional headaches are benign. In migraine or cluster headache patients, these exertional headaches may provoke an "attack" and the headaches can be difficult to distinguish from each other.

Athletes who have recently returned to training are more prone to this type of headache.

Treatment: Modify training regimens so that exercise does not cause discomfort, then gradually increase intensity, whilst avoiding headache at all times. Indomethacin is often effective and, in severe cases, prophylactic medications may be prescribed (e.g., indomethacin, ergotamine, dihydroergotamine, or methysergide).

31.8 ACUTE OTITIS

See Chapter 35.

31.9 ACUTE SINUSITIS

See Chapter 37.

31.10 OTHER CAUSES OF SUDDEN SEVERE HEADACHE

Primary headache syndromes:

- Thunderclap headache
- Cluster headache
- Trigeminal neuralgia

Other secondary headache syndromes:

- Vascular—intracranial venous thrombosis; intracerebral, intraventricular, extradural, or subdural hemorrhage; ischemic stroke; arterial dissection
- Concussion (see Chapters 29 and 30)
- Infection—for example, meningitis or encephalitis
- Acute hydrocephalus
- Intracranial tumor
- Intracranial hypotension
- Metabolic disorders
- Acute glaucoma
- Iridocyclitis
- Snow blindness
- Temporal arteritis
- Dental conditions
- Side effects due to medication

The International Headache Society has defined primary headache as a condition in which the headache and its associated features are the disorder in itself. Secondary headaches are those caused by exogenous disorders. Causes of primary headache include

- Tension-type 69%
- Migraine 16%
- Idiopathic stabbing 2%
- Exertional 1%
- Cluster 0.1%

Secondary headache causes are

- Systemic infection 63%
- Head injury 4%
- Vascular disorders 1%
- Subarachnoid hemorrhage <1%
- Brain tumor 0.1%

Recommended Reading

Al Shahi, et al. Subarachnoid haemorrhage. *BMJ.* 2006;333(7561):235.

Aronin, et al. Community-acquired bacterial meningitis: risk stratification for adverse clinical outcome and effect of antibiotic timing. *Ann Intern Med.* 1998;129(11):862.

Hop, et al. Case-fatality rates and functional outcome after subarachnoid hemorrhage: a systematic review *Stroke.* 1997;28(3):660.

Huang, van Gelder. The probability of sudden death from rupture of intracranial aneurysms: a meta-analysis. *Neurosurg.* 2002;51(5):110.

International Classification of Headache disorders (http://www.americanheadachesociety.org/professionalresources/USHeadacheConsortiumGuidelines.asp).

Linn FH, Rinkel GJ, Algra A, et al. Incidence of subarachnoid hemorrhage: role of region, year, and rate of computed tomography: a meta-analysis. *Stroke.* 1996;27(4):625–629.

Practice parameter: evidence-based guidelines for migraine headache (an evidence-based review): report of the Quality Standards Subcommittee of the American Academy of Neurology.

CHAPTER 32

Epileptic Emergencies

Contributed by Geraint Fuller, Consultant Neurologist, Gloucester Royal Hospital, UK; Advisory Consultant, British Olympic Association

Reviewer: Bredo Knudtzen, Former Team Physician, Norwegian National Ice Hockey Team; Consultant, National Centre for Epilepsy, Norway

32.1 BACKGROUND

Epilepsy is common. The prevalence of active epilepsy is 5 to 10 per 1,000. Epilepsy is not a single disease but many and in broad terms can be classified into two types:

- Generalized epilepsy. Typically, this starts before the age of 21. The following seizure types occur:
  - Generalized tonic
  - Clonic seizures
  - Absences
  - Myoclonic jerks
- Focal-onset or localization-related epilepsies. This can start at any age. The type of seizure will depend on which part of the brain it arises from, for example, olfactory hallucinations and déjà vu at onset indicate a temporal lobe seizure onset. The severity is categorized as simple partial (if consciousness is preserved), complex partial (if consciousness is impaired), and these may go onto to a secondary generalized tonic–clonic seizure. This type of epilepsy is also categorized according to the cause, for example, post head injury or, if no cause is found, cryptogenic.

Most patients with epilepsy gain good control of their seizures on anticonvulsants.

A minority will have ongoing seizures of varying frequency.

Having active epilepsy may prevent or limit the participation in some sports, particularly water sports or climbing, depending on the seizure type and frequency and safety rules of the sport.

32.2 DIFFERENTIAL DIAGNOSES OF SEIZURES

The most common situation an event physician will face is a competitor (or member of the public) having a tonic–clonic seizure.

These need to be differentiated from other causes of loss of consciousness (Table 32.1).

Concussive convulsions are an important differential diagnosis for loss of consciousness in sport—indeed, they were first characterized in sport (Australian rules football)—and are usually easily recognized as they occur on head impact and are brief. Immediate management is as for seizures. It is important to know of their existence as they have a very good prognosis, do not predispose to epilepsy, and will not prevent driving.

Syncope can be difficult to distinguish from a seizure, especially if the patient is supported when he or she may develop a convulsive syncope (also referred to as a reflex anoxic seizure). The importance in recognizing syncope is twofold. Recognition of syncope allows one to initiate appropriate investigations, particularly if the syncope occurred during exercise (which may be more sinister). Secondly, it will prevent an inappropriate investigation for seizures and all the associated lifestyle restrictions that this often entails (driving, etc.).

Nonepileptic attacks (also referred to as pseudoseizures or dissociative seizures) are psychologically induced events that can be difficult to distinguish from epileptic seizures. Investigation during an attack shows no significant abnormalities, with, for example, normal oxygen saturation as well as normal EEG. *A normal EEG does exclude*

TABLE 32.1 Differential Diagnosis of Seizures

	Features	Comments
Tonic–clonic seizure	Tonic phase: the patient goes rigid, with arms flexed or extended. Frequently associated with a groan as air is expelled from lungs. May become cyanosed. Clonic phase: limbs jerk. Goes on for 1–2 min. Usually self-limiting. Followed by sleep and confusion.	May be preceded by complex partial seizure or features of a focal onset seizure—for example, head turning to one side or one arm extending and the other flexing.
Concussive convulsions	Occur immediately after head injury. Often involves tonic contraction of upper arms, with shoulder abduction and elbow flexion—"bear-hug" position. Lasts 2–10 s. May be followed by rhythmic jerking up to 3 min. Self-limiting	
Syncope	Usually has prodrome, typically of visual loss. Falls either flaccidly or rigidly. 80% have arrhythmic multifocal or generalized myoclonic jerks that last for <30 s. Pale. Pulse is lost in the initial phase.	More profound or prolonged hypotension, e.g., if the patient is propped up, it can trigger a convulsion.
Nonepileptic attack or functional seizure	Highly variable. Frequently involves hyperextension of the back (opisthotonus). Normal color. May actively resist those around them. Variable duration, often prolonged. Cardiovascular markers, pulse and blood pressure, are normal during the episode (a tachycardia will be commensurate with the level of physical exertion).	Initially may be difficult to distinguish from epileptic seizure. Important for those in secondary care to consider.

epilepsy. Whilst it is important to be aware of this entity, this is a diagnosis that will probably be made by a neurologist.

Seizures can be triggered by hypoglycemia and in these patients, usually patients with diabetes on insulin, correcting hypoglycemia is essential. There are other rare causes of episodes of collapse such as narcolepsy or kinesogenic dyskinesia that will not be considered further.

32.3 IMMEDIATE MANAGEMENT OF SEIZURE

The first issue is to protect the patient during the seizure and then to go through the more usual resuscitation procedures: Support or cushion the head; remove any objects that might cause injury. Check the patient's pulse. Try to establish

important past history: Is the patient known to have epilepsy or diabetes?

Once the tonic–clonic phase of the seizure is over, place the patient in the recovery position, where he or she will sleep.

As the patient comes around, he or she will often become confused. Usually, the patient is disorientated but straightforward to manage with simple reassurance.

What Not to Do

Do not try to insert anything in the patient's mouth during the seizure. This will not help and is likely to lead to dental injury.

Do not try to put the patient in the recovery position until after the tonic–clonic phase of the seizure has finished. This reduces the chance of dislocation of the shoulder during the seizure.

If the seizure has occurred while the patient is in water, it is essential to hold his or her head above water—if possible, moving to shallow water—and then moving the patient to dry land once the tonic–clonic phase is over. There is the additional concern that the patient may have aspirated.

The expectation is that after a seizure the patient should then be transferred to a hospital urgently. However, this is not necessary if the patient is known to have active epilepsy, has had one of his or her usual seizures, has recovered fully, and can be supervised.

32.4 MANAGEMENT OF MORE PROLONGED OR REPEATED SEIZURES OR STATUS EPILEPTICUS

Most seizures are self-limiting and treatment is supportive, as described above. However, if the tonic–clonic phase of the seizure lasts longer than 5 minutes or if there are repeated seizures, then more active treatment is required. This will require urgent transfer to a hospital.

General measures:

- Secure airway and resuscitate

- Give oxygen

- Check blood glucose (BM stick)

- Establish IV access

- Call emergency service for transfer to hospital

Immediate drug treatments (doses given are for adults):

- Without IV access
  - Rectal diazepam 10 to 20 mg, repeated after 15 minutes if needed, or
  - Buccal midazolam 10 mg

- With IV access
  - Lorazepam IV 4 mg bolus, repeated after 10 to 20 minutes (usual dose, 0.1 mg per kg). *Diazepam IV 5 mg initially may be repeated with 2.5 to 5 mg increments.*
  - Consider IV glucose (50 mL of 50% solution).

Benzodiazepines can cause significant respiratory depression. Monitor vital signs and use pulse oximetry if possible.

The further management of status epilepticus requires hospital support, initially using either IV phenytoin or fosphenytoin, which will usually prove successful, and if not management in intensive care with general anaesthesia and ventilation (Table 32.2).

TABLE 32.2	Classification of Risks Associated with Seizures in Some Sports[a]

High-risk Sports: Risk to Life If Seizure Occurs Even with Safety Measures

White-water kayaking

Bobsleigh

Motor sports

Downhill skiing

Hang gliding

Rock climbing

Scuba diving

Cycling

Long-distance swimming

High-risk Sports: Risk to Life If Seizure Occurs—Risk That Can Be Reduced by Safety Measures

Slalom skiing

Mountain biking

Single sculling

Water skiing

(*Continued*)

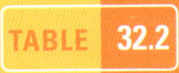

TABLE 32.2 Classification of Risks Associated with Seizures in Some Sports[a] (*Continued*)

Medium-risk Sports: Risk to Life If Seizure Occurs—Risk That Can Be Markedly Reduced by Safety Measures; Some Risk of Injury

Field hockey

Ice hockey

Ice skating

Football (soccer)

Rowing

Rugby football

Sailing (should not sail alone)

Swimming

Low-risk Sports: No Risk to Life If Seizure Occurs; Risks of Injury Equivalent to Other Daily Activities

Athletics

Baseball

Cricket

Golf

Running

Squash

Tennis

[a]Direct evidence to support this (or any other) classification is lacking.

Recommended Reading

National Institute for Health and Clinical Excellence. The epilepsies: the diagnosis and management of the epilepsies in adults and children in primary and secondary care. http://www.nice.org.uk/Guidance/CG20. Updated November 11, 2010. Accessed April 3, 2011. Excellent guidelines covering the management of all aspects of the epilepsies. The full guidelines provide references to supporting evidence.

Lemptert T. Recognizing syncope: pitfalls and surprises. *J R Soc Med*. 1996;89:372–375. Pivotal study that describes the wide range of changes that can occur during syncope.

McCrory PR, Berkovic SF. Video analysis of acute motor and convulsive manifestations in sport related concussion. *Neurology*. 2000;54:1488–1491. One of a series from these authors that defines concussive convulsions in sport.

CHAPTER 33

Acute Psychiatric Disorders

Contributed by Trygve Moe, Psychiatrist, Friskvern, Oslo, Norway

Reviewer: Are Holen, Psychiatrist, Professor of Behavioural Medicine and Vice Dean, Faculty of Medicine, NTNU, Trondheim, Norway

Event physicians will occasionally have to deal with psychiatric emergencies. Though rare, these situations represent a challenge when they occur. It may be difficult to communicate with the patient when delusions, hallucination, or strong emotions—such as anxiety, depression, or somatization—dominate the patient's condition. In order to make an adequate psychiatric diagnosis, physicians usually need to take a detailed medical history, and also to carry out a time-consuming physical and psychiatric examination. Due to the time constraints of sporting events and due to the limited investigative facilities available, a complete psychiatric evaluation and diagnosis is usually beyond the scope of the EP. Nevertheless, it is important to establish the most likely diagnosis, and to deal with the immediate situation and initiate some preliminary form of treatment, or even make a referral, when necessary.

The environment usually plays a role in the precipitation of acute psychiatric conditions. Participation at a major sports event can undoubtedly induce high levels of stress in the athletes and trigger or exacerbate their predispositions in unfortunate ways. This may result in psychiatric symptoms or manifest in a full psychiatric disorder.

This chapter will only focus on the symptoms and diagnosis of psychiatric disorders an EP may have to deal with during an event.

33.1 ANXIETY

Anxiety, along with depression, is the most common psychiatric disorder. According to the diagnostic criteria of the Diagnostic and Statistical Manual of Mental Disorders, Fourth Edition,

Text Revision (*DSM-IV-TR*), there are several subgroups of anxiety (*DSM-IV-TR*, published by the American Psychiatric Association, includes all currently recognized mental health disorders and corresponds with the International Classification of Diseases, 9th Revision [ICD-9]). There is a high degree of comorbidity within the subgroups of anxiety, and between anxiety and depression. Severe cases of anxiety are quite disabling and usually not compatible with maximum physical performance. Anxiety is one of the psychiatric conditions which is likely to be exacerbated if the patient is placed in a stressful situation.

Anxiety will often persist over time, and the patient will usually be aware of the symptoms and have some idea of how to deal with them. The EP will usually be consulted only if there is a first episode of a panic attack, or if the symptoms are particularly severe or prolonged. Anxiety disorders may affect around one quarter of the adult population, being more common amongst females.

There are two kinds of anxiety-related attacks: panic attacks and anxiety attacks. Panic attacks are perceived as very dramatic, and it is common for the patient to fear that he or she will lose control, become insane, or even die. A feeling of asphyxiation, pressure, or pain in the chest may often lead the patient to believe that he or she is experiencing a heart attack. A panic attack usually evolves quickly and reaches its peak within 10 minutes. The panic attack is dominated by a strong feeling of anxiety, often accompanied by unpleasant somatic symptoms. There is often a lack of predisposing factors, which makes an attack difficult to predict. This lack of sentinel signs and ability to predict or foresee attacks may enhance the athlete's feeling of anxiety, fearing that an attack can occur just before or during competition, particularly when he or she is exposed to large crowds or placed in situations which may be hard to escape from. This will often lead to patients dreading competition and public attention.

Anxiety attacks develop much more slowly, after hours of arousal, and the patient is usually aware of the circumstances that precipitate the attack. Always test vital equipment before the start of an event. In particular, check that oxygen tanks are working and full, check all equipment containing batteries and bulbs, make sure that there are no leakages from splints and ensure that the right pumps are available, ensure that all medications are available and not outdated, and ensure that infusion fluids are intact and have the correct temperature. (Some should have room temperature and some very cold. Note on infusion liquids and cold climates: liquids can and do freeze.)

According to *DSM-IV-TR*, four of the following criteria will have to present to cause a panic attack:

- Palpitations or increased heart rate
- Sweating
- Trembling or shaking
- Shortness of breath
- Choking sensation
- Chest pain
- Nausea or stomach discomfort
- Dizziness, unsteadiness, giddiness, or loss of consciousness
- Derealization or depersonalization
- Fear of losing control or sanity
- Fear of dying
- Numbness or tingling sensation
- A feeling of being too cold or too hot

Treatment

1. Calm the patient; make him or her sit down and breathe normally.

2. If the patient is hyperventilating, make the patient breathe into a paper bag to prevent unnecessary carbon dioxide loss. Hyperventilation and a low CO_2 will cause physical sensations that may potentiate the feeling of anxiety.

3. Pharmacological treatment: Panic attacks will usually recede before the anxiolytic medication,

such as benzodiazepines, take effect. However, both benzodiazepines and SSRIs have been shown to prevent attacks. Due to the potentially addictive nature of benzodiazepines, SSRIs are usually the drug of first choice in the prevention of future attacks, though several weeks may pass before optimal effect is experienced. Benzodiazepines will usually have a more rapid effect, often within half an hour. If benzodiazepines need to be used, then medications with longer half lives are recommended.

4. After a first-time attack, the patient should be examined for diseases of the heart and the thyroid gland as well as for neurological conditions.

5. If the attacks are repeated, the patient should be referred for psychiatric assessments.

33.2 PSYCHOSIS

Psychosis is a dramatic and major psychiatric disorder. According to *DSM-IV-TR*, a psychosis is described as presenting with delusions or hallucinations or major deviations in mood without the patient having insight into the pathological nature of these symptoms. The patient is conscious and in many instances capable of giving an account of time, place, and personal data. However, there can be some confusion in acute psychiatric psychotic states, and the patient's ability to give this account may be lost. Confusion is rarely of the same degree as found when the delirium is caused by a somatic condition, intoxication, or withdrawal reactions.

Many psychotic disorders are of a chronic nature and will often affect an athlete's level of functioning to such a degree that a sporting career is unlikely. Accordingly, we will only mention the most common acute psychotic disorder.

A brief psychotic episode (*DSM-IV-TR* criteria 298.8) is present if

- At least one of these symptoms appears:
  - Delusions
  - Hallucinations
  - Disorganized speech with frequent derailments or incoherence
  - Grossly disorganized or catatonic behavior
- The condition persists for at least one day, but less than a month, and with full remission to a premorbid level
- The disorder is not better explained as an emotional suffering with psychotic symptoms, schizoaffective suffering, or schizophrenia

■ The disorder is not caused by drugs or a somatic disorder

The EP will only be able to adjudge the first category of symptoms above and will therefore be unable to make a complete diagnosis due to a lack of investigative tools or time for adequate observation. For the sake of future treatment and diagnosis, it is desirable that the EP finds out, if possible, whether the patient has had similar stress or episodes in the past.

33.3 DELIRIUM

Delirium is a state of mental confusion. Psychotic states with a sudden onset are often associated with milder confusion. However, when the delirium is more pronounced, organic causes, including drug intoxication, side effects of drugs, physical trauma, hypoxia, severe infections, exhaustion, dementia, and metabolic disturbances, are far more likely.

Delirium (293.0) due to a general medical condition is present if

■ There is a disturbance in the level of consciousness, with a reduced ability to focus and maintain alertness

■ There is a cognitive change—such as the loss of memory, disorientation, or speech interference

■ The suffering develops quickly and has a fluctuating progress

■ There is a history pointing to intoxication, withdrawal symptoms, ingestion of other compounds, or a somatic medical condition

For the EP, it is important to assess the patient's state and degree of confusion. A delirium will tend to fluctuate during the course of the day. If the athlete is not highly confused, the condition is more likely to be of a psychotic nature.

Treatment

1. Reduce sensory stimulus by behaving calm yourself, by reducing the number of people around the patient, and by reducing noise levels.

2. Avoid confrontation; do not contradict the patient, even if his or her utterances are based on delusions.

3. Cooperate, if possible, with persons who are known to the patient.

4. Attend to your own safety and that of the medical team. One should not be alone with a confused or psychotic patient.

5. Pharmacological treatment—if the condition is related to a mental disorder, and not caused by a somatic condition: The choice will often be between antipsychotic drugs or benzodiazepines. The use of early antipsychotic treatment, as soon as possible, is recommended. Haloperidol, for example, may be used. In some cases, the treatment of choice will be to calm the patient by giving benzodiazepines and rapidly to expedite the patient to hospital. A delirium caused by withdrawal may often be treated by giving the same drug; however, the cause of the delirium should be established first. If the delirium is caused by a somatic condition such as a bacterial infection, the patient should be brought under adequate medical care as soon as possible.

Recommended Reading

American Psychiatric Association. *Diagnostic and Statistical Manual of Mental Disorders*, 4th ed. Text Revision. Washington, DC: American Psychiatric Association; 2000.
Sadock BJ, Sadock VA. *Kaplan and Sadock's Concise Textbook of Clinical Psychiatry*. 3rd ed. Baltimore, MD: Lippincott Williams & Wilkins; 2008.

Eye Conditions

Contributed by David McDonagh, Deputy CMO, Lillehammer 1994 Olympic Winter Games

Reviewer: Kjell Løfors, Consultant Ophthalmologist, St. Olavs Hospital, Trondheim; Member, Norwegian Boxing Union Medical Committee, Norway

Deep-penetrating foreign bodies should not be removed as the whole orbit may collapse. The patient should be sent to a hospital by ambulance. Cover the other eye to prevent unnecessary ocular movement—the athlete should try to focus his or her vision on one point. If the penetrating object is unstable, then endeavor to stabilize it as best you can.

Blunt trauma occurs when the eye is struck with a tennis ball, a golf ball, a racquet, a thumb (gouging), a fist, or other solid object. Damage to ocular structures is due to sudden compression and indentation of the eye and may produce bleeding in the anterior chamber, scarring of the lens (traumatic cataract), lens subluxation/dislocation, retinal tears with bleeding into the vitreous gel, or retinal tears that may lead to retinal detachment. If the external force is large enough, then a blowout fracture can also occur.

Depending on the scale of the injury, symptoms may vary from mild eye pain with or without blurred vision to intense pain, loss of vision, or diplopia.

34.1 BLACK EYE

Periorbital hematomas are common in sport, and it is not an unusual event in the United Kingdom or Ireland to meet junior doctors sporting handsome "shiners" on a Monday morning after a good weekend rugby match. The danger with this injury is that there may also be intraocular damage, so visual acuity must be tested, double vision must be inquired about, eye movements must be tested, and the eye must also be ophthalmoscoped for hemorrhage and retinal damage.

A periorbital hematoma (Fig. 34.1) is associated with a fracture of the infraorbital region, so this must be excluded when examining the athlete. Fractures are rare with mild trauma; however, the feared blowout fracture must also be examined for (see Chapter 34.11). Loss of sensation or hyperparesthesia under the eye on the cheek can imply damage to the infraorbital nerve, as seen in maxillary fractures.

34.2 EYELID INJURIES

These injuries can be serious if eyelid integrity is disturbed. The eyelids protect the eyes and keep them moist, famously described as "windshield wipers" washing away foreign matter. If the injured eyelid loses its ability to adequately cover the eye, then drying of the eye may occur, often leading to chronic infection and corneal inflammation. Tear ducts may also be damaged, so, if in doubt, refer the athlete to an eye department for surgical repair (Fig. 34.2).

34.3 OCULAR FOREIGN BODIES

In sport, the usual guilty objects are dust, dirt, grass, small stones, and even small metal particles (when polishing/sharpening skates, blades, etc.). The vast majority are nonpenetrating, but this possibility

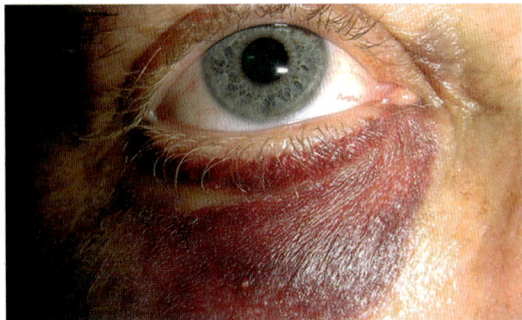

FIGURE 34.1. Periorbital hematoma.

must not be forgotten. For dust and small particles, simply rinsing the eye may be enough, but one should always invert the upper eyelid using a Q tip to inspect for entrapped objects, having applied a local anesthetic first, and then gently wipe the foreign body away using a second Q tip. Dripping the eye with flourescein followed by ophthalmoscopic inspection may reveal a foreign object or a conjunctival/scleral sore. This procedure is best conducted in the dark, so withdraw to the medical room.

If the combination of high-velocity metal foreign body and a conjunctival rift is present, then the possibility of an intraocular foreign body cannot be ruled out. Try to ascertain what type of substance may have penetrated the eye—metal, plastic, etc. Inspect the eye with an ophthalmoscope. Check the athlete's vision. If in doubt, refer the patient to an eye specialist. A careful case history is recommended.

When removing small foreign bodies/dust a Q tip can be useful; however, they may leave behind small fibers, so inspect carefully. For larger, superficially embedded objects, first drip the eye with a topical anesthetic, and then remove the foreign body with a forceps.

If the eye is very painful after treatment, then use chloramphenicol cream and cover the eye with a patch. Peroral 500-mg paracetamol tablets can be taken if the pain is great. Chloramphenicol drops can be used in the eye that is more uncomfortable than painful. If the athlete has intense pain, then reconsider your diagnosis.

If a large, penetrating foreign body is embedded (splinters, nails, etc.), then do not remove the foreign body. Immobilize it as best you can, cover the healthy eye as well, and transfer the patient urgently to a hospital.

Do *not* give oral painkillers. Instruct the patient to refrain from eating or drinking until he or she has been evaluated by a specialist. The patient may need general anesthesia and the ingestion of food or fluids may delay surgical intervention.

If you find a large foreign body that will need removal in a hospital, do not put eye drops into the eye as they may migrate into the eye and cause further inflammation and damage.

34.4 CONJUNCTIVITIS

Conjunctivitis may or may not have a traumatic origin but can often be preceded by irritation of the conjunctiva, fingernail contact, small foreign bodies, dust, etc., followed by an infection. When treating, make sure that foreign bodies

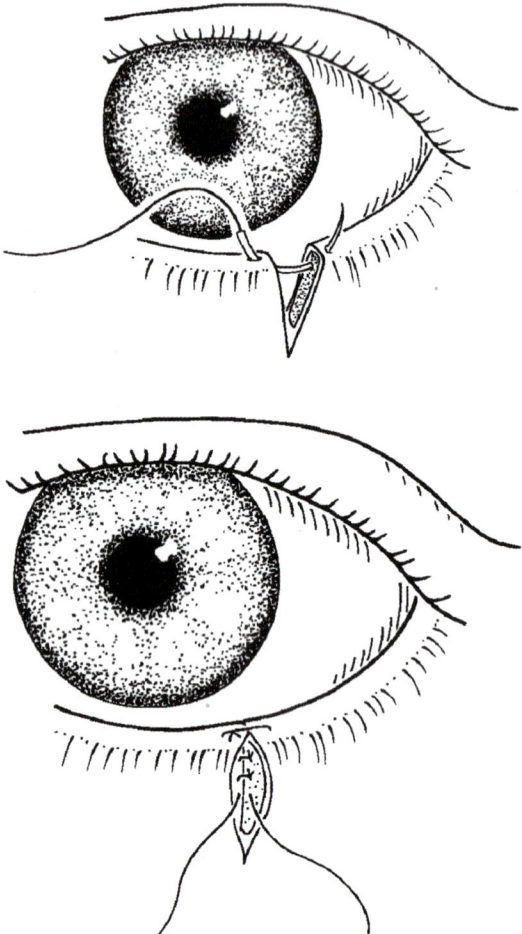

FIGURE 34.2. Suturing an eyelid injury.

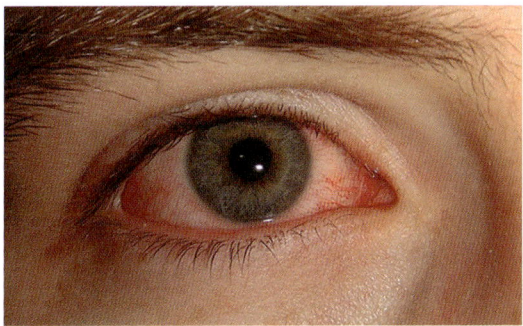

FIGURE 34.3. Viral conjunctivitis.

have been removed. Start with chloramphenicol cream and eye drops, 1 drop, five times daily, and cream at nighttime. In some countries, salt water drops and rinsing are recommended for 2 to 3 days before initiating local antibiotic treatment (Figs. 34.3 and 34.4).

34.5 SUBCONJUNCTIVAL HEMORRHAGE

This is due to capillary bleeding between the sclera and conjunctiva, often creating a bright red hemorrhage (though they can also be dark). The blood will always stay within the white sclera; it will not cross over into the clear cornea and may be limited to a small sector of the eye or may be more extensive, affecting most of the sclera. They can occur after direct trauma to the eye, after lifting heavy weights, or after coughing but also due to hypertension or bleeding disorders. Measure the athlete's blood pressure and enquire about bleeding tendencies. The benign variants are self-limiting conditions that disappear after—1 to 2 weeks. A subconjunctival hemorrhage does not cause loss of vision (Figs. 34.5 and 34.6).

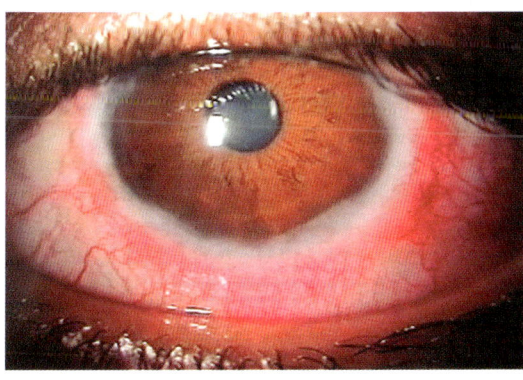

FIGURE 34.4. Allergic conjunctivitis.

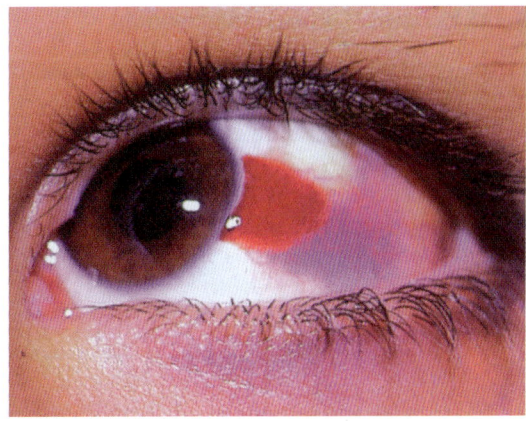

FIGURE 34.5. Subconjunctival hemorrhage.

34.6 CORNEAL CONDITIONS

Abrasions

A fingernail scratch can be very painful and can cause a corneal abrasion. Many athletes use contact lenses, and these may scratch the cornea if they are not removed on time, or if removed roughly, but also if carelessly inserted on the field of play, when small foreign bodies may be introduced behind the lens. The primary symptom is pain and redness often followed by infection. Treatment involves removal of any foreign body and then antibiotics and patching of the eye.

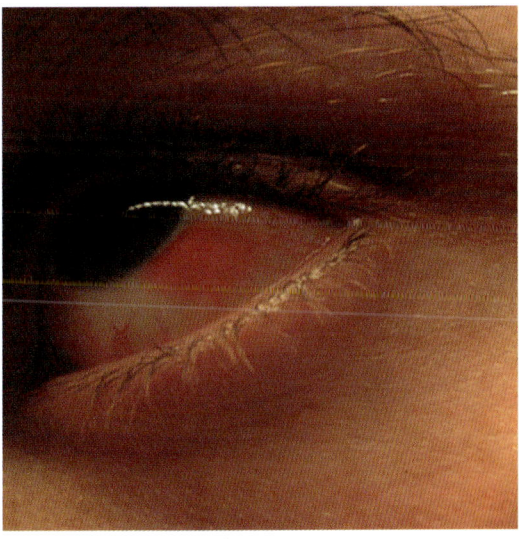

FIGURE 34.6. Small subconjunctival hemorrhage.

Acute Keratitis (Corneal Inflammation)

Inflammation can be caused by one or a combination of factors, trauma being common in sport. A typical corneal infection is the potentially serious herpes simplex keratitis, which may cause dendritic ulcers or lesions. Keratitis may also occur secondarily to other inflammatory conditions such as scleritis or episcleritis. Keratitis symptoms include

- Moderate to severe eye pain
- Red eye
- Moderate to severe foreign body sensation
- Blurred vision
- Watery eye discharge
- Photophobia

Keratitis findings:

- Conjunctival injection and possibly ciliary flush
- Corneal vascularization
- Decreased visual acuity (depending on location)
- Normal or reduced pupil size
- Fluorescein staining may reveal corneal ulcers

Treatment: These patients should be referred to an eye specialist (Fig. 34.7).

34.7 SCLERITIS

Scleritis is not very common, and an EP is not very likely to come across an acute scleritis.

Approximately 50% of all cases are idiopathic, the rest being associated with autoimmune or systemic disorders (rheumatoid arthritis, polyarte-

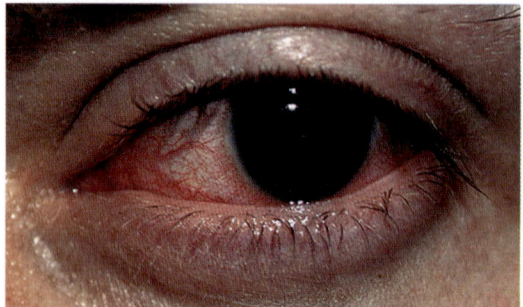

FIGURE 34.7. Acute keratitis (note ciliary flush).

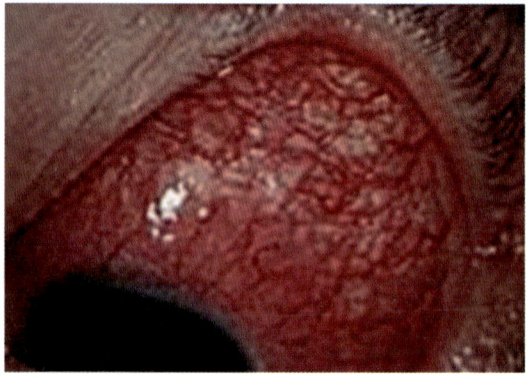

FIGURE 34.8. Scleritis.

ritis nodosa, systemic lupus erythematosus, Reiter syndrome, psoriasis arthritis, ankylosing spondylitis, inflammatory bowel disease) or herpes infections.

Symptoms:

- Significant eye pain that may radiate to the cheeks, eyebrows, or temporal region
- Red eye, may be bilateral
- Blurred vision
- Photophobia

Signs (Fig. 34.8):

- Decreased visual acuity
- Pain on palpation
- Hyperemia of sclera
- May be associated with other eye conditions

34.8 ACUTE IRITIS

Traumatic inflammation of the iris may occur after a poke in the eye or a blow from a blunt object.

Traumatic iritis usually requires treatment. Even with medical treatment, there is a risk of permanent decreased vision (Fig. 34.9).

Infection may also cause inflammation, but iritis is most often associated with systemic disorders such as juvenile rheumatoid arthritis, Crohn disease, nonspecific urethritis, and sarcoidosis.

As the iris is a part of the uveal tract, acute iritis can also be called acute anterior uveitis.

Symptoms:

- Eye pain—moderate aching pain
- Photophobia
- Vision decreased or blurred

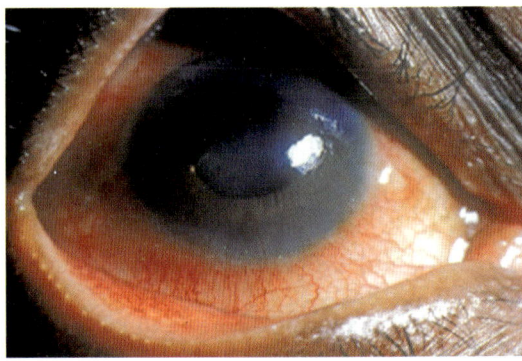

FIGURE 34.9. Acute iritis.

Findings:

- Pupil may be constricted and react poorly to light
- Flushing of bulbar conjunctiva around the limbus

Treatment: Rapid referral to an ophthalmologist is recommended.

34.9 UVEITIS

Uveitis occurs when there is inflammation of the uveal tract:

- Iris inflammation—iritis or anterior uveitis
- Ciliary body inflammation—becoming iridocyclitis or intermediate uveitis
- Choroid inflammation—choroiditis, or posterior uveitis

The causes of uveitis are many and the condition is characterized by significant sight-threatening intraocular inflammation, primarily involving the uveal tract (iris, ciliary body, and choroid), although inflammation of adjacent tissues, such as retina, optic nerve, and vitreous also occurs. Anything less than 3 months is defined as an acute lesion; longer than three months is defined as a chronic inflammation. These time frames vary around the world. Some experts use 6 weeks as a cutoff between acute and chronic lesions. Panuveitis can occur and indicates a severe inflammation involving most of the uveal tract. The International Uveitis Study Group (IUSG) also has a clinical classification of uveitis:

- Infectious—bacterial, viral, fungal, parasitic, others
- Noninfectious—known systemic association, no known systemic association
- Masquerade—neoplastic, nonneoplastic

Systemic diseases known to be associated with uveitis include sarcoidosis, multiple sclerosis, Behçet disease, the HLA-B27 positive group of diseases (sacroilitis, ankylosing spondylitis, Reiter syndrome, psoriasis, ulcerative colitis, Crohn disease, allergy), and infectious agents including

- Bacterial—tubercular, *Toxoplasma gondii*, *Borrelia*, *Streptococcus*, *Staphylococcus*, etc.
- Viral—herpes simplex, herpes zoster, CMV
- Fungal—aspergillosis, candidiasis
- Parasitic—toxoplasmosis, toxocariasis, amoebiasis

Symptoms:

- Acute anterior uveitis presents as a unilateral, painful red eye, with blurring, photophobia, and excess tear production.
- Chronic anterior uveitis presents as recurrent episodes, with minimal acute symptoms.
- Posterior uveitis causes gradual visual loss, usually bilateral. There is occasional photophobia but little or no discomfort or redness. Floaters are usually a predominant feature.

Clinical findings (Figs. 34.10 and 34.11):

- Acute red painful eye
- Reduced visual acuity
- Direct and consensual photophobia

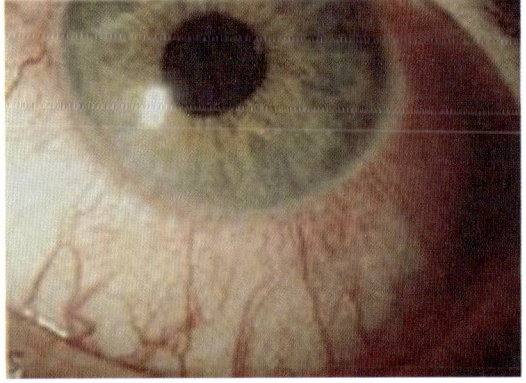

FIGURE 34.10. Iridocyclitis.

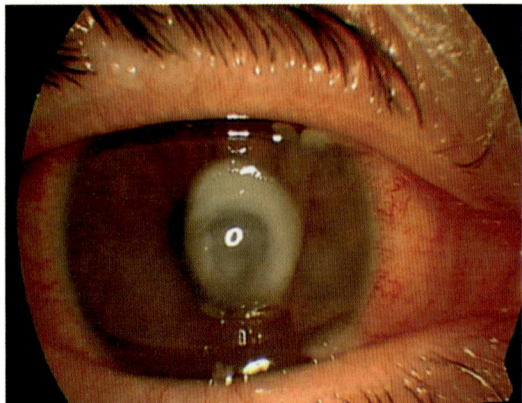

FIGURE 34.11. Acute bacterial uveitis.

■ Injection around the iris is characteristic—ciliary flushing, circumcorneal congestion due to active hyperemia of the anterior ciliary vessel

Treatment: If uveitis is suspected, immediate referral to a specialist is advised—*every hour counts*. Delay in appropriate treatment of a severe infection or panuveitis can lead to the development of significant complications and irreversible loss of vision.

34.10 SYMPTOM AND SIGN OVERVIEW (TABLE 34.1)

34.11 BLOWOUT FRACTURES

After orbital trauma—for example, a heavy punch, a baseball bat, a knee, or even a soccer ball in the face—there can be a sudden dramatic increase in intraorbital pressure that causes the eye to move backwards and then downwards through the weakest part of the orbit, the orbital floor.

Beware—fractures can occur even with minor (!) trauma.

The orbital muscle (often the inferior rectus muscle) and/or orbital fat herniates through the fracture site and the eye then becomes trapped in the fractured floor and movement is disturbed. It is of course a medical emergency, not only due to the potential eye damage, but also due to the risk of a cerebral injury, cranial fracture, and facial trauma. The patient, if conscious, may complain of diplopia and visual disturbance. On inspection, there may well be ecchymosis, deformity of the injured orbit with or without a "sunken" (enophthalmos) or rotated eye. Palpation may reveal numbness under the eye and on the cheek due to infraorbital nerve damage (Figs. 34.12 and 34.13).

34.12 VERTICAL DYSTOPIA

The classical finding on investigation is that the damaged eye fails to elevate/rotate on testing. The patient can fool the physician during testing by

TABLE 34.1	Symptom and Sign Overview					
	Red	**Pain**	**Itchy**	**Blurred Vision**	**Photophobia**	**Ciliary Flush**
Conjunctivitis	Yes	No	Yes	Maybe	No	No
Foreign body	Maybe	Yes	Yes	Maybe	No	No
Corneal abrasion Keratitis	Yes	Yes	No	Maybe	No	No
Subconjunctival hemorrhage	Yes	No	Maybe	No	No	No
Iritis	Usually	Yes	No	Yes	Yes—maybe bilateral	Maybe
Scleritis	Yes	Yes	No	Yes	Yes	Yes
Episcleritis	Yes	Yes	No	Yes	Yes	Maybe
Uveitis	Yes	Yes	No	Yes	Direct and consensual	Yes

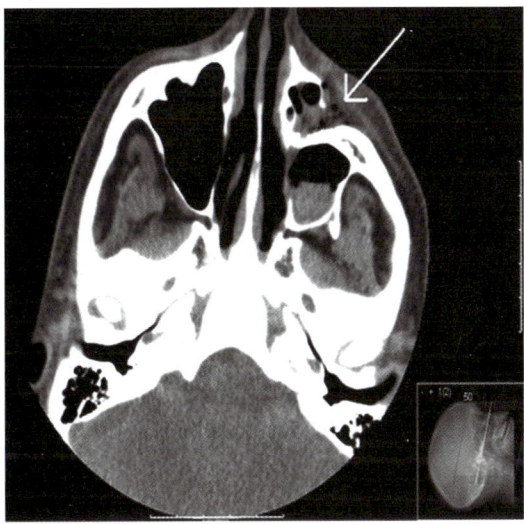

FIGURE 34.12. CT of the face, with an orbital floor fracture and maxillary sinus fracture.

moving the head, so stabilize the head with one hand while asking the athlete to follow your index finger with his eyes (Fig. 34.14). Usually, lateral movement is acceptable but is often deficient at extreme temporal rotation, but it is classically on looking upwards that the diagnosis is made. The healthy eye looks upwards, but the injured eye stares forwards, unable to move, due to entrapment (vertical dystopia—Figs. 34.15 and 34.16). The damaged orbital wall may allow air to be forced into the retrobulbar space, casing pain and even loss of vision. On occasion, crepitations may be found on palpation if periorbital subcutaneous emphysema exists.

There is always the likelihood of concomitant intracranial injury, so beware.

34.13 CHEMICAL BURNS

Chemical burns are extremely rare in sport. Should they occur, they must be treated urgently. Liquids

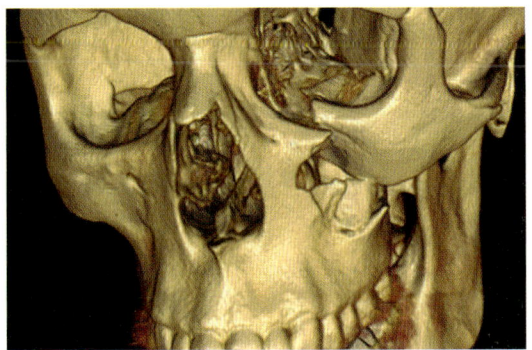

FIGURE 34.13. 3-D image of the same patient.

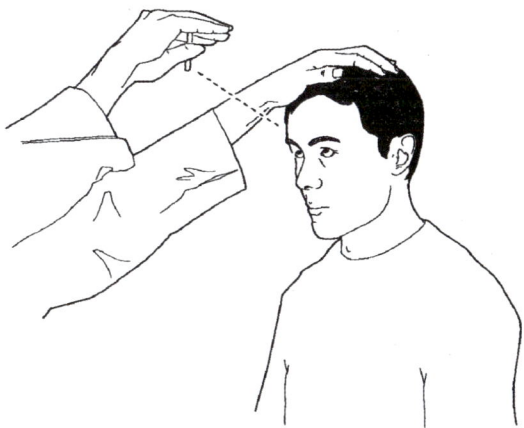

FIGURE 34.14. Examination technique.

and gases all have their own pH. Acidic agents attack the tissue, but their burning effect only lasts for some seconds. Alkaline agents, however, burn for hours and patients require continual ocular irrigation for many hours. When a chemical injury occurs, the eyes should be flooded immediately with fluid (e.g., water) to minimize burning, for as long as it takes to get to the hospital. Continuous irrigation can be difficult in an ambulance—it is possible to tape an infusion set over an open eyelid in such a way that it runs continuously during transport.

If there are visible chemical burns, always check the airway/respiration for inhalation injuries.

34.14 ANTERIOR CHAMBER HEMORRHAGE

Direct trauma to the eye—from a hockey stick, puck, tennis or squash racquet, etc.—may lead to hemorrhaging into the anterior chamber. The blood settles and forms a fluid level, so the bottom of the iris appears red like a bloody half moon (hyphema). The condition can take some hours to develop fully. Patients will complain of reduced vision, visual field defects, pain, pressure in the eye, and photosensitivity. Athletes should be hospitalized for treatment.

Hyphema may lead to the development of glaucoma (Fig. 34.17).

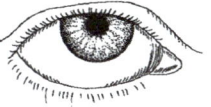 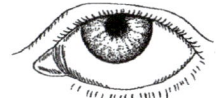

FIGURE 34.15. Normal eye.

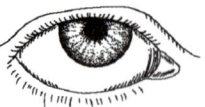 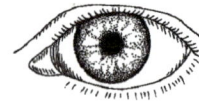

FIGURE 34.16. Dystopic eye.

34.15 POSTERIOR CHAMBER HEMORRHAGE

Posterior chamber hemorrhage is also known as vitreous hemorrhage. Once again, direct trauma to the eye may cause bleeding into the vitreous gel inside the eye due to damage to a retinal vessel. There may also be damage to the retina, and there is an increased risk of retinal detachment. Other nontraumatic causes are diabetes, sickle cell disease, and central retinal vein occlusion. The patient may complain of floaters. Rest is the key to repair, and athletes should be encouraged to rest. Sleeping with a raised pillow may facilitate drainage. Aspirin and blood-thinning agents should be avoided. I refer these athletes to an eye specialist so that he or she can decide the correct time for resumption of training.

34.16 DETACHED RETINA

Detachment of the retina, where vitreous fluid seeps through a retinal tear, can occur in sport as a result of a blow to the head or eye. This can occur immediately or may develop over some days or even weeks. The athlete will often complain of "flashing lights" and floaters before finally

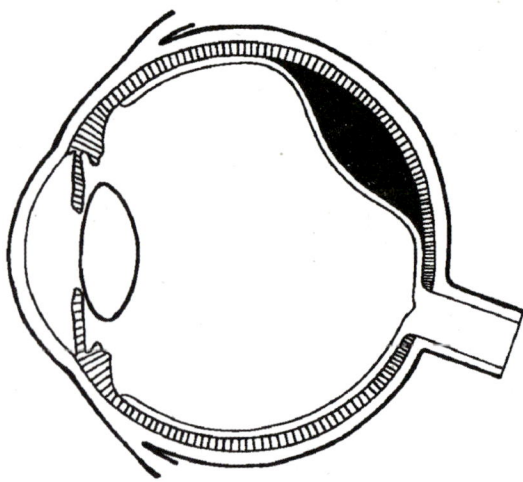

FIGURE 34.18. Detached retina.

complaining of a "curtain" falling down over the eye (this is the moment of final detachment). Referral to hospital is mandatory; if traumatic in nature, always refer the athlete to a CT of the brain and face. Retinae can detach without any obvious or known trauma (Fig. 34.18).

34.17 ACUTE LOSS OF VISION

Obviously, if an athlete presents with a sudden loss of vision, be it associated with trauma or not, urgent referral to a competent ophthalmology department is obligatory. Some causes of acute blindness include retinal vein or artery occlusion, optic neuritis, optic nerve ischemia, vitreous hemorrhage, retinal detachment, and acute glaucoma

Recommended Reading:

Barr A, Baines PS, Desai P, et al. Ocular sports injuries: the current picture. *Br J Sports Med.* 2000;34(6):456–458.

Capão Filipe J A, Rocha-Sousa A, Falcão-Reis F, et al. Modern sports eye injuries. *Br J Ophthalmol.* 2003;87:1336–1339.

Holck D. *Evaluation and Treatment of Ocular Fractures: A Multidisciplinary Approach.* Saunders; 2005.

Rodriguez JO, Lavina AM, Agarwal A. Prevention and treatment of common eye injuries in sports. *Am Fam Physician.* 2003;67(7):1481–1488.

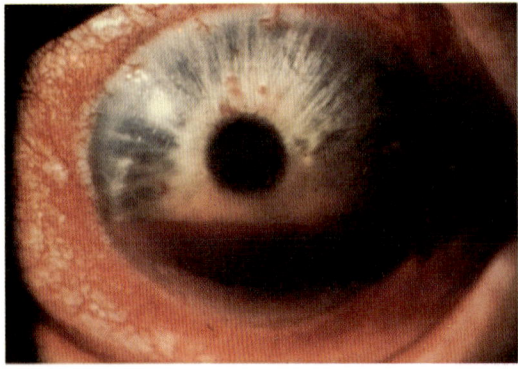

FIGURE 34.17. Anterior chamber hemorrhage.

CHAPTER 35

Ear Injuries and Illnesses

Contributed by David McDonagh, Deputy CMO, Lillehammer 1994
Olympic Winter Games

Reviewer: Vegard Bugten, ENT Consultant, University Hospital,
Trondheim, Norway

35.1 BURST EARDRUM

A fall or a blow to the side of the head can cause the tympanic membrane to rupture. This is a not uncommon finding in boxers, rugby players, etc. Loud noises (shooting) or explosions can also damage the eardrum (acoustic trauma). Barotraumatic injuries to the ear may result in perforation or rupture of the tympanic membrane and may occur in as little as 2 m of water. Generally, there is pain, bleeding or discharges from the ear, hearing reduction or loss, and tinnitus, but this is not always the case (Figs. 35.1 and 35.2).

Treatment: Inspect the ear to ensure there is no other pathology such as fracture or infection causing severe and violent vertigo. Do not put drops of any kind in the ear. Do not attempt to equalize the middle ears.

35.2 EXTERNAL EAR CANAL SUPERFICIAL VESSEL RUPTURE

This may occur alone or as part of a ruptured eardrum process and may cause some minor bleeding. Drops of blood may be found on the athlete's pillow. If the cause is diving barotrauma, further activity is not advised due to the danger of tympanic rupture. Bleeding can be followed by infection and the athlete should be warned of this. Athletes with colds seem to be more prone to injury.

35.3 BAROTRAUMA

Atmospheric pressure changes can cause swelling and obstruction of the eustachian tube and thus pressure increase in the middle ear. This lesion is commonly seen in water sports, such as diving and water skiing, but may also occur during a long flight, and athletes may arrive at a sports event with ear or sinus problems (e.g., barotitis media or barosinusitis). The increase in pressure in the middle ear may cause tympanic vessel damage, accompanied by bleeding and later by infection, and this may eventually lead to a rupture of the eardrum. Athletes may present with earache, discharge, tinnitus, decreased hearing, and even nausea and vertigo. Treatment is based on rest and the use of antibiotics and nasal decongestants. If these initial symptoms do not clear up within 2 days, referral to a specialist is recommended. The eustachian tube usually recovers, and pressure imbalances disappear. A ruptured eardrum usually grows back to normal; however, chronic tears often require surgical intervention.

35.4 CARTILAGE TRAUMA AND LACERATIONS

The ears are of course susceptible to cuts, bruising, and scrapes.

Consistent bruising of the ear may lead to the development of an auricular hematoma, the so-called cauliflower ear, which is particularly predominant in rugby. An acute hematoma should be treated with ice compression and possibly

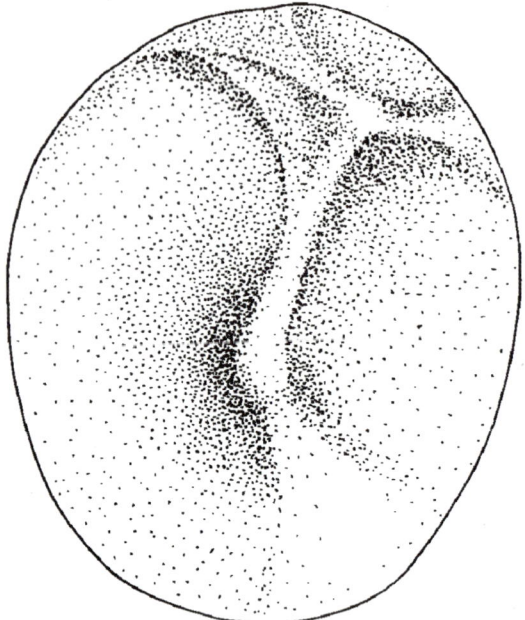

FIGURE 35.1.   Normal eardrum.

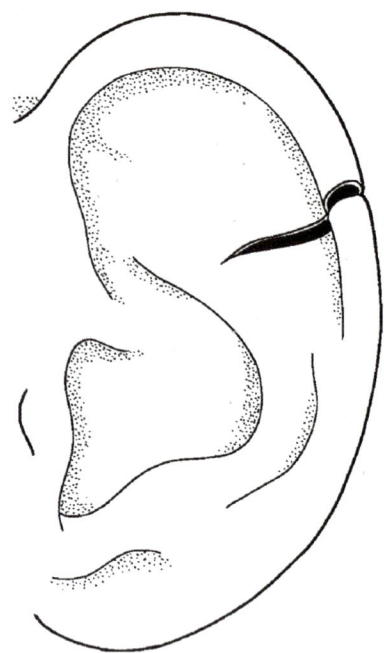

FIGURE 35.3.   Ear cartilage trauma.

needle aspiration as the hematoma may cause baronecrosis of the ear cartilage (similar to the processes involved in a nasal septal hematoma).

Cuts to the ears are treated in the same manner as cuts elsewhere in the body. However, if there is an open wound involving a small tear of the cartilage, I try to suture the skin only, using the folds of the ear as alignment landmarks. For these smaller, nongaping, well-aligned cartilage tears, I try to avoid suturing the cartilage in the hope of avoiding cartilage destruction and resorption. The dressings play an important splinting role and should support the pinna on both sides; the dressings may also help prevent the formation of a hematoma (Figs. 35.3–35.5).

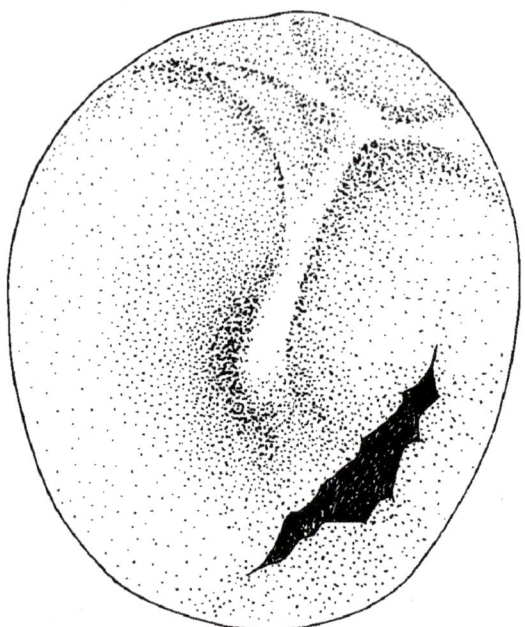

FIGURE 35.2.   Ruptured eardrum.

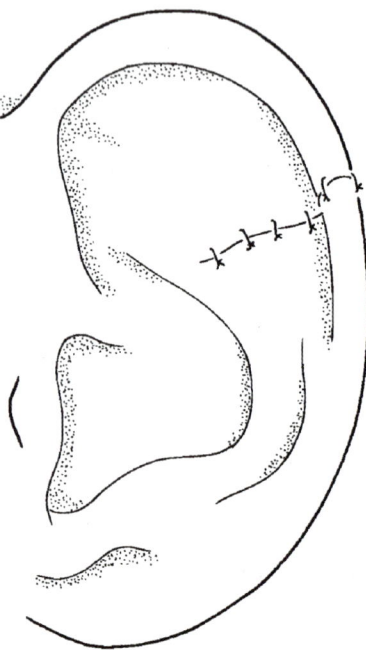

FIGURE 35.4.   Ear cartilage suture technique.

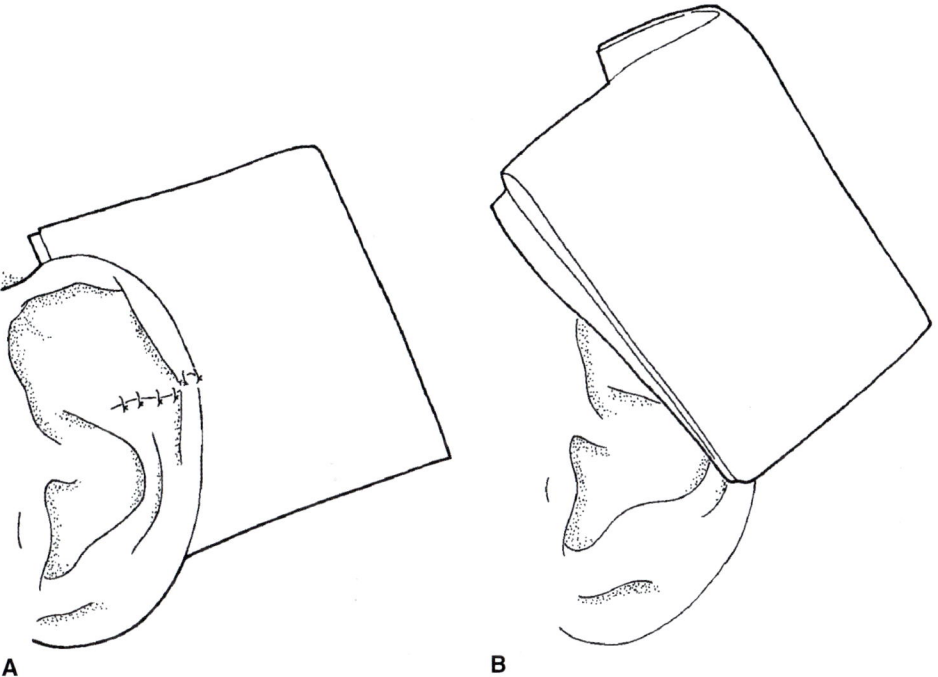

A **B**

FIGURE 35.5. Postsuture compression and bandaging.

For larger cartilage tears, the cartilage must be sutured. Wounds to the ear are commonly irregular, and if there is cartilage exposure due to skin loss, refer to a specialist.

35.5 AVULSED EAR

In the unlikely event of finding an athlete with an avulsed ear, is important to locate and save the avulsed parts by placing them in a cold, clean saline solution. The injured ear should be covered with a saline bandage and circular elasticized bandage (turban) around the head. Bleeding can be profuse, so prepare to give IV fluids. The patient should be transported to a hospital with the head elevated.

35.6 FOREIGN BODIES

Again, the main rule of foreign body management is to leave them be until one can be treated at a medical center. Some objects are tiny and can easily be removed, so go ahead. However, impaled objects must never be removed due to the risk of profuse bleeding. Try to immobilize the impaled object using bulky sterile dressings, which hopefully prevent movement under transport. Immobilize the patient, if necessary.

Some foreign bodies may be difficult to visualize and may be embedded in the ear tissue or may not be easily accessible. Obviously, one should try to avoid pressing an object further into the ear. Place a bulky dressing over the injured ear and transfer the athlete to a hospital.

35.7 BURNS

Again, rare in sport. Treat as with any other burn lesion; however, if there is sign of a grade 2 burn injury, then referral to a specialist would be a good idea due to the risk of cartilage infection and necrosis.

35.8 FROSTBITE

As burns, above. See section on frostbite.

35.9 SWIMMER'S EAR

Swimmers ears are often submersed in water, and adequate drying is not always possible. If the ear canals are not dried properly, there is a risk of infection, particularly of fungal origin.

If the ear canals are dried too often and too forcefully (with a cotton swab, fingernail) microtrauma can occur to the skin and infections can arise (otitis externa). I often take a bacterial swab from the discharge before commencing antibiotic treatment. If it turns out to be a fungal infection, I usually refer to an ENT specialist.

35.10 FLUID OR BLOOD DISCHARGE FROM THE EAR

Remember, these discharges may occur when there is an underlying cranial fracture; however, they usually reflect a blood vessel injury, otitis externa or media, tympanic rupture, or infection.

An acute discharge may be associated with

- Acute otitis media—typically very painful, with relief after drum rupture and purulent discharge

- Acute otitis externa
  - Infectious, often associated with trauma, dermatitis, painful ear traction
  - Allergic, often itchy, but less painful than infectious lesions as above
  - Combined, often swollen, red, pus, skin flakes

- Cranial fractures—to the base of the skull, with clear or bloody discharge

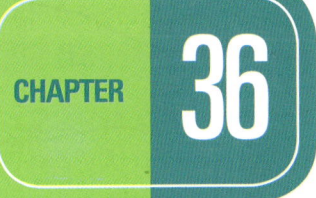

CHAPTER 36

Nasal Injuries

Contributed by David McDonagh, Chair, FIBT Medical Commission

Reviewer: Vegard Bugten, ENT Consultant, University Hospital, Trondheim, Norway

36.1 NASAL FRACTURES

When examining for nasal injuries the event physician must think of the following:

- Is there a fracture? If so, is it cartilage, nasal bone, or nasoethmoidal fracture?

- Is there a septal hematoma?

- Are there patent airways and is the athlete ventilating adequately?

- Is there an isolated nasal fracture or are there associated facial or cervical spine injuries?

- Are there any symptoms or signs of concussion and associated head injury?

Most nasal fractures are the result of minor trauma such as being punched or elbowed in the face. After ensuring that the athlete has patent airways, is breathing adequately and has no spinal injury, the event physician should examine all bony structures of the face, including the orbits, zygomatic arches, mandible, teeth and palate. Any swellings, cuts, bruises and deformities should be noted and the eyes should be examined for ocular injury, diplopia and blow-out fractures.

If a facial or mandibular fracture is suspected, then the athlete should be referred to hospital.

Similarly, if there are inadequate airways and inhibited ventilation, the athlete should be stabilized, given oxygen by mask, and transferred to hospital. The presence of a concomitant spinal injury will demand another level of care with immobilization and respiratory/hemodynamic stabilization (see Chapter 41).

Clinical findings:

- A deformity of the nose

- Epistaxis, with or without obvious nasal deformity

- Edema and bruising of the nose and periorbital structures

- Palpation of the nasal structures may reveal indentation or fracture sulcus of the nasal bone (Fig. 36.1).

Persistent epistaxis without deformity must cause the event physician to suspect a nasal fracture or, worse, a nasoethmoidal or basal cranial fracture.

Similarly, the finding of subcutaneous emphysema or clear rhinorrhea (CSF) should raise the suspicion of a maxillary or cranial fracture.

Treatment of an uncomplicated acute nasal fracture includes the application of ice, the maintenance of head elevation, rest, and appropriate pain medication. If the nose is cosmetically unchanged, no reduction will be required and nasal x-rays are not usually necessary. X Ray and CT investigations are usually only indicated with a facial or sinus fracture. Once the bleeding has stopped (see "Epistaxis" below), the nose should be inspected to rule out a septal hematoma.

If the nose is crooked or deformed, it is safe to suspect a fracture, and reduction may be required. Most ENT specialists accept that there is no indication for early fracture reduction so the athlete can be discharged but instructed to contact an ENT specialist within 3 to 5 days for reevaluation.

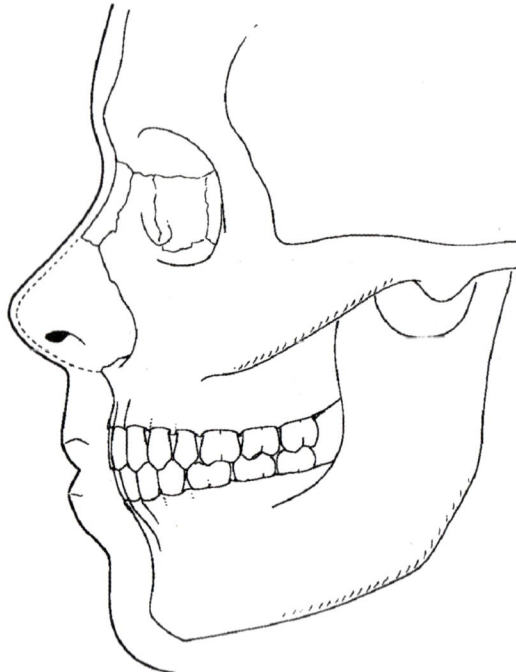

FIGURE 36.1.   Nasal bones.

36.2 SEPTAL HEMATOMAS

After receiving a blow to the nose, an athlete may develop a septal hematoma. Failure to identify and treat a septal hematoma may result in collapse of the nasal cartilage and lead to the

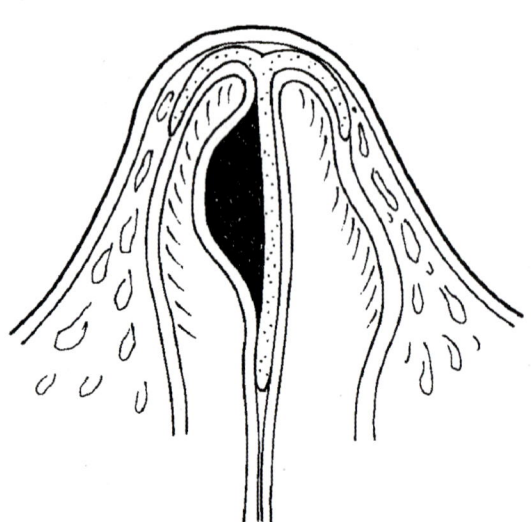

FIGURE 36.2.   Right-sided septal hematoma.

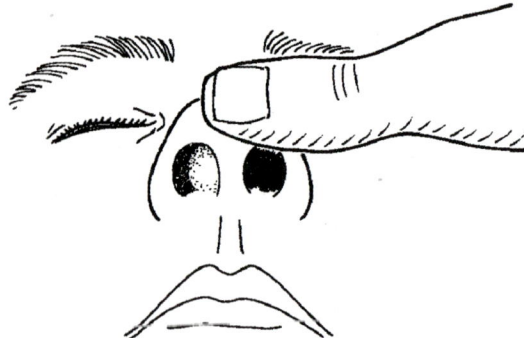

FIGURE 36.3.   Right-sided septal hematoma.

"Popeye" or saddle deformity of the septum, which can be quite disfiguring and affect nasal respiration.

The initial internal inspection usually will reveal the presence of large blood clots. If there is clot blocking inspection, ask the patient to blow the nose gently, one nostril at a time.

The septa may appear to bulge unilaterally or bilaterally and slightly discolored areas may appear on one or both sides of the nasal septum (Figs. 36.2 and 36.3). The hematoma often obstructs the nasal passage. It is soft and fluctuant on palpation, unlike a normal septum, which is hard.

During the internal examination, the physician should assess nasal airway patency and should determine if ongoing epistaxis or septal deformities are present.

Any mucosal lacerations should be noted because they may suggest an underlying fracture.

A thorough internal examination is important and referral to a hospital is necessary if a septal hematoma or arterial bleed is suspected. Hematomas may become infected.

36.3 NASOETHMOID FRACTURES

This results from a frontal blow of high energy at the level of the nasal bones. There is collapse and telescoping of the nasal bones and anterior ethmoids, and there may be a fracture of the cribriform and fovea ethmoidalis (Figs. 36.4 and 36.5). This is a complex area and fractures may be difficult to diagnose. These fractures may occur as isolated injuries or as part of the more complex LeFort fractures, so beware. Swelling of the medial canthal areas should increase awareness. Look for associated ocular injury, with enophthalmos,

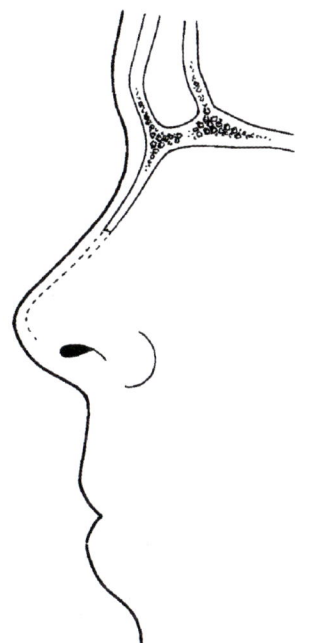

FIGURE 36.4. Nasoethmoidal structures.

diplopia, entrapment, and vertical dystopia. CSF leaks should be examined for. If in doubt, a CT scan should be requested, though x-ray can be ordered if CT is unavailable.

36.4 EPISTAXIS

Nosebleeds usually occur due to injuries to the plexus of veins in the anterior nasal septum mucosa and underlying blood vessels (anterior nose bleeds). In sport, epistaxis is usually traumatic but may signal underlying pathology, such as a coagulation disorder, hypertension, or even a juvenile angiofibroma, so take a good case history and make a relevant examination.

Inspect the face for bruising and signs of nasal and maxillary fractures. Gently palpate the facial bones. The mouth and oropharynx should be visualized with a tongue depressor and light source for hematomas, deformities, and bleeding. Examine the nose, with the patient in a sitting position, with a torch and speculum; if there is clot blocking inspection, ask the patient to blow the nose gently, one nostril at a time. Inspect Little's area for injuries (Fig. 36.6). Look for signs of septal deviation, septal hematoma, septal swelling, and bony deformity.

If these are not present, then one should start treatment. I usually ask the athlete to pinch the nostrils against the septum for 5 minutes. This usually works, but it can take up to 20 minutes on rare occasions.

If bleeding does not stop, suspect an arterial bleed, a fracture or a posterior nosebleed (rare but serious—with the nostrils squeezed shut, the

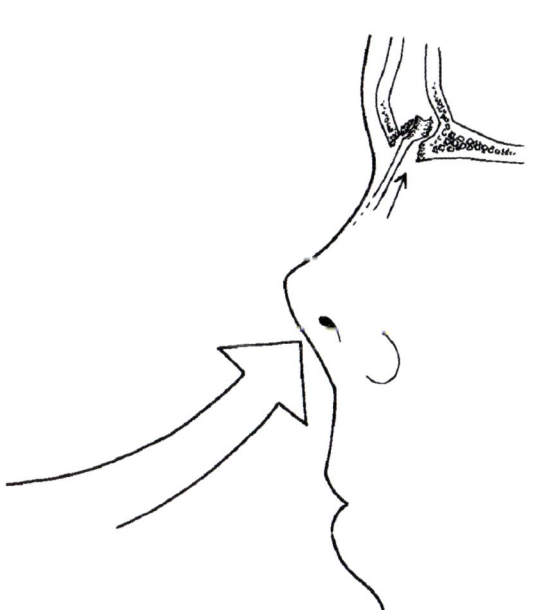

FIGURE 36.5. Nasoethmoidal fracture.

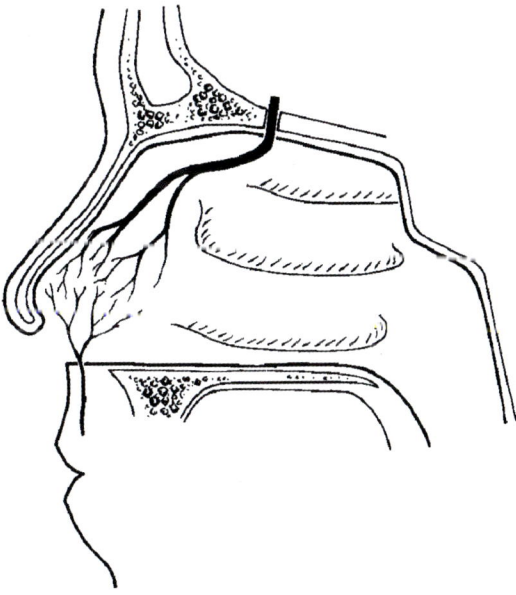

FIGURE 36.6. Little's area.

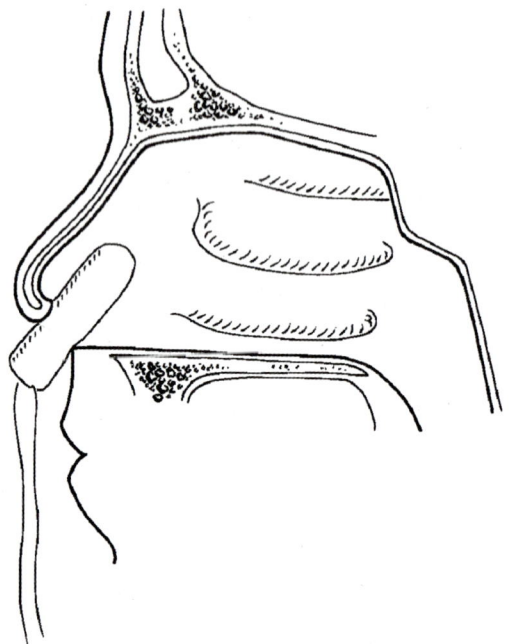

FIGURE 36.7. Anterior tamponade.

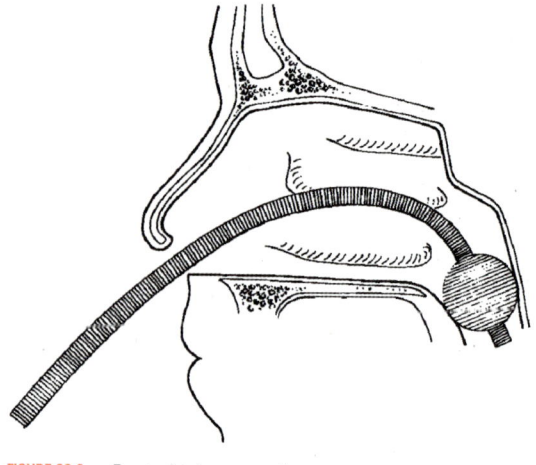

FIGURE 36.8. Posterior tamponade.

bleeding does not stop but blood runs down the back of the throat [post nasal drip]; when the nostril pinching is discontinued, bleeding continues anteriorly). At this time, one can consider using an anterior nasal packing (Fig. 36.7) unless there is a gross nasal deformity. There are several products available. I prefer to use an intranasal tampon coated with lubricant. Some physicians use a topical anesthetic and vasoconstrictor first; however, one must be aware of antidoping rules. While adrenaline is a prohibited stimulant, in 2010, the use of adrenaline in local anesthetic agents is not prohibited.

If the anterior nasal pack does not stop bleeding, then refer the athlete to hospital. If a posterior nosebleed is suspected, then the patient should also be referred to hospital where posterior packing (Fig. 36.8) is usually attempted. Arterial bleeds require hospital referral.

CHAPTER 37

Sinusitis—Maxillary, Ethmoidal, Frontal

Contributed by David McDonagh, Deputy CMO, Lillehammer 1994 Olympic Winter Games

Reviewer: Vegard Bugten, ENT Consultant, University Hospital, Trondheim, Norway

Acute maxillary sinusitis is an infectious or inflammatory process in which paranasal sinus drainage and ventilation are impaired as a consequence of mucosal edema. The commonest cause of acute sinusitis is viral. It is estimated that only 0.5% to 2% of cases of acute viral sinusitis are complicated by an acute bacterial infection of the sinuses. If symptoms increase after 5 days or continue longer than 10 days, bacteria are likely to be involved.

Major Symptoms

- Nasal obstruction and difficulty breathing through the nose
- Reduction or loss of smell and taste
- Purulent rhinorrhea with anterior discharge and postnasal drip
- Facial pain or pressure (often worsened by leaning forward)

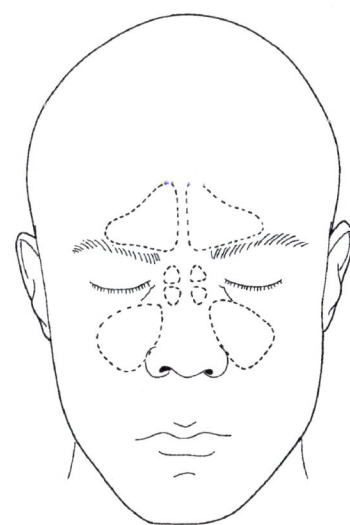

FIGURE 37.1. Sinuses.

Other Minor Symptoms

- Fever
- Headache
- Fatigue
- Dental pain
- Cough
- Bad breath (halitosis) and sore throat

Conditions that can contribute to inflammation in the mucous membranes of the nose and sinuses are

- Allergies
- Nasal polyps
- Pollution
- Smoking
- Other medical conditions—cystic fibrosis, gastroesophageal reflux, or HIV/immunodeficiency diseases

Treatment

The treatment of acute sinusitis should focus on reducing symptoms by restoring communication between the nose and the sinuses. This is most rationally achieved by mild pain-relieving medication, topical decongestive nose spray, or nasal steroids. Saline irrigation may also have favorable effects.

Antibiotics are usually first indicated if symptoms increase after 5 days or last longer than 10 days. A combination of nasal steroids and antibiotics relieves symptoms faster than antibiotics alone. In the acute phase, there may be some variation in the pain site depending on which sinuses are affected, but symptoms are often present to a varying degree in the maxillary, ethmoidal, and frontal sinuses.

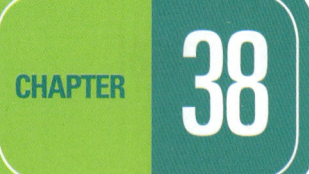

CHAPTER 38

Facial Fractures and Lacerations

Contributed by David McDonagh, Deputy CMO, Lillehammer 1994 Olympic Winter Games

Reviewer: Vegard Bugten, ENT Consultant, University Hospital, Trondheim, Norway

Injuries to facial bones are not uncommon in sport. Facial fractures are usually caused by blows to the face (low energy blows by clubs, bats, elbows, knees) but also crashes, collisions, and can cause injuries. Traditionally, injuries have been classified as low-energy fractures (nasal, zygomatic) and high-energy fractures (mandible, maxilla, and orbit). Both types of fractures can occur in most sports, however. If there is a high-energy accident, such as in skiing, ice hockey, rugby, American football, diving, or boxing, then fractures to the orbit, mandible, and maxilla may be seen.

38.1 MAXILLARY FRACTURES

Maxillary fracture lines often follow the Le Fort classification and it is obvious that an athlete must receive immediate treatment if such fractures occur. Hospital referral and CT of the face and caput should be mandatory (Fig. 38.1–38.3).

A Le Fort I fracture can be diagnosed by

- Bruising of upper lip and lower half of midface
- Mobility of whole of tooth-bearing segment of upper jaw
- Disturbed occlusion
- Hematoma in palate
- Palpable crepitation in upper buccal sulcus

A Le Fort II fracture can be diagnosed by

- Periorbital bruising
- Infraorbital nerve damage, including hyperesthesia of the cheeks

- May have bilateral subconjunctival hematomas and diplopia
- Symmetry/deformity with palpable step deformities of orbital rims, zygomatic arches, nose, maxilla
- Movement of dental arches and mobile maxilla
- Fractured/avulsed/mobile teeth

A Le Fort III fracture can be diagnosed by

- Severe facial deformity—the so-called dish-face appearance, with a flat, elongated face. Deformity with palpable step deformities of orbital rims, zygomatic arches, nose, maxilla
- Facial bruising
- The patient may be unconscious and have breathing difficulties
- Often infraorbital nerve damage including hyperesthesia
- May have bilateral subconjunctival hematomas and diplopia
- Often movable palate/dental arches
- Palate hematoma
- Always nasal discharge with CSF
- The patient has often a bloody nasal discharge (epistaxis)

Treatment

The first priority is to ensure adequate airway and ventilation. If this cannot be achieved then cricothyroidotomy/tracheostomy may be required.

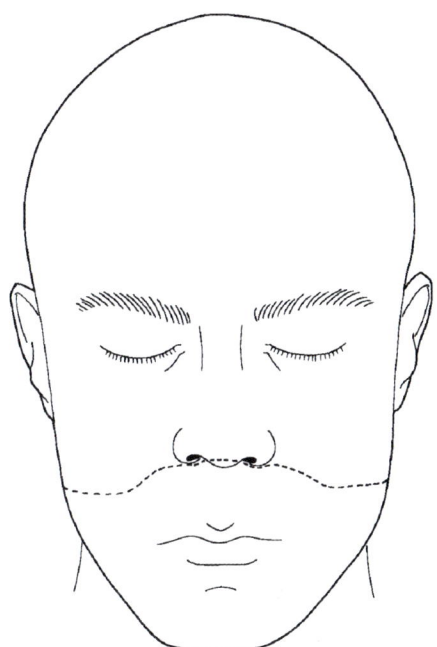

FIGURE 38.1. Le Fort I fracture.

Ensure adequate circulation. Look for and expect to find signs of cranial injury with Le Fort III fractures and possibly in Le Fort II fractures. Continuous neurological evaluation is necessary. Rapid transportation to hospital is indicated with all Le Fort fractures but especially grade 2 and 3 fractures.

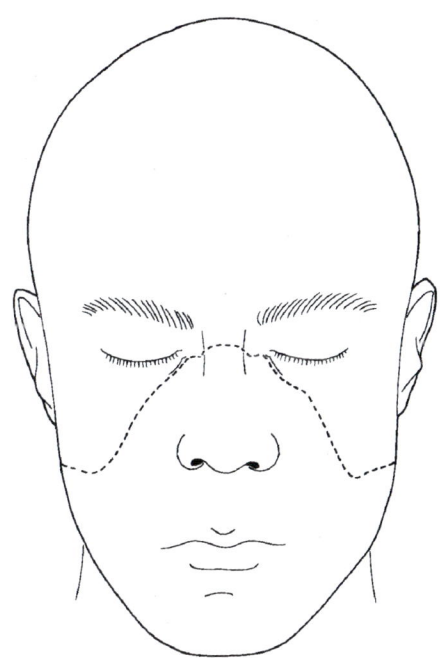

FIGURE 38.2. Le Fort II fracture.

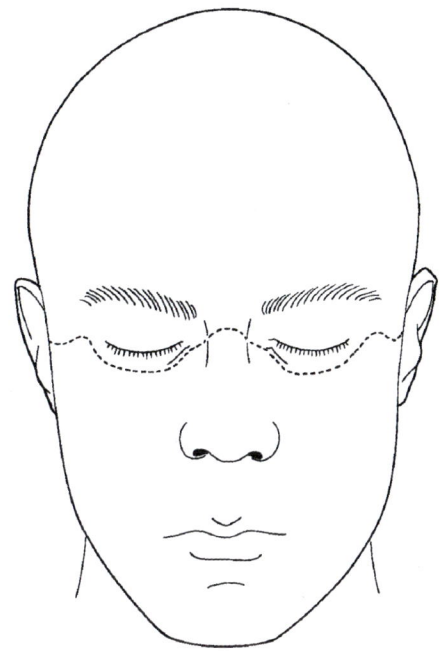

FIGURE 38.3. Le Fort III fracture.

38.2 ORBITAL FRACTURES

Trauma to the upper face may result in fractures of the orbit. These may vary from small defects in the orbital floor, blowout fractures, complex facial fractures or even fractures involving all four orbital walls.

Blowout fractures usually occur after a blow to the eye from a ball or a bat, or after a knee, elbow, or kick to the face. Disruption of the bony orbital wall results often in decompression, typically sparing the orbital rim (pure

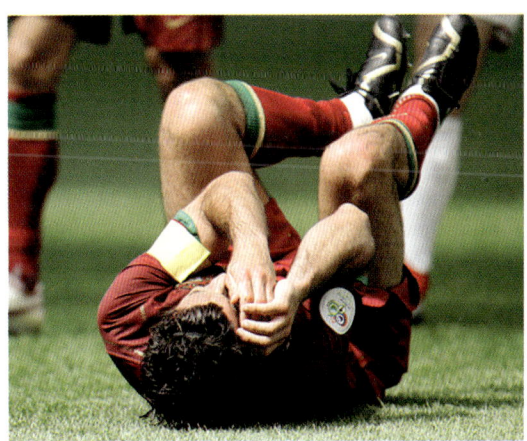

FIGURE 38.4. Luis Figo, Portugal. (Photo courtesy of FIFA.)

blowout fracture). Not all orbital fractures are blowout fractures. Blowout fractures occur when the eye sustains a direct blunt force. There are two reported injury mechanisms: The first is where there is a blow to the infraorbital area, thus causing a fracture of the orbital floor. This type of injury is less often associated with orbital entrapment than with the second type of injury, where there is a direct blow to the eye (and not the orbital rim), thus causing the true or pure blowout fracture. The eye is relatively elastic and forces may be transmitted downward to the thin orbital floor or medially through the ethmoid bones, thus causing a fracture. This type of injury—often caused by a golf ball, squash ball, handle of an ice hockey stick, or fist—is more likely to be associated with entrapment and injury to the eye itself.

Patients with blowout fractures have eyelid swelling and periorbital ecchymosis; they may have infraorbital nerve damage that leads to numbness under the eye over the maxillary sinus. They may also have symptoms and signs of eye damage such as eye pain, double vision, reduced vision, damage to the lens, anterior chamber bleeding (hyphema), posterior chamber hemorrhage, detached retina, chemosis enophthalmos, or subconjunctival hemorrhage and orbital tenderness.

As mentioned above, these lesions may also be seem as a part of the more complex Le Fort II or III facial fractures.

Isolated blow-in fractures of the superior orbital roof, inferior orbital floor, medial orbital wall, and lateral orbital wall have also been described, but are rare.

Treatment

If a fracture is suspected, then the athlete must not return to play. Melting ice can be applied gently to the infraorbital area but pressure must not be applied to the eye. Nose blowing should be avoided to prevent pressure displacement of sinus contents into the orbit.

Radiological referral is advised, and the athlete should be evaluated by an eye specialist or facial surgeon. Analgesia may be required. Antibiotics are usually employed, but seldom in the prehospital environment.

Grossly displaced fractures or fractures with persistent double vision, ocular entrapment, or pain are usually candidates for surgical repair. Timing of the repair varies, but usually is within 1 week of the injury.

38.3 ZYGOMATIC FRACTURES

Isolated fractures may occur, but they may also be associated with serious midface trauma.

If there is an isolated fracture with no or minimal displacement of the zygoma (Fig. 38.5) with no complications, then conservative treatment is recommended. The athlete should be sent to a hospital for radiological evaluation. The athlete should avoid blowing his or her nose (to avoid subcutaneous and orbital emphysema).

However, zygomatic trauma is also associated with cranial lesions, orbit and ocular injuries, facial fractures, and cervical injury, so the event physician must be alert and examine and observe these potential injuries. It is essential to ascertain that the airway is not compromised.

Examination

- Swelling and bruising over the zygoma

- Pain on palpation of the zygoma and palpable deformity if a depressed fracture is present.

- Palpation of the orbit

- Posterior displacement of the fractured fragment may cause pain on chewing.

- Examine the eye, checking for damage to the globe and enophthalmos.

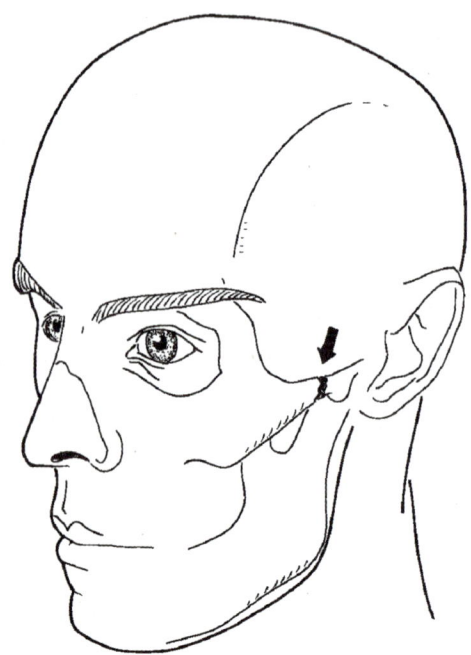

FIGURE 38.5. Zygomatic fracture.

- Diplopia is common and may be due to a blowout orbital fracture, entrapment of a muscle, neural injury, or a hematoma in an external ocular muscle.

- Periorbital and subconjunctival hemorrhage is common.

- Check for impairment of sensation below the eye (infraorbital nerve—maxilla fracture?).

- Trismus can occur (spasm of the masseter muscle), making chewing difficult and painful.

- The mucosa of the maxillary sinus may be lacerated and cause ipsilateral epistaxis.

Treatment

If a fracture is suspected, then the athlete must not return to play. Radiological referral is advised and the athlete should be evaluated by an ENT or facial surgeon. Analgesia may be required. Antibiotics are usually employed, but seldom in the prehospital environment.

38.4 MANDIBULAR FRACTURES

Mandibular fractures are not infrequent and often occur after falls or high-energy blows to the chin. Clinical findings include facial distortion, bruising, malocclusion of the teeth, or abnormal mobility of portions of the mandible or teeth. When examining the teeth, there may be gaps between the teeth or a step if there is dislocation of the fractured segment. The patient may have difficulty in opening his or her mouth. The tongue blade test is still regarded as a useful test. Ask the patient to bite on and grip a tongue blade with his teeth. If the examiner can break the blade with the patient gripping with his teeth, a radiograph is unnecessary. In my experience, this is often true, but always? I use the positive blade test: If the patient cannot hold the blade, then an x-ray is definitely needed.

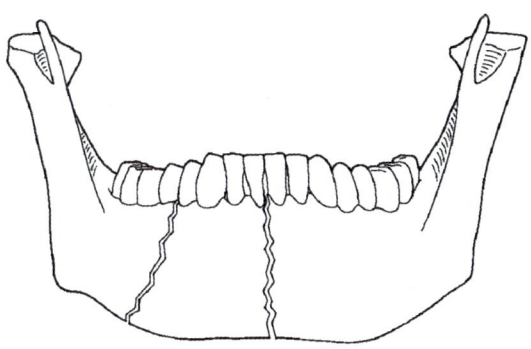

FIGURE 38.6. Mandibular fractures 1.

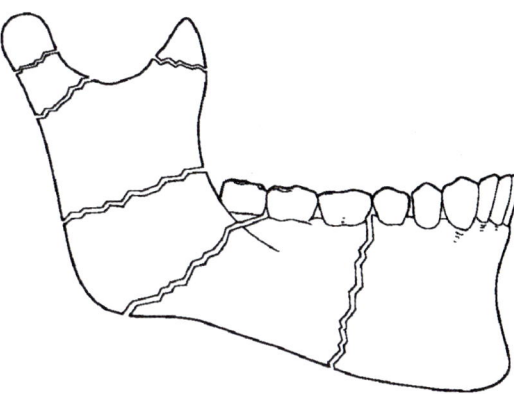

FIGURE 38.7. Mandibular fractures 2.

Mandibular fractures occur at any of the following sites (Figs. 38.6 and 38.7):

- Body: 35%

- Angle: 25%

- Condyle: 15%

- Symphysis: 10%

- Ramus: 5%

- Others: approximately 5%

Double fractures can occur; they are usually on contralateral sides of the midline symphysis. Traumatic temperomandibular dislocations may occur but are unusual. Reduction is necessary, but this should normally be carried out after radiological evaluation at a hospital.

Treatment of mandibular fractures: Prehospital treatment is conservative. Ensure that the athlete has adequate airways and normal ventilation. Suspect concomitant facial, cranial, cervical, and throat injuries. Patients should be referred to hospital.

38.5 LACERATIONS OF THE FACE

Firstly, as with all cuts, it is important to evaluate the wound length, depth, and location; the presence of bleeding; and the proximity of important structures (tear ducts, facial nerve, etc.).

It is important to examine for underlying facial fractures; if these are present, then arterial bleeding should be stopped, if possible, by gentle compression. Wounds should be cleaned (without causing bleeding) with saline and covered with a damp saline bandage. The patient should be transferred to a specialist unit. Always remember that there is an associated increased incidence of cranial and intracranial injury, so evaluate the patient's neurological status.

If on the field of play, clean the skin and irrigate the wound with saline while protecting the patient's eyes. Gross removal of foreign bodies is recommended, followed by gentle compression with a saline bandage. Once the athlete is taken to the medical room, further evaluation and treatment can be conducted. It is also important to decide whether or not you are competent enough with facial suturing, as there are several facial areas that require precise surgical technique and experience before suturing, particularly with lacerations affecting the vermilion, nostrils, eyebrows, and lacrimal duct. You need to know what you are doing when suturing these areas.

If you decide to suture, then the wound inspection and cleaning must be repeated. Debridement may be necessary, but, if so, consider referring to a specialist clinic. Similarly, if there are damaged underlying structures, refer the athlete.

If all is well and you choose to close the wound, close with simple monofilament No. 4/0 or No. 5/0 nonabsorbable sutures. If competent, then attempt to use intradermal or subdermal sutures, as these often leave a better cosmetic result. Reinforce the sutured wound with several skin tapes. Recommend that sutures be removed after 5 days, as this reduces scarring and may avoid the "zipper" scar. Skin tapes should be applied for a further 7 days. If there is suspicion of wound contamination, then prophylactic antibiotics may be recommended.

Larger facial lacerations, and particularly those associated with tissue loss, should be referred to a specialist unit. Attempt to stop bleeding, clean and irrigate the wound, remove all foreign material, and either cover the wound with a sterile saline bandage or gently pack the wound with sterile saline dressings.

Lacerations of the Lip

Most buccal lacerations should be sutured; however, some smaller lacerations can be left alone. You should advise the athlete to rinse the mouth frequently, and to try a liquid diet for a few days to avoid food particle entrapment. If the lip needs to be sutured, then inject local anesthesia with adrenalin into the cut on each side—avoid piercing the lip again, as this often causes more bleeding. Wait 5 minutes to allow the swelling from the injection to disappear; this facilitates correct realignment. Rinse the wound thoroughly. If possible, place sutures on the buccal aspect of the lip for better cosmesis.

If the cut goes through the labial vermilion, then careful adaption and proper anatomical realignment is important. I achieve this by placing the first suture through the vermilion on each side of the cut; the borders can be marked with a pen before suturing.

Then, close the rest of the wound in layers, starting deep and becoming superficial before suturing the outer lip mucosa/skin. I use interrupted No. 4/0 absorbable sutures with the smallest needle internally (Vicryl Rapide) and usually close the wound using a No. 5/0 nonabsorbable (nylon) suture, to be removed after 7 days (Fig. 38.8).

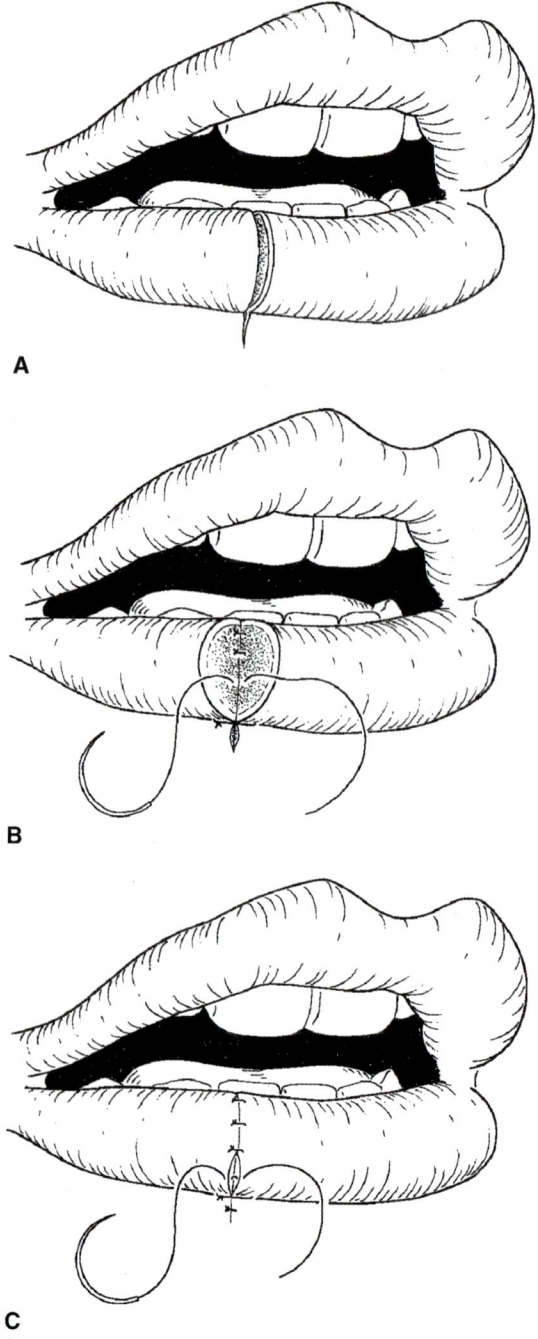

A

B

C

FIGURE 38.8. Suturing lip lacerations.

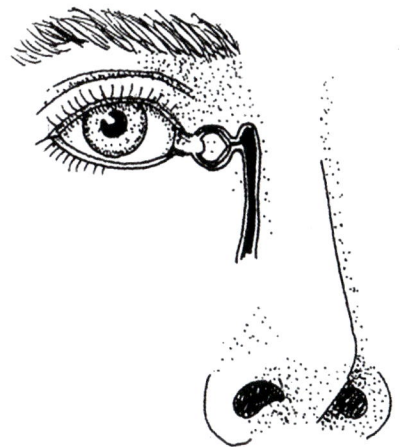

FIGURE 38.9. Lacrimal apparatus.

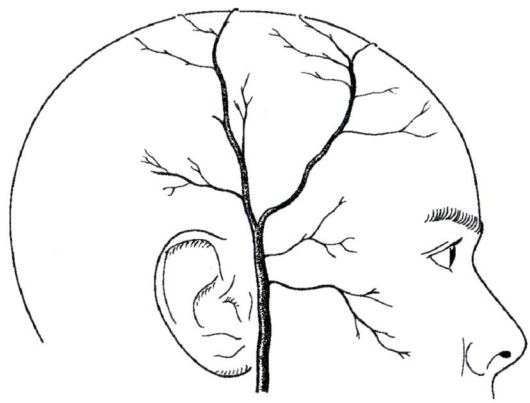

FIGURE 38.10. Temporal artery.

With "stable wounds," external closure can be achieved using adhesive tape. This gives even better cosmesis, though you must ensure that there is no bleeding, as the tape may loosen and cause an ugly scar; however, most athletes prefer a suture as this allows for early return to play. The athlete should avoid pressing the tongue against the wound in the recovery phase.

Lacerations Around the Eye

Beware cuts around the eyes and nose. Cuts involving the eyelids should be referred to a specialist. Similarly, cuts medial to the eye may encroach upon the lacrimal apparatus, so these should also be referred to specialist treatment (Fig. 38.9).

Lacerations in the Temporal Region

These cuts are usually not a problem; however, lacerations that affect the superficial temporal artery may cause profuse bleeding. This artery, which is the smaller of the two terminal branches of the external carotid artery, begins in front of the ear, almost behind the neck of the mandible, in the substance of the parotid gland, crossing over the posterior root of the zygomatic process before dividing into the frontal and parietal branches. As anyone who has performed a temporal artery biopsy knows, these arteries bleed profusely when incised. There are two courses of action—either use external compression (often the best choice) or try to ligate the artery proximal to the bleed by placing a broad suture (using No. 3/0 nonabsorbable thread) through the skin, onto the bone, under and around the artery, and then out through the skin again and knotting the suture. This closed ligating suture, that is performed without a skin incision, may help stop profuse bleeding but requires skill, experience, and luck (Fig. 38.10).

Other Deep Lacerations

Once again, if there are deep lacerations that may involve the parotid gland, facial or trigeminal nerves, or deep muscles, it is better to compress the wound with a salt water bandage and refer the patient to a hospital.

Recommended Reading

Ceallaigh PO, Ekanaykaee K, Beirne CJ, et al. Diagnosis and management of common maxillofacial injuries in the emergency department. Part 3: orbitozygomatic complex and zygomatic arch fractures. *Emerg Med J* 2007;24(2):120–122.

Patel BC, Hoffmann J, Management of complex orbital fractures. *Facial Plast Surg.* 1998;14(1):83–104. [abstract]

Ward NJ, Okpala E. Analysis of 47 road traffic accident admissions to BMH Shaibah. *J R Army Med Corps.* 2005;151(1):37–40. [abstract]

Echlin P, Upshur R, Peck D, et al. Craniomaxillofacial injury in sport: a review of prevention research. *Br J Sports Med.* 2005;39(5):254–263.

CHAPTER 39

Oral/Dental Injuries and Conditions

Contributed by Paul Piccininni, IIHF (Ice Hockey) Medical Committee, IOC Medical Commission, York University, Toronto, Canada; Anthony F. Clough, Dental Lead, London 2012 Olympic Summer Games, University College, London, British Alpine Team, British Rowing Squad, UK; Ray Padilla, Team Dentist, Los Angeles Galaxy, UCLA Athletics, USA National Men's and Women's Soccer, Dental Staff, Los Angeles 1984 Olympic Summer Games; Jean-Luc Dion, Team Dentist, Quebec Nordiques (NHL), Dental Consultant, 2008 IIHF World Championship, Quebec City; Rene Fasel, President, IIHF, Executive Member, IOC, Coordination Commission Chair, Vancouver 2010 Olympic Winter Games, President, Association of Olympic Winter Sports

Sport dentistry is the prevention and treatment of oral/facial athletic injuries and related oral diseases and manifestations that may prevent the athlete from competing and excelling at elite levels.

In sports, the main challenge to the medical and therapy staff is to maximize the benefits of competition and to minimize injuries and loss of training time. Immediate and timely treatment is a necessary part of training and competing at the elite level. Prevention and adequate preparation are the key elements in minimizing injuries. Included are the teaching of proper preventive hygiene skills, the timely treatment of hard- and soft-tissue pathosis, and certainly, whenever possible, the wearing and utilization of properly fitted protective equipment.

The National Youth Sports Foundation for the Prevention of Athletic Injuries reports several interesting statistics. Dental injuries are the most common type of oral/facial injuries sustained during participation in sports. Victims of tooth fractures and avulsions who do not have the teeth properly stored or replanted will face lifetime dental costs estimated from $10,000 to $20,000 per tooth, the inconvenience of hours spent in the dental chair, and the possibility of other dental problems. Treatment of oral/facial injuries—simple or complex—includes not only the treatment of injuries at the dental office, but also preferably timely treatment at the venue site to increase the positive prognosis.

Preseason screenings and examinations are essential in preventing injuries. Examinations should include health histories, identification of at-risk dentitions, diagnosis of caries, maxilla/mandibular relationships, orthodontics, loose teeth, dental habits, crown and bridge work, missing teeth, artificial teeth, and the possible need for extractions for orthodontic concerns or extraction of wisdom teeth to help prevent pericoronitis and reduce the incidence of traumatic jaw fractures. If possible, these extractions should be done for these athletes months prior to playing competitive sports so as to not interfere with their competition or weaken their jaws during contact. A determination of the need for a specific type and design for protective mouth guards may be made at this time.

Mouth guards may be the single most effective piece of protective equipment in sport. It is essential to educate the athlete that poorly fitted mouth guards bought at sporting good stores do not provide the optimum protection expected by the athlete, nor can they be worn without interfering with speaking and breathing. Only custom-made mouth guards, made with the pressure lamination technique from a model of the athlete's mouth, fit with the precision necessary to not interfere with the athlete's ability to perform at elite levels.

Smokeless tobacco usage should also be included as a part of any preparticipation examination (PPE), and the athlete should be educated on the dangerous properties and consequences of using smokeless tobacco and the potential oral manifestations.

It is not uncommon to recognize the symptoms of anorexia and bulimia during a dental PPE.

Erosion patterns in the teeth, caused by gastric acids, often help in the differential diagnosis of eating disorders. These patients need to be referred to the proper medical and psychological health professional.

39.1 FRACTURES OF THE TEETH

Dental fractures can involve either the crown or the root of the tooth. Root fractures are difficult to diagnose at the field of play, as there may not be any mobility. *Any* blow to the teeth should be radiographed at the earliest possible opportunity in order to detect and manage a possible root fracture.

The severity of crown fractures depends on the structures involved. Fractures of the enamel only, or of the enamel and dentin, might require no immediate management and the athlete might be able to return to play if there are no sharp edges or loose fragments present.

Fractures that involve the pulp (nerve) of the tooth require immediate treatment to both eliminate discomfort and to possibly retain the vitality of the nerve. The treatment at the field can include extirpation of the pulp or placement of a bonded dressing over the nerve area.

In all cases, an attempt should be made to locate the fractured segment. Often, these pieces can be reattached at a later time, and the long-term prognosis of fragment reattachment is excellent. As well, if the athlete has at any time lost consciousness, the risk of aspiration must be considered. Also, these fractured segments can show up in lips and have been reported in the fists of opponents after a fight.

39.2 DENTAL AVULSIONS AND LUXATIONS

While there are different philosophies on the management of avulsed teeth, there are a number of simple rules that can be followed. Avulsed teeth should be located as soon as possible, and, as with fractured dental segments, if the athlete lost consciousness, the possibility of aspiration should be eliminated with appropriate diagnostic images.

An avulsed tooth should be replanted as quickly as possible back into the tooth socket. The tooth should be gently rinsed but the periodontal ligament attached to the root of the tooth should not be damaged or removed. The socket should be gently irrigated if any clot has begun to form, and the tooth should be replaced directly into the socket. In most cases, the socket will retain the tooth, but if the alveolar bone has been damaged, the tooth may need to be held in place with moistened cotton or by the athlete.

If the athlete is unconscious, or if there are other more pressing medical issues that do not allow immediate replantation, the tooth may be placed in saline or one of the tooth preservation systems available (usually Hank's Balanced Salt Solution or similar). However, the success of the replantation decreases significantly with the amount of time the tooth is out of the socket. The best results are achieved if the tooth is replanted within 5 minutes, and there is a reduced potential for success after 30 minutes.

Tetanus prophylaxis should be considered if indicated. Return to play is not possible, and immediate splinting and radiographs are required, along with long-term follow-up.

Luxation injuries result in the teeth becoming mobile within the socket as a result of a blow. In some cases, the alveolus may also be fractured. Luxation injuries can be identified by the mobility of the tooth (mild, moderate, or severe); by a small area of bleeding around the gingival margin of the tooth; or by the athlete advising that the teeth are "out of position" or the "bite" does not feel normal.

On occasion, the athlete can return to play with a minor luxation; however, more significant luxation injuries require removal from play and splinting for an appropriate period of time. Dental radiographs and follow-up are also indicated. If the athlete returns to play with a splint in place, this area must be protected with either a mouth guard, face mask, or both.

39.3 GINGIVAL TRAUMA

"Degloving" injuries of the gingival tissue must be managed with careful irrigation of the traumatized area (under local anesthesia) followed by reattachment of the degloved area using either or both sutures and tissue adhesive. These areas must not be allowed to heal by secondary intention due to the risk of permanent damage to the periodontal tissues.

Care must be taken with other gingival and mucosal injuries—especially those in the vestibule or crevice around the upper and lower teeth—to not reduce or eliminate the depth of the vestibule when closing a traumatized area. This vestibule is necessary for proper chewing and speech and must not be reduced in size due to improper closure or scarring.

For more information about lip lacerations, see Chapter 38.)

39.4 LACERATIONS OF THE TONGUE

Either the teeth or another object may cause significant trauma to the tongue. While there are some who feel these lacerations do not require closure—or that closure is inappropriate due to the risk of sealing oral bacteria into the wound—the risk of disfigurement, speech impediment, and/or food impaction in these sites makes proper closure imperative.

39.5 BRACES AND ORTHODONTICS

As previously noted, athletes with any removable appliances should not wear these for training or competition. Athletes in contact sports with braces should be protected with a properly fitted mouth guard that accommodates the tooth movement being encouraged by the braces. Lost wires should not be replaced, but broken brackets or wires can occasionally be covered with orthodontic wax to allow an athlete to return to competition without risk of aspiration.

39.6 WISDOM TEETH

Wisdom teeth can become infected or inflamed, often due to bacteria or food debris collecting in the pocket or operculum around the tooth. Careful use of an irrigating syringe can sometimes dislodge some of this debris and help to stabilize the area until definitive treatment can be sought. Any lymphadenopathy should invite immediate assessment and treatment with appropriate antibiotics.

39.7 LOST FILLING

Lost restorations do not usually create a situation that requires immediate attention, and most commercially available temporary restorations are unstable and could result in swallowing or aspiration. A loose or lost cap or crown should be removed and retained for proper recementation as temporary replacement may also lead to swallowing or aspiration.

39.8 EMERGENCY DENTAL ANESTHESIA

In most dental and oral situations, local anesthetics with vasoconstrictors are recommended in order to maximize both duration and hemostasis. Potential allergies should be investigated prior to injection. While effective anesthesia of most areas of the maxilla can be achieved by infiltration owing to the innervation and porosity of the maxilla, mandibular anesthesia usually requires a nerve block, which should only be attempted by an experienced practitioner.

Peritonsillar Abscess

These abscesses usually start as a tonsillar cellulitis before spreading deeper into the tonsillar and peritonsillar tissues. The organisms most commonly associated with these abscesses are *Streptococcus pyogenes*, *Staphylococcus aureus*, *Haemophilus influenzae*, and *Fusobacterium*. As with most abscesses, however, there is usually a mixture of various aerobic and anaerobic bacteria.

Always enquire about the possibility of there being a foreign body in the throat. Clinically, the patient presents with fever, unilateral pain in the throat, dysphagia, difficulty in swallowing, difficulty in opening the jaw, difficulty in speaking properly (sometimes described as talking with a mouth full of marbles), the ipsilateral tonsil or its surrounding tissue appearing swollen or red, and, classically, contralateral deviation of the uvula (which may also be red and swollen).

Sometimes, diagnosis is difficult and it is not always to distinguish between mononucleosis, infectious tonsillitis, or a peritonsillar abscess.

Treatment: There is little the EP can do here. Athletes need referral to an ENT specialist for definitive diagnosis, abscess drainage, and antibiotic treatment (Figs. 39.1 and 39.2).

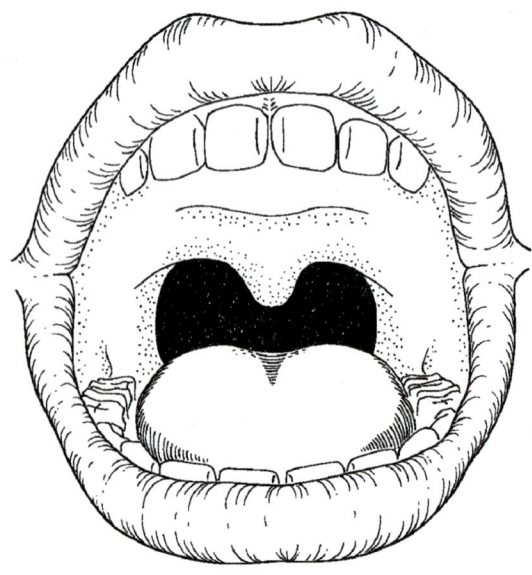

FIGURE 39.1. Normal fauces.

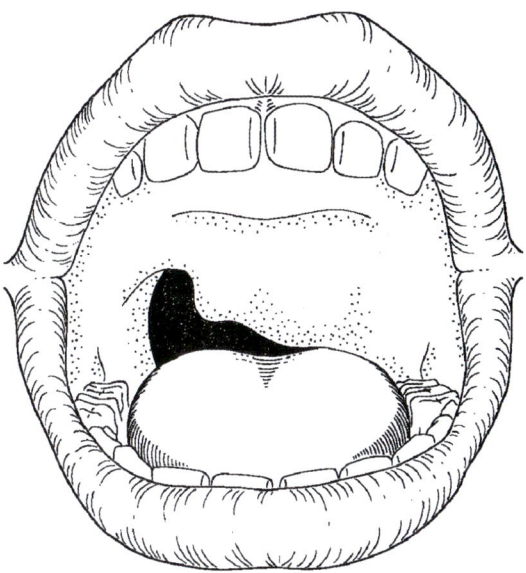

FIGURE 39.2. Left-sided peritonsillar abscess.

39.9 MOUTH SORES

There are many types of mouth sores and many causes: the commonest being cold sores (herpes sores) and aphthus or aphthus-like sores.

Aphthus

One type of common mouth sore is an aphthus. These are often recurrent, small (only 3 to 4 mm in diameter), round, or ovoid ulcers with circumscribed erythematous edges and a floor that is yellowish initially and later grey. There is often a positive family history and there may be some relationship with various HLA types, though there does not appear to be one causative infectious

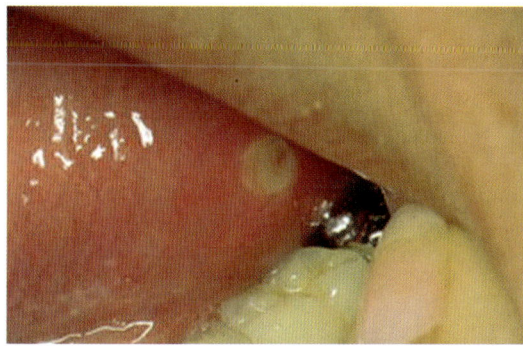

FIGURE 39.3. Aphthus of the tongue.

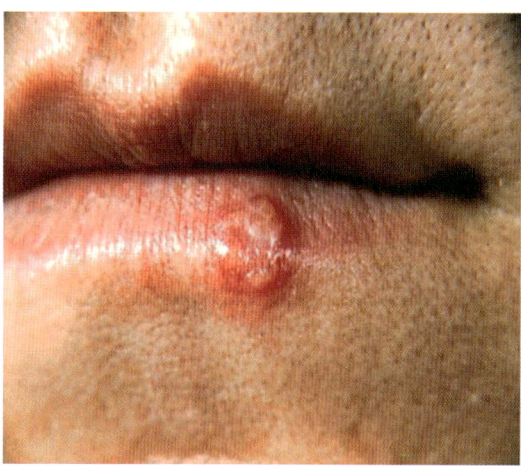

FIGURE 39.4. Cold (herpes) sore.

agent or agents. Microtraumas from mouth guards may be a cause among athletes; ulcers seem to be more common in the latter phase of a menstrual cycle and stress and food allergies may also be a factor. Thermal injuries from ingestion of hot fluids can occur.

The vast majority of aphthus sores are classified as being minor, and only 20% or so as being major. Minor ulcers usually heal within 7 to 10 days but can be quite sore when active. Larger sores (up to 10 mm or more) take much longer to heal and are usually painful.

Treatment: Mouthwashes can be effective, as can topical steroids or analgesics (lignocaine swabs). These are stop-gap measures and should only be used for short periods if pain is intense. Intense pain should cause one to suspect other conditions, such as herpetic ulcers, which must not be treated with hydrocortisone creams.

Aphthus-like sores are also seen with a number of systemic disorders, such as celiac disease, Crohn's disease, Behçet syndrome, iron/B_{12} deficiencies, HIV (Kaposi's sarcoma), and many other conditions. Candida fungal infections may occur alone or secondarily colonize existing mouth sores.

An aphthus does not have a vesicular phase, whereas a cold sore (herpes simplex virus 1) almost always does (Figs. 39.3 and 39.4).

Cold Sore

Most herpetic sores (see Fig. 39.4) around or in the mouth are caused by the herpes simplex virus 1 (HSV-1), although some maybe due to genital herpes simplex virus 2 (HSV-2). Similarly, not all genital herpetic lesions are due to HSV-2. Cold sores usually start with some prodromal symptoms, such as pain or tingling in the affected area before the debut of blisters a day or two later. The blisters usually burst and then become crusty or scabby before disappearing after 7 to 10 days, leaving pink-colored skin that normalizes after a week or so. Clinical findings may take up to 3 weeks to develop, from exposure to clinical debut.

Blisters are usually small, painful, fluid-filled blisters on a raised, erythematous area around the mouth or on the lips; on occasion, blisters can occur in the mouth (gums or hard palate), nostrils, chin, or fingers.

Recommended Reading

Flores MT, Andersson L, Andreasen JO, et al. Guidelines for the management of traumatic dental injuries. I. Fractures and luxations of permanent teeth. *Dent Traumatol.* 2007; 23(2):66–71.

Ljungqvist A, Jenoure P, Engebretsen L. The International Olympic Committee (IOC) Consensus Statement on periodic health evaluation of elite athletes March 2009. *Br J Sports Med.* 2009;43(9):631–643.

Ma'aita J, Alwrikat A. Is mandibular third molar a risk factor for mandibular angle fracture? *Oral Surg Oral Med Oral Pathol Oral Radiol Endod.* 2000;89(2):143–146.

Milosevic A. Eating disorders and the dentist. *Br Dent J.* 1999;186(3):109–113.

CHAPTER 40

Throat Injuries and Foreign Bodies

Contributed by David McDonagh, AIBA, Medical Commission

Reviewer: David Mulder, Professor, McGill University, Montreal, and Team Physician for Montreal Canadiens Ice Hockey Team

40.1 BLUNT TRAUMA

Blunt trauma to the throat is rare but has the potential to be immediately life threatening. They may also cause serious injuries that may not present before some time after the injury—hence, they can be difficult to assess and difficult to predict. Rarely, the athlete presents with acute choking-like symptoms immediately after being struck in the throat. There are many potential causes including being hit on the throat by a ball (baseball, tennis, hockey) or a stick (ice hockey, field hockey, tennis, hurling, lacrosse); even by a swinging arm (soccer, American football, rugby—the dreaded "clothesline tackle"); by a blow from a fist, knee, head, etc.; or by a choking grab from a hand or elbow. In boxing and the martial arts, trauma to the throat is not uncommon. Obviously, throat injuries may also occur in motor sports, in particular with seatbelts or due to contact with handle bars, etc.

Remember also that foreign bodies can be swallowed *or aspirated* and include chewing gum, chewing tobacco, betel leaves, even mouth guards, causing great discomfort, even respiratory distress.

Danger Signs

- Hoarseness or change in voice ("bass to tenor")
- Dysphagia
- Breathing difficulties, dyspnea, stridor
- A feeling of fullness in the throat
- Speech difficulties
- Anterior neck swelling
- Subcutaneous emphysema
- Hemoptosis and oropharyngeal bleeding

Practical Treatment

The patient should desist all activity and sit down (it is easier to breathe in the seated position than when lying on the back). Be careful when placing ice around the neck: It must rest against the skin and no force should be used. Never give the patient anything to eat or drink as this may aggravate the injury.

Basic life support techniques such as the jaw thrust and chin lift may be used. Effective suctioning of nasal and oropharynx can be critical.

In the conscious and breathing athlete, give supplemental oxygen—as high a concentration as you can—as soon as possible. Inspect, gently palpate, and auscultate the neck. Exclude cervical injury. If the patient has even the mildest form of choking or gasping symptoms, or findings, then he or she should be transferred to a hospital posthaste. ("Scoop and run" always trumps "stay and play.")

In an unconscious patient, CPR must be attempted but may be unsuccessful if the airway is blocked. Intubation may be necessary and may be either impossible or dangerous, or both. Cricothyroidotomy may be necessary. Tracheostomy should only be attempted in a controlled environment after the patient has been stabilized.

40.2 LARYNGEAL AND TRACHEAL INJURIES

Blunt injuries to the larynx are not uncommon in boxing, rugby, American football, or ice hockey, whereas cervical trachea injuries are rare and also very dangerous as the force needed to cause a tracheal fracture or rupture is also likely to cause an associated cervical vertebrospinal injury. Both structures can be damaged by direct blows or impact to the neck or may occur during high-velocity falls with abrupt deceleration. Injuries to the larynx may vary from mild inflammations to fractures, dislocations, laryngeal collapse, or lacerations. The more serious the injury, the greater is the likelihood of associated tracheal and cervical spine injury. So if you have a patient with a laryngeal or tracheal injury, always look for/expect an associated cervical injury. Similarly, if you have a patient with a cervical injury, always look for an associated laryngeal/tracheal injury.

Laryngeal Injuries

Clinical Findings: Firstly, one must be aware of the possibility of a cervical vertebral or spinal injury and one must be extremely careful when examining the throat. If the injury is serious, then the patient may well be unconscious.

History If Conscious:
- "Choke sign" coming off the playing field
- Describe incident—hoarseness, dysphonia, or aphonia indicate trauma
- Pain in the larynx and chest, particularly on inspiration
- Pain or difficulty swallowing
- Sudden cough with or without blood

Inspection:
- Look for wounds in the throat region
- Are there laryngeal deformities?
- Is the throat swollen? Is the swelling spreading?
- Respiratory distress with stridor, cyanosis
- On airway inspection you may find blood in the throat or mouth

Palpation:
- Laryngeal swelling
- Subcutaneous emphysema—crepitus
- Laryngeal deformity
- Laryngeal tenderness

Auscultation:
- Inspiratory or expiratory stridor over the lungs and over the throat
- Noisy breathing
- Stertorous breathing

Tracheal Injuries

Patients with tracheal lacerations or ruptures are usually acutely ill, irrespective of whether or not the spinal cord has been injured. Clinical findings may demonstrate the findings found with a laryngeal injury above, but the patient is often more ill and maybe unconscious with or without a concomitant cervical spinal lesion. As the airways may be damaged, it is difficult to oxygenate and ventilate these patients. It may also be extremely difficult to intubate such athletes and an anesthetic expert may be required. Some experts believe that inexperienced intubators should not even attempt intubation for fear of causing irreparable damage, whereas others maintain that this may be the only option if death is imminent. If endotracheal intubation is not possible, then one should consider inserting a surgical airway.

Clinical Findings: Firstly, one must be aware of the possibility of a cervical vertebral or spinal injury and one must be extremely careful when examining the throat. If the injury is serious, then the patient may well be unconscious. History, inspection, palpation, and auscultation findings are often similar to those with laryngeal trauma—but worse.

Treatment
One can be fooled clinically, but treatment is pretty much the same for all of the alternative diagnoses. The patient can have an airway obstruction either in the larynx or trachea or even a tracheobronchial obstruction, so one must ensure that the mouth is *suctioned* or explored digitally. Place a tongue deppressor in the mouth and administer maximum oxygen. One usually has to ventilate the patient, auscultate, and check O_2 saturation to see if there is adequate ventilation. Use basic life support techniques such as jaw thrust and chin lift (takes advantage of mandibular musculature reducing anatomic deformities of larynx and cricoid fracture). If airway damage is suspected, then intubation must be considered, with all the difficulties this may bring. Cricothyroidotomy may be an option if the injury is above the thyroid cartilage; remember the usual incision point is between the thyroid cartilage and the cricoid cartilage, that is, through the cricothyroid membrane. One should try to control hemorrhage as best one can and establish an intravenous line. Always use optimum care regarding the cervical spine.

If there is an obstruction below the level of cricothyroidotomy then adequate oxygenation is very difficult to achieve.

40.3 CAROTID ARTERY CONTUSIONS OR DISSECTIONS

Carotid artery contusions or dissection can occur after major (and in some cases relatively minor) injuries (one such case of carotid artery injury was Gareth Thomas, the then Welsh rugby captain). Dissections can occur spontaneously. It is well nigh impossible to diagnose an arterial contusion or dissection on the field of play as the full spectrum of symptoms may not present until days later. Patients may present with neck trauma and an array of nonspecific complaints. Maintaining a high index of suspicion is important after an athlete has received a blow to the neck, and patients should be referred if they develop subsequent symptoms, particularly unusual focal neurological complaints involving the cranial nerves. There is a real danger of an ischemic cerebral episode. Similarly, "healthy" athletes should be advised to contact a physician should symptoms develop later (Thomas developed "migraine" symptoms). The event physician should be alert to the possibility of arterial dissection when the athlete has been injured with the neck in hyperextension, flexion, and/or rotation. As mentioned, dissection of the internal carotid artery can occur with seemingly minor trauma.

History

- As the patient may be unconscious, a description of the accident may help alert the EP.

- A tackle in rugby or American football or a blow to the neck from a fist, knee, ball, or stick may cause an injury.

Symptoms

Symptoms may include

- The athlete will complain of pain in the neck due to the initial trauma.

- Later, the patient may complain of ipsilateral jaw pain, facial pain, or headache.

- The headache can mimic migraine or cluster headaches.

- Tinnitus

- Ocular symptoms include transient visual field defects (amaurosis fugax) or scintillating scotoma. Facial pain with ptosis and miosis may occur.

- Decreased taste sensation has also been described.

- Symptoms of cervical spinal injury *may be asymptomatic.*

Clinical Findings

- Neck swelling with a hematoma, ecchymosis, "seat belt" mark in motor sports

- Look for signs of cervical spine, facial, cranial, thoracic injuries

- Look for other signs of injury

- Neurological deficit—hemiparesis or focal deficit due to cerebral ischemia or even stroke (it is difficult/impossible to know if the injury has been caused by a cerebral and/or spinal lesion)

- Cranial nerve lesions often affecting the facial, trigeminal, and oculomotor nerves

- Visual field defects

- Auscultation of the neck may reveal a cervical bruit

Treatment

Treatment should follow airway injury in the ABC concept.

Airways:
- Stabilize the neck and spine due to the high risk of spinal cord injury

- Beware—semirigid/rigid neck collars may compress the injured artery, so manual support may be necessary.

- Tongue depressor

- Maximum oxygen supply

- Ventilation, if necessary

- Intubation if necessary (may be extremely difficult and dangerous due to pharyngolaryngeal injury)

- Cardiac resuscitation if necessary

- IV line—attempt to keep the blood pressure within the normal range

- Rapid transfer to a hospital

For less dramatic cases, always refer if in doubt.

40.4 LACERATIONS OF THE THROAT

During an NHL ice hockey game in February 2008 between the Florida Panthers and the Buffalo Sabres, Richard Zednik's carotid artery was cut by an opponent's skate (http://www.youtube.com/watch?v=vjoByuFt1_8). Even worse was the injury to the Buffalo goalie Clint Malarchuck who miraculously survived a dramatic common jugular vein laceration (http://www.youtube.com/watch?v=nWatxWBnKVw).

Whilst all lacerations to the throat are potentially fatal, different structures may be injured, depending on the localization of the laceration. Similarly, penetrating injuries to the throat may damage some of the same structures as well as the spinal cord.

In the NATO handbook, neck injuries are classified based on two criteria: (a) localization and (b) the presence or absence of major bleeding (hemodynamically stable or hemodynamically unstable)—this is a very important concept. Localization of neck lacerations:

- Zone 1—between the clavicle and cricoid cartilage
- Zone 2—between the cricoid cartilage and the mandibular angle
- Zone 3—between the mandibular angle and the base of the skull (Fig. 40.1)

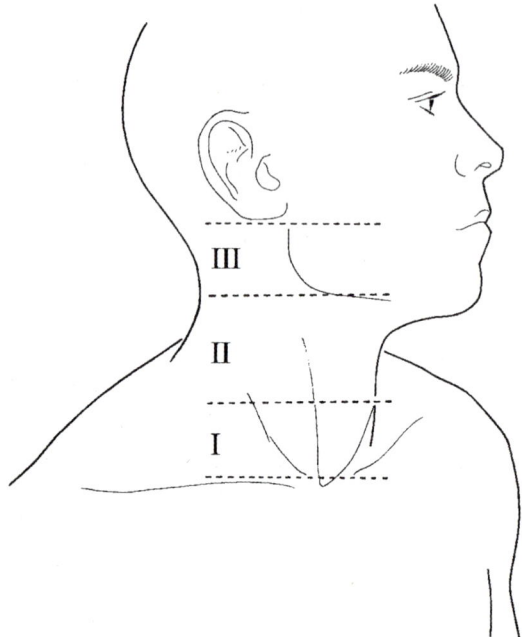

FIGURE 40.1. Throat laceration zones.

Zones 1 and 2—potential for

- Hemopneumothorax (see Chapter 43)
- Vessel injury, mediastinal injury
- Esophageal injuries
- Tracheal injuries
- Beware—these structures may be damaged even if they appear normal on first inspection
- Never, ever explore the wound

Zone 3—potential for

- Carotid artery injuries
- Other injuries

As these injuries are often fatal, patients are classified as either being hemodynamically unstable or hemodynamically stable. Any patient with a penetrating neck wound and significant hemorrhage needs emergency surgical intervention. Bleeding may be arterial or venous and one must be alert for the possibility of an air embolism. This is not usually available, so the event physician has to do the best he or she can before the urgent transfer of the patient to a hospital. This includes attempts to compress the bleeding site, using direct or indirect digital compression—not easy as blood spurts out of the wound. There should be no attempt at exploration or blind clamping. With arterial laceration at other sites, digital compression is usually followed by indirect mechanical compression, for example, a cravat with a knot placed over the course of the artery; however, this is not recommended in the neck for obvious reasons, as it will cause choking and may compress the healthy contralateral carotid artery. If it is impossible to compress the bleeding artery, then attempt to place a bandage over the wound, clear the airways (whilst protecting the cervical spine), ensure maximal oxygenation and ventilation, intubate (may be difficult or impossible due to laryngeal injury), perform cricothyroidotomy, establish an IV line, and initiate fluid replacement (see Chapter 25), all the time endeavoring to protect the spine.

40.5 PENETRATING THROAT INJURIES

Due to the seriousness and potentially fatal nature of these injuries, injuries can be initially classified as

- Hemodynamically unstable—often with massive bleeding, an expanding hematoma, hemomediastinum, hemothorax, and hypovolemic shock

■ Hemodynamically stable—regrettably, a hemodynamically stable patient may be only temporarily so and there is always a danger of dramatic deterioration. These patients must be stabilized as best as you can (ABCDE) *and transferred to a hospital as soon as possible.* In such cases, a helicopter should be called for, preferably with trained anesthetic staff onboard.

40.6 FOREIGN BODY IN THE THROAT

An athlete may present with a foreign body in the throat. This may occur at any time before, during, or after a sporting event, with a wide variety of objects such as mouth guards, *teeth,* prosthetic dental plates, chewing gum, or food that can become lodged in the throat or even the trachea or a bronchus. The presence of a pharyngeal foreign body is a potentially life-threatening situation as it may lead to partial or complete airway obstruction.

The patient may present with an array of symptoms and signs including cyanosis, unconsciousness, choking, stridor, unusual breathing sounds, inability to speak or cry out, desperately holding his or her throat, "choke sign," dysphagia, or a combination of these findings, all depending on the anatomical site of obstruction and the extent of lumen blockage. Physicians should have a high degree of suspicion in patients with a foreign body history or acute debut of unexplained coughing and upper respiratory symptoms.

Treatment

Foreign body removal attempts can be extremely difficult in the prehospital environment due to lack of proper medical equipment, gravitational forces, the gag reflex, and the distinct danger of pushing the foreign body even further into the hypopharynx, esophagus, or trachea.

If conscious, try to get the patient to cough out the foreign body. If this does not help, a hard slap on the back may assist the patient. Using your finger, it may be possible to "sweep" the oral cavity for foreign bodies, but beware the digital induction of vomiting as this may just make things worse. Heimlich maneuver is still used and can be effective. Instrumentation of the throat may lead to tissue damage, hemorrhage, laryngeal edema, vomiting, even, and pushing the foreign body into the subglottic space, esophagus, or trachea. Many patients require sedation and endoscopic removal.

Do not rely exclusively on x-ray diagnostics as many foreign bodies will be missed on radiology due to their radiolucency. Indirect laryngoscopy and fiberoptic bronchoscopy are far more reliable, so refer the patient to an ENT department/specialist if the foreign body is not visible or readily accessible for removal or if in doubt.

Recommended Reading

Bowen TE. *Emergency war surgery: second United States revision of the emergency war surgery NATO handbook.* Washington, DC: US Government Printing Office, 1988.

Karlsson T. Homicidal and suicidal sharp force fatalities in Stockholm, Sweden. Orientation of entrance wounds in stabs gives information in the classification. *Forensic Sci Int.* 1998;93(1):21–32.

Cervical Spine Injuries

Contributed by David McDonagh, Chair, FIBT Medical Committee

Reviewer: Tomm Müller, Neurosurgeon, St.Olavs Hospital, NTNU, Trondheim, Norway

Sports injuries after motor vehicle accidents are the commonest cause of SCI. In the United States, there is approximately 1 spinal cord injury per 45,000 head of population, and 1 per 90,000 head of population in the United Kingdom where 11% of spinal injuries are sports associated (9% in the United States). Serious spinal cord injuries are rare but more common in high-energy sports. Acute traumatic cervical disc herniation may also occur.

Spinal column trauma may result in spinal cord injury with a varying degree of neurologic injury.

It is essential that the EP knows when to suspect a traumatic, unstable spinal column condition and how to diagnose a spinal cord injury in an emergency situation. This may be especially difficult in an athlete with an altered state of consciousness due to concomitant head injury.

41.1 EXAMINATION OF A PATIENT WITH A POTENTIAL CERVICAL SPINAL INJURY

When arriving at the scene, always initiate your examination by evaluating

- Respiration
- Perfusion
- Mental status

If the patient is unconscious, assume that there is both a head injury and a spinal injury. Carefully expose the chest and abdomen, and perform an initial inspection: Are there any deformities of the neck or other body parts? Is the patient breathing normally and is there normal chest movement? Is there abdominal muscle movement during respiration?

Ensure a patent airway, give oxygen, apply a cervical collar, give oxygen, assist ventilation if necessary, ensure adequate circulation, immobilize the whole spine using a backboard, and transfer the patient to an ambulance or helicopter.

If the patient is conscious, evaluate the patient to see if he or she follows simple commands. If the patient does not, this may be due to a cerebral or spinal lesion. Make a simple neurologic evaluation: Superficially palpate the extremities for gross deformities/fractures/dislocations whilst simultaneously asking the patient about sensation and testing motor function. Ask the patient to move the various joints in each extremity. Get the patient to squeeze your fingers and to extend and flex the elbow with and without resistance. Get the patient to lift his or her leg, then arms, hold them elevated, and then apply resistance. Grade each extremity by using a motor scale. The American Spinal Injury Association recommends the following motor strength scale for evaluation of SCI:

- 0: No contraction or movement
- 1: Minimal movement
- 2: Active movement, but not against gravity
- 3: Active movement against gravity
- 4: Active movement against resistance
- 5: Active movement against full resistance

Assessment of sensory function helps to identify the different pathways for light touch, proprioception, vibration, and pain. The use of a pinprick to evaluate pain sensation is considered a useful tool; however, this may be time-consuming and may not be appropriate in such an emergency setting. Differentiating between a nerve root injury and an SCI

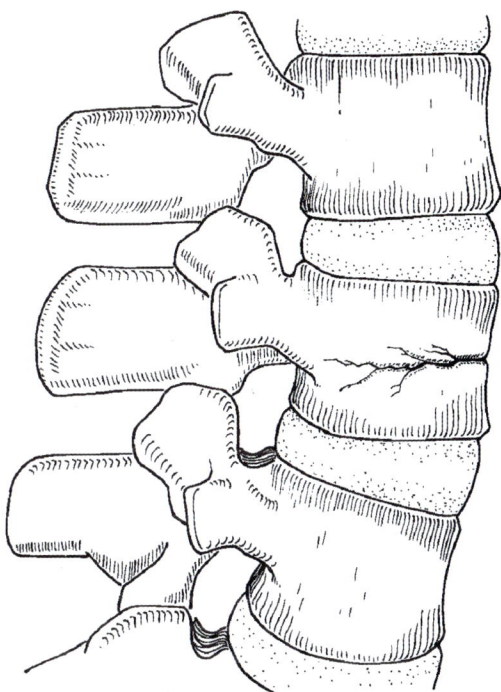

FIGURE 41.1. Vertebral fracture without dislocation.

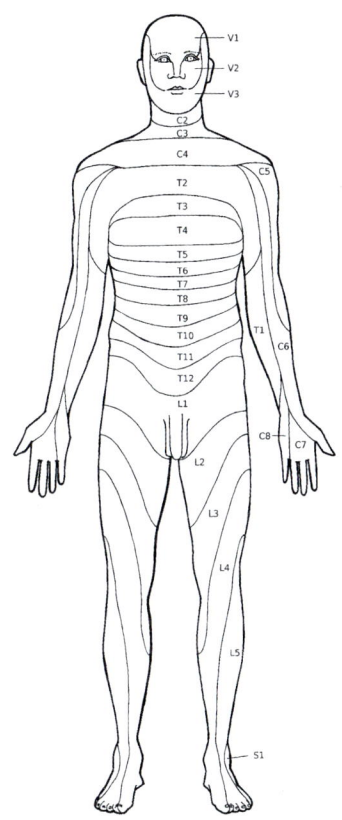

FIGURE 41.3. Dermatomes front.

is difficult. The presence of multilevel neurologic deficits may indicate an SCI rather than a nerve root injury. In the absence of spinal shock, motor weakness with intact reflexes may indicate an SCI,

while motor weakness with absent reflexes may indicate a nerve root lesion (Figs. 41.3 and 41.4).

If, at any stage, you find a neurologic deficit, then immobilize, stabilize, and transfer the patient urgently to a neurosurgical unit.

If you suspect a cervical injury, always assume that there is a concomitant head injury. Remember the unholy triad of high-velocity injuries—head, chest, and pelvic injury (adults); head, chest, and femur (children)—and always initiate your inspection with airway, breathing, and circulation investigation. Once other life-threatening conditions have been excluded, or treated, evaluate the neck for spinal cord injury and fracture.

In the absence of positive findings after a rudimentary motor and sensory examination, carefully palpate the back of the neck for midline tenderness, if present, immobilize the neck and spine, stabilize, and transfer. If there is no pain on palpation, ask the patient to gently flex, extend, and laterally flex the neck. If, at any stage, the patient experiences pain or difficulty, then the patient needs to be immobilized, stabilized, and transferred to a hospital, preferably to a neurosurgical unit.

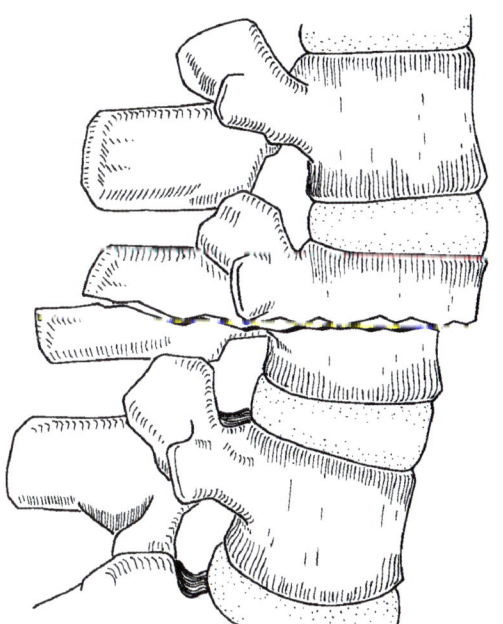

FIGURE 41.2. Vertebral fracture with dislocation.

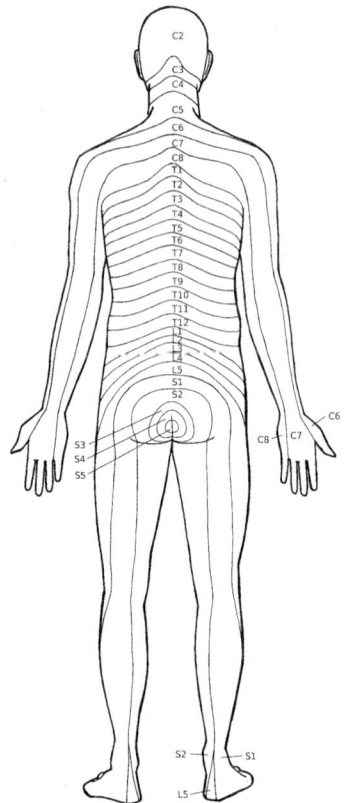

FIGURE 41.4. Dermatomes back.

If the patient is conscious and has no pain, no midline tenderness, normal neurology and pain-free, normal neck movements, then the likelihood of a cervical fracture or dislocation (Figs. 41.1 and 41.2) being present is minimal (see Canadian C-Spine Rule). However, clinical evaluation of the cervical spine in a prehospital environment is notoriously difficult, and if one suspects a spinal column or cord injury, then the patient must be immobilized, stabilized, and transferred to a hospital for further investigation.

41.2 TRAUMATIC SPINAL CORD INJURY

Trauma to the spinal column may cause structural damage, resulting in an unstable spine. This may be due to fractures and/or dislocations, traumatic disc herniation, or other types of soft-tissue injury. There are several classification systems for spinal fractures/dislocations, but these are of minimal relevance in an emergency situation. Sometimes, SCI may be seen without apparent traumatic structural changes, but then, often a degenerative or congenital spinal stenosis may be found.

Spinal cord injury may be complete or incomplete and occur at different levels. A complete cord lesion is characterized by a complete loss of motor and sensory function below the level of disrupted cord. Incomplete lesions may present with a variety of "syndromes" such as

- Central cord syndrome: Injury of the cervical medulla with greater loss of function in upper than in lower limbs, with varying degrees of sensory loss, typically after a hyperextension. This syndrome may occur in the absence of a spinal fracture/dislocation, but then a spinal stenosis or traumatic cervical disc herniation is usually present.

- Brown-Séquard syndrome: Ipsilateral (to the injury) weakness and proprioceptive loss with contralateral loss of pain and thermal sensation—more often seen with penetrating injuries of the cord.

- Anterior spinal syndrome: Damage to the anterior part of the spinal cord, resulting in weakness, loss of pain, and thermal sensations below the injury site but intact proprioception (due to intact posterior spinal cord).

- Cauda equina syndrome: Often caused by an acute lumbar disc herniation and often presents with loss of bladder or bowel control. There may be partial loss of motor and sensory function in the lower limbs.

41.3 SYSTEMIC COMPLICATIONS OF SPINAL CORD INJURY AND TREATMENT

Patients risk developing spinal shock (up to 50%) and/or neurogenic shock.

Spinal shock may occur immediately after a spinal injury and may last for months.

Findings with spinal shock are

- Flaccid paralysis, with an absence of neurologic function (motor, sensory, autonomic, reflexes) below the lesion

- Limbs may be atonic

- Loss of anal sphincter tone and incontinence

- Priapism

- Even spinal cord reflex arcs immediately above the level of injury may also be severely depressed

Neurogenic shock may also occur due to the loss of sympathetic stimulation of smooth muscle in vessel walls and, thus, lead to vasodilation and hypotension with paradoxical bradycardia. The skin may become flushed, dry, and warm.

It is not always easy to differentiate between hemorrhagic shock and neurogenic shock.

Prof. Donald Schreiber of Stanford University offers some hints that may be useful:

a) Neurogenic shock occurs only in the presence of acute SCI above T6. Hypotension and/or shock with acute SCI at or below T6 is caused by hemorrhage

b) Hypotension with a spinal fracture alone, without any neurologic deficit or apparent SCI, is invariably due to hemorrhage.

c) Patients with an SCI above T6 may not have the classic physical findings associated with hemorrhage (e.g., tachycardia, peripheral vasoconstriction). This vital sign confusion is attributed to autonomic dysfunction and is common in SCI, but the high incidence of associated injuries requires a diligent search for occult sources of hemorrhage.

So look for the following problems:

- Respiratory dysfunction can occur depending on the level of spinal lesion. If the lesion affects the diaphragm, intercostal muscles, or abdominal muscles, then respiration will be compromised. Patients with suspected SCI need 100% oxygen and may need assisted ventilation.

- Cardiovascular problems:
  - Tachycardia and hypotension—suspect hypovolemia/hemorrhage; treat with IV fluids
  - Bradycardia and hypotension (decreased cardiac output, peripheral dilatation)—suspect neurogenic shock (the patient needs IV fluids but must not be overloaded)

- Urologic: Bladder distension—also increases pressure on veins from the legs and may reduce venous flow; urine retention—patients should be catheterized.

- GI tract: Similarly, autonomic dysfunction may lead to gastric and bowel relaxation, ileus, and the reversing of normal movement of fluids in the tract, allowing fluid to be aspirated into the oropharynx and lungs. Rectal tone should be examined for. A rigid abdomen may indicate intraperitoneal bleeding. A nasogastric tube should be inserted.

- Skin care: Remove keys or metal from pockets; this may help prevent decubitus sores in the spinally injured patient.

- Temperature changes with loss of normal temperature control.

Note: Follow local guidelines regarding methylprednisolone bolus and acute spinal cord injury. Many centers no longer recommend the administration of corticosteroids in the acute posttraumatic phase.

41.4 CORRECT IMMOBILIZATION OF THE NECK

The goal of immobilization is to achieve neutral anatomical position, as this position gives the spinal cord optimal space within the spinal canal. A rigid cervical collar should then be applied to hold the neck in this neutral position. Once the collar has been fitted, the rest of the spine must be immobilized.

However, what do you do with a fixed deformity—a fixed fracture-dislocation deformity?

This is an extremely difficult situation. If the neck is rigid and fixed in one position and cannot be returned to the neutral anatomical position, this implies that there is a fracture dislocation that prevents neck movement. If one attempts to move the neck in this situation, one may further compromise spinal cord integrity with catastrophic result. The neck must be supported in that fixed position, and you cannot release that hold until you get the athlete to a hospital or have another assistant to carefully take over this supporting role. The consequence of this is that you cannot use a rigid cervical collar, as this will merely force the neck into the neutral anatomical position. You have to use some sort of support that can be molded into position to support the neck in this pathologically fixed position. I use a vacuum splint—usually a leg splint as this allows you to mold the splint around the head, neck, shoulders, and upper back.

The splint must not interfere with respiration.

41.5 CANADIAN C-SPINE RULE FOR RADIOGRAPHY IN ALERT AND STABLE TRAUMA PATIENTS

Ian G. Stiell et al. have produced many important articles on the need for x-ray in the emergency room. The Canadian C-Spine Rule was based on research carried out on 8,924 adults (mean age,

37 years) who presented to the emergency department with blunt trauma to the head/neck, stable vital signs, with a Glasgow Coma Scale score of 15. They concluded that the Canadian C-Spine Rule is a highly sensitive (approaching 100%) decision rule for use of C-spine radiography in alert and stable trauma patients.

The Canadian C-Spine Rule comprises three main questions:

- Is there any high-risk factor present that mandates radiography (i.e., age ≥ 65 years, dangerous mechanism, or paresthesias in extremities)?

- Is there any low-risk factor present that allows safe assessment of range of motion (i.e., simple rear-end motor vehicle collision, sitting position in ED, ambulatory at any time since injury, delayed onset of neck pain, or absence of midline C-spine tenderness)?

- Is the patient able to actively rotate neck 45 degrees to the left and right?

By cross validation, Stiell claims that this rule had 100% specificity. Though this study was carried out in a hospital, it can also be a useful tool for the event physician in the prehospital environment.

Children—to x-Ray or Not?

Recent reviews of published papers show that cervical spine radiography is not necessary in pediatric blunt trauma victims over the age of nine if they

- Are fully alert
- Are conversant
- Show no signs of intoxication
- Have no neurologic deficit
- Have no midline cervical tenderness
- Have no painful distracting injury

41.6 SPINAL NERVE INJURY—STINGERS AND BURNERS

A "stinger" (or "burner") occurs when there is trauma to the upper trunk of the brachial plexus and/or fifth or sixth cervical nerve roots (traumatic radiculopathy or radiculitis), resulting in burning pain radiating down the arm and may be accompanied by numbness, paresthesia, or weakness.

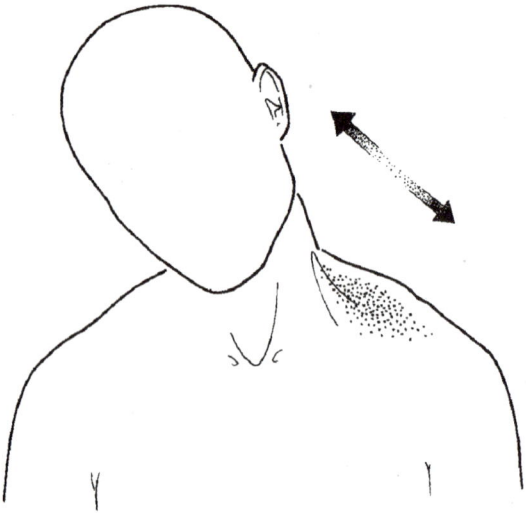

FIGURE 41.5. Stinger injury site.

This usually occurs when an athlete is struck over the midsupraclavicular region (Erb's point), particularly if the neck is laterally flexed away from the injury. Stingers may also occur due to nerve stretching with forced contralateral hyperflexion and hyperextension of the neck or nerve compression with ipsilateral hyperflexion and hyperextension of the neck (Fig. 41.5). The symptoms are usually transient but weakness may persist for several weeks. Some athletes have a tendency to repeat injuries and symptoms can become chronic. Stingers are most often seen in American football, rugby, wrestling, gymnastics, and ice hockey players. Stingers are unilateral. Bilateral symptoms are something completely different and one must suspect spinal cord damage.

Important

Symptoms and signs are not unlike those seen with a cervical fracture/dislocation or spinal cord contusion/lesion. Until these conditions have been excluded, an EP should advise against further participation until spinal cord injury or a traumatic disc herniation has been excluded. The athlete should be immobilized and transferred to a hospital if symptoms persist. If symptoms disappear during examination, the athlete will often want to resume play. Field side examination will not exclude a fracture or spinal lesion. There is also the possibility of carotid artery dissection (see Chapter 40). This is a difficult decision with possible medicolegal consequences (see Chapter 12).

Brachial Plexus Innervation

Innervation of the brachial plexus includes the upper trunk (C5 and C6), middle trunk (C7), lower trunk (C8 and T1).

Clinical Findings

History: The usual cause is injury in a tackle in American football or rugby. Immediately after contact, the injured player classically feels a burning pain in the supraclavicular area, which radiates down the arm, usually in a circumferential pattern. It is a unilateral phenomenon. The player might also note numbness, paresthesia, or weakness in the extremity. Frequently, the discomfort resolves spontaneously in 1 to 2 minutes. Information on previous burners and their treatment is also useful.

Inspection: On the field, the athlete may shake the arm or hold it against the body to relieve pain and discomfort. Signs of chronic injury should be looked for, such as shoulder depression and atrophy of the deltoid and supraspinatus muscles.

Palpation: Usually reveals local tenderness in the supraclavicular area with swelling if there is a contusion.

Motility: Do not test the neck if the patient complains of pain or limited motion in the neck. The presence of stinger symptoms may indicate a cervical fracture, and the athlete should thus be treated with cervical immobilization, a patent airway, oxygen, etc. If the injury has been caused by a direct blow to the supraclavicular area (e.g., a hockey stick), then one can be more liberal with motility testing; if the injury was caused by a knee blow or shoulder tackle, then cervical injury is not unlikely. Once assured of the absence of a cervical fracture (!), range of motion in the neck and the shoulder should be evaluated.

Sensory and Motor Tests: First, test for intact sensation (dermatomes), then motor function (see above), then Spurling's test and even Tinel's sign. As stingers usually affect the fifth and sixth cervical nerves, there may be a weakness in the ipsilateral biceps and deltoid muscles, and there may be reduced shoulder abduction strength, reduced elbow flexion, and reduced wrist extension strength. The onset of weakness is usually immediate; however, weakness can also develop hours or days later. Immediate onset weakness usually disappears within a few minutes of the injury but may on some occasions last for days, weeks, and even months. Frequent reexamination of patients is recommended initially.

Treatment: As for cervical fracture above, refer to a hospital for further investigation. If cervical fracture, spinal cord injury and disc herniation have been excluded, the athlete can resume training but should avoid contact sports and weightlifting until symptoms disappear and normal function is restored.

A return-to-play decision must never be taken before cervical fracture and spinal cord injury have been excluded. The athlete must be pain-free and have pain-free and normal motion and strength. The athlete should consider using protective shoulder pads as recurrence is common.

41.7 REMOVING AMERICAN FOOTBALL HELMETS

There is still a lack of agreement on this issue, particularly in emergency sports scenarios. In US textbooks, is a tendency to recommend leaving the football helmet on, and studies seem to show no significant difference between removing or retaining the helmet in the prehospital environment. In most other emergency scenarios helmets are removed. Everyone (!) agrees that the face mask should be removed carefully. The question is not if the helmet and shoulder pads should be removed (they will be sooner or later) but *when* they should be removed and by *whom*. If helmet removal will benefit the athlete, then the helmet should be removed. If not, the helmet should stay on. If the athlete is conscious and breathing normally, then there are good arguments for not removing the helmet and pads. The removal of the helmet and pads will inevitably cause movement of the cervical spine and the cervical collars, which will undoubtedly be used after a helmet removal, and may not give optimal immobilization. If the athlete who is breathing normally can be adequately stabilized using lateral supports on a backboard, then the helmet and pads do not need to be removed until the athlete has been x-rayed in a hospital. If the athlete is not breathing normally and there is a need for a jaw thrust, airway management, or intubation, then the helmet should be removed in a careful and safe manner.

41.8 MOTOR SPORTS AND BOBSLEIGH HELMETS

In high-velocity sports, motor bike races, car races, or bobsleigh, athletes use a full-face impact helmet with a chin bar. There are several systems available for judging the helmet impact-resistance such as DOT, Snell, or BSI. These helmets, while giving good head protection, may prevent visualization of serious wounds and may interfere with optimal oxygenation and respiration—hence the tendency to remove these helmets at the injury location. After bobsleigh accidents, we recommend helmet removal before transfer to a hospital.

Recommended Reading

Anderson RC, Scaife ER, Fenton SJ, et al. Cervical spine clearance after trauma in children. *J Neurosurg.* 2006; 105(5 Suppl):361–364.

Bell RM, Krantz BE, Weigelt JA. ATLS: a foundation for trauma training. *Ann Emerg Med.* 1999;34(2):233–237.

Domeier RM, Swor RA, Evans RW, et al. Multicenter prospective validation of prehospital clinical spinal clearance criteria. *J Trauma.* 2002;53(4):744–750.

Stiell IG, Wells GA, Vandemheen KL, et al. The Canadian C-spine rule for radiography in alert and stable trauma patients. *JAMA.* 2001;286(15):1841–1848.

Ummenhofer W, Scheidegger D. Role of the physician in prehospital management of trauma: European perspective. *Curr Opin Crit Care.* 2002;8(6):559–565.

42 Low Back Pain

Contributed by Scott Kincade, Professor, University of Texas Southwestern, Dallas, Texas

Reviewer: Richard Budgett, IOC Medical Committee, Chief Medical Officer, London 2012 Olympic Summer Games

You are seeing a 32-year-old soccer player for back pain. He is otherwise healthy. During practice yesterday, he experienced intense lower back pain that prevented him from playing any longer. He used some ibuprofen for pain relief and spent the remainder of the day resting. The next morning, he had increased muscle stiffness and was not feeling any better so he came to see you. He describes the pain as dull and burning. There is some radiation into the left buttock. He does not have any fever, chills, dysuria, abdominal pain, bowel, or bladder problems. The pain is aggravated by prolonged sitting and moderate activity. He can get relief when he lies down. He denies any trauma and has never had back pain like this before. On your focused exam, the abdomen is benign. There is limited forward flexion of the back due to pain and tender muscles in the lumbar area. There is no spine or sacroiliac joint pain. The neurologic exam and straight leg raising test are normal.

Low back pain is a common complaint in athletes. The incidence of back pain in athletes is similar, if not higher, than the general population. Some sports with an increased incidence of back pain include golf, gymnastics, swimming, tennis, American football, wrestling, and throwing.

Because it can be difficult to determine a precise etiology in the majority of back pain cases, the goal of the clinical examination is to identify patients who require immediate surgical evaluation and those whose symptoms suggest a more serious underlying condition such as malignancy, infection, or fracture (Table 42.1). After screening to rule out serious etiologies, we then decide whether the athlete's activity should be restricted and what treatments and recommendations can return him or her to play in the shortest amount of time. A conservative approach to back pain is warranted as most cases are self-limited.

42.1 DIFFERENTIAL DIAGNOSIS

The key components of the spine are the vertebral bodies that articulate via posterior facet joints and the intervertebral disc, the spinal cord and nerves that exit via the neural foramina, and ligaments that stabilize the vertebral bodies. In the athlete, almost all causes of back pain have a mechanical etiology such as

- Lumbar strain or sprain/idiopathic low back pain
- Degenerative disc/facet process
- Herniated disc
- Degenerative disease of the spine
- Spondylolysis and spondylolisthesis
- Fracture or stress fracture

Nonmechanical spinal conditions (infection, tumor, inflammatory arthritis) and nonspinal visceral disease (pancreatitis, aneurysms, etc.) are the cause in athletes in less than 1 to 2% of cases. Mechanical back pain is made worse by activity and relieved by rest. Nonmechanical back pain is constant, often worse in the morning and not affected much by activity.

TABLE 42.1	Red-Flag Findings Concerning for More Severe Conditions			
Red-Flag Finding	**Cauda Equina**	**Fracture**	**Cancer**	**Infection**
Age > 50		X	X	
Significant trauma		X		
History of cancer or strong suspicion for current cancer			X	
Unexplained weight loss			X	
Failure to improve after 6 wk of conservative therapy			X	X
Unrelenting night pain or pain at rest			X	X
Progressive motor or sensory deficit	X			
Saddle anesthesia, difficulty urinating, fecal incontinence	X			
IV drug use				X
Fevers, chills, recent urinary tract or skin infection, penetrating wound near spine				X
Immunosuppression				X
History of osteoporosis		X		
Chronic oral steroid use		X		X
Substance abuse		X		X

The incidence of spondylolysis is increased in athletes. There also seems to be an increased incidence of lumbar disc degeneration as well. Other degenerative conditions are less likely due to athletes typically being younger than the general population.

Lumbar strain or sprain is the most common cause of back pain and presents with pain in the lower back that can radiate into the buttocks or proximal lower extremities. There may be a history of overuse, but usually there is no obvious mechanism of injury. The neurologic exam should be normal. There may be decreased range of motion in the back and tenderness in the soft tissues of the lower back. The pain is worse with activity and better with rest. Degenerative disc disease presents and is managed similarly to lumbar strain. The pain from degenerative disc disease is localized pain without radiculopathy and may be worse with increases in intradiscal pressure (Fig. 42.1).

Herniated disc or herniated nucleus pulposus (HNP) that causes pain radiating in a dermatomal pattern down the leg and below the knee is also known as sciatica. The distinction of whether symptoms radiate past the knee is a key distinguishing feature of sciatica. Pain is usually worse with maneuvers that increase the intradiscal pressure (leaning forward and Valsalva maneuvers). Often, the leg pain is more bothersome to the patient than the back pain. There may be associated muscle

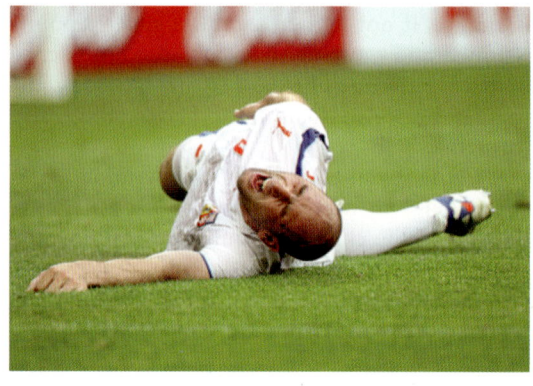

FIGURE 42.1. Jan Koller, Czech Republic. (Photo courtesy of FIFA.)

weakness, sensory loss, or diminished reflexes. The L4–L5 disc and L5–S1 disc account for 95% of herniations, and the L3–L4 disc accounts for about 5%. Herniation is very rare in discs above L3.

Cauda equina syndrome is a surgical emergency that requires urgent diagnosis and referral. Patients present with an acute radiculopathy that features bladder dysfunction (typically urinary retention with overflow incontinence), possible bowel incontinence with decreased rectal tone, saddle anesthesia, and bilateral neurologic deficits or pain. The most common causes are large paracentral disc herniations and tumors. Even with prompt decompression, some patients do not recover completely.

Vertebral compression fractures are typically related to osteoporosis. Amenorrheic female athletes or those who have a history of prolonged corticosteroid use are at increased risk. Anterior vertebral wedge compression fractures can be seen with trauma or activities that cause significant axial loading or flexion of the spine. Pain is typically worse with direct palpation of the spine, flexion, and activity. There may be nerve root involvement and associated findings. Plain radiographs identify most of these fractures.

Stress fractures occurring in the spine are usually due to spondylolysis (stress fracture of the pars interarticularis along the posterior vertebrae). Spondylolysis is more common in younger athletes. The prevalence varies according to the sport but can be the cause of low back pain in up to 30% to 40% of the cases in sports such as gymnastics, weightlifting, and wrestling. Spondylolysis can be unilateral or bilateral. Spondylolisthesis refers to subluxation of an affected vertebral body posteriorly, which can occur in bilateral spondylolysis. About half of symptomatic athletes with spondylolysis also have spondylolisthesis. On exam, the pain from spondylolysis may be localized to the spine and may be worse when the patient is standing on one foot with the spine hyperextended. There may be a palpable step-off along the vertebrae in the case of spondylolisthesis. Both of these entities can typically be diagnosed with x-ray of the lumbar spine (including oblique views).

Less common causes of back pain include stress fractures of the sacrum or pelvis, fractures of the transverse processes or spinous processes, neoplasms, infections, inflammatory conditions such as Reiter's syndrome or ankylosing spondylitis, and referred pain.

42.2 PHYSICAL EXAM

One can start with a quick assessment for fever, abdominal pain or masses, and other nonspinal conditions. Inspect the back for obvious deformity and assess the range of motion. Palpate along the spine for bony tenderness or a step-off that could indicate spondylolisthesis. Also, palpate the paraspinal muscles and the sacroiliac joints. The straight leg raising test should be performed with the patient supine to see if radicular pain occurs when the affected or contralateral leg is elevated between 30 and 60 degrees. Pain with flexion of the spine can be seen with lumbar disc disorders and anterior vertebral compression fractures. Pain with extension, particularly standing on one leg in a hyperlordotic position can aggravate structures in the posterior spine, such as a spondylolysis. The neurologic exam should assess sensation, strength, and deep tendon reflexes (Table 42.2).

TABLE 42.2 Neurologic Exam Findings

Level of Disc Herniation	Nerve Root Affected	Sensory Loss	Motor Weakness	Screening Exam	Reflex
L3–L4	L4	Medial foot	Knee extension	Squat and rise	Patellar
L4–L5	L5	Dorsal foot	Dorsiflexion ankle/great toe	Heel walking	None
L5–S1	S1	Lateral foot	Plantarflexion ankle/toes	Walking on toes	Achilles

42.3 DIAGNOSTIC TESTING

Since the vast majority of low back pain is not due to a serious underlying condition and since most cases are self-limited, diagnostic testing can be used sparingly. Diagnostic imaging options in back pain include plain radiographs, CT, MRI, and radionuclide bone scans. Plain radiographs are not highly sensitive or specific. They are reasonably useful to identify compression fractures, spondylolysis and spondylolisthesis, and degenerative changes of the spine. CT scanning is relatively good for revealing most bony spinal pathology. MRI, because it provides the most detailed images of the soft tissues of the disc and nerve roots, is the most commonly used advanced imaging modality. MRI and CT scanning, because they provide such good detail, also show many abnormalities that are not causing clinical symptoms, a factor that diminishes their specificity. In the case of MRI, studies in asymptomatic adults show herniated discs in about 30% to 40% of patients, bulging discs in about 50% of patients, and degenerative changes in up to 90% of patients. Radionuclide bone scanning is helpful in detecting osteomyelitis, bony metastases, and occult fractures. Single photon emission computed tomography (SPECT) is the most accurate test for identifying acute fractures of the pars in spondylolysis.

If the patient has significant trauma or any red-flag symptoms or risk factors, a plain radiograph with or without a complete blood count and erythrocyte sedimentation rate (ESR) is an appropriate first step. If there is strong suspicion for serious underlying pathology and initial imaging is non-diagnostic, consider obtaining advanced imaging with MRI, CT, SPECT, or radionuclide bone scan. Patients who have abnormalities on imaging or complications of a herniated disc (cauda equina syndrome, intractable pain, progressive neurologic deficits) should be referred to a spine specialist. Assuming the patient does not have any red flags, conservative management for several weeks is appropriate.

42.4 MANAGEMENT

Acute lumbar strain, which accounts for most cases of acute back pain, has a good prognosis and can be treated conservatively. The goal of treatment is to provide pain relief and, thus, improve function. Acetaminophen, (NSAIDs, mild opioids, and skeletal muscle relaxants are all effective for acute low back pain. The most common side effect of NSAIDs is gastrointestinal toxicity. If this becomes a problem, a COX-2 specific NSAID or acetaminophen can be used. Muscle relaxants are effective in the short-term treatment of acute LBP. If drowsiness is a problem with muscle relaxants, patients can take a lower dose, use them only at bedtime, or try metaxalone, which is less sedating. Ice applied to the area does not seem to be as effective as heat therapy. Severe low back pain may require 1 or 2 days of rest, but generally, patients should be advised to stay active. There is strong evidence that bed rest for more than 2 or 3 days does not decrease pain intensity or improve function. Back braces, steroids, anticonvulsants, or tricyclic antidepressants are not recommended.

Sciatica due to a herniated disc is treated similarly to acute lumbar strain, with analgesics, NSAIDs, and/or muscle relaxants, and a recommendation for physical activity as tolerated. Specifically, patients with sciatica who are advised to rest in bed have no significant difference in pain or functional status compared with patients advised to stay active. Most patients will improve over 4 to 6 weeks. Patients with severe or intractable pain or progressive neurologic deficits should be reevaluated earlier and may need referral to a spine specialist.

More significant injuries including compression fractures and spondylolysis will need to be removed from activity and evaluated by a spine specialist. Return to activity for any spinal condition depends on the underlying etiology and the sport. For most sprains, strains, and overuse injuries, the athlete can return when he or she has regained his or her normal functional range of motion and the pain is improving. For fractures, including spondylolysis, definitive evidence of healing is required prior to return to participation.

42.5 DISCUSSION OF THE INTRODUCTORY CASE

1. What is the most likely etiology of his back pain?

   The patient has acute low back pain likely from an acute lumbar strain. He does not have any red-flag conditions that would warrant a search for serious underlying pathology. Since he only reports pain into the buttock and not true sciatica (pain radiating below the knee) he most likely does not have a herniated disc.

2. What diagnostic testing is indicated at this point?

Because there is almost no concern for a serious underlying condition (red-flag condition) and because he has no abnormal neurologic findings, his can initially be managed conservatively. If his condition worsens or he continues to have moderate to severe pain, reevaluate him with consideration of appropriate imaging. Assuming he does not develop any neurologic abnormalities and does not develop any new symptoms that might suggest a serious underlying disorder, plain AP and lateral x-rays would be appropriate.

3. What are the best recommendations for his treatment?

Tell the patient his diagnosis and that his prognosis is very good. It is common for patients to be confused about the cause of their back pain and believe that they are very likely to worsen things with normal activities. If bed rest is necessary, it should only be for a few days. Encourage him to stay active and resume normal activities as tolerated. He should avoid heavy lifting, significant flexion and twisting motions (especially while lifting), and high-impact activities while he is recovering. Pain can be alleviated with ice or heat, acetaminophen, NSAIDS, opioids, or short-term use of muscle relaxants.

Recommended Reading

American Academy of Physical Medicine and Rehabilitation Guidelines, www.aapmr.org

White book on physical and rehabilitation medicine in Europe. *Eura Medicophys*. 2006;42(4):292–332.

Contributed by David McDonagh, Emergency Department, St. Olavs University Hospital, Trondheim, Norway.

Reviewer: David Mulder, Professor, McGill University, Montreal, and Team Physician, Montreal Canadiens, Montreal, Canada

Serious thoracic injuries, though rare in sports, occur mainly in high-velocity sports (motor sports, alpine skiing, freestyle skiing, ski jumping, horse riding, hockey, ice hockey) and in sports with intrinsic penetration danger (javelin, water skiing, fencing, injuries from tree branches, etc.). Minor thoracic injuries are seen in almost every sport.

Many multitraumatized patients have serious thoracic injuries. The combination of thoracic and cerebral lesions is particularly serious.

Deceleration injuries arise from falls or violent contact with fixed obstacles such as goalposts, trees, etc. Compression in a vehicle or between a vehicle and the ground is also possible. Such injuries, though rare, are reported in bobsleigh and luge. It is still useful to think of thoracic injury as blunt or penetrating. Virtually all thoracic traumas in contact sport are blunt.

As a rule, treatment of serious thoracic injury focuses on maintaining oxygenation, ventilation, and circulation (ATLS basics), administering analgesia, and ensuring safe transportation to the nearest qualified hospital.

43.1 MUSCULAR INJURIES

Pectoralis majoris muscle injuries vary from strains to partial ruptures to complete tears. Major muscle tears are relatively rare and seem to primarily affect athletes lifting heavy weights during a bench press. Complete ruptures are usually avulsions at or near the humeral insertion but can also be due to injury at the musculotendinous junction. Tears may also occur in the muscle body. The patient may complain of hearing a snap at the time of injury and report pain, weakness, swelling, or muscular deformity. Physical examination can reveal ecchymosis, a palpable defect, asymmetric webbing of the axillary fold, and weakness on resisted shoulder adduction and internal rotation. A detailed history and physical examination can be augmented by radiologic studies, including MRI. Nonsurgical treatment is now recommended only for the older, sedentary patient or for proximal muscle belly tears. Surgery, whether early or delayed, consistently yields superior results compared with nonsurgical management. Prompt diagnosis and timely intervention likely will produce improved results (Fig. 43.1).

43.2 FEMALE BREAST INJURIES

Females may experience injuries to their breasts when involved in contact or collision sports such as contact martial arts, rugby, and football. The use of sports bras may afford some protection, but contusions of mammary tissue, including fat tissue, may lead to hematomas and fat necrosis, which need to be appropriately managed early on to minimize morbidity. Nipple trauma from friction in sports and activities that involve running can be reduced by using appropriate dressings to cover the nipples and by using sports bras.

43.3 RIB FRACTURES

Always look for a pneumothorax, hemothorax, and tension pneumothorax. Isolated fractures of the ribs can impair breathing—there may be indications for giving analgesics.

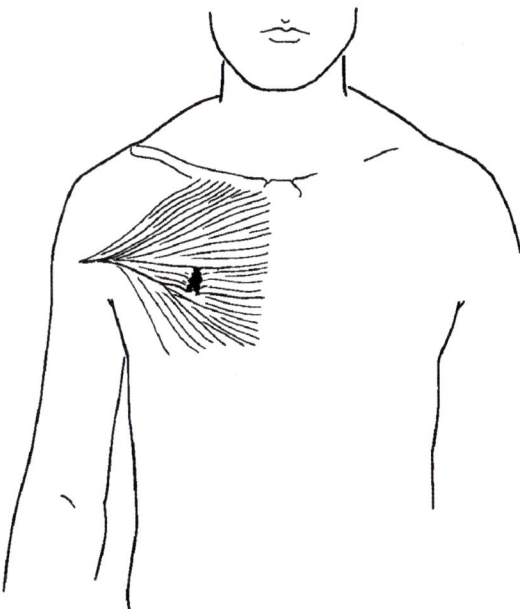

Partial tear of right pectoral muscle.

Multiple rib fractures can lead to a flail chest (causing asymmetrical respiratory movement), pneumothorax, or lung contusion (observe signs of low oxygen saturation). In children, significant intrathoracic injury may be present without rib fracture due to rib cage elasticity. Fracture of the 1st rib indicates significant force, and the underlying brachial plexus and arteries maybe damaged, causing a brachial plexus deficit, absent radial pulse, or even pulsating supraclavicular mass.

Classical symptoms of a simple rib fracture are pain on coughing, pain on deep inspiration, and pain on laughing. There is tenderness with or without crepitus with palpation of the fracture site. In exceptional circumstances, pain-relieving taping of the fractured rib with sports tape may be considered, and this may give temporary pain relief; however, taping is not generally recommended as prolonged or exaggerated taping may cause atelectasis and is not therefore generally not recommended. Many practitioners immobilize the arm on the affected side. Others use no form of bandaging or taping at all.

Stress fractures can occur in the ribs and these have been reported in golfers and rowers.

Undislocated fractures are difficult to visualize on radiographs. Sternal stress fractures can occur in weightlifters. Traumatic sternal fractures are rare in sport as these are usually associated with high-energy injuries. Some cases of sternal fractures have been reported in wrestlers. Sternal fractures are most often seen in deceleration injuries and/or direct blows to the chest, with transverse midbody fractures predominating. Manubrial fractures can also occur.

43.4 COSTOCHONDRAL INJURIES

These injuries are not uncommon in sport. Injuries around the costochondral joint may cause osseous fractures, muscle contusion or tear but also injuries to the costal cartilage. The term *costochondral separation* is also used to describe subluxations or dislocations at the costochondral junction, but separation can also occur at the chondrosternal junction. These separations have been reported in American football, *ice hockey*, rugby, wrestling, and weightlifting. It can be quite difficult to clinically differentiate between these various conditions, particularly in the prehospital environment. If the patient complains of a popping-like sensation over the costochondral or chondrosternal junction, then a separation may be suspected. There is usually local tenderness over the injured bone cartilage area. Further investigation is often required, but imaging does not always clarify the cause of the pain. X-rays are useful in the detection of osseous injury. CT, sonography, and MRI may be useful in muscle, soft-tissue, and cartilage diagnostics. Treatment is usually conservative, based on rest and avoidance of provocatory movements. Taping may help as a temporary short-term solution but should not be used over time. The displaced costal cartilage with underlying visceral injury (liver) or the chronic costochondral separation with chronic pain may require surgical treatment (Fig. 43.2).

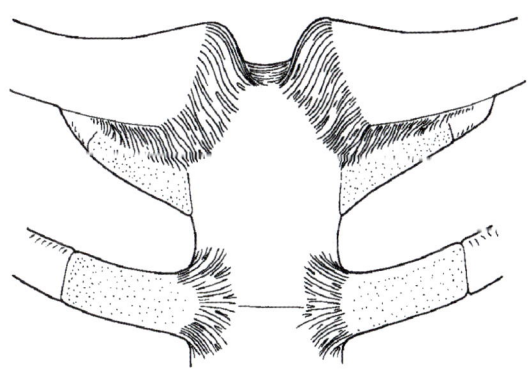

Costochondral joint.

43.5 STERNOCLAVICULAR JOINT INJURIES

The sternoclavicular (SC) joint can be contused like any other joint, either by direct force to the joint or by injuries to the shoulder. It is the least commonly injured joint of the shoulder girdle. The joint is the only direct bony attachment of the shoulder to the axial skeleton. Its stability is due to the costoclavicular ligaments, sternoclavicular ligaments/capsule, intra-articular disk, and interclavicular ligament. The medial end of the clavicle is the last epiphyseal plate to ossify. The joint is injured either by the clavicle dislocating anteriorly or posteriorly. The mechanism is usually a blow to the anterior shoulder leading to anterior instability or a blow to the posterior shoulder leading to posterior instability. The importance of this injury is in the direction of dislocation/instability. Posterior SC instability can be life threatening due to compression of mediastinal structures and lung injury. Anterior SC instability is disfiguring but of little functional significance (Figs. 43.3 and 43.4).

Clinical findings include local pain and tenderness and discomfort on movement of the shoulder joint. An athlete with a posterior SC dislocation will complain of breathing and swallowing difficulties; there may also be a palpable or visible hollow at the joint. If suspected, the athlete should be transported immediately to a hospital. A reduction should not be attempted on the field because of potential injury to the mediastinal structures and the potential need for thoracic surgical assistance.

Most injuries do not cause dislocation and are treated conservatively with ice, compression, and rest. Capsular and ligament injuries may take up to four or six weeks to heal. Anterior dislocations are rarely treated surgically. Posterior dislocations are potentially more serious and require further investigation, so a CT scan is usually advised,

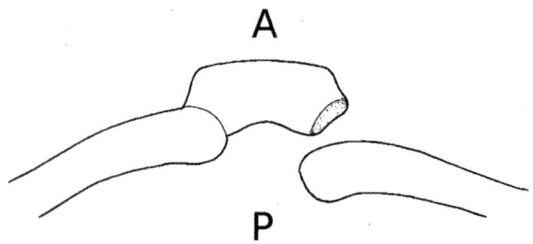

FIGURE 43.4. Posterior dislocation of right clavicle.

particularly if there is a visible dislocation or compression symptoms. There may be associated great vessel injury with hemorrhage on reduction.

An anterior dislocation can be managed with supportive care. The athlete is not usually able to return to play on the same day of injury due to pain. Return to play can occur when the athlete has full range of motion and strength. Athletes under the age of 22 years with an SC injury are likely to have had an epiphyseal fracture, which is usually treated conservatively; they require fracture healing time. Return to play must wait until full fracture healing has occurred.

The athlete with a posterior dislocation can return to play, usually six weeks after reduction, when the capsule has healed and full range of motion and strength has returned.

43.6 STERNUM FRACTURES

These fractures are most unusual in sport, great energy being needed to fracture a healthy sternum. The main concern with sternal fractures is that the energy needed to fracture a sternum is also enough to cause cardiac or pulmonary contusions and even aorta and diaphragmatic damage. For this reason, sternal fractures should be urgently referred to a hospital once oxygen has been administered and an IV line established.

43.7 CLAVICULAR FRACTURES

These are common injuries and are easy to treat with RICE principles, x-ray referral, and Collar'n'Cuff or Gilchrist bandage. They are often seen after a fall in sports and are easily diagnosed by inspection and particularly by palpation. Always start palpation at the sternoclavicular joint and continue in a lateral direction with bidigital palpation of the clavicle, using both the thumb and index finger, all the way

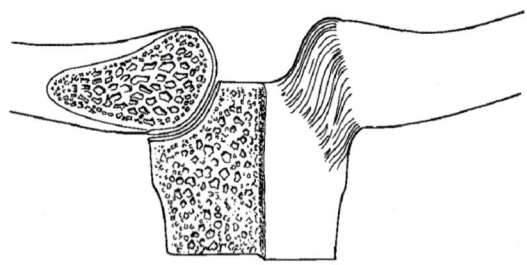

FIGURE 43.3. Sternoclavicular joint.

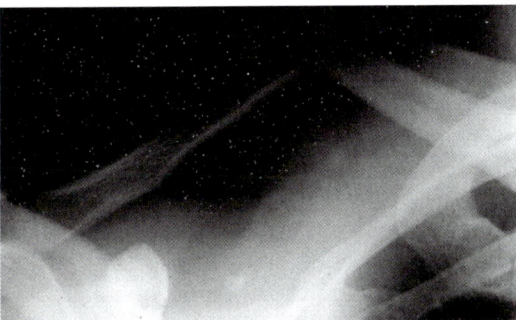

FIGURE 43.5. Midshaft clavicle fracture with concomitant acromioclavicular separation. (Reprinted from Bucholz RW, Heckman JD. *Rockwood & Green's Fractures in Adults*. 5th ed. Philadelphia, PA: Lippincott Williams & Wilkins; 2001, with permission.)

to the acromion. These fractures are almost always treated conservatively, unless there is a spiky bone fragment threatening the skin or causing major bleeding. A fractured clavicle can theoretically puncture the apex of the lung (Fig. 43.5).

43.8 SCAPULAR FRACTURES

Fractures of the scapula are also associated with high-energy or high-velocity and are thus not common in sport. The body of the scapula is the commonest site of injury. Due to the trauma forces involved, always look for associated pulmonary injuries, contusions, pneumothoraces, and other fractures.

43.9 FLAIL CHEST

Flail chest is rarely seen in sport—I have never seen one in 30 years as a sports doctor. It is usually associated with high-energy/high-velocity injuries, such as car accidents, explosions, etc. Flail chest occurs when a portion of the rib cage is separated from the rest of the chest wall. Usually this is defined as a minimum of two fractured ribs with at least two fractures per rib. A "loose" segment is created, which does not move in symmetry with the rest of the rib cage, thus lung expansion is compromised. Large flail segments will disrupt pulmonary mechanics and patients will most likely require ventilation (even the use of a CPAP unit).

Patients with flail chest have often an underlying lung contusion. Pulmonary contusions are difficult to diagnose clinically and particularly in the prehospital situation (Figs. 43.6–43.9).

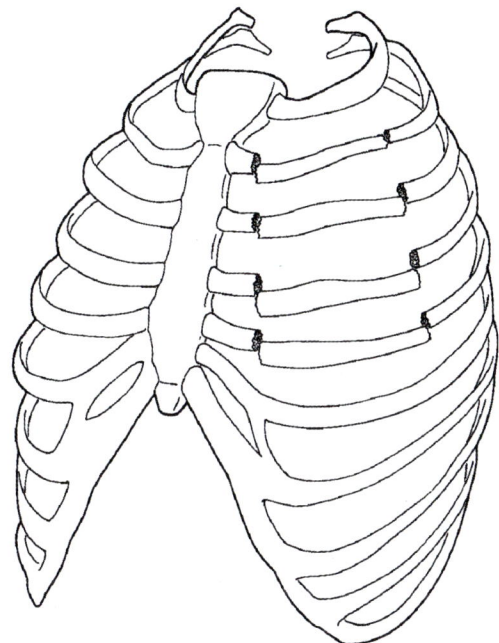

FIGURE 43.6. Left-sided flail chest.

Diagnosis

Expect to find bruising and/or grazing of the chest wall. Conscious patients may complain of pain, particularly with inspiration. On palpation, there may be tenderness and crepitus over broken ribs. Classically, there is paradoxical respiration with the flail segment moving in the "wrong" direction—i.e., the flail segment moves in or does not move on inspiration and moves outward when the rest of the chest relaxes during expiration. This paradoxical movement may be palpated or visualized in the coronal plane. There are often impaired respiratory sounds over the damaged lung due to presence of a lung contusion and/or hemothorax.

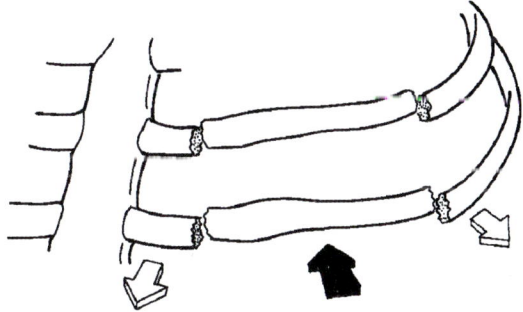

FIGURE 43.7. Flail chest during inspiration, paradoxical respiration.

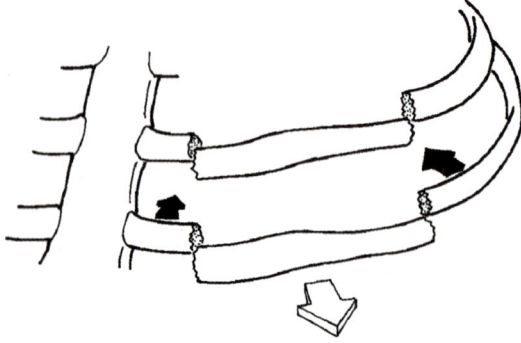

FIGURE 43.8. Flail chest during expiration, paradoxical respiration.

Treatment

Concentrate on protecting the injured chest wall and the potentially damaged underlying lung. The patient needs oxygen and probably ventilation. Intubation should be considered in serious cases. If the rib cage is severely damaged, then intubation and CPAP are usually required. Rapid transportation to a hospital is required if the patient is hypoxic. The patient should be transported with the injured side down to reduce eventual paradoxical movement (however, the patient should not lie on the injured ribs; this may cause further bleeding and lung damage). Circulation should be ensured so insert an intravenous canula but do not overload the patient with fluid, as this can lead to a hemo/hydrothorax. Effective pain control with epidural anesthesia and treatment of the underlying lung contusion are essential.

43.10 FALLS AND THORACIC INJURIES

An autopsy study of fall deaths carried out by the Institute of Legal Medicine, Hamburg, Germany, from 1998 to 2002, showed that cardiac injuries

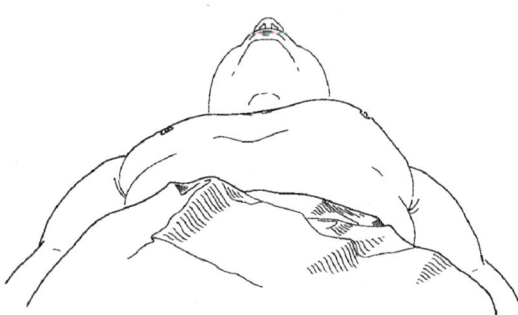

FIGURE 43.9. Left-sided flail chest during expiration, coronal plane.

were found in 54% of cases where falls from heights exceeded 6 m. The most frequent finding was pericardial tearing (45%). Tears caused by stretching of the epicardium in the area where the inferior vena cava leads into the right atrium and epicardial hematoma were present in 33%. Endocardial tears of the atria were found in 18%, transmural tears to the right atrium were present in 39%, and to the left atrium in 18% of cases.

Sternal fractures were seen in 76% of all cases involving heart injuries. In 16% of these cases, the fractures were multiple. Thus, the presence of severe sternal fractures can be used as an indicator of possible cardiac trauma.

43.11 PENETRATING THORAX INJURIES

As with all major penetrating injuries, the foreign body should not be removed until the athlete is at a hospital. The removal of foreign bodies is often accompanied by extreme bleeding and shock—blood transfusion may be necessary. The EP does not have blood units available so avoid removing impaled objects. If injury is caused by an impaled penetrating foreign body then the right ventricle is the most commonly injured part, followed by the left ventricle. Hypotension that does not respond to rapid volume replacement suggests significant injury. The only thing an event physician can do is

- ABC with rapid volume replacement
- Stabilize the foreign object, preventing further internal damage
- Rapid transportation to hospital

For these patients, surgery is usually necessary.

When considering damage caused by penetrating objects, one must consider two things: blood loss and structural damage. In the case of the thorax, these structures are the lungs, heart, aorta, great veins, spinal cord, esophagus, and diaphragm. But one can also expect to find signs of pneumothorax, hemothorax, subcutaneous emphysema, pneumomediastinum, hemoptysis, vascular damage, and breathing difficulties. Do not forget to examine the abdomen as puncture wounds in the chest may involve the upper abdominal organs such as liver, spleen, and stomach.

It is important to remember that any penetrating injury to the fourth intercostal space or below may well have damaged the diaphragm and intra-abdominal organs.

Laceration of intercostal or internal mammary arteries can cause serious bleeding. Digital compression of these arteries is critical until operative intervention is available.

43.12 BLUNT THORAX INJURIES

These include injuries to the chest wall, in particular

- Rib fractures
- Pulmonary contusion occurs to a varying degree in almost all major thoracic injuries, in particular with a flail chest
- Pneumothorax and tension pneumothorax can occur
- Subcutaneous emphysema (which should lead one to suspect pneumothorax or tracheal injury).
- Hemothorax should be suspected with thoracic injury—particularly with open wounds
- Tracheal injuries, bronchial injuries
- Cardiac injury
- Great vessel injury
- Diaphragmatic rupture
- Visceral injury with lower rib fractures (liver, spleen, kidney)

When the heart is damaged in blunt trauma, myocardial contusion is the most common injury and this may lead to ECG changes and enzyme elevation. Trauma to the coronary artery can result in thrombosis and myocardial infarction. Atrial or ventricular rupture is usually fatal, though in some occasions, if the pericardium is intact, bleeding and leakage may be restricted. Aortic rupture is usually fatal.

43.13 COMMOTTIO CORDIS

This poorly understood, rare, but potentially life-threatening condition typically affects young male athletes who receive a sudden blunt (and often innocent looking) blow to the sternum or left anterior chest, causing collapse, ventricular fibrillation, and sudden cardiac arrest. The timing of the blow in relation to the T wave may be of consequence and further research needs to be carried out on this area. Suffice it to say that as death is usually due to ventricular fibrillation, early defibrillation is the only tool available to the EP, though resuscitation rates are not good. Early resuscitation and defibrillation—within 1 to 3 minutes—seem to improve the survival rate, though treatment is often delayed by the sheer surprise of a patient with an innocuous injury becoming so ill.

43.14 CARDIAC TAMPONADE

Cardiac tamponade is seldom seen in sports as it is associated with major trauma or prolonged serious illness (e.g., lung cancer, advanced cardiac disease). Occasionally it can be seen with penetrating chest injuries or after a viral or bacterial pericarditis. Symptoms include chest pain that is sharp or stabbing, is worsened on deep inspiration, and often radiates to the neck, shoulder, back, or abdomen.

The patient may go into shock with falling blood pressure and rapid pulse. The respiratory rate increases and the patient may be dyspneic or cyanotic. The patient may be dizzy and wander in and out of consciousness. Neck veins may be distended. Classically, heart sounds are muted on auscultation and an ECG will reveal small, faint signals due to the presence of fluid in the pericardium.

Cardiac tamponade is a potentially life-threatening condition and requires hospitalization. If qualified to do so, pericardiocentesis may be performed by inserting a large bore needle under the xiphoid process into the pericardium and aspirating the collected blood (the angle of insertion is at 45 degrees to the skin in the direction of the left shoulder). Full emergency ABCDE must be performed (Fig. 43.10).

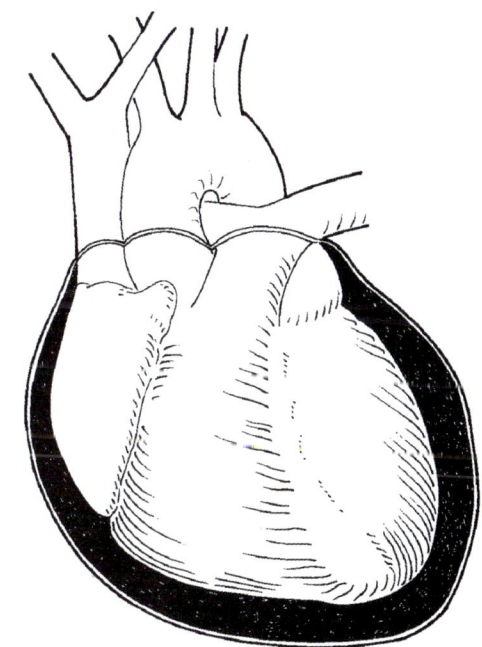

FIGURE 43.10. Cardiac tamponade.

43.15 PNEUMOTHORAX

A pneumothorax occurs when there is a collection of air in the pleural space. Air may come from an internal injury (e.g., a bronchial tear) or from an external chest wall injury or diaphragmatic injury, thus allowing air to enter through a pathologic opening. This collection of air, unless extremely small, usually impedes lung expansion and therefore reduces lung function. In a simple pneumothorax, this collection of air is nonexpanding and relatively static initially. In a tension pneumothorax, the volume of air increases continuously, there is a rapid reduction in lung function, there is rapid clinical deterioration, and the athlete is ill and getting worse (Figs. 43.11–43.13).

Suspected Pneumothorax

Pneumothoraces can be very difficult to diagnose in a sporting environment. It is often impossible to detect deficient respiratory sounds and hyperresonant palpation sounds at a sporting event due to noise from spectators, loudspeakers, other athletes, wind and rain, traffic, etc. The case history is often the most important indicator, so suspect a pneumothorax if the athlete has received a strong blow (e.g., shoulder charge to the chest), has a rib fracture, has subcutaneous emphysema, and is showing signs of dyspnea. Treatment for a stable athlete is ABC with oxygenation, analgesia if necessary (or intercostal blockade), and oxygen on mask.

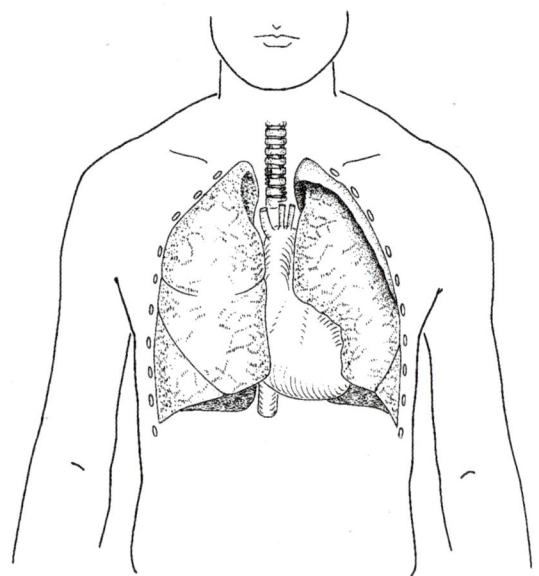

FIGURE 43.12. Lungs and heart, left-sided pneumothorax.

Closed Pneumothorax

Case history as above. The patient may have dyspnea, chest pain (often worse on inspiration), impaired respiratory sounds on the injured side and inequality between the two sides, hyperresonant percussion sounds (dullness with hemothorax), no penetrating injuries, even increasing dyspnea, subcutaneous emphysema with crepitations, asymmetrical respiration, cyanosis, and signs of shock.

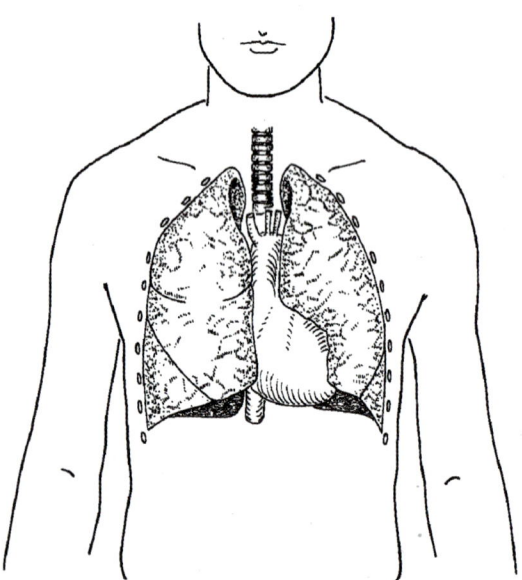

FIGURE 43.11. Lungs and heart, normal.

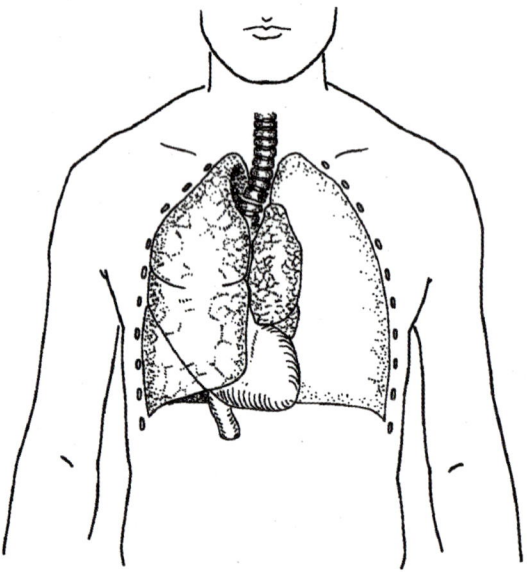

FIGURE 43.13. Tension pneumothorax with collapsed left lung, cardiac and tracheal deviation.

Always evaluate the jugular veins. Extended veins may indicate a tension pneumothorax.

Treatment: Treatment depends on the size of the pneumothorax: Minor lesions require adequate oxygen treatment, cessation of activity, and referral to a hospital.

Major lesions require oxygen treatment and the insertion of a thoracic drain, but this is seldom necessary at a sporting event.

There are several possible drain insertion points but most practitioners utilize the second, third, or fourth intercostal space in the anterior or midclavicular line. Connect the drain, if possible, to a Heimlich valve.

Open Pneumothorax

History and diagnosis as above, except that we expect to find a wound; however, these are not always visible. If you find a wound, there may be sucking air sounds from the wound.

Treatment: Cover the wound, preferably taped on three sides, leaving the fourth side open and thus preventing a valve effect that could induce a tension pneumothorax. Ensure that the airway is patent, administer oxygen/ventilate/intubate if necessary, maintain adequate circulation, and organize rapid transportation to a hospital.

Tension Pneumothorax

Pneumothorax findings as above, but accompanied by a dramatic clinical deterioration in a short period of time with increasing dyspnea, deteriorating consciousness, neck–vein congestion, tachycardia, hypotension, tracheal deviation, mediastinal displacement, and absent breathing sounds over the injured lung.

Treatment: The treatment for tension pneumothorax is immediate needle thoracostomy with immediate depressurization of the tension pneumothorax. Several needles can be inserted if necessary.

Needle Thoracostomy

See Figure 43.14.

- Wash the skin with alcohol swabs and use an aseptic technique
- Insert a 14-gauge intravenous catheter with a syringe attached

- Insertion site: At the top of the 2nd, 3rd or 4th rib in the intercostal space in the midclavicular line
- Insert the catheter/needle until air escapes; if in doubt, aspirate air into the syringe or remove the syringe and you may hear a gush of air
- Remove the trocar from the catheter and tape the catheter to the chest wall
- If available, attach the tubing from the Heimlich valve to the hub of the catheter
- Use tape to securely fasten the catheter hub and Heimlich valve to the patient
- Maintain a patent airway and adequate oxygenation; intubate or ventilate, if necessary; ensure adequate circulation. If this procedure fails, repeat on the contralateral side
- Rapid transportation to hospital is mandatory—the patient still has a pneumothorax

Treatment: By Surgical Drain Insertion

The tube end outside the pleural space should be placed in an underwater seal or have a valve that allows unidirectional flow of air out of the pleural space only.

- Identify the point of incision: Third or fourth intercostal space, in the anterior or midaxillary line.
- Clean the skin with antiseptic and infiltrate the skin, muscle, and pleura with 1% lidocaine.

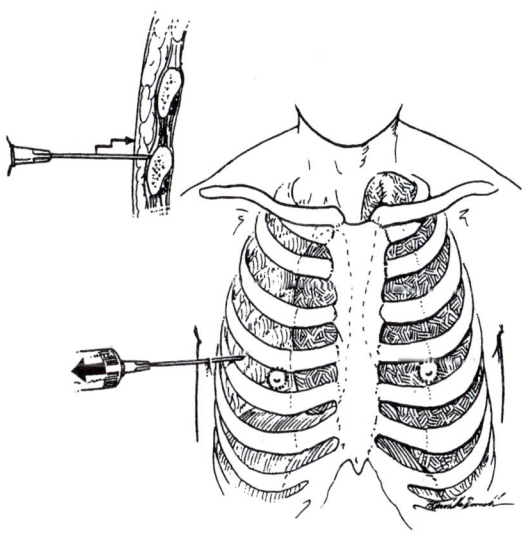

FIGURE 43.14. Needle thoracostomy.

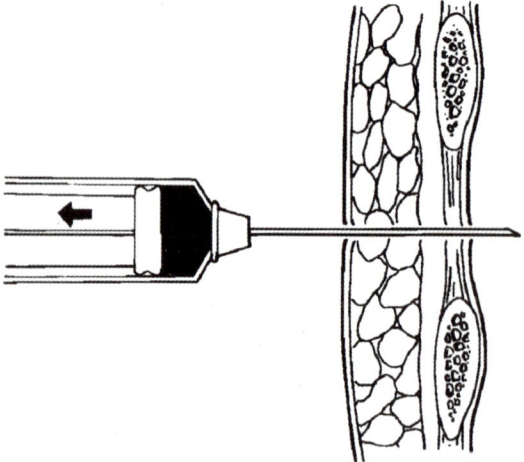

FIGURE 43.15. Anesthesia.

- Note the length of needle needed to enter the pleural cavity; this will help when inserting the drain (Fig. 43.15).

- Attempt to aspirate any fluid from the chest cavity.

- Make a small transverse incision just above the rib to avoid damaging the intercostal vessels and nerves just under the rib. In children, it is advisable to keep strictly to the middle of the intercostal space (Fig. 43.16).

- Using a pair of large, curved artery forceps, penetrate the pleura and enlarge the opening (Fig. 43.17).

- Use the same forceps to grasp the tube at its tip and introduce the tube into the chest (Fig. 43.18).

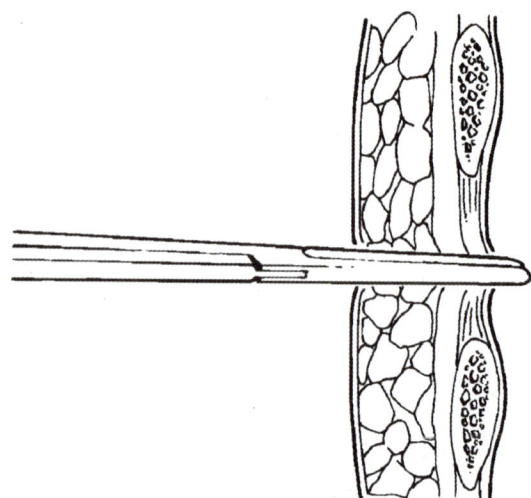

FIGURE 43.17. Enlarge incision opening.

- Close the incision with interrupted skin sutures, using one stitch to anchor the tube (Fig. 43.19).

- Leave an additional suture untied adjacent to the tube for closing the wound after the tube is removed. Apply a gauze dressing. Finally, connect the tube to the underwater-seal drain.

Conclusion: To Decompress or Not to Decompress; That is the Question

Clinical practice varies around the world, but the general consensus for prehospital emergency needle thoracostomy seems to be that if you are able to diagnose a pneumothorax (i.e., history, dyspnea, increased respiratory rate, tachycardia, tympanitic

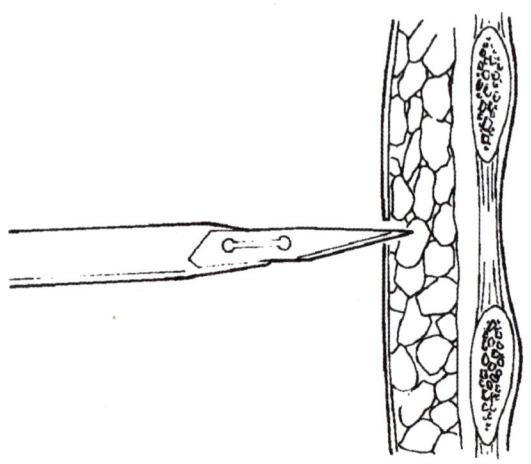

FIGURE 43.16. Incision.

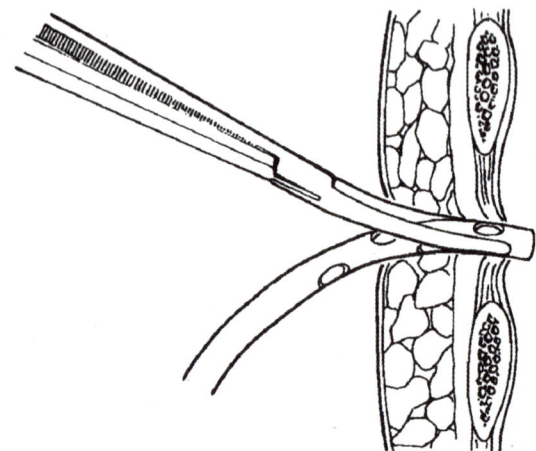

FIGURE 43.18. Tube insertion.

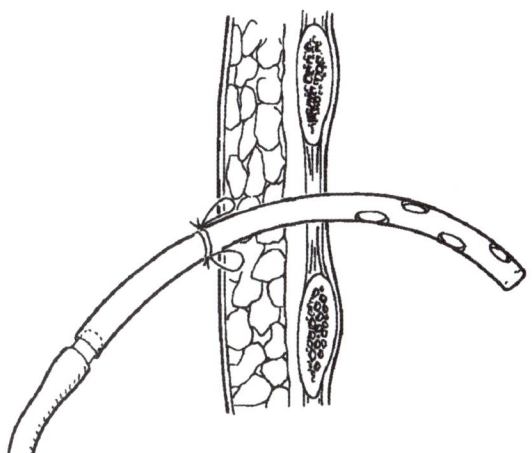

FIGURE 43.19. Tube stabilization.

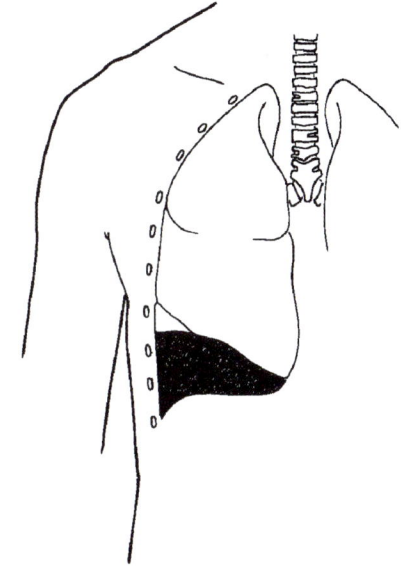

FIGURE 43.20. Right-sided hemothorax.

percussion sounds, absent respiratory sounds, etc.) in the often noisy prehospital environment, then there is probably a relatively large pneumothorax present and decompression should be attempted.

Things are slightly different in a hospital (with a stable, conscious patient, no respiratory distress, and a small pneumothorax); conservative treatment with controls may be considered. However, the sports field is a different environment where we have little else but our clinical skills to aid us in making a diagnosis. It goes without saying that if you insert a needle, you must leave it in and continue to check its patency while the athlete is under your care and that the athlete will require transfer to a hospital setting.

A tension pneumothorax should always be decompressed immediately.

43.16 HEMOTHORAX

A hemothorax occurs when there is a collection of blood in the pleural space. Blood comes from a torn vessel and may be caused by blunt or penetrating trauma. Most hemothoraces are the result of rib fractures, lung parenchymal injuries, and minor venous injuries and are often self-limiting. Arterial injuries are less common but they are more likely to require surgical repair. A hemothorax can be found accompanying a closed pneumothorax and almost always with an open pneumothorax.

Most small to moderate hemothoraces are not detectable by physical examination and will be identified only on chest x-ray or CT scan. However, larger and more clinically significant hemothoraces may be identified clinically and should be treated promptly.

Chest examination may indicate the presence of significant thoracic trauma with external bruising and/or lacerations, or palpable crepitus indicating the presence of rib fractures. There may be evidence of a penetrating injury over the affected hemithorax. Do not forget to examine the back. The classic signs of a hemothorax are decreased chest expansion, percussion dullness, and reduced breath sounds over the affected hemithorax. Mediastinal or tracheal deviation is absent unless in the presence of a massive hemothorax. All these clinical signs may be subtle or absent in the supine trauma patient and most hemothoraces will only be diagnosed after imaging studies. Beware of the patient with hypotension after rib fractures. He may have occult bleeding into the chest or abdomen (ruptured spleen, liver, or kidney).

Treatment: With shock symptoms without neck–vein congestion: Volume therapy and oxygen. With increasing dyspnea, intubation may be necessary and thorax drainage may be required. If the patient is deteriorating, reevaluate the need for circulation—are you flooding the lungs? Rapid transportation is essential (Fig. 43.20).

43.17 LUNG CONTUSIONS

A pulmonary contusion occurs after lung parenchyma has been injured, leading to swelling of the lung tissue and bleeding into the alveolar spaces, thus causing a loss of normal lung function. Often occurring after blunt trauma to the chest, it often develops over a 24-hour period; the effect is poor gas exchange locally, increased pulmonary vascular resistance, and decreased lung compliance. It is believed that the presence of blood components in the alveolar spaces may cause a significant inflammatory reaction in the lung. This may be a causal force in the development of acute respiratory distress syndrome (ARDS); as many as 50% of patients with significant pulmonary contusions can develop bilateral ARDS.

Pulmonary contusions are rarely diagnosed on physical examination but must be suspected with blunt chest trauma, particularly with obvious signs of chest wall trauma or hemoptysis. This is one reason why the event physician should be restrictive in his return-to-play evaluation of chest injuries. If an athlete has had two or more costal fractures, I advise against sporting participation for at least three weeks whatever the situation—Olympics or not. A "second impact" effect on the lungs—a second trauma within a few days—can also cause life-threatening pulmonary contusions.

Diagnosis: Pulmonary contusions often occur in combination with other thoracic injuries, such as multiple costal fractures, flail chest, hemothorax, pneumothorax. Signs are seldom present on initial examination but, if present, look for bloodstained expectorate, dyspnea, and crackles on auscultation.

Treatment: Airway, oxygen, hospitalization; intubation may be necessary with increasing dyspnea and signs of falling oxygen saturation.

Complications: ARDS is particularly common in thoracic trauma and typically begins a few hours after injury. Progress is often rapid. Patients require ICU treatment often with ventilation. Failure of ARDS to improve within 4–6 days is associated with a high incidence of death (Fig. 43.21).

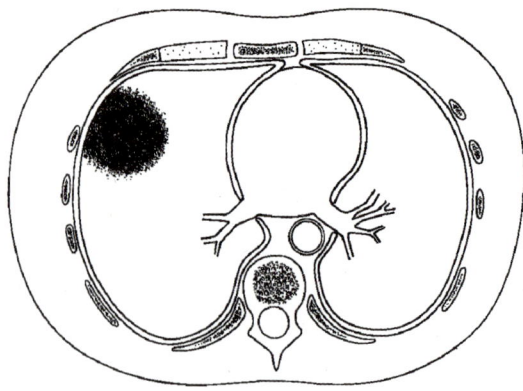

FIGURE 43.21. Contusion of the left lung.

43.18 CONCOMITANT ABDOMINAL/ DIAPHRAGMATIC INJURIES

With penetrating injuries, in particular, the diaphragm and abdominal organs can be affected. These injuries must not be overseen.

Recommended Readings

Manes N, Hernandez-Rodriguez H, Lopez-Martin S, et al. Pneumothorax—guidelines of action. *Chest.* 2002; 121(2):669.

Miller AC, Harvey JE. Guidelines for the management of spontaneous pneumothorax. Standards of Care Committee, British Thoracic Society. *BMJ.* 1993;307(6896): 114–116.

Molnar TF, Hasse J, Jeyasingham K, et al. Changing dogmas: history of development in treatment modalities of traumatic pneumothorax, hemothorax, and posttraumatic empyema thoracis. *Ann Thorac Surg.* 2004;77(1): 372–378.

Nolan JP, Soar J, Zideman DA, et al. European Resuscitation Council Guidelines for Resuscitation 2010 Section 1. Executive summary. *Resuscitation.* 2010;81(10): 1219–1276.

CHAPTER 44

Cardiac Emergencies

Contributed by Fabio Pigozzi, Professor, IUSM, Rome, UIPM Modern Pentathlon Chair MC, President, FIMS, Italy; and Maria Rizzo, Department of Health Sciences, IUSM, Italy

Reviewers: Gary Mak, Consultant Cardiologist, Hong Kong Sports Institute, Hong Kong; Johan-Arnt Hegvik, Consultant Anesthesiologist, NTNU, Trondheim, Norway

Traumatic injuries of the musculoskeletal system are common in most sporting activities and are almost considered an integral part of the sport itself. On the other hand, cardiac emergencies on an athletic field would appear to be something of a paradox. Compelling epidemiologic and clinical evidence accumulated over the past two decades indicates that regular physical training is associated with manifold health benefits, cardiovascular in particular. Exercise is today seen as one of the most important means of maintaining good health and, conversely, the lack of regular physical activity is considered an independent cardiovascular risk factor.

Athletes are therefore usually considered the healthiest members of our society and sporting champions personify the ideals of health, strength, and invulnerability. Nevertheless, the sudden cardiac death of elite athletes during a sporting event has alerted the general public to the fact that even well-trained athletes are not immune to cardiac diseases. Exercise-related cardiac episodes generally occur in individuals with underlying congenital or acquired cardiac diseases, the recognition of which is the main target of preparticipation screening programs, which have recently been implemented in most European countries.

Unfortunately, not all competitive athletes undergo an adequate cardiovascular evaluation and, regrettably, not all life-threatening cardiac conditions can be excluded by screening so sudden cardiac deaths in athletes will continue to occur. This shows the need for therapeutic equipment at sporting events and the need for trained medical staff to be present.

Cardiac emergencies at sporting events are not as infrequent as we would like to believe, and their prompt recognition and treatment are essential for saving lives.

This chapter deals with the most important cardiac emergencies that may occur in athletic settings. We focus, in particular, on the recognition and treatment of sudden cardiac arrest, the main cause of death in sport.

The most important cardiac emergencies present with two symptoms:

- Exertional chest pain (with related symptoms and signs)
- Sudden collapse with syncope and cardiac arrest

44.1 EXERTIONAL CHEST PAIN

Chest pain is an uncommon symptom in active subjects but, if present, demands immediate concern and attention.

The causes of chest pain in athletes are numerous and are usually of noncardiac origin.

Among young athletes (<35 years), chest pain is generally due to musculoskeletal strain, pleuritis, bronchitis, and pneumonia and is not related to physical exertion.

However, up to 6% of athletes <35 years who present with acute, serious, exercise-related chest pain have an underlying primary cardiac or pulmonary pathology.

The most frequent causes are

- Pneumothorax (traumatic or spontaneous)
- Pulmonary or cardiac contusion secondary to blunt chest trauma.

Young individuals with chest pain symptoms, especially *when accompanied by syncopal or near-syncopal episodes,* should alert one to the possibility of underlying severe cardiac diseases, such as

- Coronary artery anomalies/diseases
- Aortic stenosis
- Hypertrophic cardiomyopathy
- Premature ischemic heart disease
- Connective tissue defects such as Marfan's syndrome

Chest pain in these conditions is due do myocardial ischemia, except for Marfan's syndrome where aortic rupture is generally the cause.

In older athletes (>35 years), exertional chest pain is more frequently of cardiac origin such as

- Coronary artery disease (CAD)—leading cause of sport-related sudden cardiac death in this age group
- Acquired valvular diseases
- Aortic dissection
- Pulmonary thromboembolism

When should acute chest pain in athletes be considered a cardiac emergency?

A cardiac emergency should always be considered when an athlete (whatever age) complains of

- Chest pain or discomfort lasting more than 3 to 5 minutes
- Chest pain that goes away and then returns
- Chest pain not relieved by rest, by changing position, or by medication, which may spread to shoulders, arms, back, neck, or jaw
- Shortness of breath
- Dizziness
- Palpitation
- Nausea
- Sweating or changes in skin appearance

When these symptoms are recognized, the athlete should immediately stop all activity and rest. Restrictive clothing has to be removed. Vital signs (breathing, pulse, and arterial blood pressure) and movement should be monitored closely, and medical staff should be prepared to give CPR and to use an AED, if available.

Once the athlete has become clinically stable, he or she must undergo a complete and thorough cardiovascular examination to identify the causes of the chest pain episode. Athletes should be sent to a hospital.

44.1 SUDDEN COLLAPSE WITH SYNCOPE AND SUDDEN CARDIAC ARREST

Cardiac arrest (CA) is the most important cardiac emergency on a sports field, presenting with collapse that may be sudden (as generally occurs in

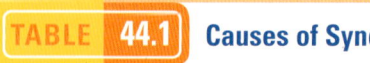

TABLE 44.1 **Causes of Syncope**

Some Noncardiovascular Causes of Syncope

Reflex mechanism

Vasovagal and vasodepressor syncope (neutrally mediated syncope)

Situational syncope

Blood drawing

Urinating (micturition syncope)

Defecating

Coughing

Orthostatic hypotension

Dysautonomies

Fluid depletion, hyponatremia, hyperkalemia/hypokalemia

Illness, bedrest, deconditioning

Drugs

Hypoglycemia

Head injury

Anaphylaxis

Psychogenic

Some Cardiovascular Causes

Arrhythmic causes

AV block with extreme bradycardia

Sinus pauses (sick sinus syndrome, negative chronotropic drugs)

Ventricular tachycardia (VT) associated with structural cardiac disease or channelopathies

Nonarrhythmic causes

Hypertrophic cardiomyopathy

Aortic stenosis

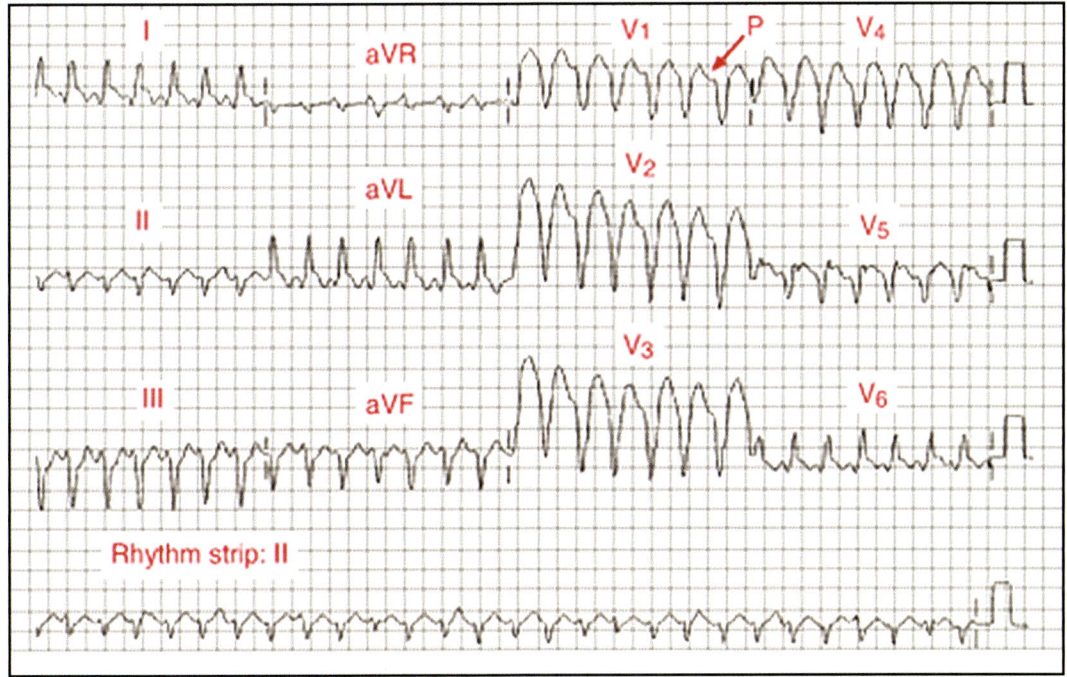

FIGURE 44.1. Ventricular tachycardia.

the young athletes) or proceeded by premonitory symptoms (palpitations, chest pain, dizziness). Fortunately, most athletes who collapse during or immediately after exertion have not had a cardiac arrest. Other frequent causes are hypoglycemia, exercise-associated collapse, exertional heat stroke, heat exhaustion, hyponatremia, and seizures.

However, an unresponsive collapsed athlete should always be treated as a potential cardiac arrest. Open the airway and see if spontaneous breathing occurs. If the patient is breathing normally, do not start CPR. If there is abnormal breathing, start CPR.

Syncope is the abrupt and transient loss of consciousness associated with the absence of postural tone and awareness of oneself and one's surroundings, followed by a rapid, spontaneous, and complete recovery. Syncope is the consequence of a transient reduction of blood flow to the brain, causing a transient hypoxia of the brain itself. Syncope is usually benign and self-limited but there are many possible causes, generally divided into cardiac and noncardiac disorders (Table 44.1).

When a syncopal episode occurs during or immediately after an exertion, further thorough investigation is always required due to the high probability of an underlying life-threatening cardiac disease (even if reported episodes of exercise-induced neurocardiogenic or vasodepressor syncope have tempered the clinical dictum that

exercise-induced syncope is a malignant arrhythmia until proven otherwise).

Nevertheless, the pathologic disorders associated with life-threatening arrhythmias in young athletes are

- Congenital cardiomyopathy (hypertrophic cardiomyopathy or arrhythmogenic right ventricular cardiomyopathy)

- Coronary artery anomalies

- Primitive arrhythmogenic conditions: Conduction system anomalies or channelopathies (e.g., the long- or short-QT syndrome)

In all these cases, syncope is often the only symptom preceding sudden cardiac death. Thus, evaluation of athletes with exertional syncope in a specialist setting should specifically exclude the pathologic substrates associated with sudden death before a complete return to activity is permitted.

44.2 LIFE-THREATENING TACHYARRHYTHMIAS IN ATHLETES

The most common tachyarrhythmias observed in athletes, usually associated with cardiac diseases, are

- Ventricular tachycardia (VT, Fig. 44.1)

- Supraventricular tachycardia (SVT) with aberrancy and preexcited tachycardia associated with an accessory pathway (Fig. 44.2)

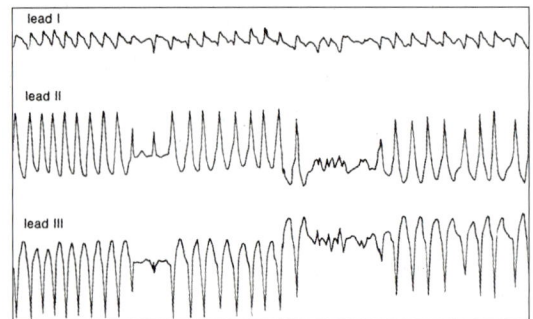

FIGURE 44.2. Supraventricular tachycardia (atrial fibrillation) in an athlete with WPW syndrome.

Treatment depends on associated clinical conditions.

If the athlete is stable, breathing should be supported and blood pressure monitored until an ECG has been taken.

If the athlete has collapsed and is unresponsive, then he or she requires an immediate SCA assessment, as discussed, and usually requires ACLS.

44.3 EXERCISE-RELATED SUDDEN CARDIAC ARREST

Sudden cardiac arrest (SCA) is a frequent event in the general population and one of the commonest causes of death. It has been estimated that in the United States, the annual number of deaths due to cardiac arrest is approximately 250,000, greater than those due to prostate cancer, breast cancer, and automobile accidents considered altogether (~118,500).

In Italy, there are approximately 50,000 SCA a year, 5% (2,500) of which occur during recreational activities.

The true incidence of SCA and sudden cardiac death (SCD) in athletes is not easily estimated due the lack of a mandatory national reporting or surveillance systems. The general perception is that over the past few years, a growing number of cardiac disasters have occurred on athletic fields, the most recent of which affected the professional soccer players Marc Vivien Foe, Antonio Puerta, and Miklo Feher.

SCA and SCD in athletes are generally considered very rare events, especially in the young individuals. However Maron et al., have recently reported a frequency of SCD in young US competitive athletes of about 110 cases per year, corresponding to one death every 3 days. In Italy, Corrado reported an incidence of 2.3 cases in 100,000 young athletes per year, which is about twice the incidence previously reported in other series. Collectively, these data suggest that SCD in athletes has been an underestimated problem for a long time.

Sport, also the most strenuous activity, does not increase the risk of cardiac events in healthy subjects. However, compelling evidence indicates that vigorous exercise increases the risk of cardiovascular events among subjects with underlying cardiac diseases. The pathologic substrate of sport-related sudden cardiac arrest is age dependent.

Among young individuals (<35 years) the most frequent pathologic findings are the inherited cardiomyopathies (hypertrophic cardiomyopathy and arrhythmogenic right ventricular cardiomyopathy) and congenital coronary artery anomalies, followed by a number of various diseases, including myocarditis, Marfan's syndrome, valvular heart diseases, dilated cardiomyopathy, premature coronary artery disease (CAD), and channelopathies, a group of primary electrical heart diseases caused by mutations in genes encoding for cardiac ion channel proteins such as the long- or short-QT syndrome and the catecholaminergic polymorphic ventricular tachycardia (CPTV).

In contrast, in older athletes over 35 years, CAD is the leading cause of exercise-related sudden cardiac death, as reported in publications.

Independently of the specific pathologic substrate, the final common pathway is usually that of an electrical instability resulting in a fatal arrhythmia (ventricular fibrillation in most cases) and cardiac arrest. The only exception is represented by the Marfan's syndrome in which the mechanism of death is generally aortic rupture. All other mentioned pathologic substrates share a marked arrhythmogenicity—that is, the propensity for potentially lethal arrhythmias—that is further increased by exercise as a consequence of increased sympathetic drive and the associated transient alterations in blood volume and hydroelectrolyte balance.

Finally, cardiac arrest may also occur also in young athletes without cardiac abnormalities. This typically happens in commotio cordis, caused by a blunt, nonpenetrating blow to the chest that produces a ventricular fibrillation without structural injury to the ribs, sternum, or heart. Commotio cordis is responsible for about 20% of SCD in the youngest athletes (<21 years), 70% of which occur in subjects younger than 16 years.

Unfortunately, cardiac arrests that occur on athletic fields are often fatal due not only to the severity of the pathologic substrate but also due the lack of prompt and effective cardiopulmonary resuscitation and defibrillation.

44.4 RECOGNITION AND MANAGEMENT OF CARDIAC ARREST

The prompt recognition of SCA is critical for athlete survival. SCA that occurs on an athletic field is always witnessed but, unfortunately, its recognition is not always immediate. Rescuers who have not received intensive training in emergency management may mistake agonal or occasional gasping for normal breathing or falsely identify the presence of a pulse or misdiagnose SCA as a seizure due to the presence of myoclonic activity after collapse.

In order to avoid threatening delays in the activation of the so-called Chain of Survival, the first rule for all the bystanders is that any collapsed, unresponsive athlete requires an immediate assessment for SCA, even if seizure-like activity is present (it has been reported in 3 of 10 athletes with SCA).

44.5 THE CHAIN OF SURVIVAL

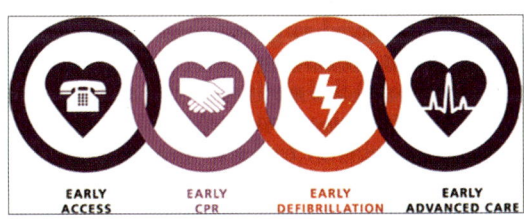

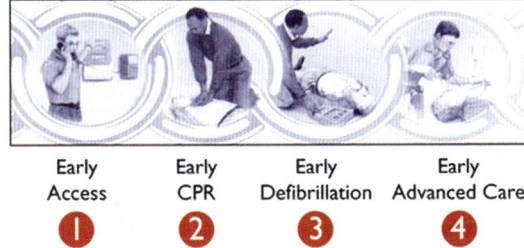

The *Chain of Survival*, defined by the American Heart Association (AHA), is composed of four fundamental steps required to improve the survival of out-of-hospital cardiac arrest victims.

- Early recognition of an emergency and telephone activation of the local emergency response system

- Early bystander CPR: Immediate CPR can double or triple the victim's chance of survival from ventricular fibrillation SCA

- Early delivery of defibrillator shock: CPR plus defibrillation within 3 to 5 minutes of collapse can produce survival rates as high as 49% to 75%

- Early advanced life support followed by postresuscitation care delivered by health care providers.

44.6 CARDIOPULMONARY RESUSCITATION AND AUTOMATIC EXTERNAL DEFIBRILLATION

The first responder should first quickly check the victim's response by both tapping on the forehead and calling to him or her for two or three times. The unresponsive athlete should be positioned lying supine on a firm, flat surface to prepare for the eventual CPR.

CPR is composed of three key components of the ACB:

- A: opening the **A**irway

- C: applying external **C**hest **C**ompressions 30:2

- B: providing artificial respiration with mouth-to-mouth **b**reathing

If you do not have access to an AED, continue until more help is available

If you do have access to an AED, connect up to the patient and access status, either shocking if ventricular fibrillation (VF) (Fig. 44.3) or continuing with CPR

The rescuer should check breathing by opening the airway using the head tilt–chin lift maneuver to lift the tongue away from the back of the throat. If normal breathing is present, the collapsed athlete does not require CPR. But if the athlete is unresponsive and has only agonal gasps or no breathing activity, then chest compressions should

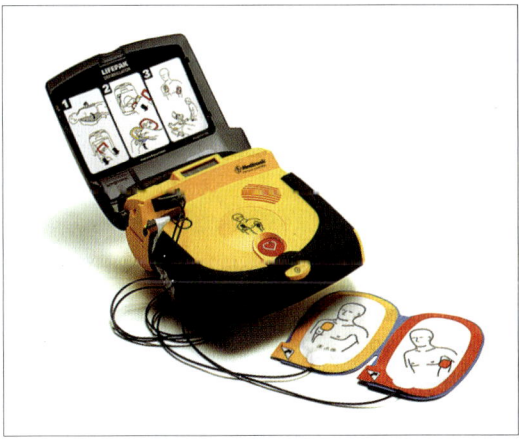

FIGURE 44.3. Medtronic LIFEPAK CR Plus.

be initiated while another bystander calls the local emergency medical services (EMS) and retrieves the AED, if available.

Effective chest compression in adults is performed by compressing the lower half of the sternum, using the bases of the hands, and depressing the chest to a depth of minimum 5 cm (2 in or more). Rescuers should *push hard and push fast* (rate of 100 compressions per minute), allow complete chest recoil between compressions, and minimize interruptions in compressions. According to the latest European Resuscitation Council, guidelines (https://www.erc.edu) a compression–ventilation ratio of 30:2 is recommended. When multiple rescuers are present, they should rotate the compressor role about every 2 minutes or earlier if fatigue develops.

Thus, CPR is a combination of compressing the chest wall, which squeezes the heart and pushes blood out to vital organs—in particular to the brain and the heart itself—and breathing to supply oxygen to the blood. Unless breathing and circulation are established within 4 to 6 minutes of a cardiac arrest, irreversible brain damage occurs. CPR, however, cannot preserve life indefinitely, but it can keep a person alive until more effective medical intervention is available to restore normal heart function. If bystanders provide immediate CPR, many adults in ventricular fibrillation can survive with intact neurologic function, especially if defibrillation is performed within about 3 minutes after SCA. For more detailed information regarding CPR, see Chapter 22.

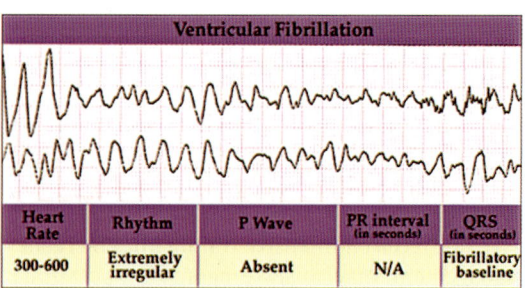

Heart Rate	Rhythm	P Wave	PR interval (in seconds)	QRS (in seconds)
300-600	Extremely irregular	Absent	N/A	Fibrillatory baseline

FIGURE 44.4. Ventricular fibrillation.

An AED should be attached to the victim for rhythm analysis as soon as possible, minimizing all interruptions in chest compression. If several responders are present, CPR should be continued while attaching the AED leads. AEDs are computerized devices that analyze a victim's rhythm, determinate if a shock is needed, charge to an appropriate shock dose, and use audio and visual instructions to guide the rescuers. They are easy to use and extremely accurate in recommending a shock only when VF or rapid ventricular tachycardia (VT) is present.

Most cardiac arrest victims demonstrate VF on first rhythm analysis. This lethal arrhythmia is characterized by chaotic rapid repolarizations and depolarizations, which cause the heart muscle to quiver and lose its ability to pump blood effectively. Rapid VF (Fig. 44.4) or VT (Fig. 44.5) are the most common arrhythmias at the time of collapse, but these rhythms frequently deteriorate to asystole, absence of electrical activity, before the first rhythm analysis.

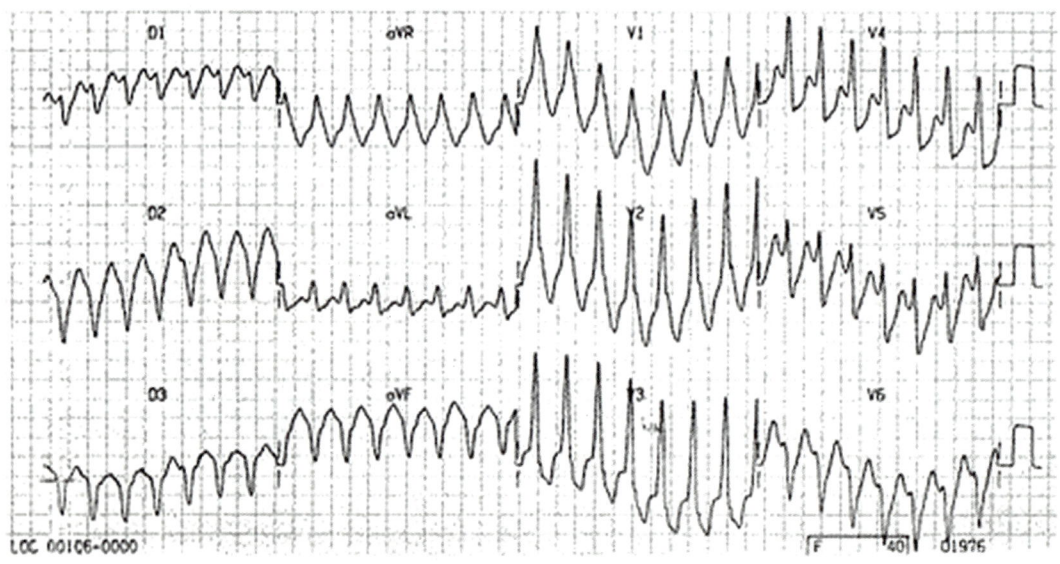

FIGURE 44.5. Rapid ventricular tachycardia.

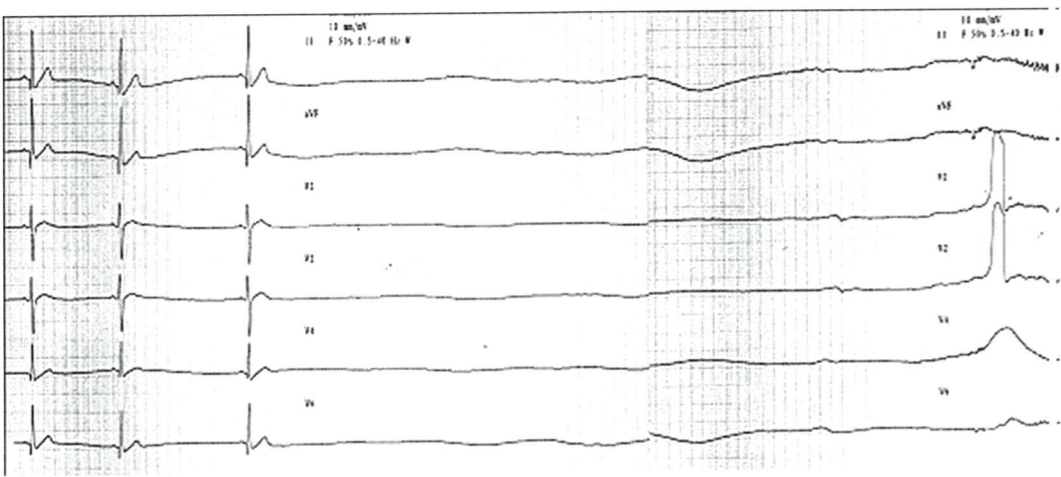

FIGURE 44.6. Asystole.

The probability of successful defibrillation for VF SCA diminishes rapidly over time, with survival rates declining 7% to 10% per minute for every minute that defibrillation is delayed. Survival after SCA is unlikely once VF has deteriorated to asystole (Fig. 44.6).

CPR is of critical importance both before and after defibrillation.

In the first phase of cardiac arrest (the first 4 minutes) CPR provides a small but critical amount of blood flow to the heart and brain and increases the likelihood that defibrillation will restore a normal rhythm in time to prevent neurologic damage. When CPR is initiated, survival declines by 3% to 4% per minute for every minute defibrillation is delayed. After shock delivery, CPR is also critical to provide perfusion as many victims are in a pulseless electrical activity or asystole for several minutes after defibrillation. Thus, CPR can greatly improve survival from SCA, but, unfortunately, it has been estimated that CPR is initiated in less than one-third of cases of witnessed SCA and, in about 40% of cases, chest compressions are not effective. Thus, it is vital for all medical staff at a sporting event to be trained in CPR and AED.

Survival of Athletes after SCA

Available data on the survival rate of young athletes after SCA indicate a low resuscitation rate (between 11% and 46%), despite timely CPR and prompt defibrillation. To explain this disturbing data, it has been postulated that ventricular arrhythmias associated with structural heart disease, especially cardiomyopathies, may be more resistant to even short delays in defibrillation than those occurring in a structurally normal hearts. However, as the single greatest factor affecting survival of out-of-hospital cardiac arrest remains the time interval from the cardiac arrest to defibrillation, there will always be a compulsion on the event physician to make a speedy diagnosis and initiate correct treatment as soon as possible.

Recommended Readings

American College of Sports Medicine (ACSM) and American Heart Association (AHA). Exercise and acute cardiovascular events: placing the risk into perspective. *Med Sci Sport Exerc.* 2007;39(5):886–897.

European Resuscitation Council. *European Resuscitation Council Guidelines 2010.* http://www.cprguidelines.eu/2010/. Accessed April 5, 2011. Guidelines developed by Europeans and been written with European practice in mind.

Field JM, Hazinski MF, Sayre MR, et al. 2010 American Heart Association guidelines for cardiopulmonary resuscitation and emergency cardiovascular care science. *Circulation.* 2010;122(18 suppl 3):S640–S946.

Drezner JA, Courson RW, Roberts WO, et al. Inter-association task force recommendations on emergency preparedness and management of sudden cardiac arrest in high school and ollege athletic programs: a consensus statement. *J Athl Train.* 2007;42(1):143–158.

Perron AD. Chest pain in athletes. *Clin Sports Med.* 2003;22:37–50

Pigozzi F, Rizzo M. Sudden death in competitive athletes. *Clin Sports Med.* 2008;27:153–181.

Williams RA. *The Athlete and Heart Disease: Diagnosis, Evaluation & Management.* Philadelphia, PA: Lippincott Williams &Wilkins; 1999.

CHAPTER 45

Respiratory Emergencies

Contributed by Joseph Cummiskey, President, EFSMA, IOC Medical Committee, Modern Pentathlon Medical Committee, Ireland

Reviewer: Richard Budgett, IOC Medical Committee, Chief Medical Officer, London 2012 Summer Olympic Games

There are many different respiratory diseases and many ways of classifying these disorders. Respiratory diseases can be divided on the basis of spirometry into either obstructive conditions where disorders impede the flow of air into and out of the lungs (e.g., asthma) or restrictive lung diseases where there is a decrease in ability to expand the lungs (e.g., pulmonary fibrosis).

Respiratory diseases can also be classified anatomically as upper or lower respiratory tract disorders such in the case of respiratory infections. As spirometry is not readily available at most sports events, it is probably better to use another anatomical classification—that is, the use of various anatomical parts:

Airway

- Trauma
- Allergy—anaphylaxis
- Asthma
- Aspiration/foreign body
- Acute and chronic bronchitis—air pollution and smoking
- Respiratory tract infections

Parenchyma

- Pneumonia
- Pulmonary edema

Pleura

- Pneumothorax
- Hemothorax

Pulmonary vasculature

- Pulmonary embolism

Airways

45.1 TRAUMA

(See Chapter 43.)

45.2 ALLERGY—ANAPHYLAXIS

(See Chapter 25.)

45.3 ASTHMA

Definition

Two main definitions of asthma have been used. The first is the classification of asthma as a manifestation of atopy, thereby including eczema and raised levels of IgE in the definition.

The second approach is by defining asthma in the form of induced bronchial hyperreactivity, without reference to atopy.

Exercise-induced bronchoconstriction (EIB) is defined as the acute transient airway narrowing that occurs during, but more often after, exercise, often arbitrarily defined as a fall in FEV_1 of > 10% (FEV_1 = forced expiratory volume in one second).

This definition includes the objective fall in lung function associated with exercise that occurs in persons with known preexisting asthma where exercise "triggers" exacerbation in otherwise asymptomatic persons without a known history of asthma (often athletes). EIB is more frequent and severe in persons with an atopic form of asthma.

Diagnosis

The diagnosis of asthma in sport is based on both a clinical evaluation and a pulmonary function test/tests (PFT). These PFTs should comply to European Respiratory Society (ERS) and/or American Thoracic Society (ATS) standards. PFTs are usually not readily available to the EP, nor are previous test results, unless at the Olympic Games or major sport World Championships. An athlete can present with an acute, serious, previously undiagnosed asthma. One should always exclude trauma, acute infection, or allergy/anaphylaxis reactions before even considering acute asthma.

Clinical findings with a severe asthmatic attack in adults:

- Hunched forward
- Agitated or drowsy
- Exhausted
- Confused or coma
- Wheeze is loud or absent
- Respiratory rate of 25 or more
- Heart rate of 110 or more
- Inability to complete sentences—talks only with a few words
- If you have the ability to measure PEF, a peak flow between 33% and 50% of best for the patient or predicted

Diagnosis of a *life-threatening* asthmatic attack in adults

- The same findings as above
- $SpO_2 < 92\%$
- Silent chest
- Cyanosis
- Poor respiratory effort
- Bradycardia or hypotension
- Confusion or coma
- Peak flow less than 33% of expected or best
- Remember, anaphylaxis can present with asthma symptoms and findings only

Differential Diagnosis of Asthma

- Other lung obstructive diseases
- Chronic bronchitis, emphysema, bronchiectasis, bronchiolitis
- Interstitial lung disease
- Swimming-induced pulmonary edema
- Exercise-induced hypoxemia
- Vascular lung disease
- Hyperventilation with exercise
- Upper airway disease
- Vocal cord dysfunction—paradoxical movement
- Laryngeal prolapse
- Laryngomalacia with inspiratory stridor
- Gastroesophageal reflux

If available, percentage changes in PFT should show

- Resting pulmonary function tests
  - 12% bronchodilation above the athlete's resting FEV_1 after an inhaled bronchodilator
- Nonpharmacological, indirect challenge
  - 10% bronchoconstriction
  - Exercise or eucapnic voluntary hyperventilation
- Pharmacological stimulation tests
  - 20% bronchoconstriction at a methacholine dose of 4 to 16 mg per mL or less
  - 15% bronchoconstriction after inhalation of a Mannitol test of cumulatively 636 mg
  - 15% bronchoconstriction to a 4.5% saline challenge

Assessment

Symptoms include dyspnea, chest tightness, or wheeze after exercise. Physical examination usually reveals wheeze or rhonchi. A silent chest may be a sign of severe pathology due to the air entry failure. This may be accompanied by cyanosis and other effects of hypoxemia.

PFT in the form of a peak flow or FEV_1 may reveal a reduction from the athlete's normal values or accepted general population values. A drop of 50% is considered severe and should be managed in an emergency department, where blood gases can be used to access and monitor severity.

A low oxygen tension or widened arterial-alveolar (A-a) oxygen gradient is the first sign. This may be accompanied by a low carbon dioxide tension. A normal carbon dioxide value may be a normal sign or a sign of progression if accompanied by a widened A-a oxygen gradient. High carbon dioxide tension or a severely widened A-a oxygen gradient is a late and severe sign.

Treatment

Therapy can usually start with the use of the athlete's own inhalers. This will usually be a beta-2 sympathomimetic. Two puffs every hour until relief or side effects (usually tachycardia or tremor of hands) may be used. A useful devise for delivering the drug to the lower airways is a spacer device or a nebulizer (Fig. 45.1). Nebulizers are the most efficient way of delivering drugs to the distant airways. The addition of an anticholinergic and a steroid by inhalation may assist with therapy.

Remember: Beta-2 sympathomimetics require a TUE on the WADA 2010 list.

IV steroids may be a last resort, depending on the severity. Their effect is seen within 60 minutes and is believed to be an effect on the permeability of the blood vessels to the lung. Their longer term effects are on the inflammatory system. Their use requires a TUE.

Severe attack (GINA Guidelines):

- Oxygen—the goal of treatment is to restore SpO_2 to at least 94%
- Glucocorticosteroids, either
  - Hydrocortisone 100 mg IV over 30 seconds (alternatively, IM, but slower onset)
  - Prednisolone 40 to 50 mg per os
- Beta-2 agonists—salbutamol 5 mg. preferably via a nebulizer and pressure-dose inhaler
- Short-acting bronchodilator—ipratropium 0.5 mg, preferably via nebulizer and pressure-dose inhaler; if you do not have a nebulizer, then inhale two to four puffs every 20 minutes; if milder attack, two to four puffs every 3 to 4 hours

Factors Contributing to Asthma Severity

- Increased patient exposure to inhalant allergens
- Increased tobacco smoke exposure
- Increased air pollution exposure of particular matter, SO_2, NO_2
- Poor control (brittle asthma)
- Rhinitis/sinusitis
- Gastrointestinal reflux
- Some medications
- Viral RTI

Training as a Cause of Asthma in Elite Athletes

Long-term, intense endurance training may be associated with an increased risk of development of airway hyperresponsiveness and asthma in elite athlete.

Environmental factors, such as allergens, chlorine derivatives, pollutants, or cold air exposure may contribute to the development of airway inflammation and functional changes. Their penetration into the airways will be enhanced by the high ventilation required during intense exercise.

The final common pathway of all these insults on the airways is probably through the production of reactive oxygen free radicals. The best management of these insults, especially tobacco use, is avoidance. In polluted environments, this would involve training indoors at times of poor air quality. An additional approach is the use of oxygen free-radical scavengers like vitamins E and C.

The changes in lung function and airway responsiveness are normally reversed after cessation of long-term endurance training.

After an episode of bronchoconstriction, there is often a refractory period where subsequent exercise causes less airway narrowing due to the degranulation of mast cells in the bronchioles and so a lower dose of inflammatory cytokines. Athletes with poor control may be aware of and use this refractory period.

The danger of worsening hyperresponsiveness over time means athletes who need any more than the occasional inhaled beta-2 agonist should be given a preventative inhaler (corticosteroid) and compliance checked. Known asthmatics should be treated using a therapeutic escalator consisting of use of short-acting beta-2 agonists as required, low-dose inhaled corticosteroids, long-acting beta-2 agonists, and higher dose inhaled corticosteroids and/or systemically administered corticosteroids.

More research is necessary on how to prevent or minimize the adverse effects of long-term training on the airways, particularly the effects of environmental exposure on airway structure and function.

45.4 ASPIRATION

Definition

Aspiration is defined as the passage of a foreign body or the contents of the stomach or mouth into the laryngopharynx, larynx, or main airway. The commonest substance aspirated is chewing gum. The use of chewing gum should be banned in sport activity. Other substances that can be aspirated include the teeth, bridges, portions of a gum shield, aspirated chunks of meat, and, reportedly, the tongue (though the existence of such a condition is disputed by many).

Symptoms and Signs

The athlete usually cannot speak when aspiration occurs because the foreign body may be lodged at the vocal cords. The vocal cords are the narrowest part of the airway. The athlete may therefore point to his or her throat in a distressed, cyanotic manner. Collapse may occur if the condition is left for too long.

Treatment

The only appropriate treatment is immediate removal of the foreign body from the pharynx either with a finger or a Magill forceps. Only if any attempt for direct removal is not successful, the Heimlich maneuver should be applied. This maneuver is designed to raise intra-abdominal pressure by pressing vigorously and in a sustained manner over the epigastrium. The pressure ideally will be transferred up the esophagus to the pharynx and dislodge the foreign body. This can be done with the athlete standing and leaning forward over a solid object about four feet high (back of a chair or a railing). It can also be attempted in the left horizontal position. If successful, the athlete will experience immediate relief and will commence talking. Cyanosis will be relieved within minutes.

If this maneuver is unsuccessful, too, an emergency cricothyroidotomy or tracheostomy may be necessary. This is a dangerous procedure even in the experienced hands outside the operating theatre (see Chapter 21.4). The site of entry for a sharp object would be just below the cricoid bone. The orifice may be kept open with a tube or, in an emergency, with a Bic pen. Immediate transfer to a hospital is required as secondary bleeding is a possibility.

45.5 ACUTE AND CHRONIC BRONCHITIS

Definition

Acute or chronic bronchitis is defined as an inflammation of the respiratory tract. The major environmental factors that could influence airway function in elite athletes are allergens and ambient conditions such as temperature, humidity, and air quality. Because of the high minute ventilation during exercise, the effects of these exposures may be more marked in athletes. Exposures of importance to the athlete include seasonal and perennial allergens, dry/cold air, chlorine derivatives in swimming pools, airborne ultrafine particulate matter emitted from ice resurfacing machines in indoor ice rinks, ozone, and combustion-derived pollutants, such as oxides of nitrogen and particulate matter.

Symptoms and Signs

Inflammation is manifested by increased secretions in the upper or lower respiratory tract. This may lead to cough, sputum, wheeze, blocked nasal passages, and dyspnea when severe.

Treatment

Remove patient from the adverse environment or source of pollution. An anti-inflammatory inhaler will relieve symptoms and over time may reverse the acute effects of inflammation.

45.6 RESPIRATORY TRACT INFECTIONS

Definition

A respiratory tract infection (RTI) is defined as infection of the upper or lower respiratory tract.

In an athlete, upper and lower respiratory tract infections occur on average about 1.7 times a year. These are one of the commonest causes of acute bronchitis.

Symptoms and Signs

The symptoms of a RTI are runny nose, post nasal drip, cough, sputum, wheeze, dyspnea, and possible systemic symptoms of fever or shivering. The signs of a RTI are increased secretions from the nose or lower respiratory tract that are expectorated or swallowed. Rhonchi or crackles may be heard with the use of a stethoscope.

Treatment

A rule of thumb is that training and competition should be curtailed or stopped if there are below-the-neck symptoms or systemic symptoms (lower RTI). The indications for an antibiotic have to be carefully weighed against the disadvantages (e.g., resistance) and may include the appearance of lower respiratory tract symptoms, the presence of green or yellow sputum, and systemic symptoms. Raised C-reactive protein and/or leucocyte count may also indicate bacterial infection. Antibiotics are not indicated in viral disease.

Prevention

Mild training regimes decrease the incidence of RTI. Severe training without adequate recovery increases the incidence of RTI.

Parenchyma

45.7 BRONCHOPNEUMONIA

Definition

Bronchopneumonia is an extension of a bronchitis (acute bacterial or viral infection of the larger airways) to include the parenchyma of the lung. The causational bacteria are similar. The usual source of the organism is from airborne particles in a crowded external environment via the proximal airways.

Symptoms and Signs

Bronchopneumonia usually presents with a degree of severity greater than bronchitis (cough, mucus, fever, chills, chest pain, and fatigue). Classically, rales or crackles can be heard in bronchopneumonia together with the wheeze or rhonchi of bronchitis.

Treatment

Similar treatment to bronchitis is usually given to the patient. In addition, an antibiotic is more likely to be indicated. In a community-acquired infection, a macrolide antibiotic may be started empirically to cover gram-positive bacteria and atypical microorganisms. If the infection is severe, an additional broader spectrum antibiotic to cover gram-negative bacteria may be added.

45.8 INTERSTITIAL PNEUMONIA

Definition

This is defined as infection or inflammation in the interstitium of the lung tissue.

Symptoms and Signs

Interstitial pneumonia appears more linear than fluffy on chest radiograph as opposed to the more fluffy appearance of bronchopneumonia. There are over 200 forms of chronic interstitial pneumonia. The acute form is an intermediary between bronchitis and alveolar pneumonia.

Treatment

This is similar to bronchopneumonia but with less or no coverage for bronchitis. A diuretic may be considered in the acute stages.

45.9 HIGH-PRESSURE PULMONARY EDEMA

Definition

High-pressure edema is, as the name implies, secondary to high pressure in the left atrium and pulmonary veins. The fluid is low in protein. There are mainly two forms:

- *Cardiogenic pulmonary edema* is the commonest form of pulmonary edema and is cardiogenic in origin. Any cause of left heart failure can lead to pulmonary edema.

- *Neurological pulmonary edema* occurs usually secondary to trauma to the brain. A surge of sympathetic activity results in systemic hypertension that causes heart failure and pulmonary edema. Often, at the time of examination, the blood pressure has returned to normal but the effects of the hypertension cause persistent pulmonary edema.

45.10 HIGH-PERMEABILITY PULMONARY EDEMA

Definition

High permeability edema is seen in septic shock. There is a high content of protein in the edema fluid, which tends to prolong this more severe form of pulmonary edema.

Symptoms and Signs

Edema in the lung is manifested by dyspnea, cyanosis, wheeze (secondary to the edema around airways), and crackles.

Treatment

Treatment is management of the cause of the high permeability, which is most commonly an infection. In the acute situation, symptoms are usually managed by the administration of an oral or intravenous loop diuretic.

Pleura

45.11 PNEUMOTHORAX AND HEMOTHORAX

Definition

Pneumothorax is the presence of air in the pleural space. It causes symptoms because the air fills the pleural space, raising intrapleural pressure, thus preventing maximal lung expansion, thus compromising lung function. Pneumothorax occurs most commonly with blunt trauma to the chest (a shearing lesion), after a penetrating lesion of the lung (unusual in sport), or spontaneously (in tall, thin individuals). Severe forms of pneumothorax may have bleeding into the pleural space (hemothorax).

Symptoms and Signs

The symptoms are sudden onset of dyspnea. A wheeze or cyanosis may occur. The signs are rhonchi or, more commonly, a decrease in breath sounds. In the presence of tension pneumothorax, there may be a shift of the mediastinum away from the affected side. This is manifested clinically and on the chest x-ray by a shift of the trachea.

Treatment

The occurrence of a tension pneumothorax is a medical emergency. Relief of the tension is achieved by placing a needle or tube in the pleural space (see Chapter 43).

Pulmonary vasculature:

45.12 PULMONARY EMBOLISM AND DEEP VEIN THROMBOSIS

Definition

Deep venous thrombosis (DVT) and pulmonary emboli (PE) are caused mainly by stagnant flow in leg or pelvic veins. DVT is more common in smokers; in women who take the contraceptive pill; after long-haul flights (more than 4 hours); in hereditary Factor V Leiden thrombophilia; in patients aged over 40 and with occult malignancy. Varicose veins, surgery within the previous 10 days, and other medical conditions can be predisposing factors.

Symptoms and Signs of Pulmonary Embolism

Symptoms can vary greatly, depending on clot size, how much of the lung is affected, and the presence of underlying lung or heart disease. Common signs and symptoms include

- Acute resting dyspnea
- Cyanosis
- Chest pain that may radiate to the shoulder, arm, neck, or jaw; the pain may be sharp and stabbing or aching and dull
- The chest pain may be pleuritic (may become worse on breathing deeply or coughing) or be exaggerated by eating or bending; pain is often worse with exertion but still present during rest
- There may be bloody or blood-streaked sputum
- There may be wheezing
- Tachycardia
- Ankle edema
- Excessive sweating and anxiety
- Depending on severity, there may be light-headedness or syncope to sudden death

Symptoms and Signs of DVT

- Leg pain, but can also be asymptomatic
- Acute cramp-like pain in the calf with possible radiation to the ankles and feet
- Swelling in the affected leg; this can include swelling down to the ankles and feet

- Redness and warmth over the affected area

- Palpation tenderness over the thrombosis, often on the posteromedial aspect of the calf

- Homans' sign: The patient's knee should be in the flexed position. The examiner should forcibly and abruptly dorsiflex the patient's ankle and observe for pain in the calf and popliteal region (a positive sign). The accuracy of Homans' sign has been researched intensively. Most authors now agree that Homans' sign is unreliable, insensitive, and nonspecific in the diagnosis of DVT.

Beware: DVTs are often notoriously difficult to diagnose. For example, it can be extremely challenging to differentiate between a partial calf muscle tear and a DVT. Venography is the gold standard in establishing a correct diagnosis although ultrasound may be sufficient. D-dimer may also be elevated.

Treatment

If in doubt, do not take any chances. Once a suspicion of DVT or PE arises, then rapid hospital assessment is recommended. Having made a definite diagnosis of DVT or PE, treatment is with anticoagulants for months. Low molecular weight heparin and warfarin are the most commonly used agent. A new group of antifactor agents is now available, need no laboratory monitoring, and should replace the two latter agents over the coming years. The only common side effect of all these agents, if not properly monitored, is internal bleeding (hemorrhage).

Prevention

Incidence can be reduced by exercising the leg muscles for five minutes every hour during long flights. Wearing elastic stocking assists with venous return from the legs. Adequate systemic hydration, by drinking non–diuretic-inducing fluids liberally, also helps to reduce the likelihood of thrombi. In athletes who have experienced thrombi, the use of preventive low molecular weight antifactor X, heparin, warfarin, or aspirin is helpful.

Recommended Reading

Carlsen K-H, Cummiskey J, Delgado L. Diagnosis, prevention and treatment of exercise-related asthma, respiratory and allergic disorders in sport. *Eur Respir Mon.* 2005;33.

Fitch KD, Sue-Chu M, Anderson SD, et al. Asthma and the elite athlete: summary of the International Olympic Committee's Consensus Conference, Lausanne, Switzerland, January 22–24, 2008. *J Allergy Clin Immunol.* 2008;122(2):254–260.

Flaherty KR, King TE, Raghu G. Ideopathic interstitial pneumonia: what is the effect of a multidisciplinary approach to diagnosis? *Am J Resp Crit Care Med.* 2004;170:904–910.

Geerts WH, Bergqvist D, Pineo GF, et al. Prevention of venous thromboembolism: American College of Chest Physicians evidence-based clinical practice guidelines (8th edition). *Chest.* 2008;133(6 suppl);381S–453S.

Henry M, Arnold T, Harvey J. BTS guidelines for the management of spontaneous pneumothorax. *Thorax.* 2003;58(suppl 2):ii39–ii52.

Mandell LA, Bartlett JG, Dowell SF, et al. Update of practice guidelines for the management of community-acquired pneumonia in immunocompetent adults. *Clin Infect Dis.* 2003;37:1405–1433.

Acute Respiratory Infections

Contributed by Shane Brun, Professor, James Cook University, Queensland; Team Physician, Australian National Soccer Team; previously, Australian Cricket Team, Bangladesh Cricket Team, and Australian Olympic Swimming Team

Infections affecting the respiratory tract of athletes present themselves not infrequently to the physician responsible for the care of athletes. All too often, the athlete succumbs to a respiratory tract infection (RTI) just prior to or just after a major event or competition. The timing tends to coincide with intense training leading up to the competition and the competition itself; this is particularly true for the endurance athlete, and recent epidemiologic evidence is consistent with this observation. The time the athlete is most at risk of RTI is at the peak intensity of training and for 1 to 2 weeks following competition.

There appears to be a J-curve relationship between the amount of physical activity and risk of RTI (this relationship has mostly been demonstrated for upper RTI [URTI]). These data support the relationship and the hypothesis that moderate levels of physical activity are associated with a reduced risk for URTI and intense and prolonged activity results in immunosuppression and the increased risk of infection.

The observed immunologic basis for this is that intense and prolonged activity suppresses concentration of lymphocytes, suppresses natural killer and lymphokine-activated killer cytotoxicity and secretory IgA in mucosa, and increases adrenaline and cortisol, whereas moderate amounts of exercise may decrease an athlete's risk of URTI through favorable changes in immune function without the negative effects of the stress hormones, adrenaline and cortisol.

Common Pathogens of RTIs

Respiratory tract infections can be classified as upper respiratory tract infections (URTI) and lower respiratory tract infections (LRTI). To some degree, there is crossover of pathogens in that, in a significant proportion of patients with URTI and LRTI, there is serologic evidence of infection with more than one pathogen, although there are also pathogens that have a particular predilection to either the upper or lower respiratory tract.

The vast majority of RTIs are spread by droplet infection, either directly or by way of fomites. The dilemma for the clinician is of diagnosis. For the event physician and team physician, particularly when traveling, it is often the case that appropriate and easily accessible pathology and radiology services are difficult to access. The taking of an accurate and focused history with an appropriate and focused examination is, in most cases, all an experienced and practiced team physician needs to arrive at the correct diagnosis. Although there may be multiple single and combined pathogens causing an RTI, often the diagnostic criteria are similar whether it is an LRTI or URTI. Determining the particular organism is much more difficult and an awareness of what pathogens are common to the geographic region and are being transmitted at the time will assist greatly in coming to a more accurate diagnosis, so utilizing epidemiologic and travel medicine data prior to arriving at a destination is essentia.

The treatment of RTIs comprises two sections: one is the treatment of the individual infected, and the other is to contain the infection and prevent spread among other team members or accompanying staff. Quarantining, although a very effective way of preventing transmission of infection, is not always practicable; therefore, the implementation of as many appropriate public health measures as possible to contain the spread is essential. Making players aware of how viruses and bacteria are spread is an important role of the team physician.

It is the physician's responsibility to enforce strict hand washing; avoiding the sharing of personal objects, clothing, and bedding, which may act as fomites; and coughing and sneezing away from other people and preferably into the patient's own arm folded across his or her face, into the region of the cubital fossa, or into a disposable tissue.

In all cases of either an URTI or LRTI, the athlete will experience fevers and possibly rigors; fever in itself is not always a reliable indicator as to severity of infection. The physician must be aware that associated with fevers and rigors is the increased risk of dehydration, in which case, every athlete with fever should ensure increased fluid intake to compensate for the potential increase in fluid loss.

It is the physician's responsibility to be fully aware as to the WADA classification of every drug that is prescribed for the athletes under his or her care. Under no circumstances should patient care and safety be compromised by withholding a drug that is indicated for the treatment of a diagnosed medical condition. It is the physician's responsibility to ensure appropriate authorities are notified, either by way of a TUE or by other means as outlined by the organizing committee or sporting authority. The physician must also be aware that many over-the-counter and "natural" cold and flu remedies lack evidence as to their efficacy and may contain substances that are banned or restricted under WADA guidelines (see http://www.wada-ama.org/en/).

It should be noted that the drug therapy outlined in this section has been refined and condensed. It is the assumption that the team physician, when traveling with athletes, will have available for his or her use only a limited selection of medications. It should be noted that in many circumstances other medications may be appropriate to use, in which case, the appropriate authorities and drug guidelines should be referred to; although for the purposes of this chapter, the drugs selected are those that have the broadest cover for the most common RTIs thereby streamlining the number of drugs the team physician needs to have at his or her disposal.

The team physician must be aware if any of the athletes for whom he or she is responsible has had a previous drug hypersensitivity reaction, in which case, it is the physician's responsibility to ensure appropriate alternative drug therapy is available.

When prescribing analgesia, the physician should be aware that the use of aspirin is not indicated in those aged 16 years and under, especially those in this age group with fever or influenza.

46.1 UPPER RESPIRATORY TRACT INFECTION

We will classify URTIs as essentially those involving the facial sinuses (sinusitis), the nasal cavity (rhinitis), the pharynx (pharyngitis), and the middle ear (otitis media).

Rhinitis (Common Cold)

Coronavirus, rhinovirus (which has over 100 different serotypes), and influenza and parainfluenza viruses are the most common agents that cause acute viral rhinitis. Influenza is caused by influenza A and B viruses.

During influenza epidemics, patients with early influenza symptoms (fever > 38°C plus at least one systemic symptom, such as myalgia, and one respiratory symptom) have a 60% to 70% chance of influenza.

Of increasing concern is avian influenza, which is caused by a subtype of influenza A virus. It is occasionally transmitted to humans via close contact with infected birds (especially chickens, but also ducks and geese). Occasional cases of human-to-human transmission have been reported. It is the responsibility of the team physician to know the current action plan for suspected avian influenza and the risk associated with the area in which the team is traveling.

In most cases, symptomatic treatment is all that is required with athletes with the common cold. It is prudent to consider

- Simple analgesia

- Oral or topical decongestant (check WADA classification before prescribing certain decongestant medications) in combination with antihistamines may provide increased symptomatic relief

- Steam inhalations and nasal irrigation with normal saline to help relieve thick nasal mucus production

- Currently there is no evidence that zinc lozenges or echinacea are effective in the treatment of the common cold

Sinusitis

Acute bacterial sinusitis follows upper (usually viral) RTI in 0.5% to 5% of cases. It is usually caused by *Streptococcus pneumoniae* or *Haemophilus influenzae* and less frequently by *Moraxella catarrhalis*.

In up to 50% of cases, sinusitis is a self-limiting condition. The patient often describes a biphasic illness whereby he or she experiences an initial URTI that seems to settle, only to have the congestion and discomfort return.

Bacterial sinusitis may be suspected if the patient presents with at least three of the following:

- Persistent mucopurulent nasal discharge (>7 to 10 days)
- Facial pain
- Poor response to decongestants
- Tenderness over the sinuses, especially unilateral maxillary tenderness
- Tenderness on percussion of maxillary molar and premolar teeth that cannot be attributed to a single tooth

Appropriate initial management includes

- Simple analgesia
- Oral or topical decongestant (check WADA classification before prescribing certain decongestant medications) in combination with antihistamines may provide increased symptomatic relief
- Steam inhalations and nasal irrigation with normal saline to help relieve thick nasal mucus production
- If antibiotics are indicated: Amoxicillin 500 mg three times daily for 5 to 7 days

Pharyngitis

For the clinician, it is often quite difficult to distinguish between viral and bacterial causes of pharyngitis. A bacterial cause of acute pharyngitis is more common in children aged 3 to 13 years (30% to 40%), than in adults (5% to 15%).

Although most URTIs comprise a fairly standard array of pathogens, the physician must be mindful of other infections that may cause exudative pharyngitis including Epstein-Barr virus (glandular fever) and gonococcal infection. Vesicular or ulcerative eruptions may occur with infection due to some types of enterovirus and herpes simplex virus (HSV) types 1 and 2; the primary infection with HSV may result in a mild to severe pharyngostomatitis with associated systemic features.

The most common bacterial pathogens in pharyngitis are *S. pneumoniae*, *H. influenzae*, and *M. catarrhalis*.

Indeed, for patients with pharyngitis, laboratory testing is often not indicated, and after conducting a concise and focused history, all adults should be screened for the following:

- History of fever
- Lack of cough

- Tonsillar exudates
- Tender anterior cervical adenopathy

The purpose of attempting to arrive at a diagnosis with pharyngitis is to rule in or out the possibility of infection with group A β-*hemolytic streptococci* (GABHS). The reason behind initiating treatment in those infected by GABHS is to prevent rheumatic fever; it is estimated that 3,000 to 4,000 patients with GABHS must be treated for every case of acute rheumatic fever prevented.

Appropriate symptomatic treatment if indicated may include

- Simple analgesia
- Salt water gargles
  - If the patient fulfills the criteria for a bacterial tonsillitis: Phenoxymethylpenicillin 500 mg orally twice daily for 10 days
  - If the patient is unable to swallow: Benzathine penicillin 900 mg as a single IM dose

Epstein-Barr Virus (Glandular Fever)

As has been previously mentioned, primary infection with Epstein-Barr virus (EBV; glandular fever) may be associated with severe pharyngitis. Antibiotics are not indicated for the treatment of glandular fever, and symptomatic treatment should be instituted. The physician must be aware that infection with EBV is often associated with varying degrees of splenomegaly, which may take several weeks to resolve following infection. It is prudent that the physician does not clear the athlete to resume contact activities until the spleen has returned to its usual size and is again protected by the rib cage.

The physician must also be aware of other more serious causes of apparently exudative pharyngitis including diphtheria (*Corynebacterium diphtheriae*), which presents as gross membranous pharyngitis, with or without airway obstruction, associated with features of severe systemic illness.

Otitis Media

The most common bacterial pathogens in otitis media are *S. pneumoniae*, *H. influenzae*, and *M. catarrhalis*.

Visualizing the tympanic membrane is a vital component; pain alone is not an adequate or reliable diagnostic feature.

The diagnosis is considered certain if there is

- A history of acute onset of symptoms and signs

AND

- A demonstrable middle ear effusion characterized by any of the following:
  - Bulging of the tympanic membrane
  - Limited or absent movement of the tympanic membrane
  - An air–fluid level behind the tympanic membrane
  - Perforation of the tympanic membrane with otorrhea

AND

- Signs and symptoms of middle ear inflammation, characterized by
  - Distinct erythema of the tympanic membrane
  - Distinct otalgia (pain clearly originating from the ear)

If the athlete fulfills the criteria for bacterial otitis media, along with symptomatic treatment, antibiotic therapy may be indicated and includes amoxicillin 500 mg three times daily for 5 days.

46.2 LOWER RESPIRATORY TRACT INFECTION

In addition to *S. pneumoniae*, *Mycoplasma pneumoniae* and *Chlamydophila* (*Chlamydia*) *pneumoniae* are the common causative organisms in patients with LRTI. In younger adults, *M. pneumoniae* is the most frequently identified causative agent. Other, less common agents include *Legionella pneumophila*, influenza viruses, adenoviruses, and Chlamydia. Although in some parts of the world these pathogens are now recognized as a significant cause of acute LRTIs, group A β-hemolytic *streptococci* is also occasionally implicated.

LRTI is suspected in a patient because he or she presents with at least two of the following symptoms:

- Fever
- Rigors
- New-onset cough
- Change in sputum color if there is chronic cough
- Pleuritic chest pain
- Dyspnea

Then a more detailed history and examination should be performed, and a diagnosis of LRTI should be made if the patient fulfills the following criteria:

- The identification of chest rales
- Dullness to percussion over a segment of the chest

- New onset of purulent sputum or change in character of sputum

The physician must at all times be mindful of severe acute respiratory syndrome (SARS), which is caused by the SARS-associated coronavirus and is primarily transmitted via respiratory droplet transmission and by fomite contact.

In the majority of cases, athletes encountered with the diagnosis of LRTI will have a Pneumonia Severity Index risk of Class I; in the rare cases, an athlete presents with more severe signs and symptoms, and hospital care should be immediately sought.

If the patient fulfills the above criteria, an appropriate oral antibiotic dosing regimen would be amoxicillin 1,000 mg orally, three times daily for 7 days. If there is suspicion of *M. pneumoniae or C.* (*Chlamydia*) *pneumoniae*, add roxithromycin 300 mg daily for 5 days.

If the patient has had a prior hypersensitivity reaction to either of these medications, a suitable substitute medication must be provided.

Bronchitis

Bronchitis is often considered an LRTI. In the majority of the athletic population, acute bronchitis is most often viral and antibiotics are not indicated. It has been demonstrated in randomized controlled trials that antibiotic therapy at most provides marginal benefit (<1 day for symptom resolution) and may cause harm, in which case, the physician must be able to justify the use of antibiotics.

Influenza

The physician should consider recommending the administration to all athletes under his or her care the current influenza vaccine before winter, which provides protection against the disease and its complications in up to 70% of vaccinees.

Neuraminidase inhibitors may have a role in prophylaxis. Following brief exposure to known influenza, 5 days of antiviral drug is adequate. Prolonged courses of up to 42 days may be considered in those likely to be subjected to repeated exposure during a major epidemic or pandemic.

Participating in Competition/Training

This is indeed a chapter on its own, although when the physician is considering whether to allow the infected athlete to compete or train, the risks needing to be considered include

- Transmitting infection to the other players
- Prolonging or worsening the illness

■ The infected athlete performing poorly especially in competition and therefore jeopardizing the outcome for himself or herself, or the team

Recommended Reading

Acute viral rhinitis: common cold [Revised June 2006]. In: *eTG Complete* [CD-ROM]. Melbourne: Therapeutic Guidelines Limited; 2008.

Influenza [Revised June 2006, amended November 2007]. In: *eTG Complete* [CD-ROM]. Melbourne: Therapeutic Guidelines Limited; 2008.

Avian influenza (including H5N1) [Revised June 2006, amended November 2007]. In: *eTG Complete* [CD-ROM]. Melbourne: Therapeutic Guidelines Limited; 2008.

Sinusitis [Revised June 2006]. In: *eTG Complete* [CD-ROM]. Melbourne: Therapeutic Guidelines Limited; 2008.

Pharyngitis and/or tonsillitis [Revised June 2006]. In: *eTG Complete* [CD-ROM]. Melbourne: Therapeutic Guidelines Limited; 2008.

Otitis media [Revised June 2006]. In: *eTG Complete* [CD-ROM]. Melbourne: Therapeutic Guidelines Limited; 2008.

Severe acute respiratory syndrome (SARS). In: *eTG Complete* [CD-ROM]. Melbourne: Therapeutic Guidelines Limited; 2008.

Community-acquired pneumonia in adults: risk classes I and II [Revised June, 2006]. In: *eTG Complete* [CD-ROM]. Melbourne: Therapeutic Guidelines Limited; 2008.

Bisno AL. Diagnosing strep throat in the adult patient: do clinical criteria really suffice? *Ann Int Med.* 2003;139(2):150–151.

Blasi F. Atypical pathogens and respiratory tract infections. *Eur Respir J.* 2004;24(1):171–181.

Cooper RJ, Hoffman JR, Barlett JG, et al. Principles of appropriate antibiotic use for acute pharyngitis in adults: background. *Ann Int Med.* 2001;134(6):509–517.

Garibaldi RA. Epidemiology of community-acquired respiratory tract infections in adults: incidence, etiology, and impact. *Am J Med.* 1985;78(6B):32–37.

König D, Grathwohl D, Weinstock C, et al. Upper respiratory tract infection in athletes: influence of lifestyle, type of sport, training effort, and immunostimulant intake. *Exerc Immunol Rev.* 2000;6:102–120.

Lieberman D, Lieberman D, Korsonsky I, et al. A comparative study of the etiology of adult upper and lower respiratory tract infections in the community. *Diagn Microbiol Infect Dis.* 2002;42(1):21–28.

McKinnon LT. Immunity in Athletes. *Int J Sports Med.* 1997;18(Suppl 1):S62–S68.

Nieman DC. Exercise and resistance to infection. *Can J Physiol Pharmacol.* 1998;76(5):573–580.

Spurling GK, Del Mar CB, Dooley L, Foxlee R. Delayed antibiotics for symptoms and complications of respiratory infections. *Cochrane Database of Systematic Reviews.* 2004(4):CD004417.

CHAPTER 47

Acute Abdominal Pain

Contributed by Abel Wakai, St. James's Hospital, Dublin; and John M. Ryan, St. Vincent's University Hospital, Dublin, and Medical Officer, Leinster Rugby Football Team, Irish Rugby Football Union, and Irish Hockey Union

Reviewer: Katharina Grimm, Head of Medical Office, FIFA, Zurich, Switzerland

Abdominal pain in an athlete may be due to a sports-related intra-abdominal injury, non–sports-related abdominal conditions, or referred pain from adjacent anatomical structures. A systematic evaluation is mandatory in the assessment of acute abdominal pain by the EP. The principal characteristics of acute abdominal pain include location, quality, severity, onset, duration, radiation, and aggravating and alleviating factors. By combining a thorough history, assessment of hemodynamic stability, and a systematic four-quadrant abdominal examination, the EP can reach a clinically valid working diagnosis.

47.1 CLINICAL EVALUATION

History

The diagnoses of many causes of abdominal pain can be made by history alone. Key points in the history include the following:

- Time of onset
- Mode of onset (sudden or gradual onset)
- Type of sporting activity if sports-related (e.g., lower abdominal pain due to athletic pubalgia or "sports hernia" is more likely with running, basketball, soccer, American football, and baseball)
- Location (e.g., flank pain after a direct blow is suggestive of renal trauma)
- Radiation (e.g., to the back)
- Character

- Duration
- Progression
- Aggravating or relieving factors
- Past medical history
- Travel history (e.g., typhoid)
- Menstrual history
- Associated symptoms (e.g., fever, anorexia, nausea, vomiting, change in bowel habit, dysuria, hematuria, hesitancy, melena, dyspnea, or chest pain)

Physical Examination

The principles of the physical examination are

- To confirm the diagnoses suggested by the history
- To localize the pathology
- To avoid missing extra-abdominal causes of abdominal pain

Key points in the physical examination include the following:

- Vital signs (heart frequency, blood pressure, breathing, temperature)
- Abdominal examination (auscultation, inspection, palpation)
- Genitalia, respiratory system, skin, spine, and hips (if referred pain and an extra-abdominal cause is a possibility)

Rectal examination (for blood, masses, and tenderness) and pelvic examination (for blood, masses, tenderness, and discharge) may be clinically indicated but not practical in the out-of-hospital setting.

47.2 SPORTS-RELATED INTRA-ABDOMINAL INJURY

Exercise-Related Transient Abdominal Pain

This condition, often loosely referred to as "side ache" or "stitch in the side" or "side cramp" by athletes, characteristically occurs during running, early in an exercise regimen of an unconditioned athlete. Although the etiology of exercise-related transient abdominal pain (ETAP) is unknown, several etiologic factors, including muscle cramping, have been postulated (Table 47.1). Recent evidence, however, suggests that pain associated with ETAP is not the result of muscle cramping. When an athlete warms up appropriately, the incidence of this phenomenon decreases (Table 47.2). Meanwhile, ETAP does not preclude participation in most sports because most athletes learn how to deal with it. The only treatment required for ETAP is therefore reassurance and advice to the athlete regarding the importance of appropriately warming up by the event physician.

Blunt Abdominal Trauma

Abdominal injuries are rare in sports and EPs may not see them frequently. Because of this, the early signs of sports-related intra-abdominal injury may be missed, even in cases that progress to shock or collapse. However, with the increasing popularity of

TABLE 47.1	Etiologic Factors in ETAP

- Diaphragmatic ischemia
- Visceral connective tissue stress
- Local skeletal muscle cramp
- Acute increase in venous return from the lower extremities to the liver
- Inhibition of the movement of intestinal contents

TABLE 47.2	ETAP Treatment Modalities

1. Reassurance
2. Offer advice regarding warming up appropriately

TABLE 47.3	Symptoms of Intra-abdominal Visceral Injury

- Severe abdominal pain
- Thirst
- Hematuria

snowboarding and extreme skiing, the rate of abdominal injuries is beginning to rise slightly. Sports injuries account for 10% of all abdominal injuries, with the spleen being the most commonly injured organ. Though the liver is the most frequently injured abdominal organ in general, the spleen is the most frequently injured organ in sport, and spleen injuries are the most common cause of death due to abdominal trauma in athletes. The kidney is also commonly injured from blunt abdominal trauma. American football, hockey, and martial arts are the sports associated with the greatest risk for renal injury.

It is therefore important that the EP is alert to the warning signs of potentially life-threatening injury to solid (liver, spleen) or hollow abdominal viscera. Patients with evolving major intra-abdominal injuries may be relatively asymptomatic initially and may manifest minimal physical signs. Though the EP may not always provide definitive treatment of many of these conditions, he or she should be familiar with the preferred diagnostic modalities and latest treatment options so that he or she can appropriately triage the patient. This information is also important in making return-to-play decisions.

Athletes who sustain a direct blow to the abdomen that results in injury to spleen, liver, or kidney may have immediate severe pain and can rapidly develop signs of shock and peritonism (Tables 47.3 and 47.4). The EP always needs to be aware of this

TABLE 47.4	Signs of Intra-abdominal Visceral Injury

- Pallor
- Diaphoresis
- Prolonged capillary refill time
- Rapid and thready pulse
- Hypotension
- Peritonism

possibility. In addition, athletes who have sustained a direct blow causing slower bleeding may collapse later on the field, at the sideline, or at home. They will be pale and sweaty and will complain of thirst, and their pulse will be rapid and thready (Table 47.4). If blunt abdominal trauma is associated with abdominal pain, the athlete should be given nil by mouth (no liquids to drink). If the athlete collapses or has clinical peritonism, he or she should be placed in a recumbent position, and their legs elevated in order to assist blood in returning to the heart (Trendelenburg position) (Table 47.5).

47.3 NON–SPORTS-RELATED INTRA-ABDOMINAL CONDITIONS

Surgical Causes

These arise from pathology in gastrointestinal, genitourinary, gynecologic, and vascular structures. The "quadrantic approach" is most practical (Table 47.6).

It is also possible to have right-sided pain as an early sign of acute appendicitis. A so-called typical or classical course in acute appendicitis is the following and occurs in about half of the patients: Initially, the athlete will have a loss of appetite, followed by periumbilical or generalized abdominal pain. With progressing inflammation, the chief complaint of the athlete with acute appendicitis might be severe pain in the lower right quadrant. At times, this pain will be excruciating. The athlete will experience nausea, possibly vomiting, and develop a fever that increases over time. The athlete will be point tender to palpation in the lower right quadrant and should be taken to the hospital immediately.

However, presentation of appendicitis is, in fact, notoriously inconsistent with protean manifestations, and no single sign, symptom, or diagnostic test accurately confirms the diagnosis of appendicitis in all cases. The main findings on examination of the abdomen are rebound tenderness, pain on percussion, rigidity, and guarding. With diagnostic or therapeutic delay, or without medical attention, perforation rate increases and an athlete may die from the complications associated with a ruptured appendix.

Nonsurgical Causes

Most cases of acute abdominal pain do not arise from surgical pathology. The abdominal pain due to these nonsurgical causes is typically diffuse in nature. Despite sophisticated modern diagnostic technology, for patients presenting to emergency departments with abdominal pain, undifferentiated abdominal pain remains the commonest diagnosis for both discharged (25%) and admitted (35% to 41%) patients. Other less common nonsurgical causes of abdominal pain based on etiology are metabolic, infectious, inherited, and neurogenic (Table 47.7).

Extra-abdominal Conditions (Referred Pain)

Pain from adjacent anatomical regions can be referred to the abdomen and present as abdominal pain (Table 47.8). For example, diaphragmatic inflammation resulting from pneumonia may present as right upper quadrant abdominal pain; acute myocardial infarction and pericarditis may present with epigastric pain. Furthermore, upper gastrointestinal conditions such as acute cholecystitis or a perforated peptic ulcer are frequently associated with intrathoracic complications; for example, hemoperitoneum associated with solid visceral abdominal injury may present as supraclavicular or shoulder tip pain. Similarly, acute distension of the extrahepatic biliary tree may present as subscapular pain.

Abdominal pain of extra-abdominal origin can present a diagnostic challenge to the EP because it is substantially less common than that of intra-abdominal origin. The EP should consider the possibility of referred pain in every athlete with abdominal pain, especially if the

TABLE 47.5	Immediate Management of Intra-abdominal Visceral Injury if in Shock or Collapsed

- Keep in recumbent position
- Trendelenburg position
- Rapid transport to a hospital (preferably to a center with advanced trauma life-support capabilities)

TABLE 47.6 — Quadrantic Approach to the Differential Diagnosis of Acute Abdominal Pain

Quadrant	Common Causes of Acute Abdominal Pain
Right upper quadrant	Atypical acute appendicitis
	Biliary tract disease (e.g., acute cholecystitis)
	Inflammatory bowel disease
	Liver disease
	Meckel diverticulum
	Subphrenic abscess
Left upper quadrant	Pancreatitis
	Perforated peptic ulcer
	Splenic rupture
	Subphrenic abscess
Right lower quadrant	Acute appendicitis
	Bowel obstruction
	Diverticulitis
	Ectopic pregnancy
	Endometriosis
	Hernia
	Inflammatory bowel disease
	Irritable bowel syndrome
	Meckel diverticulum
	Mesenteric adenitis
	Mittelschmerz
	Ovarian cyst
	Pelvic inflammatory bowel disease/tuboovarian abscess
	Spontaneous/threatened abortion
	Urolithiasis
Left lower quadrant	Acute diverticulitis
	Bowel obstruction
	Ectopic pregnancy
	Endometriosis
	Hernia
	Inflammatory bowel disease
	Irritable bowel syndrome
	Mittelschmerz
	Ovarian cyst
	Pelvic inflammatory bowel disease/tuboovarian abscess
	Psoas abscess
	Spontaneous/threatened abortion
	Urolithiasis

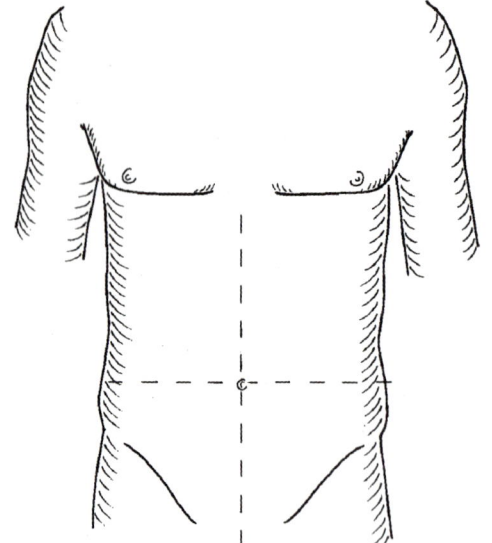

FIGURE 47.1.   The four abdominal quadrants.

presenting complaint is upper abdominal pain and if there are no obvious correlating signs on physical examination. This should prompt the search for an extra-abdominal cause of the abdominal pain. In particular, clinical assessment should be aimed at determining the presence of intrathoracic

pathology (e.g., myocardial infarction, pulmonary infarction, pneumonia, or pericarditis).

Case Histories

Case History 1: You are the EP at a European athletic meeting and are called to see a 22-year-old female athlete complaining of severe abdominal pain. She states that she was well until 48 hours previously when she developed abdominal pain while on a flight from India where she had been on holiday. She has tried to "stick it out" but the pain has progressively worsened and is presently unbearable. Her past medical history is unremarkable. She is taking no regular medication. She also complains of high fever and constipation for the previous 48 hours. On examination, she is unwell and dehydrated, with marked central and hypogastric abdominal rebound tenderness and guarding. Psoas sign, obturator sign, and Rovsing's sign are all negative. What is your differential diagnosis and disposition of the patient?

Case History 2: A 20-year-old male rugby player collapses on the pitch while running. As the EP, you immediately run onto the pitch to find him conscious but distressed and clutching his abdomen.

TABLE 47.7	**Nonsurgical Causes of Acute Abdominal Pain**	
Etiology	**Clinical Condition**	**Clinical Condition**
Infectious	Gastroenteritis	Urinary tract infection
	Acute hepatitis	Pelvic inflammatory disease
	Typhoid	Henoch-Schonlein purpura
		Acute rheumatic fever
Metabolic	Addison disease	Diabetic ketoacidosis
	Uremia	Hypercalcemia
		Lead toxicity (e.g., secondary to herbal remedy ingestion)
Hematologic	Sickle cell crisis	Leukemia
Neurogenic	Herpes zoster	Tabes dorsalis
	Referred spinal pain (see below)	
Inherited	Acute intermittent porphyria	Familial Mediterranean fever
	Hereditary angioedema (C1 esterase deficiency)	
Miscellaneous	Drug-related (e.g., alcohol, cocaine)	Irritable bowel syndrome
	Psychogenic	

TABLE **47.8**	**Referred Acute Abdominal Pain**
Origin of Pain	**Clinical Condition**
Thoracic cavity	Lobar pneumonia
	Pulmonary infarction (secondary to pulmonary embolism)
	Acute myocardial infarction
	Acute pericarditis
	Dissecting thoracic aortic aneurysm
Genitalia	Testicular torsion
Spine	Prolapsed intervertebral disc
	Facet joint dysfunction
Hip	Osteoarthritis

He received a blow to his abdomen while playing rugby 4 days previously but denies any trauma today. He has been taking some paracetamol for abdominal pain for the previous 3 days. He looks pale and diaphoretic. His radial pulse is rapid (130 per minute) and thready. On abdominal examination, he has some bruising over his left upper quadrant associated with rebound tenderness and guarding. What is the most likely diagnosis? Describe your immediate management of this player.

Case History 3: At an athletic meeting, a 16-year-old male athlete presents to you, as the event physician, complaining of sudden-onset lower abdominal pain and scrotal pain 1 hour previously. He denies any other gastrointestinal symptoms. He is sexually active and admits to some dysuria but no urethral discharge over the last couple of days. His past medical history was unremarkable and he was not taking any regular medications. On physical examination, his abdomen is soft and nontender. But he has obvious generalized scrotal erythema with bilateral testicular tenderness. What is the differential diagnosis? What disposition is required for this patient?

Case History 4: A 30-year-old female athlete preparing for a triathlon the next day consults you with a 2-day history of dull lower abdominal pain, nausea, and urinary frequency. She has a past history of endometriosis. Other than this, her more recent medical history is unremarkable

and she was taking no regular medications. She has no other urinary or gastrointestinal symptoms. Her vital signs are normal. Abdominal examination is unremarkable. What is the differential diagnosis? What disposition is required for this patient?

Discussion of Case Histories

Case History 1: Differential diagnosis includes acute appendicitis and typhoid. Appendicitis often causes vague central abdominal pain that localizes to the right iliac fossa. Nausea, vomiting, and diarrhea may be associated features. Psoas sign (extend the patient's leg at the hip with the patient in the lateral decubitus position, to move the psoas muscle), obturator sign (flex and externally and internally rotate hip), and Rovsing's sign (palpation in the left lower quadrant causes pain in the right lower quadrant) are all suggestive of appendicitis but are only present in a fraction of patients. The EP must maintain a high index of suspicion for unusual infectious causes of abdominal pain when there is a history of recent foreign travel, especially to the tropics. Meanwhile, typhoid and malaria are the first diseases to consider if fever develops after a visit to the tropics. Typhoid (caused by *Salmonella typhi*) causes severe abdominal pain and tenderness. If there is a change in bowel habit, it is toward constipation, but diarrhea may occur. A high fever, other constitutional symptoms, and recent foreign travel should alert the EP to the possibility of typhoid. This patient has to go to a hospital immediately for further investigation, including blood cultures for *S. typhi*, because intestinal perforation can complicate typhoid.

Case History 2: The most likely diagnosis is delayed presentation of splenic trauma. Traumatic splenic rupture usually occurs as a result of direct blow to the left lower chest wall or left upper quadrant of the abdomen. With the exception of splenic avulsion or shatter, lesser degrees of splenic trauma classically result in delayed presentation. This patient is hemodynamically unstable. He should be kept recumbent in the Trendelenburg position and rapidly transported to the care of a surgeon in a hospital.

Case History 3: Differential diagnosis includes testicular torsion and epididymitis. Testicular torsion should be considered in any adolescent patient presenting with a painful or swollen testis. Symptoms of testicular torsion include sudden, severe testicular pain, which may radiate to the groin and be referred to the lower abdomen (hypogastrium). There may be nausea and vomiting and, occasionally, a history of similar but self-limiting pain. There are no specific or pathognomic clinical signs that permit precise differentiation of testicular torsion from epididymitis. The patient should therefore be referred for urgent surgical review to prevent testicular infarction.

Case History 4: Differential diagnosis includes a urinary tract infection, endometriosis, or ectopic pregnancy. Urinary tract infection can account for all the symptoms (lower abdominal pain, nausea, and urinary frequency) this athlete has. Meanwhile, endometriosis can cause urinary tract symptoms (hematuria, dysuria, and urinary frequency) as a result of endometriosis lying on the outside of the bladder or irritation from endometrial implants lying anterior to the uterus. However, an ectopic pregnancy needs to be ruled out in any female of childbearing age with abdominal pain. Failure to make prompt and correct diagnosis of ectopic pregnancy could result in tubal or uterine rupture, depending on the location of the pregnancy, which could lead to massive hemorrhage, shock, disseminated intravascular coagulopathy, and death. A high index of suspicion is necessary to make a prompt and early diagnosis, and avoid the complications of ectopic pregnancy. The EP should therefore refer the patient to a hospital for investigations to rule out an ectopic pregnancy.

Recommended Reading

Ahumada LA, Ashruf S, Espinosa-de-los-Monteros A, et al. Athletic pubalgia: definition and surgical treatment. *Ann Plast Surg.* 2005;55(4):393–396.

Brewer RJ, Golden GT, Hitch DC, et al. Abdominal pain. An analysis of 1,000 consecutive cases in a university hospital emergency room. *Am J Surg.* 1976;131:219–223.

Davenport M. ABC of general surgery in children: acute problems of the scrotum. *Br Med J.* 1996;312:435–437.

Diamond DL. Sports-related abdominal trauma. *Clin Sports Med.* 1989;8(1):91–99.

Finkler JH. Abdominal pain: myths and misdiagnosis. Parkhurst Exchange. 2008;16(3), http://www.parkhurstexchange.com/clinical-reviews/mar08-p70. Accessed April 6, 2011.

Flik K, Callahan LR. Delayed splenic rupture in amateur hockey player. *Clin J Sport Med.* 1998;8:309–310.

Gross H. Evaluation of abdominal pain in the emergency department. http://www.google.com/search?hl=en&q=Gross+H%2C+evaluation+of+abdominal+pain&btnG=Search. Accessed November 3, 2008.

Irvin TT. Abdominal pain: a surgical audit of 1190 emergency admissions. *Br J Surg.* 1989;76(11):1121–1125.

Morton DP. Exercise related transient abdominal pain. *Br J Sports Med.* 2003;37(4):287–288.

Morton DP, Callister R. EMG activity is not elevated during exercise-related transient abdominal pain. *J Sci Med Sport.* 2008;11(6)569–574.

Powers RD, Guertler AT. Abdominal pain in the ED: stability and change over 20 years. *Am J Emerg Med.* 1995;13(3):301–303.

Rifat SF, Gilvydis RP. Blunt abdominal trauma in sports. *Curr Sports Med Rep.* 2003;2(2):93–97.

Walter KD. Radiographic evaluation of the patient with sport-related abdominal trauma. *Curr Sports Med Rep.* 2007;6(2):115–119.

Waninger KN, Harcke HT. Determination of safe return to play for athletes recovering from infectious mononucleosis: a review of the literature. *Clin J Sport Med.* 2005;15:410–416.

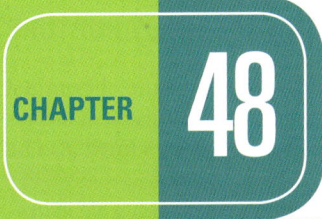

CHAPTER 48

Abdominal Injuries

Contributed by David McDonagh, Chair, FIBT Medical Committee

Reviewer: John Ryan, Leinster Rugby Football Club, Irish Hockey Union, Dublin, Ireland

48.1 ABDOMINAL WALL INJURIES

Blows to the abdominal wall are not infrequent in sport and can be seen with "winding" or "solar plexus" punches. They may result in contusions in the abdominal wall muscles (usually the rectus abdominis muscle). As with other contusions, early icing, NSAID treatment, and rest are the usual modalities. Some athletes may need several days rest, others several weeks. Other injuries, such as lateral and rotatory stretching, sudden explosive weight lifting, and hyperextension of the spine, can cause partial muscle tears and contusions. Similarly, tennis players are commonly afflicted with myalgia in the rectus and transversus muscles—probably due to the rotations involved in serving.

Diagnosis is usually straightforward as the pain is usually superficial and can be easily provoked by stretching the affected muscle. One can also ask the athlete to tighten the abdominal muscles, and this usually causes pain if the lesion is in the abdominal wall. Palpation will further enhance the discomfort.

One must always be aware of the possibility of underlying organ injury or injuries when examining the abdomen, and minor organ injuries can be overseen.

48.2 BLUNT ABDOMINAL INJURIES

Serious abdominal injuries are caused by blunt or penetrating trauma. The most common trauma mechanism is when an athlete who is moving at speed has a sudden, rapid deceleration due to being hit by another athlete or crashing into an object. This rapid deceleration can cause intra-abdominal organ contusion, hemorrhages, or even laceration. Obviously, the greater the initial speed, the greater the deceleration, and the greater the injury potential. The organs most commonly involved in sport are the spleen, liver, and small intestine. One must be aware of these potential injuries particularly in high-velocity sports such as bicycling, alpine skiing, ski jumping, and motor sports, as well as in contact sports such as rugby, American football, soccer, boxing, and other martial arts, as well as injuries from bicycle and motorbike handlebars.

Evaluation and Examination

- Blunt injuries may cause external injuries, such as abrasions, contusions, and lacerations. Abdominal tenderness, guarding, and rigidity, even abdominal distension may be found.

- Percussion of the abdomen may offer some important information in this prehospital environment—such as tympanitic sounds with gastric distension or dull sounds with hemoperitoneum. Auscultation of the abdomen may reveal the presence or absence of bowel sounds. Rupture of the spleen, liver, and kidneys can occur in various degrees, but the finding of signs of shock with low blood pressure, rapid pulse, pale skin, and constriction of peripheral vessels combined with pain and guarding over the liver and spleen should give cause for alarm. With major bleeding, abdominal distension may occur, and this is obviously a critical situation requiring immediate intervention and patient evacuation.

- Hematuria can indicate kidney rupture or kidney injury. Treatment is discussed below.

48.3 PENETRATING ABDOMINAL INJURIES

Penetrating injuries occur when the abdominal region abruptly comes into contact with sharp objects. These objects can be part of the sporting apparel such as in fencing or gymnastics but can also be any kind of stationery object such as picket fences, camera equipment, or glass windows. Remember, there may be accompanying thoracic and diaphragmatic injury.

Evaluation and Examination

The presence of a penetrating object must be noted and an assumption made over which internal organs may be injured. There is always the possibility of a foreign body having entered the abdomen, but this is unlikely in a sporting environment. The adage "Never remove a foreign body" applies, as removal almost always increases bleeding (an exception being penetrating injury to the cheeks). Penetrating foreign bodies should be left in place and immobilized to prevent further damage to internal organs (movement may cause a sawing-like effect) during transport. Open wounds should be covered with saline-dampened bandages. There may be increasing abdominal swelling. Guarding and pain may be present if the patient is conscious. There may be dull percussion sounds due to internal bleeding. Auscultation of the abdomen may reveal the absence of normal intra-abdominal sounds.

Treatment

Secure adequate oxygenation and ventilation; evaluate the need for intubation.

Blood volume should be restored by giving intravenous solutions such as Ringer's lactate/saline or plasma expanders; however, rapid infusion is not advised as the sudden rise in blood pressure may disturb the natural wound hemostasis. A slow infusion is advised. If possible, use wide-bore intravenous catheters; two portals are better than one.

If the patient is becoming hemodynamically unstable, then rapid transportation to the nearest hospital is required. In-flight treatment may also be necessary, so the athlete may be accompanied by a physician. Intravenous analgesia may be considered in conscious patients. Nitrous oxide should be avoided. The use of antishock trousers is usually contraindicated due to the risk of intra-abdominal bleeding.

48.4 GASTROINTESTINAL TRACT RUPTURE

In high-energy trauma injuries to the abdominal region, severe intra-abdominal lesions must always be suspected. Asymptomatic patients must also be evaluated.

Rupture of the small intestine can give symptoms similar to those of peritonitis. Rupture of the colon often causes pain and guarding initially. Injuries of the pancreas are often overseen due to lack of clinical findings in the initial phase.

Treatment

Routine stabilization treatment with free airway, oxygen, and intravenous infusion.

Analgesia if necessary. Due to the risk of occult injury, all high-energy abdominal injuries should be admitted to a hospital for observation and/or advanced diagnostic imaging.

48.5 DIAPHRAGMATIC RUPTURE

Most lacerations occur on the left hemidiaphragm and result from automobile accidents. The stomach can herniate into the thorax and may undergo volvulus, causing the stomach to dilate, thus compressing the left lung. There is often a mediastinal shift to the right. Gastric distension can also result in perforation and should be prevented by inserting a nasogastric tube.

Splenic and liver injury are also common with penetrating diaphragmatic injuries.

Diagnosis

Dyspnea, hypoxia, and abdominal pain may be present. Impaired respiratory sounds, loss of resonant percussion sounds over the lower lung region may be found. Diaphragmatic injury is often associated with other severe thoracicoabdominal injuries.

Treatment

Secure oxygenation and ventilation. The patient may often require intubation before transportation. Hypovolemia must be corrected. Nasogastric tube insertion may be necessary to prevent gastric distension. Severe pain must also be treated.

48.6 SPLENIC INJURIES

Blunt trauma, often after a direct blow from a knee, shoulder, or kick to the upper left abdomen, may cause bruising, tearing, or even rupture of the spleen. The spleen has a rich blood supply so trauma to the spleen may also cause varying degrees of internal bleeding. Splenic injury can be classified in several ways, but for the event physician, the most critical issue is to decide whether or not there is damage to the splenic blood vessels—in other words, is the athlete hemodynamically stable or not?

In milder injuries, there may be small capsular tears and small subcapsular hematomas, without any significant damage to the splenic parenchyma, where bleeding is limited and local.

Contusions of the spleen may occur, so there is bruising and bleeding, affecting larger areas of the spleen.

Finally, lacerations can occur, and if these involve the main splenic blood vessels of the spleen (which they often do), there may be serious internal bleeding. The spleen filters between 500 and 750 mL of blood per minute. With penetrating injuries, great care must be taken in avoiding infection as the spleen produces white blood cells.

The main challenge for the event physician is to detect these serious splenic lacerations, offer correct treatment, and admit patients urgently to a hospital. With minor injuries, there is also concern regarding return-to-play issues, as undiagnosed capsular tears and contusions may worsen if reexposed to trauma, especially if there is an underlying mononucleosis or splenamegaly.

Field-Side Diagnosis

The history of blunt trauma to the upper left abdomen, such as a knee or shoulder tackle in rugby or American football, or a stick in ice hockey, should raise concern. (Always ask about previous or current Epstein-Barr infections and other illnesses.)

In the hemodynamically stable athlete, there may be localized or general abdominal pain, tenderness, swelling, or localized guarding. Surrounding ribs may be fractured.

If there is splenic vessel damage, then the patient may present with symptoms of shock or, more commonly in sport, gradual onset of shock symptoms and findings such as dizziness, vomiting, fainting, sweating, pale or clammy skin, rapid heartbeat and weak pulse, falling blood pressure, dyspnea and generalized deterioration of vital signs and eventually loss of consciousness.

Always consider other causes of shock.

Field-Side Treatment

With severe splenic injury, treatment is obvious but extremely demanding: ABC, stabilize as best you can, load, and go. Obviously, ensure that the airway is patent, give 100% oxygen, ventilate if necessary, insert a venous catheter—preferably two, if you can—and administer fluid. Accompany the athlete to a hospital if the medical staff in the ambulance does not have sufficient emergency training. If there are time or distance factors involved, order a helicopter.

With moderate splenic injury, the athlete should be withdrawn from sporting activity, stabilized, and transferred to a hospital for a CT/ultrasound investigation. Ensure that the airway is patent, give 100% oxygen, insert a venous catheter just in case, and administer IV fluid, if in doubt.

If you are unsure of the presence of splenic injury and choose not to refer the athlete for further investigation, then it is important to evaluate the athlete's status, observe for a period, and reevaluate the situation. Remember that athletes can appear to be in reasonably good form for some hours after injuring their spleen, before suddenly deteriorating. The athlete or his or her coaching team should be informed of this possibility so that plans can be adapted (e.g., long air flights, return to remote locations).

Predisposing Factors

Splenic trauma is more common in children than in adults, probably due to the fact that they are more active than adults, but also because their abdominal organs are less protected by bone, muscle, and fat.

In adults, ruptured spleens are sometimes associated with splenomegaly caused by infections such as infectious mononucleosis, immune system disorders, malignancy, and other splenic diseases. Atraumatic ruptures have been reported.

48.7 KIDNEYS

The kidneys are usually well protected deep in the abdomen by the lower rib cage and back muscles. Blunt trauma can however damage the kidneys, and injuries are seen in American Football, ice hockey, rugby, soccer, lacrosse, bicycle accidents, and equestrian sports. Some athletes have transplanted kidneys, and these are to be found lower in the abdomen often under the normal position.

Clinical Features

First, look for abrasions or bruising over the loin or abdomen. There should also be pain and tenderness in the same area. There may be a loss of loin contour and look for the presence of a loin mass. Fractured ribs may also be found. Often, blood is found in the urine if there is renal damage; however, the absence of hematuria does not exclude kidney injury (as seen when there is disruption between the kidney and ureter). Bleeding can range from microscopic to macroscopic hematuria to profuse bleeding. In some cases, there is significant blood loss and hypovolemic shock can develop. The combination of macroscopic hematuria and hypotension is potentially serious. Severe renal trauma is often accompanied by other intra-abdominal organ trauma. It is impossible to correctly classify a damaged kidney in the prehospital environment.

Classification of Kidney Injuries

- Class I: Renal contusion or contained subcapsular hematoma

- Class II: Cortical laceration without urinary extravasation

- Class III: Parenchymal lesion extending more than 1 cm into renal substance

- Class IV: Laceration extending across the corticomedullary junction

- Class V: Renal fragmentation or renovascular pedicle injury

Treatment

If you suspect renal trauma, then the patient should be stabilized and transferred to a hospital for CT examination—ultrasound examination alone is not sufficient. As renal trauma is often associated with other abdominal organ injury, it is a good idea to refer symptomatic athletes to further evaluation. A urine sample should test negative for blood before an athlete is allowed to return to play.

Almost all class I and II blunt renal injuries and most class III and IV injuries—are treated conservatively with strict bed rest until hematuria has resolved. Surgical repair is seldom needed after blunt sports trauma.

Penetrating trauma is often much more serious. Stabilize the patient and the foreign body, check ABC set up an intravenous line, and transfer the patient to a hospital as soon as possible. Such trauma often requires surgical exploration, although accurate CT injury staging may allow conservative treatment if the patient is hemodynamically stable and has no other associated intra-abdominal injuries. Late complications of renal injury include hypertension, arteriovenous fistula, hydronephrosis, pseudocyst or calculi formation, chronic pyelonephritis, and loss of renal function.

48.8 LIVER INJURIES

Injuries to the liver, bile duct, and pancreas are not uncommon and pose a significant challenge to the event physician in terms of both diagnosis and management. In the prehospital setting, these injuries require a high index of suspicion, rapid diagnosis and treatment of hemorrhagic conditions, referral, and transport protocols.

Despite being relatively well protected, the liver is the most frequently injured intra-abdominal organ in nonsporting accidents. Liver injuries can be classified in many ways: anatomically, by the extent of vascular injury (subcapsular vessel injuries, transcapsular vessel injuries, and in-/outflow–vessel injuries), by organ injury scale (AAST) classification, or by CT classification.

For the event physician, the challenge is to find out if there is any injury at all and, if an injury is present, to try to evaluate the extent of the injury. The most serious risk is that of hemorrhage, so defining the patient's hemodynamic status—stable or unstable—is the correct clinical starting point. The hemodynamically unstable patient requires rapid treatment and transportation. Findings include local signs of injury as well as rapid heartbeat and weak pulse, falling blood pressure,

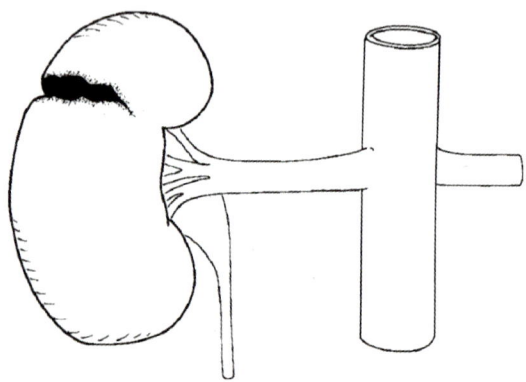

FIGURE 48.1. Kidney rupture.

dyspnea, generalized deterioration of vital signs, and eventually, loss of consciousness. Always consider other causes of shock.

The hemodynamically stable patient with a probable liver injury should be given oxygen, an intravenous portal should be established, and the patient should be rapidly transferred to a hospital.

If the patient has normal and stable pulse and blood pressure but is dizzy, vomiting, fainting, malaise, or sweating, or has pale or clammy skin, then there is a serious possibility that there is some form of bleeding—again, rapid airway/circulation intervention and hospital transportation are required. The patient with abdominal tenderness and any other symptom (dizzy, vomiting, fainting, malaise, sweating, or pale or clammy skin) should be withdrawn from the event and referred to a hospital. The need for referral of a patient who has abdominal tenderness but no other symptoms or signs (and who is, of course, hemodynamically stable) has to be made on an individual basis—but if the pain and tenderness are moderate and the case history does not suggest major impact trauma, then the patient can be observed and reevaluated after 10 to 15 minutes. Once again, the importance of taking an accurate and detailed case history cannot be emphasized enough.

Pancreatic trauma is rare but is seen with injury to other organs.

48.9 WINDING

Winding is a relatively common injury in contact sports, resulting from a blow to the abdomen. The exact pathophysiologic mechanism is unknown; however, it is thought that the force causes vagal stimulation and temporary diaphragmatic spasm. Typically, the winded athlete doubles up and has difficulty breathing. The situation resolves itself quickly without any residual symptoms. If symptoms persist, there may be internal injury requiring examination, observation, reexamination, and even hospital referral.

Recommended Reading

As with Chapter 47.

CHAPTER 49

Genital/Venereal Conditions and Injuries

Contributed by David McDonagh, Deputy CMO, Lillehammer 1994 Olympic Winter Games

Reviewer: Jan Mjønes, Head of Urology Department, St. Olavs University Hospital, Trondheim, Norway

Trauma

Genital trauma is more common in men and includes injury to the testes, scrotum, and penis. Penetrating injuries can occur, though these are very rare in my experience. Minor lacerations can occur in the penis or scrotum, as well as bites, burns and zipper injuries. Blunt trauma is the commonest cause of testicular injury and can lead to testicular contusion, even ruptures if the tunica albuginea is damaged.

Penile injuries are rare, though an athlete may present with problems that arose during sexual intercourse—for example, penile fractures (corpus cavernosum rupture) and strangulation.

Clinical Findings

A direct blow to the scrotum (knee, fist, foot) can cause intense pain, nausea, and even scrotal swelling. The scrotum may be discolored and tender. If there is bleeding, one may be able to palpate a hard scrotal mass or hematocele, but examination is usually limited by pain. The scrotum may fail to transilluminate. In these cases, it is wise to refer the patient to scrotal ultrasound in case there is a need for surgical repair.

Zipper injuries can be corrected by injecting local anesthetic into the affected area and attempting to unzip the zipper. If this does not work, try to cut the bar on the top of the zipper slider using a wire cutter; the zipper then breaks in two and usually comes apart.

49.1 ACUTE TESTICULAR PAIN

Acute, nontraumatic testicular pain can occur at any age, and the commonest causes are

- Testicular torsion
- Acute epididymitis
- Acute epididymo-orchitis

Differentiating among these entities is almost impossible in the prehospital environment, so I recommend that all patients be referred to a specialist surgical unit quickly. Always take a good medical history: Is this an acute episode, or have there been similar episodes or inflammation or pain in nearby structures? Inquire about possible trauma episodes, recent or past, mild or severe. Inquire about previous genitourinary infections and symptoms of these. Ultrasound is a useful diagnostic tool but *do not* refer suspected testicular torsions to x-ray departments: Refer them to a surgical unit and let the surgeons order the ultrasound. Why? Sometimes patients can wait for hours at an x-ray department—hours that may be important in relation to spermatogenesis and the future vitality of the testicle.

49.2 TESTICULAR TORSION

Testicular torsion is a surgical emergency, and if suspected, patients must be urgently transferred to a hospital. Failure to operate within an appropriate time may lead to reduced spermatogenesis (4 hours) in the affected testicle or even infarction (6 hours), resulting in amputation. If you suspect torsion, I repeat, do not send the athlete to radiology first; send him straight to the surgeon/urologist.

Torsion can occur at any age but is most frequent in adolescent males. There is usually a predisposing congenital abnormality (often called the "bell-clapper" anomaly) that allows the testicle to rotate on the spermatic cord within the tunica vaginalis, causing venous and arterial occlusion, with subsequent arterial ischemia and possibly infarction of the testicle.

The bell-clapper abnormality is reportedly present in 12% of males, of which almost 40% have a bilateral anomaly. Torsion may be categorized as complete, incomplete, or transient.

History

- Sudden onset of unilateral scrotal pain, usually intense and usually in the absence of trauma

- Pain can occasionally build up slowly

- Some patients have a previous history of intermittent testicular pain that resolved spontaneously (intermittent torsion and detorsion)

- Scrotal swelling

- Nausea and vomiting

- Abdominal pain

- Fever

- Urinary frequency

Clinical Findings

Due to pain and discomfort, clinical examination is not always easy, but the patient's extreme tenderness or discomfort should in itself alert one to the possibility of a torsion. Common findings are

- Tender testicle on palpation

- Edematous swollen testicle—sometimes swollen scrotum

- The affected testicle may be elevated and may have a horizontal lie

- Enlargement and edema of the testicle

- Scrotal erythema

- Ipsilateral loss of the cremasteric reflex

- Fever has been described

Treatment

Prehospital treatment requires diagnostic alertness and urgent referral to a surgical unit.

49.3 ACUTE EPIDIDYMITIS

Epididymitis can present with a relatively acute inflammation of the epididymis and can thus mimic a testicular torsion. Usually, the onset is more insidious with pain and swelling of the epididymis being the dominant signs and symptoms. Patients are usually youngish, from the late teens to the middle 30s. The condition is usually caused by a bacterial infection and is often, but not always, transmitted sexually—so gonorrhea or chlamydia must be examined for. On occasions, viruses or fungi may be the cause. Not all inflammations have organic origins; cyclists can have discomfort due to constant pressure, and some sources postulate "reverse flow" urine irritation as the cause of "Weight lifters' epididymitis." On occasion, the patient may also present with orchitis, where the testicle also becomes inflamed.

History

A history of recent sexual contact, penile discharge, urethritis symptoms, or prostatic symptoms may be indicative of an infectious condition. Patients complain of testicular pain and may complain of pain during intercourse or ejaculation. The pain may radiate to the lower abdomen or pelvis. There may be blood in the semen. The condition can last for weeks or months if untreated.

Clinical Findings

Clinical findings may include

- A swollen, red, or warm scrotum

- Tender, swollen epididymis/testicle

- Enlarged inguinal lymph nodes

- Discharge from the penis

Treatment

If the patient has a painful scrotal swelling or tenderness, then he should be referred to a specialist center to exclude a torsion or testicular cancer. If the patient has a classic sexually transmitted disease (STD), then tests should be taken and correct antibiotic treatment should be initiated.

Try to ascertain the presence of a causative organism and treat thereafter, but if none is found or suspected, then athletes may be treated with oral antibiotics (tetracyclines, trimethoprim/sulfamethoxazole, or ciprofloxacin are often effective). Padded jockstraps may be of assistance.

49.4 ACUTE ORCHITIS

Orchitis may be caused by number of different types of bacteria and viruses and often occurs secondarily to an infectious epididymitis. Bacterial causes include STDs such as gonorrhea and chlamydia, as well as bacteria seen with recurrent urinary tract infections and chronic prostatitis. Mumps is the most common viral cause of orchitis, often occurring 4 to 6 days after the mumps clinical debut.

Clinical findings may include

- Painful, tender, swollen testicle, scrotum, and groin
- Mumps findings
- STI findings with penile discharge, dysuria, pain with intercourse or ejaculation
- Tender and enlarged inguinal lymph nodes
- Enlarged or tender prostate gland on rectal examination

Testing

Testing may include urinalysis and culture, chlamydia and gonorrhea tests (urine and/or urethral sampling), and Doppler ultrasound. As ultrasound is not commonly available at a sports venue, the patient will usually need referral.

Treatment

Viral orchitis can only be treated by analgesics or NSAIDs, as well as ice packs (for short periods of time) and bed rest. Bacterial conditions should be treated with the appropriate antibiotic.

Other Causes of Testicular Pain

As with all other body parts, chronic conditions may have an acute presentation, so a good medical history is important; inquire about previous wounds, trauma, infection or inflammation of the epididymis, testicle, or pelvis; urinary tract infection; and STD (orchitis). Epididymitis is the most common cause of testicle pain in adult men. Other conditions:

- Varicocele—spermatocele or hydrocele
- Testicular cancer
- Referred pain from abdominal or groin pathology (e.g., inguinal hernia, urethral stone)

49.5 ACUTE PROSTATITIS

Though not very common, cases do occur. In many cases, no bacterial agent can be held responsible, either because of the difficulty of taking adequate samples or due the fact that no bacteria are present. The cause of inflammation in these nonbacterial cases is postulated to be due to incomplete relaxation of the urinary sphincter, dyssynergic voiding, elevated urinary pressure causing reverse flow of urine into the prostate—as seen with "Weight lifter's epididymitis"—and urine-induced mucosal inflammation. Bacterial prostatitis is usually caused by urinary pathogens such as *E. coli* and *Klebsiella*, but may also be due to *Chlamydia* infections.

Differentiating between the two types of conditions is not easy. Patients usually need further investigation. The patient may complain of frequency, urgency, incomplete bladder emptying, the need to void again shortly after urinating, or nocturia. Pain is usually felt in the perineum but may radiate to the testes, penis, or back. Some patients experience painful ejaculations. In severe cases, patients may have fever and feel quite ill.

Rectal examination of the inflamed prostate will reveal an enlarged and tender prostate.

Diagnosis is based on the history and clinical findings. Samples can be taken for microscopic examination and culture, but this falls outside of what is normally expected of an EP. Bacterial inflammations are best treated with antibiotics; nonbacterial conditions can be treated with muscle relaxants and/or NSAIDs.

49.6 URETHRITIS—CHLAMYDIA AND GONORRHEA

In men, urethral inflammation is usually caused by a sexually transmitted agent, most commonly chlamydia, gonorrhea, and herpes viruses. Symptoms include dysuria, urge, frequent urinations, and possibly urethral discharge associated with—or independent of—urination. Gonorrhea can cause some men to develop a sore, red urethral opening. Oral or rectal sex can lead to lesions in the mouth or anus/rectum. Some patients are asymptomatic.

Other sexually transmitted agents can also be causal, including *Trichomonas*. Temporary irritation can be caused by soaps and other chemical substances.

In women, the commonest agents are lower intestinal bacteria such as *E. coli* but also sexually transmitted organisms and fungi. Urethritis in women is often associated with cystitis. Women may also experience urethral discomfort if they have vaginitis, as urine (which is acidic) can seep into the inflamed vulva and vagina, thus exacerbating symptoms. Gonorrhea in females can also affect the whole of the genital tract (pelvic inflammatory disease) with the vagina, cervix, uterus, fallopian tubes, and ovaries involved in severe cases. Discharge is less common in females than in men.

If the athlete has a discharge, then swabs should be taken and sent to a laboratory. These tests take some days to analyze, so it is difficult to give a precise diagnosis initially. If you take a swab sample, try to do so when there is discharge present. Gonorrhea discharge is usually thicker and more profuse with a yellow–green coloration and tends to appear 3 to 10 days after contact, whereas chlamydia discharge tends to be a clearer, watery solution. Early-morning, full-bladder urine samples may also be used for testing for chlamydia but, again, take 3 to 4 days before a result is forthcoming.

Treatment is dependent on the results of the microbiologic tests. Antibiotics are usually prescribed. Oral azithromycin or doxycycline is usually effective against acute chlamydia infections. Azithromycin may also be effective against gonorrhea, though many prefer to treat with cephalosporin antibiotics.

If tests show neither chlamydia nor gonorrhea in patients without discharge, I usually start with an oral trimethoprim-sulfamethoxazole cure. If tests are negative and the athlete still has a discharge, I usually take a new swab and start the patient on antibiotics, 1 g of oral azithromycin. The patient needs to be followed up until a diagnosis has been made and treatment successfully concluded; if not, chronic infections may occur and complications may occur (gonorrhea:urethral diverticula, urethral stricture, urethral fistula, Reiter syndrome, arthritis, uveitis). Trichomonas can also cause urethritis and can be treated with oral metronidazole.

Note: Patients with gonorrhea may have other STDs, such as chlamydia, syphilis, or HIV infection.

49.7 VAGINITIS

Vaginitis is a common complaint among young females and is often infectious in nature. There maybe a disruption in the normal vaginal flora (bacterial vaginosis—with an overgrowth of normal bacteria that replace the protective lactobacilli) or the presence of foreign pathogens such as candidiasis or trichomonal vaginitis. In some cases, the vulva is infected as well or alone. Patients complain of a vaginal discharge, vaginal and vulval irritation, and pruritus; some complain of pain and local bleeding. There may be burning during micturition and discomfort during sex. The vulval region may be redder than normal.

One can usually guess what the cause is by examining the discharge. Candida gives a white, thickish, sticky, cheese-like discharge. There may be traces of discharge on the vulva. There is often itching. With *Trichomonas*, the discharge is a yellow–green color. In PID, the discharge is usually purulent. In bacterial vaginosis, the discharge is slightly colored and more watery in consistence, with a characteristic fishy smell.

Treatment recommendations vary slightly around the world. Candidiasis is usually treated with a mixture of creams, vaginal suppositories, or oral medication; clotrimazole (Canesten) is widely used in Europe. Oral metronidazole or clindamycin can be effective for bacterial vaginoses.

49.8 PELVIC INFLAMMATORY DISEASE

This serious infection occurs when the upper female genital tract becomes infected by microorganisms ascending from the vagina and cervix into the endometrium, fallopian tubes and ovaries. It is most commonly seen between ages 18 and 35. Chlamydia and gonorrhea are common causes of PID, but not all cases are sexually transmitted, some cases being only associated with vaginoses caused by supposedly innocent pathogens such as *Gardnerella vaginalis*. The use of intrauterine contraceptive devices seems to increase the risk of infection.

Common symptoms and signs include lower abdominal pain, cervical discharge, and irregular vaginal bleeding. Symptoms and findings are, of course, dependent on which part of the genital tract is affected: Cervicitis often presents with a yellow–green mucopurulent discharge, and the cervix is red and bleeds easily. Salpingitis and endometritis may have an acute or chronic presentation; acute episodes tend to be associated with intense, bilateral lower abdominal pain and are often accompanied by nausea, vomiting, and even fever. In less acute cases, pain may be less severe and the patient complains of pain, discharge, irregular bleeding, and fever.

Treatment

Swabs should be taken, but if symptoms are mild to moderate, it is not unusual for physicians to prescribe azithromycin empirically to cover both *N. gonorrhoeae* and *C. trachomatis* until laboratory results are available. More serious episodes demand hospitalization and athletes are unfit to participate in sport.

49.9 GENITAL HERPES

This is a contagious condition usually caused by contact with HSV-2 virus–infected sores or skin, but can also be caused the more common "cold sore" HSV-1 virus. While the disorder is most contagious when blisters and ruptured blisters are present, transmission can occur during sex without the presence of blisters in some chronically infected patients. Genital herpes sores can be found around the mouth just as cold sores can also be found in the genital region. The primary genital herpes infection is usually the most pronounced and usually lasts longer and is more painful than subsequent attacks. Patients classically present with multiple painful blisters in the genital area but may also have fever, malaise, dysuria, difficulty urinating, or pain during defecation. Some people have blisters but few other symptoms.

Unfortunately, genital herpes can strike many times, but subsequent episodes are often less intense and present initially with a local discomfort or ache, followed by the eruption of painful reddish skin or mucosal blisters hours or days later. Mucosal blisters in the vagina and cervix may not be so painful, whereas vulval blisters tend to be most uncomfortable. While a primary herpetic episode may last several weeks, subsequent episodes usually subside after a week.

Primary diagnosis is usually relatively easily made based on clinical findings, but diagnosis can be confirmed by sending a swab sample from the sore for culture. Again, it can take several days to get test results.

Herpes encephalitis is a known complication.

As a general rule, the earlier one starts treatment, the quicker one experiences symptomatic relief—preferably before the blisters appear—hence, medication does seem to be more effective for subsequent attacks than with the primary episode, though patients should be treated for both primary and subsequent episodes. The usual drug of choice is acyclovir, and in Norway, we use 800 mg × 4, for 5 to 10 days, depending on the severity of the attack.

Athletes with acute infections should be isolated from other athletes to prevent multiple infections, and gentle washing of the genitalia with soapy water and regular and effective hand washing are recommended, particularly after going to the toilet. Patients should avoid sharing glasses and food utensils, as well as kissing or oral sex, when the blisters are active. Condoms should be used at all times, as the herpes 2 virus can be transmitted in the clinically dormant phase.

49.10 SYPHILIS

Patients still present with syphilis (*Treponema pallidum* bacteria), though the incidence has fallen dramatically in Western Europe in the last 20 to 30 years. Regrettably, there has been a marked increase in the countries of the ex–Russian Federation and Baltic states. Other countries that have high incidence rates are Cameroon, South Africa and the Central African Republic, Oceania, Cambodia, Papua New Guinea, Djibouti, and Morocco.

Ulceration of the urogenital tract, mouth, or rectum are usually the first clinical signs, which if left untreated may lead to a more generalized infection with disseminated mucocutaneous lesions, fever, malaise, alopecia, and hepatitis. Tertiary syphilis is rare and one will not expect to see this in athletes. Ulceration usually appears about 3 to 4 weeks after exposure, often starting as a red papule that quickly develops into a painless, firm-based ulcer (chancre). The ulcer may seep fluid, particularly when rubbed. There are usually enlarged lymph nodes in the drainage areas and these are often firm and nontender.

There are several blood analysis tests available but most rely on the detection of antibodies, and as antibody production can take between 3 and 4 weeks from the time of infection, early testing may produce negative results. Bacteria can also be found on microscopic analysis of chancre secretions.

Treatment for primary syphilis is with penicillin G injections, usually administering 1.2 to 1.4 g intramuscularly in each buttock as a one-off dosage. Patients should be referred to a specialist.

49.11 GENITAL WARTS

These warts usually appear within 1 to 6 months after exposure to the human papillomavirus, often beginning as small, soft growths. Genital warts can mature rapidly and become quite large if ignored and may grow in clusters. In men, warts usually grow on the penis, foreskin, or even in the urethra. In women, genital warts occur on the vulva, vaginal wall, cervix, and skin around the vaginal area. Genital warts may develop in the area around the anus and in the rectum, especially in people who engage in anal sex. Warts are usually asymptomatic but can cause occasional burning pain in some patients.

Warts may grow more rapidly and spread in pregnant women and in immunosuppressed patients. As with all warts, treatment is not always effective. Once infected, one can expect repeated outbreaks, even if the initial warts are successfully treated. Several methods can be used—applying podophyllin solutions or Aldara cream, cryotherapy, surgery, electrocautery, or laser therapy.

Recommended Reading

Centers for Disease Control and Prevention, http://www.cdc.gov/

Julius Schachter, ed. Journal of the American Sexually Transmitted Diseases Association, International Union Against Sexually Transmitted Infections, and the Scandinavian Society for Genito-Urinary Medicine. [ISBN/ISSN: 01485717 Published monthly].

Shah KH, Egan D, Quaas J. *Essential Emergency Trauma.* Philadelphia, PA: Lippincott Williams & Wilkins, 2010.

Sweet RL, Gibbs RS. *Infectious Diseases of the Female Genital Tract* (5th Ed.). Philadelphia, PA: Lippincott Williams & Wilkins, 2009.

CHAPTER 50

Menstrual Conditions

Contributed by Julia Alleyne, Canadian Skating Team, FIMS Executive Committee, University of Toronto, Canada; and Demitri Constantinou, Director, FIFA Medical Centre, University of Witwatersrand, Johannesburg, South Africa

Reviewer: Talia Alenabi, Secretary General, Asian Federation of Sports Medicine, Tehran, Iran

50.1 VAGINAL BLEEDING

One of the challenges in assessing vaginal bleeding in athletes is determining what is normal, nonurgent, and urgent, and then deciding if athletic participation is advised. This chapter will provide you with some tips on clinical assessment for event-related diagnosis and management.

Normal Menstrual Bleeding

The average age of menarche in westernized countries is 12.2 years; however, over the last century, we have witnessed advancement in onset of menses to as early as 9 years of age in some subsets of the population. This is theorized to be related to improved nutrition, increased peripheral estrogen in higher body fat, and increased exposure to environmental estrogens through food and water supply. In the athletic subset, we are still observing that some female athletes have a delay in onset to ages 15 to 17 years due to lack of primary pubertal development or an exercise-induced energy deficit. Usual flow is for 3 to 5 days and can vary from light to heavy, producing a red color consistent with fresh blood. The time between cycles can vary from 21 to 42 days.

Normal menstrual bleeding can occur unexpectedly after amenorrhea or as a primary menstrual cycle. This is usually accompanied by mild cramping, and flow starts within hours of initial red or pinkish spotting. Although flow increases, pain and cramping subsides within the first 12 to 24 hours. Athletic participation is recommended.

Menstruation itself does not have known specific effects on sports performance, and any effects appear to be dependent on the psychological and cultural attitude of individual females. Some will report no change in physical performance; some report a reduction in performance, while others report improved performance. Discomfort and pain may affect a female athlete's ability to train and participate in sport optimally for short time periods. If this occurs, then anti-inflammatory and analgesic medications should be considered prophylactically when the menstrual cycle starts.

Abnormal Menstrual Bleeding—Nonurgent

Menstrual dysfunction is defined as unexpected bleeding occurring in the early, mid, or late phase of the menstrual cycle. This bleeding is usually light to moderate in flow and may look more like brownish spotting. This bleeding is not usually accompanied by cramping or pain and often resolves in 1 to 3 days. The cause of abnormal menstrual bleeding is often related to hormonal imbalance, contraceptive dosage, or stress. There frequently is a previous pattern of abnormal cycles or bleeding. Medical evaluation including examination and investigations can be delayed for a month to observe the cycle pattern. Athletic participation is recommended.

Abnormal Vaginal Bleeding—Urgent

The four main clinical characteristics that indicate abnormal vaginal bleeding are

- Heavy flow (menorrhagia)
- Significant pain

- Dark brown or dark color

- The presence of noticeable clots

Athletic participation is not recommended in the presence of these symptoms until a diagnosis is identified.

Heavy menstrual flow can be estimated by measures required to maintain hygiene. The flow is considered heavy if pad or tampon changes occur more frequently than every 2.5 hours or more than six changes per day. Another sign of heavy flow is unexpected soiling of clothes with regular hygiene changes. Heavy flow may be related to spontaneous abortion, vaginal lacerations, or cystic rupture.

Vaginal or pelvic pain with or without bleeding should be evaluated if the pain is sharp, persistent, and escalating in nature. The cause may be related to ectopic pregnancy, pelvic inflammatory disease, ovarian cyst, abscess, or infection. If pelvic or vaginal pain is associated with sport trauma, the differential diagnosis would include pelvic fracture, uterine rupture, or vaginal laceration.

Brownish or dark bleeding signifies that the blood has been retained and the source may be deeper in the genital tract in conjunction with internal hemorrhage. This may be seen with pelvic inflammatory disease, pregnancy loss, abscess, or tumor.

Large clots are uncommon in young women and may be related to internal bleeding, pelvic inflammatory disease, pregnancy loss, or recent pelvic trauma. This is a serious symptom in a young woman and should be assessed.

50.2 AMENORRHEA

Once conditions requiring medical intervention have been ruled out, most delays or lack of menstruation can be reversed with nutritional and exercise counseling aimed to achieve energy balance. This will often take 6 months to resume or initiate menstruation with an initial modification in exercise intensity combined with graduated caloric intake. Weight gain is minimal but energy resumption and performance improvement is noted within weeks. Athletic participation may need to be modified for an amenorrheic athlete for energy balance to be achieved, but if the athlete is medically stable, then participation should not be completely restricted.

Amenorrhea may be a part of the female athlete triad, which can occur in all sports and is associated with significant short- and long-term health consequences. It is an issue that all physicians working with female athletes need to be aware of. The diagnosis is based on three criteria: (a) disordered eating, (b) amenorrhea, and (c) osteopenia/premature osteoporosis. The syndrome can result in the development of stress fractures, eating disorders, and low peak bone mineral density, which can lead to osteoporosis later in life. A cross-sectional study looking at the prevalence of female athlete triad characteristics in a club triathlon team showed that 60% had a calorie deficit, 53% had a carbohydrate deficit, 47% had a fat deficit, 40% had a protein deficit, and 33% had a calcium deficit. Forty percent reported a history of amenorrhea. Such findings are not uncommon in other sports.

Oral Contraceptives in Sport

There are many options for contraception available; however, some should be considered carefully if used in avid athletic woman. The pill must be taken accurately for effective use as a contraceptive. In many countries, the continuous oral contraceptive pill is being used safely, and this eliminates or reduces the occurrence of any menstrual bleeding. Most preparations are for 4, 6, or 12 months of continuous pills without a period. For some athletes, this is a desirable option if they are susceptible to low iron levels, premenstrual symptoms, or concern about traveling and competing during their menstrual period. The current literature suggests that this use is safe and that contraceptive error is reduced. Depo-Provera is an injection or implantation of progesterone, providing a 3-month duration for contraception, which increases the compliancy when compared to taking a daily pill. However, without estrogen, there is a risk of osteoporosis being induced or enhanced with Depo-Provera and use is not recommended if bone health is at risk.

Pregnancy

There are well-known issues that arose when human chorionic gonadotrophin (hCG) was on the prohibited list for female athletes; several athletes had tested positive for this substance, and it turned out that they were pregnant. It also speaks to the fact that often secondary amenorrhea may be from a pregnant state. Pregnancy should never be forgotten in female athletes of reproductive age and sometimes even occurs with no disruption in menstrual cycles. It would be important in the history taking to ascertain whether the athlete is sexually active or not. Numerous symptoms that an athlete may present under the guise of pathologic illness may be from underlying pregnancy; these include nausea, vomiting, fatigue, lower abdominal congestion, and discomfort. It is important to monitor pregnant athletes for possible complications and advise them appropriately as to what best exercise to continue with, what to avoid, and when to return to sport postpartum.

Recommended Reading

Benjamin HJ. The female adolescent athlete: Specific concerns. *Pediatr Ann.* 2007;36(11):719–726.

Gamboa S, Gaskie S, Atlas M, VanZant R. Clinical inquiries: what's the best way to manage athletes with amenorrhea? *J Fam Pract.* 2008;57(11):749–750.

Warren MP, Chua AT. Exercise-induced amenorrhea and bone health in the adolescent athlete. *Ann NY Acad Sci.* 2008;1135:244–252.

Warren MP, Shangold MM. *Sports Gynecology. Problems and care of the athletic female.* Cambridge, MA: Blackwell Science, 1997.

CHAPTER 51

Shoulder and Upper Arm Injuries

Contributed by Eugene Byrne, CMO, USA Bobsleigh, Skeleton, and Luge Teams

Reviewers: Christian Schneider, FIBT Medical Committee, German Bobsleigh and Skeleton Team, and Schön Clinic, Munich, Germany; and Mike Wilkinson, Deputy CMO, Vancouver 2010 Winter Olympic Games

51.1 LACERATIONS OF THE SHOULDER REGION

The management of sports-related lacerations of the shoulder is the same as for other parts of the body. It is the responsibility of the athlete to contact the medical personnel for assistance. The most important element is the control of bleeding—for the protection of both the athlete and the other participants. The medical personnel must follow universal precautions when dealing with bloody fluids to protect themselves from the athlete's potentially infectious blood. An important item to keep in your pockets on the sideline is a few pair of nonsterile gloves for care of sports-related lacerations. The medical personnel need to control the bleeding by applying pressure until the bleeding has stopped. Be careful if applying pressure over a sharp bony fracture fragment. The laceration then needs to be closed with Steri-Strips, wound glue, or a combination of these. If the bleeding is not controllable with either of these methods, then the laceration will need to be sutured prior to return to play. Once the laceration is stabilized, then a compression dressing and flexible tape needs to be applied. This should keep the laceration protected and allow return to play. In the shoulder area, it is sometimes difficult to keep a dressing in place. The medical person may need to partly immobilize the shoulder to ensure the dressing is stable prior to return to play.

51.2 CONTUSIONS

Contusions in the shoulder region are common in contact sports. The areas with the highest rate of injury are the lateral and superior shoulder. The most important element in evaluating a contusion is differentiating it from a more serious injury. This can be a difficult task. A contusion to the lateral shoulder and/or rotator cuff is usually associated with mild, diffuse swelling and tenderness more in the soft tissues and muscles then on the bone itself. If the athlete is unwilling to move the shoulder, then a more serious injury may have occurred. The shoulder contours will be maintained in contusions but often disrupted in fractures and dislocations when compared to the opposite side. The shoulder should be able to be actively moved by the athlete but may be painful. If there is a difference in shoulder contours or at the acromioclavicular joint or clavicle, then the athlete should not be allowed to return to play until cleared by an x-ray. The athlete with a contusion needs to be able to protect himself or herself from further injury prior to returning to play. The event physician should make sure that athletes have full range of motion and strength in all planes so that they can protect themselves in contact and noncontact sports.

If the athlete has tenderness over the lateral aspect of the shoulder or over the acromioclavicular joint, a pad may be placed over the tender area and taped in place under the clothing to aid in protecting the area. If more protection is required, then a thick, plastic material can be molded to the area to offer more protection and taped or strapped into place. This often is used in American football, rugby, ice hockey, and luge in my experience. It is also important to make sure that the athletes' shoulder pads are in good condition and fit appropriately. The equipment manager may have more heavy-duty shoulder pads if needed to add in the protection of the superior and lateral shoulder areas. Be aware, though, that in many sports (e.g., rugby union), hard pads and protection are against the rules and may not be used. In this case, supplemented "donut" padding to the athlete's soft shoulder pads is useful and legal.

51.3 JOINT INJURIES—DISLOCATIONS, SUBLUXATION, SPRAINS, AND INSTABILITY

There are three shoulder girdle that are prone to ligamentous injury or sprain. These are the

- Acromioclavicular joint
- Glenohumeral joint
- Sternoclavicular joint

The acromioclavicular *(AC) joint* is prone to injury during contact with the ground/playing surface or another player. There are several ways of classifying AC sprains, but we will concentrate on that of clinical observation classification, which has three subclasses. The AC joint is stabilized by two sets of ligaments: the AC ligaments and the coracoclavicular (CC) ligaments.

- Type 1: The AC ligaments are injured and there is little to any deformity.
- Type 2: The AC ligaments are disrupted but the CC ligaments are intact and a slight deformity is observed.
- Type 3: The AC and CC ligaments are disrupted and a significant deformity exists compared to the other, normal side. The athlete will complain of superior and lateral shoulder pain. The athlete will feel a popping of the clavicle, and this will give him or her the most concern.

During the evaluation on the sideline, you must be able to rule out a distal clavicle fracture, which can be misdiagnosed on the sideline for an AC separation. You must also rule out damage to the glenohumeral joint. A careful neurological and vascular evaluation must be performed to rule out a concomitant brachial plexus injury and arterial injury. An athlete

with an AC joint injury that is able to fully move the shoulder through functional range of motion can be returned to play. Taping of the joint may relieve symptoms and increase stability. A plastic or foam pad should be placed over the AC joint to protect the joint from further injury. The joint may also be taped to give additional support (see diagram).

If the athlete cannot be returned to play, then a sling should be applied, giving support to the elbow, and referral for an x-ray is recommended to fully evaluate the type and extent of injury and to exclude a fracture. The athlete can be returned to play when he or she has regained full shoulder range of motion and strength and is able to protect himself or herself from further injury.

The sternoclavicular *(SC) joint* is discussed in Chapter 43.

The glenohumeral *joint* is the second most commonly injured joint of the shoulder girdle.

The injuries range from

- Grade 1 strain
- Grade 2 subluxations
- Grade 3 dislocations

The direction of instability is most commonly anterior but posterior instability is also not unusual in contact sports. An important part of the history is that of previous shoulder instability; and the number of episodes of instability/dislocations. An athlete with ligamentous laxity and multiple subluxations/dislocations will have a much faster return to sport then an athlete with a first-time dislocation.

The evaluation of the athlete with glenohumeral luxation/subluxation starts with a comparison of the contralateral shoulder to help define the direction of instability. If the athlete has fullness anteroinferiorly, deficient deltoid contour and a coracoid process that is difficult to palpate, then anterior dislocation is likely. If the athlete has fullness posteriorly and the coracoid process is easily palpated, a posterior dislocation is more likely. The deltoid contour is often more pronounced with an anterior dislocation. The examination also needs to exclude a fracture as cause of the deformity.

If crepitus is felt or the humerus and the shoulder mass do not move as a unit, then a proximal humeral fracture must be suspected and an x-ray should be taken prior to reduction maneuvers. The athlete's neurovascular status must be assessed prior to any reduction maneuver since up to 30% of shoulder dislocations are associated with an axillary nerve injury. This is due to its course inferior to the glenohumeral joint.

The axillary nerve provides cutaneous innervation over the lateral shoulder and motor innervation to the deltoid and teres minor muscles. The athlete with an acute axillary nerve injury will present with loss of sensation or altered sensation over the lateral shoulder area and inability or weakness in shoulder abduction as compared to the contralateral side. In chronic cases, there will be observable atrophy of the deltoid with significant weakness and difficulty in early shoulder range of motion.

The athlete with a glenohumeral dislocation can be reduced on the sideline if reduced quickly after the injury prior to the muscle spasm, which makes reduction difficult without muscle relaxants and/or pain medications. There are many reduction maneuvers and these depend on the direction of instability. The hanging shoulder technique is often the least painful and may be attempted first, but it is often unsuccessful. Before attempting a shoulder reduction, the event physician must be sure of the diagnosis—following local procedure guidelines is recommended

Maneuvers should be performed quickly and, if not successful after a few attempts, should be abandoned and the athlete should be transported to a hospital where an x-ray can be taken and a fracture ruled out. The athlete can then receive pain medications and sedation to allow for glenohumeral reduction to be performed with less trauma. The more reduction attempts made, the greater the risk of cartilage damage and possible neurovascular injury.

The athlete should be placed in a sling after reduction and taken out of play. The athlete can come out of the sling as the pain decreases and begin to work on range of motion and strengthening. Return-to-play can occur when the athlete has attained full range of motion and full strength.

Before the athlete returns to play, he or she needs to be able to protect himself or herself in abduction and external rotation, especially in contact sports. A functional brace can be applied to the athlete on return to some sports to assist in preventing repeated instability. The brace works well in nonthrowing positions and for the nondominant arm on a throwing athlete. Braces containing metal are not allowed in many sports, particularly team sports, where there is an injury risk to opponents. Athletes with repetitive dislocations or recurrent instability should undergo surgical stabilization prior to return to sport. It is becoming more popular to operate on first-time dislocators in athletes. This is usually performed at the end of the season if possible to minimize time out of sport. This is dependent on the athlete regaining full range of motion, strength, and function. Make sure that the athlete can protect his or her arm in 90 degrees of abduction with external rotation.

51.4 SHOULDER REDUCTION TECHNIQUES

Early treatment of shoulder dislocation promptly eliminates the stretch and compression of nerves and muscle, and reduces the amount of muscle spasm that must be overcome to reduce the shoulder. Although some dislocations can be reduced without medication, in many instances, the patient is lightly anesthetized or given a muscle relaxant. The depth of anesthesia depends on the amount of trauma that produced the dislocation, the duration of the dislocation, how many times the patient has previously dislocated, whether the dislocation is locked, and to what extent the patient can voluntarily relax his or her shoulder muscles. Some of the main reduction techniques are described below.

Hippocratic Technique (No Longer Used in Many Countries)

When only one person is available to reduce the shoulder, the stocking foot of the physician is used as countertraction. The heel does not go into the armpit but extends against the chest wall. The traction is slow and gentle. The arm may be gently rotated internally and externally to disengage the head of the humerus. Hippocrates also described other techniques such as where a child provides countertraction.

Stimson's Technique

Appropriate weights (e.g., 5 lb) are taped to the wrist of the dislocated shoulder, which hangs free over the edge of the table. If medication is used, the patient should be monitored, as it may take 15 to 20 minutes for the reduction to occur.

Milch's Technique

With the patient lying on the back, the arm is raised by the side and externally rotated. The therapist's thumb is used to gently push the head of the humerus back in place. A modified version of this technique is applied to patients lying on their abdomen.

Kocher's Leverage Technique

This technique was first described in Egyptian hieroglyphs 3,000 years ago. For this maneuver, the humeral head is levered on the anterior surface of the shoulder cavity and the long shaft of the humerus is levered against the chest wall until the reduction is complete. This procedure is prone to complications and is no longer used in some countries.

Matsen's Technique

Matsen's preferred method of anterior reduction is where the patient lies on his or her back with a sheet around the chest and also around the assistant's waist for countertraction. The surgeon stands on the side of the dislocated shoulder near the patient's waist with the elbow of the dislocated shoulder bent to 90 degrees. A second sheet, tied loosely around the surgeon's waist and looped over the patient's forearm, provides traction while the surgeon leans back against the sheet while grasping the forearm. Steady traction along the axis of the arm usually causes reduction.

Additional simple techniques for reducing the dislocated shoulder include the forward elevation maneuver, the modified gravity method, the scapular manipulation, the crutch and chair technique, the chair and pillow technique, the external rotation method, and others.

51.5 FRACTURES

The incidence of shoulder girdle fractures in sport varies depending on the sport. The most common being a clavicle fracture, though there has been an increase in proximal humeral fractures in the winter sports. The athlete with a clavicle fracture will present with pain and often deformity. The most common clavicular fracture is a midshaft fracture, which is obvious when compared to the opposite side and on palpation. There will be pain and crepitus and the athlete will not move the arm into elevation. The sideline dilemma is differentiating a distal clavicle fracture from AC joint instability. On inspection, a grade 3 AC dislocation is often more pronounced than a fracture. The tenderness is slightly more proximal to the AC joint in distal fractures and there is usually more pain and crepitus—hence the need for x-ray with suspected AC joint instability. The athlete with a clavicle fracture should be placed into a sling and swath acutely. The athlete can then be fitted with a figure-of-eight splint to aid in pulling the scapula posterior and assist with posture. A comparison study found there to be no significant difference in results when bandaging clavicle fractures with a sling versus figure-of-eight splint. Proximal humeral

fractures are a concern due to the proximity to the neurovascular structures. The most important sideline concern is differentiating a glenohumeral dislocation from a proximal humeral fracture. This is sometimes difficult on field-side diagnosis. The athlete with a fracture usually has more pain and a different deformity, with the swelling being slightly more lateral, whereas in a dislocation there is often a depression in the subacromial area with a diminution of the deltoid contour. Anteriorly, the fractured shoulder appears more symmetric bilaterally, whereas a dislocated shoulder may protrude anteriorly when inspected from the side. Tenderness is more lateral on the fracture patients and often more pronounced than in dislocations. Thus, shoulder reductions in the first-time dislocator should be performed gently, if at all, if no x-ray is taken prior to attempted reduction. The athlete's neurovascular status needs to be documented when a proximal humeral fracture is suspected due to the potential of neurovascular injury. The athlete should be placed into a sling and swath or vacuum splint, and transported to a facility where an x-ray and definitive treatment can be undergone. The athlete with either a clavicle or humeral fracture cannot return to play until complete fracture union and full range of motion and strength. This may take from 6 to 10 weeks from injury.

51.6 LABRUM INJURIES

The labrum glenoidale shoulder joint cartilage stabilizes the head of the humerus by deepening the socket and by being the attachment site for ligaments. If injured, the shoulder may become unstable and athletes may complain of locking, subluxation experiences, grinding, etc. as well as other typical shoulder symptoms such as deep pain, limited range of motion, and decreased strength. Injuries may be caused by acute trauma such as a blow to or falls on the outstretched arm or shoulder dislocations, or they may occur due to repetitive micro injuries as occurs with javelin throwers, discus throwers, baseball pitchers, weight lifters, etc.

The term *internal impingement* is often used to describe the discomfort felt due to repetitive trauma of the rotator cuff and the greater tuberosity on the posterior labrum. Tennis players are often bothered by this impingement, as their arms are often in the overhead position during serving and returning high lobs. The pain, which is often located posterosuperiorly, is usually worsened when the arm changes direction from late cocking to forward acceleration.

The symptoms of a labrum tear are not dissimilar to many other shoulder conditions, and it is difficult to make a diagnosis on clinical findings alone. Further investigation is always necessary to make a definitive diagnosis. Tears are usually located superiorly (e.g., a SLAP lesion) or inferiorly (e.g., a Bankart lesion). A SLAP (superior labrum, anterior to posterior) tear is often extremely painful and can cause the biceps tendon to rupture. O'Brien's test, which causes pain when stretching the biceps, can be helpful in diagnosing a labral tear with biceps involvement.

A Bankart tear occurs in the anteroinferior aspect of the labrum and almost always associated with an anteroinferior dislocation of the head of the humerus.

Treatment

There is not a lot an EP can do about these injuries, not least because of the diagnostic uncertainty. Anti-inflammatory medication and rest may have a temporary effect, and physiotherapy may help stabilize the shoulder. If conservative treatment fails, then refer.

51.7 SHOULDER INSTABILITY

Shoulder instability should be tested for in athletes who present with shoulder pain. Athletes with habitual subluxation tendency may have shoulder pain that can be difficult to distinguish from biceps tendinitis, acute rotator cuff tendinitis, or microtrauma. The rotator cuff, the labrum, and the outer joint capsule stabilize the shoulder joint. A history of previous injury or instability can give valuable clues. Capsule or labrum tears are usually painful. A "dead arm" sensation, due to nerve compression during dislocation, may also be a symptom. If the pain is atraumatic and not too intense, then a detailed physical examination can be conducted and the EP can attempt to exclude specific biceps and rotator cuff pathology while also stress testing for multidirectional joint laxity.

The Apprehension Test

With the patient lying supine, grasp the patient's elbow and abduct the humerus to 90 degrees. Gently externally rotate the arm while also pushing anteriorly on the head of the humerus with your other hand. The athlete may feel that the arm is

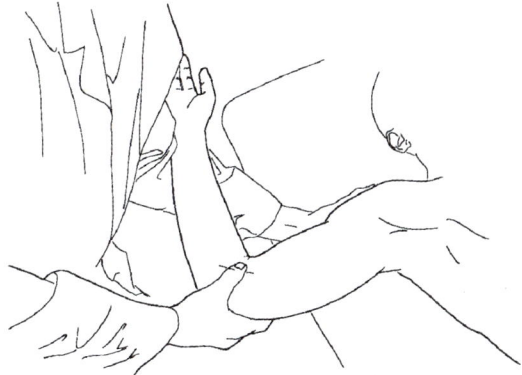

FIGURE 51.1 Shoulder instability.

about to dislocate or has partially been subluxated (Fig. 51.1). A relocation test may then be conducted.

If instability is discovered and identified as the cause of pain, the only course of action is medication and possibly taping. Correction of muscular imbalance will have to take place at another arena.

Any of these conditions may lead to secondary capsulitis.

51.8 BICIPITAL TENDINITIS

Bicipital tendinitis describes inflammation of the biceps tendon. Peritendinitis is an inflammation of the tendon sheath, and both conditions often present together (tenosynovitis). The inflammatory response in the tendon is believed to be caused by chronic overload and resulting microtears, and/or focal tendon ischemia and/or neurally mediated mast cell degranulation. Tendon sheath inflammation may be caused by direct trauma or by repetitive irritation with the sheath (and tendon) constantly gliding over a bony prominence. Tendinopathy refers to pathology in a tendon and may thus have an inflammatory, degenerative, or other underlying processes involved. Biceps tendinopathy is rarely seen in isolation. It is often seen with other lesions of the shoulder, including rotator cuff pathology, bursitis, and shoulder instability.

The biceps brachii is innervated by the C5 and C6 nerves. Because the biceps long head is both intracapsular and extracapsular, symptoms may mimic other intracapsular, capsular, and extracapsular pathological lesions.

Pain on palpation of the biceps long head in the bicipital groove may indicate biceps tendonitis. Pain may be elicited by Yergason's sign.

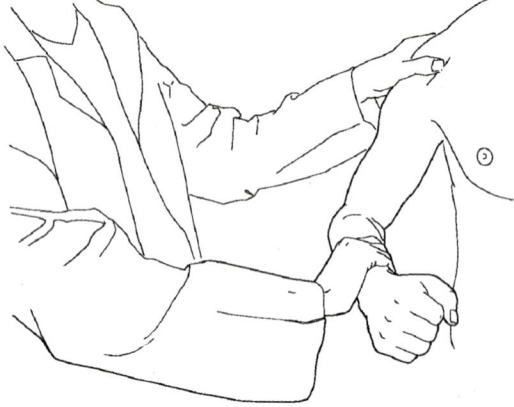

FIGURE 51.2 Yergason's sign.

Yergason's Sign

Yergason's sign is described as resisted forearm supination with bicipital tendon compression. The physician places a thumb over the bicipital groove and compresses (this alone may cause pain). Then, flex the elbow to 90 degrees with the arm held in against the body. Grasp the patient's forearm, applying resistance to both flexion and supination, and tell him or her to supinate the forearm so that the palm of the hand faces upward. Pain suggests tendinitis of the biceps (Fig. 51.2).

Speed's Test

With the examiner resisting flexion, adduction, and supination, the patient tries to flex an extended elbow. Pain in anterior shoulder indicates biceps tendinitis (Fig. 51.3).

Treatment

The EPs arsenal is pretty empty if a severe, painful inflammation occurs. Ice packs, analgesics,

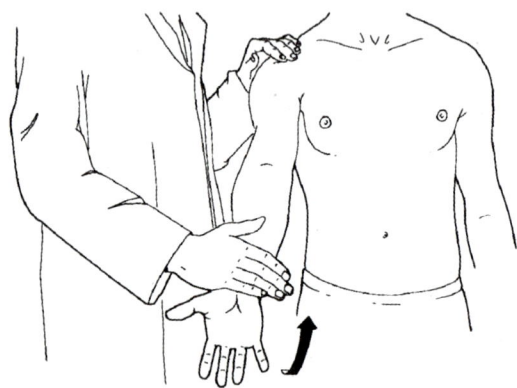

FIGURE 51.3 Speed's test.

NSAIDs, and rest may help somewhat initially. Many athletes will not accept rest as a therapeutic option and will request/demand a corticosteroid injection. If the pain is due to an inflammation, such injections may reduce the inflammation and thus pain, but they do nothing to remove the cause (microtrauma, bone irritation, etc.). Iontophoresis (the introduction of ionizable drugs through intact skin by the administration of continuous, direct electrical current into the tissues of the body) may have fewer side effects and be less painful than injecting corticosteroids, but the effect of the corticosteroid seems to be weaker than when given by a periarticular injection.

Pain and swelling will surely return if causational problems are not addressed. Is it correct medical practice to give a periarticular corticosteroid/anesthetic injection and advise rest and rehabilitation? Most sports physicians would agree that this is acceptable treatment. Is it correct medical practice to give a corticosteroid/anesthetic periarticular injection and then allow the athlete to return to play on the same or following day— without rest? Most sports physicians would disagree. How often can you give a steroid injection in the same sit? What time frame should there be between injections? All these issues are poorly documented in the literature and there are varying practices around the world.

Corticosteroid Injection: The most important consideration when injecting is to avoid causing damage. The purpose of this injection is to deposit corticosteroids inside the tendon sheath of the biceps tendon and/or around the sheath without injecting into the tendon itself. The tendon is found by palpating the bicipital groove of the humerus. Insert a needle through the skin at the point of maximal tenderness and direct it toward the bicipital groove. Many physicians then angle the needle so that fluid is deposited along or around the sheath. Resistance to flow or increasing resistance suggests that the needle is in the tendon; if experienced, withdraw the needle tip slightly and deposit the steroid fluid in the peritendous space. It is important to press gently at all times to avoid overloading tissue with injection fluid.

51.9 SHOULDER BURSITIS

Both the subdeltoid bursa and the subacromial bursa are to be found in the subacromial space and they are usually contiguous; they protect the rotator cuff tendons against friction. Inflammation of these bursae may be due to a primary injury, but more often than not, the bursae are irritated by nearby inflammation processes involving the rotator cuff (e.g., partial rotator cuff tears). The four tendons of the rotator cuff all pass underneath the acromion en route to their insertions on the humerus. The space between the acromion/coracoacromial ligament and the tendons (in particular, the supraspinatus) can become relatively narrowed for any number of reasons (e.g., the growth of an osteophyte on the under surface of the bone). This causes the tendons to become impinged upon. The resulting friction inflames the tendons as well as the subacromial bursa, which lies between the tendons and the acromion. The net result is shoulder pain, particularly when raising the arm over head (e.g., swimming, reaching for something on a top shelf, arm positioning during sleep). Over time, chronic irritation to the tendons can lead to fraying, tears, and even complete disruption.

Clinical Presentation

Typically, the athlete complains of acute, severe pain superimposed on a history of chronic milder pain. Pain is often worse at night when the patient lies on the shoulder, and athletes often complain of poor quality of sleep. Swimming or reaching for something on a shelf may cause pain. Patients may wake up several times at night due to pain. Clinically, it is very difficult to differentiate between subacromial bursitis, subdeltoid bursitis, and rotator cuff tendonitis. On examination, there may be tenderness on palpation along the lateral border of the acromion and in the subacromial area.

Patients may have a painful arc throughout the whole 180 degrees of active motion—or limited to between 60 and 120 degrees of abduction. Tests for impingement will often be positive (e.g., Hawkins' test or Neer's test). Impingement tests impinge upon all the structures in the subacromial space, between the roof (acromion/coracoacromial ligament) and the floor (head of the humerus), in other words, all the rotator cuff tendons and the subacromial bursa. So a positive impingement test may indicate tendinitis (usually supraspinatus), bursitis, or a combination of both.

Hawkins' Test: The physician stabilizes the patient's scapula from behind. Abduct the arm to approximately 90 degrees or more, and flex the shoulder forward. Internally rotate the arm so that the thumb points downward to the floor. This test elevates the greater tubercle of

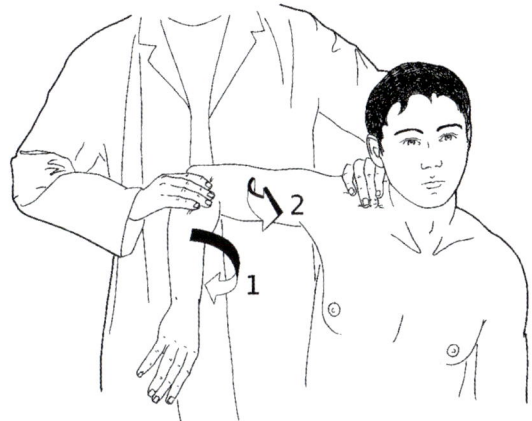

FIGURE 51.4 Hawkins' test.

the humerus and minimizes the subacromial space, thus impinging structures. Pain suggests impingement (Fig. 51.4).

51.10 ROTATOR CUFF TENDINITIS

Rotator cuff tendinitis is the most common cause of shoulder pain and secondary decreased shoulder mobility that manifests with pain on passive and active abduction. Pain is usually greater with internal rotation of the shoulder than with external rotation. The key finding is pain in the rotator cuff on active abduction, especially at 60 to 100 degrees of abduction. Ultimately, there may be impingement and a loss of mobility. Tenderness may be elicited anteriorly over the humeral head when the arm is extended (Fig. 51.5). Calcific tendinitis may also lead to impingement.

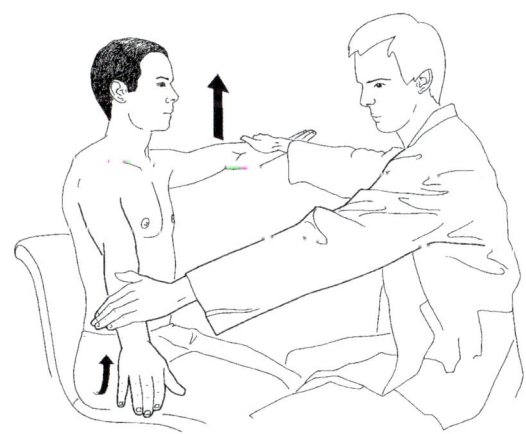

FIGURE 51.5 Rotator cuff tendinitis.

Jobe's Test

With both arms abducted to 90 degrees and flexed forward to 30 degrees of flexion, with the arm internally rotated, the patient tries to abduct the arm while the physician applies resistance. A positive test results in pain (tendonitis, peritendinitis, partial tears, or microtears) and weakness (chronic lesion with muscle atrophy or partial tear).

51.11 ROTATOR CUFF TEARS

There are many tests for tears of the rotator cuff and many are variations of the drop-arm test. In acute injuries, it is very difficult to assess rotator function as most tests require an ability to abduct the shoulder to 90 degrees. As this is usually impossible due to pain, it is important to retest the athlete's rotator cuff after 3 or 4 days when some of the pain has subsided. Tests are for complete tears (inability to hold the arm abducted) or partial tears (inability, reduced ability, or pain, when a force is applied to the arm in various abducted positions). If a rotator cuff rupture is discovered, the patient should be transferred to an orthopedic assessment relatively quickly, as most orthopedics prefer to operate within a week of rupture.

Unassisted Drop-Arm Test

Holding the arm abducted to 90 degrees with the thumb pointing downward, ask the patient to slowly lower the arm. If the arm drops suddenly, there is more than likely a rotator cuff tear.

Assisted Drop-Arm Test

Assist the patient in abducting the arm to 90 degrees (this test is usually conducted when the patient has so much pain that he or she will not voluntarily abduct to 90 degrees). Holding the arm, tell the patient that you will release the arm at the count of three. When released suddenly, the arm will either drop straight down (positive test indicative of a rotator cuff tear) or slowly sink downward with the patient grimacing with pain (probably a negative test, with functioning though partially damaged rotator cuff), or the patient has controlled adduction, implying a healthy rotator cuff.

Tests for partial tears include the patient again holding the arm abducted to 90 degrees while the physician presses the arm downward. The same procedure can be conducted with the arm in 90 degrees

of flexion with the thumb pointing downward. Failure to resist, reduced ability to resist, or painful resistance imply various degrees of rotator cuff injury. Similarly, the patient can abduct the arm to 90 degrees, flex the elbow to 90 degrees, and point the thumb toward the ceiling. The physician then tries to force the hand in toward the stomach. Failure to resist, reduced ability to resist, or painful resistance imply various degrees of rotator cuff injury.

51.12 SHOULDER CAPSULE INJURIES

The shoulder capsule is composed of interlocking tendons, capsular ligaments, and connective tissue. The capsule originates from the labrum and the surrounding glenoid bone and attaches to the shaft of the humerus (Fig. 51.6). It is strengthened by the rotator cuff tendons. The capsule is lined with synovial tissue. There are three bursae that are commonly injured in the shoulder, the predeltoid bursa, the biceps tendon bursa, and the subacromial bursa.

Injury to one of these structures will affect the capsule in some way and it is often difficult for the EP to make a precise diagnosis in the acute stage.

An athlete who presents with shoulder pain or movement restriction problems can be difficult to evaluate. Many shoulder conditions have similar symptoms, causes, precipitating factors, and treatments. Active ROM is often reduced in both articular lesions and with extra-articular conditions. However, a reduction in

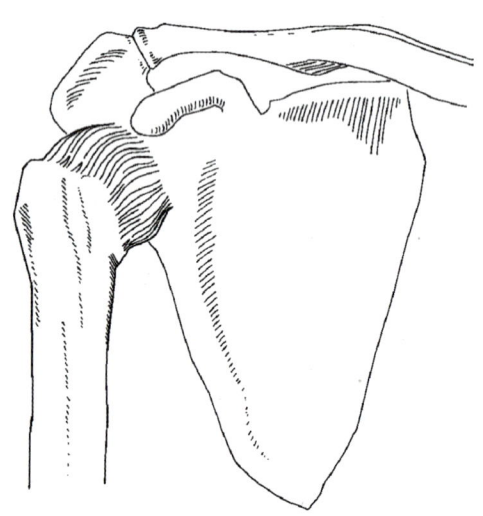

FIGURE 51.6 Shoulder capsule.

passive ROM (often with pain) usually indicates joint or capsule pathology. Conversely, normal passive ROM indicates an extra-articular lesion, such as muscle/tendon inflammation or strains, or bursitis.

A shoulder examination must always include active and passive ROM testing. It is important to make the correct diagnosis, as treatment modalities vary and the wrong choice of treatment (e.g., intensive physiotherapy on a frozen shoulder) may only make things worse.

Capsule inflammation may be traumatic in origin but may also be associated with systemic illnesses.

Conditions can be classified as

- Acute capsulitis

- Chronic capsulitis

- Frozen shoulder

- Chronic adhesive capsulitis

There is a lot of confusion regarding these terms, particularly when one uses the term "frozen shoulder." The term "frozen shoulder" was first introduced in 1934 by Codman. He described a painful shoulder condition of insidious onset, associated with stiffness and difficulty sleeping on the affected side. He also noted a reduction in shoulder flexion and external rotation that typify this disorder. Later, in 1945, Naviesar introduced the term "adhesive capsulitis."

This has made life very confusing for us humble EPs. According to *Stedmans Medical Dictionary* a frozen is a synonym for adhesive capsulitis? Having read hundreds of articles by learned colleagues, many still use the terms chronic capsulitis and frozen shouldert interchangeably as if they were the same condition, thus possibly explaining the divergent forms of treatment available for these conditions.

Clinical findings will be pretty similar, although the history may vary. Frozen shoulders are associated with a three-phase clinical pattern usually ending up with recovery—the terms freezing, frozen and thawing have been used.

Recommended Reading

Arroll B, Goodyear-Smith F. Corticosteroids for painful shoulder: a meta-analysis. *Br J Gen Pract.* 2005;55(512): 224–228.

Chapman MW. *Chapman's orthopaedic surgery.* Philadelphia, PA: Lippincott Williams Wilkins, 2001.

Codman EA. *The shoulder.* Boston: Thomas Told, 1934.

Neviaser JS. Adhesive capsulitis of the shoulder: a study of the pathological findings in periarthritis of the shoulder. *J Bone Joint Surg.* 1945;27:211–222.

CHAPTER **52**

Elbow and Forearm Injuries and Lesions

Contributed by James A. Whiteside, American College of Sports Medicine, Alabama; and James R. Andrews, Washington Redskins football team, Ladies Professional Golf Association, US Olympic Committee, USA Baseball

Reviewer: Mike Wilkinson, Deputy CMO, Vancouver 2010 Winter Olympic Games, Canada

52.1 DISTAL HUMERUS FRACTURE

Field Assessment

Following a fall, collision, or direct blow to the elbow, the athlete has severe elbow pain, with or without visible deformity. Swelling occurs rapidly. Circulation to the hand may be decreased if there is associated vascular injury. Depending on the severity of the injury and deformity, a splint is applied on the field, with the limb in its resting position, or a sling is applied and the athlete is assisted to the sideline or an examining area for further evaluation and elbow immobilization.

Diagnosis

Deformity and rapid onset of significant swelling suggest displaced fracture(s), often with intra-articular fracture extension. Examine the wrist for possible additional injury. In the case of combined elbow and wrist fractures, acute compartment syndrome is more likely to develop, so check frequently to make certain that passive extension of the fingers and thumb does not cause forearm pain, which is often the first sign of compartment syndrome.

Treatment

Initial evaluation and management focus on the neurovascular condition of the limb, including splinting the limb in a position that allows good circulation to the hand and forearm, typically 30 to 60 degrees of elbow flexion for the most common injury patterns. Frequent monitoring of the neurovascular status is necessary. X-ray evaluation is performed, followed by appropriate nonsurgical or surgical care.

Return to Play

Fractures that are treated nonoperatively may take less or more time, depending on the specific fracture pattern. With internal fixation, an athlete in the 20- to 30-year age range can anticipate approximately 8 weeks before fracture healing is complete enough to allow heavy lifting and partial return to sport activity.

52.2 RADIAL HEAD/NECK FRACTURE

Field Assessment

Following a fall onto an outstretched hand, the athlete has moderate to severe elbow pain maximal over the radial aspect, usually without visible deformity. Swelling is mild to moderate and may develop slowly. Tenderness is localized to the radial head. A sling is applied and the athlete is assisted to the sideline or an examining area for further evaluation and elbow immobilization.

Diagnosis

The elbow appears normal except for diffuse swelling. Elbow flexion and extension may be only slightly decreased, but supination is limited and causes significant pain. X-rays are required to determine the specific anatomic site and the amount of displacement.

Treatment

The majority of radial head or neck fractures are not treated surgically, even if slight displacement or up to 30-degree angulation is present. X-ray evaluation is performed urgently, followed by appropriate orthopedic management. In most cases, this consists of splinting for a few days, then applying a brace or a bulky dressing and gradually increasing the range of motion each day. Aspiration of the hemarthrosis (blood in the joint) under sterile conditions usually decreases pain and allows earlier, improved range of motion.

Return to Play

In some sports that require little use of the arms, the athlete may return to limited training as soon as a few days following the injury, with an appropriate splint, brace, or dressing for protection. Early healing typically takes 3 weeks, with complete healing by 6 to 8 weeks after the injury.

52.3 MEDIAL EPICONDYLE AVULSION FRACTURE

Field Assessment

The young athlete presents with sharp medial elbow pain after a hard throw. Voluntary elbow motion is decreased. Swelling is mild, localized immediately over the medial epicondyle. The athlete is removed from competition, and either a sling or a splint is applied for comfort until x-ray evaluation is completed and definitive management arranged.

Diagnosis

Within a few hours of the injury, a small effusion may be present. The athlete has pain with attempted active forearm pronation. The athlete may have had previous symptoms in this exact region, with throwing or weight bearing (as in gymnastics or wrestling). Elbow x-rays with comparison views of the opposite elbow may be necessary to determine the amount of displacement.

Treatment

Although once controversial, the need for near-anatomic medial epicondyle position for throwing athletes, gymnasts, and wrestlers is now generally accepted. If the epicondyle is displaced more than 2 mm, reduction and internal fixation are indicated. Ice, a sling or splint, and NSAIDs are used until surgical intervention, when appropriate. Once fixation is complete, the integrity of the ulnar collateral ligament can be evaluated.

Return to Play

Most activities are allowed by 10 to 12 weeks following the injury, provided full range of motion and good strength are present and x-rays show healing. Forceful throwing activities are discouraged for a full year.

52.4 OLECRANON FRACTURE/EPIPHYSIS AVULSION

In the skeletally immature athlete, with open secondary centers of ossification, a sudden, forceful contraction of the triceps can avulse its insertion into the olecranon epiphysis. The olecranon growth plate may not fuse until young adulthood. In other athletes, the same mechanism, often from a fall onto an outstretched hand, may cause a more proximal or more distal intra-articular olecranon fracture. Older athletes may have a fibrous union at the olecranon tip from a previous injury such as after striking the tip of the elbow on a hard surface in a fall. This fibrous union also is susceptible to disruption by a massive contraction force. True stress fractures are rare in this area, but in the early teen years before closure of the growth plate, a simple stone's throw may produce sufficient force to avulse the olecranon tip while maintaining the integrity of the triceps/olecranon relationship. Such a fracture may be complete but is more often incomplete—open at the dorsal, tension side, but hinging on the articular cartilage and the portion of the physis near the joint.

Field Assessment

The athlete has significant pain and tenderness over the olecranon after a fall directly onto the elbow or onto the outstretched hand/forearm. Swelling is diffuse, and ROM is limited by pain and effusion. The olecranon appears prominent posteriorly, and a defect may be palpable. The triceps tendon/olecranon mechanism often seems intact but weakened. The athlete is removed from play and splinted in a comfortable position, usually about 30 degrees of flexion, and sent for x-rays and further appropriate management.

Diagnosis

X-rays are necessary for a precise diagnosis. Often, particularly in the case of minimally displaced fractures, comparison views of the opposite elbow are indicated to determine the amount of displacement.

Treatment

Treatment decisions are based on the amount of displacement and the athlete's situation with regard to sport. For the young adolescent with an incomplete fracture and minimal displacement, a brief period of immobilization (until nontender) and slowly progressive rehabilitation usually lead to healing. However, complete avulsion fractures through the growth plate/fibrous union that have even slight displacement generally require surgical intervention for the athlete, since the incidence of nonunion is very high with nonoperative treatment. Very small, avulsed fragments may be excised, and the triceps insertion repaired. Otherwise, rigid internal fixation of the fracture is indicated.

Return to Play

Progressive pain-free activity is permitted once healing is complete. Typically, full range of motion is established and strength is good by 8 weeks following the injury.

52.5 POSTERIOR ELBOW DISLOCATION

Field Assessment

The athlete has severe elbow pain following a fall onto an outstretched hand with the elbow fully extended. The elbow appears deformed, with an abnormal posterior prominence. Check the neurovascular status distal to the injury. Splint the elbow in its resting position of full extension or slight flexion. If circulation to the hand is poor, splint the elbow in 30 to 45 degrees of flexion or consider performing on-field closed reduction. Observe the neurovascular status carefully. Transport the

athlete for emergent reduction and further management.

Diagnosis

The history, abnormal elbow contour, and palpable deformity suggest the clinical diagnosis of posterior dislocation of the elbow, with or without fracture of the coronoid process of the ulna. The differential diagnosis includes distal humerus fracture and fracture dislocation. Avulsion fracture of the medial epicondyle often accompanies posterior elbow dislocation in the young adolescent athlete.

Treatment

The team physician may consider reduction of the posterior dislocation on the field if appropriately trained and experienced. By an hour or so after the injury occurs, intravenous sedation is often necessary in order to facilitate manual reduction. An intra-articular fracture or medial epicondyle avulsion that is displaced more than 2 mm following reduction generally requires surgical reduction and internal fixation for the athlete.

Return to Play

Normal daily activities are permitted when arm strength is 80% of normal and ROM is functional. Sport activities are allowed when the athlete's confidence in the strength of the elbow and the required technical skills for the sport have returned. The elbow brace is continued for sports for approximately 6 to 9 months.

52.6 DISTAL BICIPITAL TENDON RUPTURE

Field Assessment

The athlete presents with the sudden onset of severe anterior elbow pain as a result of lifting or pulling a heavy object. Flexion and supination strength is reduced. To observation, there is usually a defect in the region of the distal bicipital tendon and anterior swelling without ecchymosis. Immediate treatment consists of local ice application and a sling for support.

Diagnosis

Disruption of the distal bicipital tendon is a clinical diagnosis. The distal biceps muscle belly is tender to touch with associated weakness. Beware of the partial or complete tendon tear where the tendon sheath is intact as the deformity may not be immediately apparent. When there is a history of anabolic steroid use or local steroid injections, the pathology usually is found to be confined to the tendon–bone interface. An MRI scan is quite helpful in elucidating the exact location of the pathology.

Treatment

Initial treatment consists of local ice application, sling support, and the use of oral NSAIDs for comfort. Surgical repair of the distal biceps tendon rupture is necessary to restore bicipital function, unlike the case of proximal long head of the biceps tendon rupture, which can heal with reasonable (although usually decreased) flexion strength without surgical reattachment.

Return to Play

Rehabilitation is required until there is pain-free and essentially full ROM. Resistance exercise training is continued until full strength is restored before unlimited activity is permitted.

52.7 LATERAL EPICONDYLOSIS

Tenderness and chronic pain localized to or near the lateral epicondyle after repetitive wrist extension is known as lateral epicondylosis, or "tennis elbow." Damage to the extensor carpi radialis brevis tendon that occurs with the stress of overuse/overload results from a hypoxic, degenerative tendinopathy or tendinosis with associated neovascularity.

Diagnosis

The clinical diagnosis of lateral epicondylosis is suspected by the history of repetitive eccentric/concentric motion at the wrist and/or isometric overload at the origin of the extensor tendon, often associated with racket sports. Local tenderness and swelling, and pain over the common extensor tendon origin with resisted wrist and/or finger extension, especially with pronated forearm, confirm the diagnosis.

Treatment

Initial treatment is conservative with altering or removing the factors that led to the injury, frequent local ice application, oral NSAIDs, and a forearm compression sleeve or band. If these measures are unsuccessful, then a local corticosteroid injection may be indicated for the inflammatory component. Rehabilitation must include eccentric loading exercises. Recent research has shown significant improvements with the use of topical nitroglycerine patch or cream and local sclerosant injections. Arthroscopic or minimally invasive epicondylar release should be considered when no relief is evident after the above treatments.

Return to Play

Return to activity is permitted when grip strength, pronation, supination, and hand and finger action are normal. Wearing a compressive forearm sleeve or band is suggested.

52.8 OSTEOCHONDROSIS/ OSTEOCHONDRITIS DISSECANS

Diagnosis

The young athlete presents with persistent activity-related lateral elbow pain. Swelling may be negligible, or an effusion may be present. Flexion and extension are generally limited somewhat and full supination causes pain as does throwing or upper extremity weight bearing. The capitellum and/or radiocapitellar joint are tender to palpation. The child gymnast or throwing athlete with lateral elbow pain of gradual onset sufficient to limit ROM is likely to have osteochondrosis of Panner. MRI and x-rays typically show rarefaction and partial obliteration of the ossification center of the capitellum, usually without loose body formation. In the adolescent, a similar lesion from the same mechanism of injury is generally termed osteochondritis dissecans. Osteocartilaginous fragments may become loose in the joint, and deformity of both the capitellum and the radial head are typical in the adolescent with this condition. The etiology of each disorder is unclear, but there appears to be a relationship between avascular necrosis and throwing or weight-bearing activities with lateral compression due to valgus stress on the elbow.

Treatment

In the case of osteochondrosis, cessation of the causative activity generally allows for recovery. In osteochondritis dissecans, surgical reattachment or removal of articular fragments, and stimulation of the subchondral bone to produce replacement fibrocartilage are indicated when rest and therapeutic exercise do not restore ROM and function, or if imaging studies show loose fragments.

Return to Play

Gradual return to full activity is permitted under supervision when elbow motion is pain free, arm strength is comparable to the uninvolved elbow, and the osseous lesion has healed.

52.9 MEDIAL EPICONDYLITIS

Tenderness and chronic pain localized to or near the medial epicondyle after repetitive valgus extension, especially in skeletally immature athletes, is known as lateral epicondylitis, or "tennis elbow." In skeletally mature athletes, the condition may coexist with medial collateral ligament insufficiency.

Diagnosis

Local tenderness and swelling, and pain with resisted wrist pronation or wrist flexion, confirm the diagnosis.

Treatment

Initial treatment is conservative with altering or removing the factors that led to the injury, frequent local ice application, and oral NSAIDs. If these measures are unsuccessful, then a local corticosteroid injection may be indicated.

Return to Play

Return to activity is permitted when pain free and when the demands of the sport are met.

52.10 FOREARM FRACTURES

Field Assessment

Athletic forearm fractures usually occur from a fall onto an outstretched hand or a direct bending force such as another player stepping on the athlete's forearm. Immediate severe pain is often accompanied by obvious deformity and rapid swelling. There may be a deformity (Fig. 52.1), and circulation is always a major concern. The limb should be splinted from axilla to midpalm, and the athlete transported for further evaluation and fracture care. Watch for possible development of compartment syndrome.

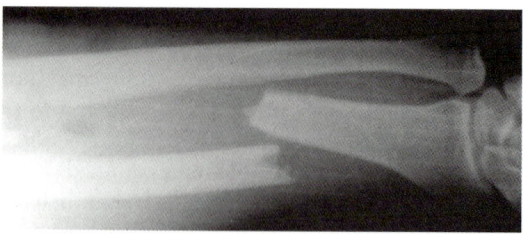

FIGURE 52.1   X-ray of a forearm fracture. (Reprinted from Bucholz RW, Heckman JD. *Rockwood & Green's Fractures in Adults.* 5th ed. Philadelphia, PA: Lippincott Williams & Wilkins; 2001, with permission.)

Treatment

Young athletes with two or more years of growth remaining are often successfully treated by closed reduction and cast immobilization. Older athletes usually require surgical internal fixation of the fracture(s) to maintain good position.

Return to Play

The athlete must have at least nearly normal range of motion and strength, and be able to perform the necessary sport-specific activities.

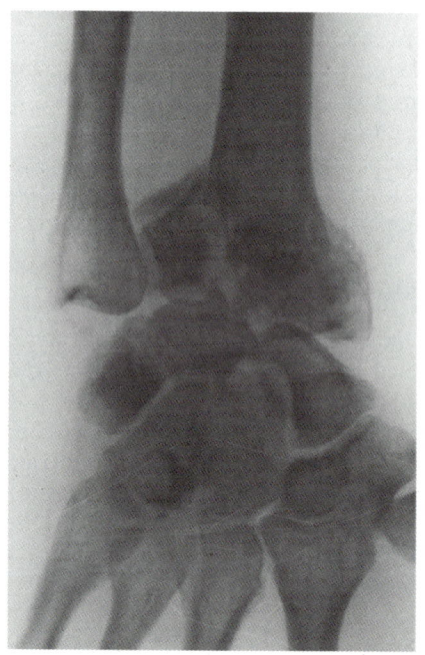

FIGURE 52.2   X-ray of a distal radius fracture. (Reprinted from Bucholz RW, Heckman JD. *Rockwood & Green's Fractures in Adults.* 5th ed. Philadelphia, PA: Lippincott Williams & Wilkins; 2001, with permission.)

52.11 WRIST FRACTURES

Field Assessment

The athlete presents with pain, with or without obvious deformity, following a fall onto an outstretched hand or a direct blow. The athlete is removed from the field, with on-field splint or sling application if deformity is noted. Emergent or urgent thorough evaluation and management are indicated, depending on the severity of the injury.

Diagnosis

There is bone tenderness, most frequently involving the distal radius (Fig. 52.2), distal ulna, and/or carpal navicular (scaphoid). In skeletally immature athletes, wrist sprain is extremely rare, so the diagnosis is almost always a fracture when wrist pain and swelling are present. Salter-Harris type I (nondisplaced) growth plate fracture is a clinical diagnosis made by tenderness that follows the line of the growth plate. With deformity and/or severe swelling, the neurovascular examination may be abnormal, indicating injury or compression of the involved structures.

Treatment

Initial treatment includes ice, splinting, and elevation. Further treatment depends on the specific fracture pattern and the athlete's age.

Return to Play

Return to action must be individualized depending on the fracture stability and the demands of the sport.

CHAPTER 53

Hand Injuries and Hand Infections

Contributed by David McDonagh, Deputy CMO, Lillehammer 1994 Olympic Winter Games

Reviewer: Mike Wilkinson, Deputy CMO, VANOC, Vancouver, Canada

53.1 HAND WOUNDS

Hand wounds can be divided into the following categories:

- Cuts and lacerations to the palm, the dorsum of the hand, or the fingers
- Fingertip wounds and amputations
- Nail injuries
- Bite wounds

Lacerations of the Hand

As with cuts elsewhere on the body, you must always inspect for underlying tissue damage, so look for muscle, tendon, capsule, and nerve/artery lesions. In the fingers, there is not a lot you can do about superficial nerve damage—these usually regenerate after a period of time.

For all wounds to the palm that are more than skin deep, it is a good idea to refer these to an orthopedic or hand/plastic surgeon—if for no other reason than to properly inspect the deeper palmar structures and to evaluate for function.

All wounds to the hand must be examined for

- Tendon injuries
- Joint capsule injuries
- Nerve injuries
- Infections

Cuts in the hand must be rigorously cleaned (with salt water, soap, Hibiscrub/povidone, and if necessary a soft, plastic surgical nail brush); do not use strong chlorhexidine as this may irritate or inflame some of the delicate structures in the hand. Put the hand in a bowl of soapy salt water for 10 to 15 minutes, then clean and examine thoroughly. Remove rings first. It can be a good idea to anesthetize the finger (ring blockade) before cleaning the wound; however, make sure that you test for nerve function, muscle and tendon function (strength and ROM) before anesthetizing. Partial ruptures should be referred to a hand surgeon. Always use sterile gloves. If referral to a hand surgeon is not deemed necessary, then primary suture should be conducted within 6 to 8 hours. Finger arterial bleeds can usually be stopped with compression, but sometimes a ligating suture has to be utilized. Use 5/0 suture material where possible, but 4/0 must usually be used over joints or in the palm. Use a short 3/8 or 4/8 needle. Remove sutures after 12 days.

Many EPs prescribe prophylactic phenoxymethylpenicillin for tissue cuts in the hand, and cephalexin or dicloxacillin for joint or tendon/ligament/capsule injuries.

Evaluate the need for tetanus vaccine based on your local tetanus guidelines.

Finger Amputations

Fingers can be traumatically amputated at any level, but most lesions involve the fingertips. Amputations have been known to occur in luge and skating sports. Some amputations require specialist treatment, particularly when replantation is considered as with the loss of a thumb, several fingers, etc. (Consult local guidelines for referral.) I would recommend referral when the amputation is below the level of the nail—even if the stump is even—not because they are so difficult to treat, but because the facilities at a sports event are not usually suitable.

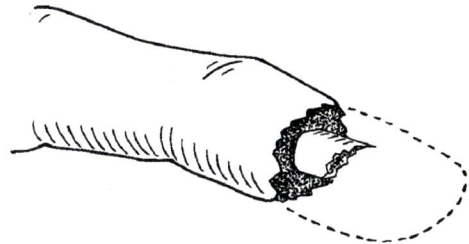

FIGURE 53.1. Open fracture/amputation, jagged bone end.

Fingertip amputations are usually pretty straight, clean cuts; by this, I mean the stump is not jagged. If the stump is uneven, particularly if the distal phalanx is prominent, then referral for surgical treatment is necessary (Figs. 53-1 and 53-2).

If the stump is even, then an occlusion bandage will often suffice. I usually get a sterile glove, squeeze silver sulfadiazine cream into the relevant glove finger, get the patient to put the glove on, and then cut away the glove at the injured finger's MCP joint, wrapping some tape around the base of this glove bandage. If the amputated finger fragment is large and clean enough, surgeons at some major centers may endeavor to replant, but results are often unsuccessful. Tetanus vaccine should be considered. Similarly, antibiotics should be used if bone has been exposed.

Fingernails

The nail is a complex structure involving three layers: the nail itself, the nail bed (the matrix, which is responsible for nail growth and support), and the cuticle (eponychium) and lateral nail folds (raised skin on the sides of the nail). Injury mechanisms include tearing or ripping actions, as when catching a fingernail or stubbing a toe; blunt force mechanisms, as when a toenail is stood upon or when hit by a field hockey stick; or when cut, from skate blades, machinery, etc.

There are various types of nail injuries:

■ Subungual hematoma occurs when blood collects under the nail and are usually caused by

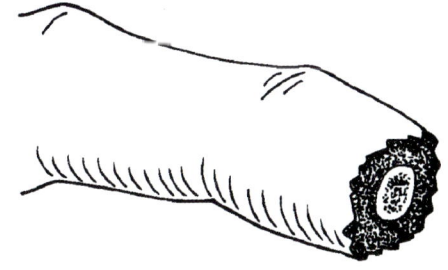

FIGURE 53.2. Open fracture/amputation, even bone end.

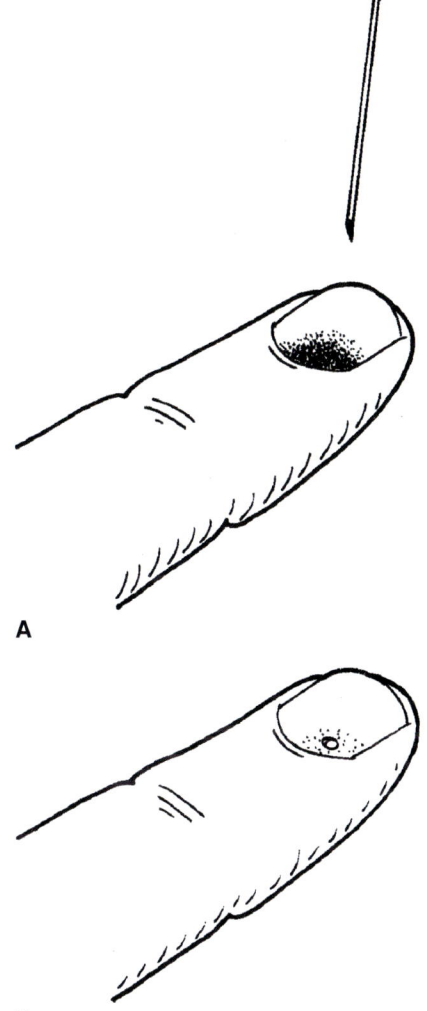

A

B

FIGURE 53.3. A, B: Subungual hematoma.

a blow to the nail. They are initially a red or red/blue, purple color, darkening to blue, and then almost black before receding to normal coloration after many weeks. The hematoma may cause a pressure swelling and the nail can become tender and quite painful. If still in the fluid state, pressure can be released by gently boring a hole in the nail at the midpoint of the discoloration (Fig. 53.3A,B). This be done by either gently rotating a needle (as with acupuncture technique) or by burning through the nail using the point end of a paper clip (having first heated it up on a spirit lamp—a useful tool for any kit is a hand drill available at any hobby store. This is even more effective and less painful than a paper clip when heated.) If the hematoma has coagulated fully, there is little point in making a hole in the nail.

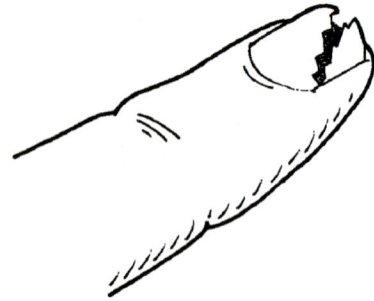

FIGURE 53.4. Nail laceration.

- Beware: A history of trauma must be present. Malignant melanomas can occur under the nail and can have the appearance of a hematoma.

- Lacerations of the nail may occur and affect the nail, the matrix, the cuticle, the lateral nail folds, or a combination of these. Lacerations or fractures of the nail may vary in presentation, from simple lacerations (simple split nails are usually left alone unless they are dislocated or there is an underlying matrix injury—then a suture may be placed through both nail parts and underlying matrix, which can be removed after a week) to multiple nail fragments often with small lacerations into the matrix and cuticle. These must be sutured as best can, and it is usually a good idea to leave isolated nail fragments alone as their removal may cause the removal of underlying matrix. The nail also acts as a splint for underlying matrix. Fractured, dislocated nail fragments that pierce the

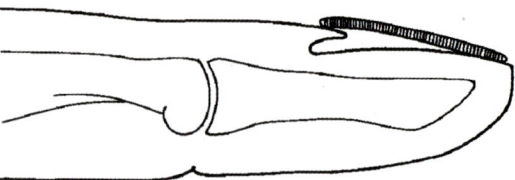

FIGURE 53.6. Avulsed nail.

matrix should be gently relocated or removed (Figs. 53.4 and 53.5).

- Nail avulsion or dislocation of the nail: These should be relocated. Usually, the nail is avulsed at its base and the nail that was under the cuticle becomes displaced so that it lies on top of the cuticle. There is usually damage to the soft tissue around the nail that requires suturing. Using a ring blockade anesthetic, lift the nail at the proximal end, bend it, causing a convexity, and then slide the nail back under the cuticle, if this is still present. Suturing of the nail is usually unnecessary, but if so, I usually just pierce the center of the nail and make a deep stabilizing suture (Figs. 53.6–53.11).

All of the above injuries may be associated with a fracture, so the need for x-ray has to be evaluated. There is usually a need for antibiotics in cases with a fracture as they are, per definition, open fractures. Antibiotics are not usually recommended in nonfracture injuries unless the wound has been caused by a bite or has been contaminated. Fingernails may take between 4 and 6 months to grow back. After an injury, permanent nail deformities are not uncommon.

Bite Wounds

As mentioned in Chapter 17, infections may arise after cuts caused by hitting an opponent's teeth with a clenched fist. Penicillinase-producing bacteria may infect these wounds, so correct antibiotics should be chosen. These wounds can be very painful and tender and may even spread into

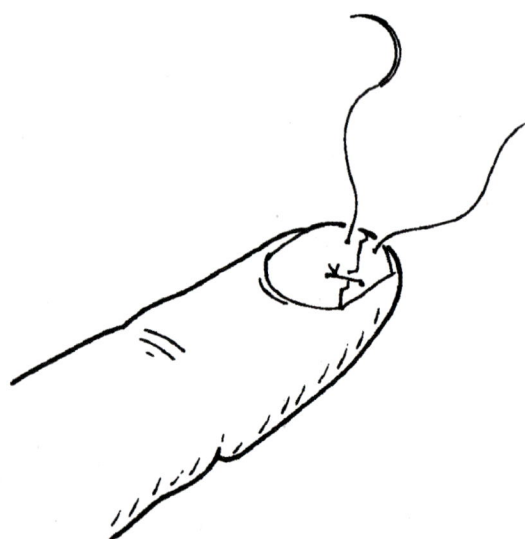

FIGURE 53.5. Nail suture.

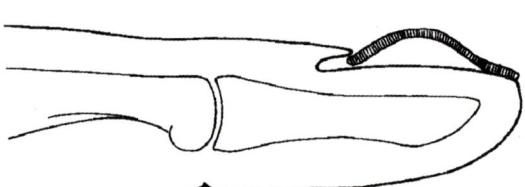

FIGURE 53.7. Bend nail before relocating.

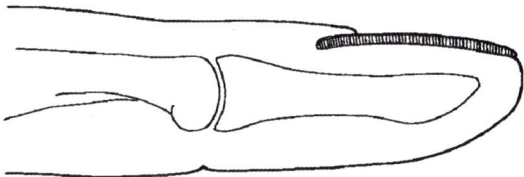

FIGURE 53.8   Relocated nail.

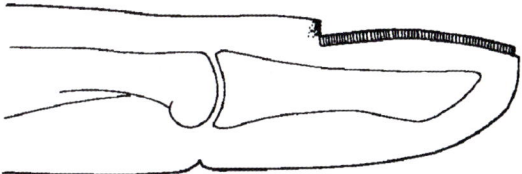

FIGURE 53.10.   Relocated nail.

nearby joints causing a bacterial arthritis with cartilage destruction. Wounds must be thoroughly cleansed and athletes with possible joint infections should be admitted to a hospital for treatment including arthrotomy, joint lavage, antibiotics, and joint elevation. Mobilization of the joint should be initiated as soon as possible.

53.2 HAND INFECTIONS

The number of organisms that can infect the hand is legion, and while making the diagnosis is often easy (i.e., infection or no infection), guessing the causative organism can be extremely difficult in the absence of microbiological culture results. As it often takes 3 or more days before bacteria typing of swabs is available, and 5 or more days to get drug sensitivity reports, it is essential to take a culture and send this to the lab as soon as possible and also to initiate treatment with the right antibiotic. As a general rule, superficial infections are caused by streptococci and deep infections by staphylococci.

Streptococci are the usual causative bacteria with

- Cellulitis
- Erysipelas
- Impetigo
- Necrotizing fasciitis
- Paronychia

Staphylococci are the usual causative bacteria with

- Phlegmonas
- Carbuncles
- Furuncles
- Abscesses
- Paronychia

Panaritium (pulp infections) are deep infections and can have multiple causes. Admission to a hospital or referral to a specialist is a good idea as these infections can erode into bone or joints causing osteomyelitis or infectious arthritis. Untreated paronychias may also be the source of deep infections—milder paonychias often respond to treatment with soapy water baths (immerse the affected finger in a solution of 10 mL green surgical soap diluted in 1 L of lukewarm water for 10 minutes twice daily).

Also of major concern are untreated or poorly treated infections on the volar aspect of the fingers as infection may spread down toward the flexor ligaments and their fascia causing a bacterial or purulent tendovaginitis that may require admission to hospital, IV antibiotics and surgical toilet. Untreated, these may lead to tendon destruction and spread proximally into the palmar aponeurosis with abscess formation and major disturbance of hand function. Thus, the presence of a warm thenar, palmar, or hypothenar swelling should cause immediate concern, and the presence of an abscess requires admission to a hospital. Therefore, be extremely alert for this particularly nasty infection (Fig. 53.12).

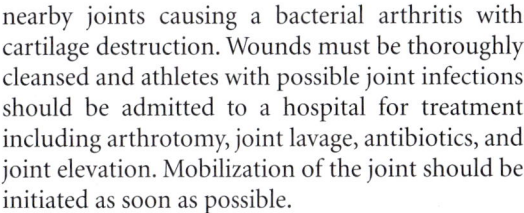

FIGURE 53.9.   Avulsed nail with damaged cuticle.

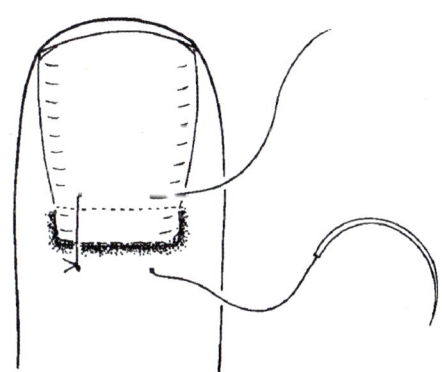

FIGURE 53.11.   Suturing of relocated nail.

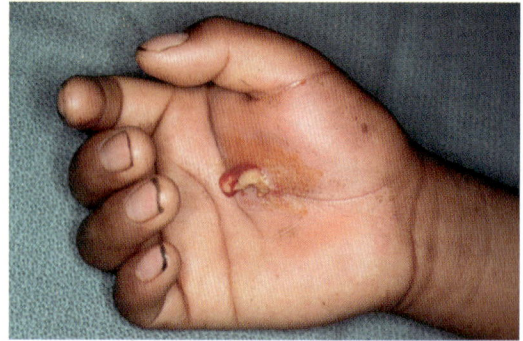

FIGURE 53.12.   Thenar abscess.

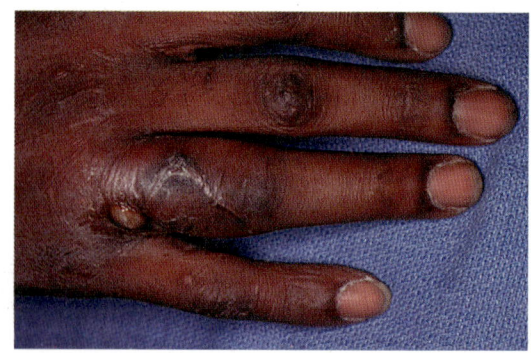

FIGURE 53.13.   Osteomyelitis.

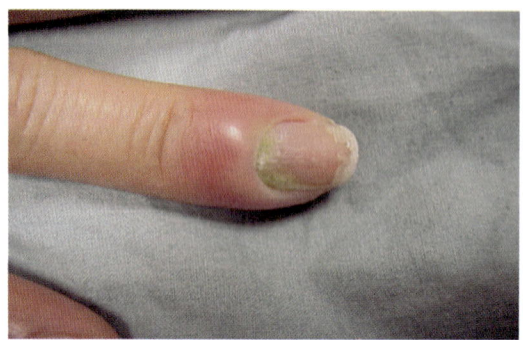

FIGURE 53.14.   Paronychia.

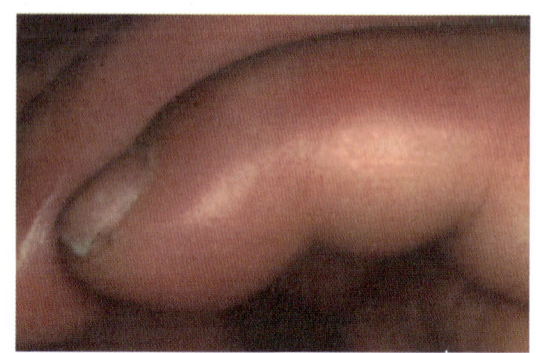

FIGURE 53.15.   Panaritium.

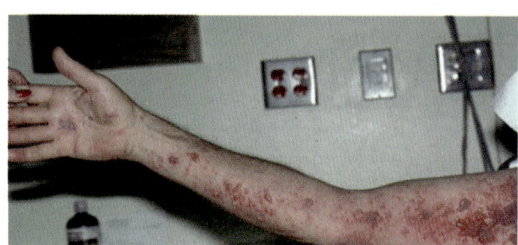

FIGURE 53.16.   Herpes simplex.

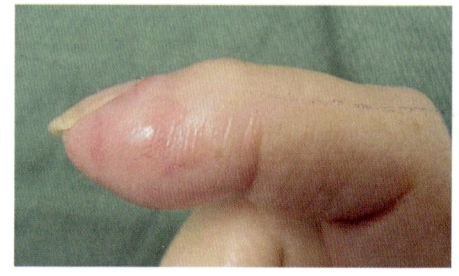

FIGURE 53.17.   Metastases from breast cancer.

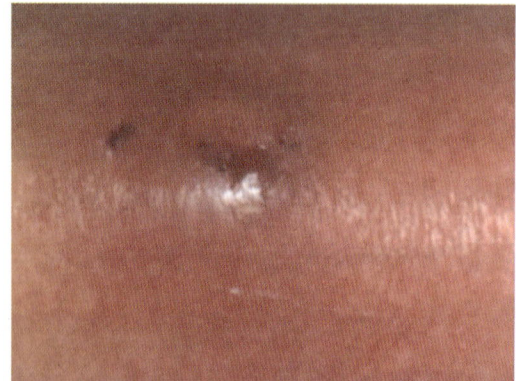

FIGURE 53.18.   Erysipelas.

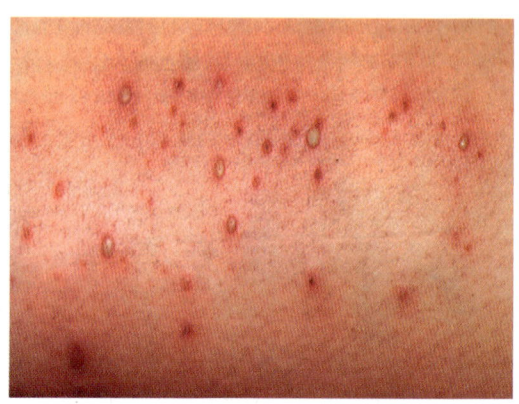

FIGURE 53.19.   Impetigo.

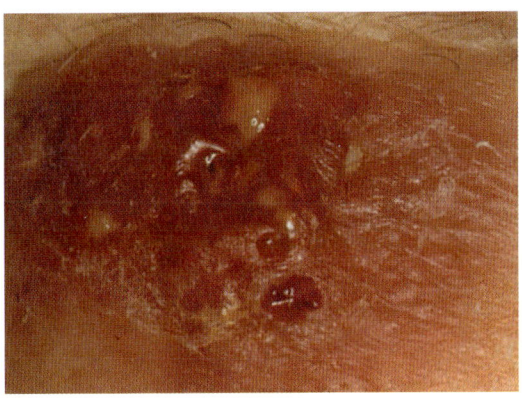

FIGURE 53.20. Carbuncle.

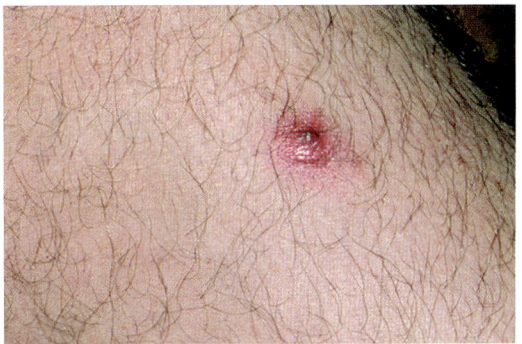

FIGURE 53.22. Furuncle. (Reprinted from Goodheart HP. *Goodheart's photoguide of common skin disorders.* 2nd ed. Philadelphia, PA: Lippincott Williams & Wilkins; 2003:126, with permission.)

Other Conditions

- Pyoderma gangrenosum—an idiopathic, painful, ulcerative condition associated with disorders such as Crohn's disease, ulcerative colitis, arthritis, myeloproliferative conditions, and chronic hepatitis

- *Mycobacterium marinum*—seen in swimmers, fishermen, and aquarium employees

- Erysipeloid—unusual disorder in sport, but most often seen in fishermen and butchers

- Dentist's finger—a painful herpes simplex lesion of the finger

- Orf—a zoonotic disease, contracted through direct contact with infected sheep and goats, causing a purulent-appearing papule, usually on the fingers, hands, and arms

- Fungal infections of the nails

- Subungual malignant melanomas including the amelanotic malignant melanoma

53.3 OPEN LIGAMENT AND TENDON INJURIES

As a rule, all tendon, ligament, and capsule injuries should be sent to a hand surgeon. An open dorsal DIP joint drop finger injury, in the third, fourth, and fifth finger may be attempted sutured if you have the necessary competence and experience; if not, refer. I would recommend referral of DIP joint injuries in the second finger and IP thumb joint injuries due to the importance of these joints in ensuring grip function. Open wounds on the palmar surface of the fingers should be inspected for and tested for flexor tendon injury. Flexor tendon injuries, if found or suspected, should be referred to an orthopedic surgeon.

53.4 CLOSED LIGAMENT AND TENDON INJURIES

There are numerous variations of these closed ligament ruptures. Some need surgery; some do not. As a general rule, rupture of flexor tendons require surgical repair. If a flexor tendon has ruptured, there is a loss of flexion and thus pronounced extension at either the PIP or DIP joint.

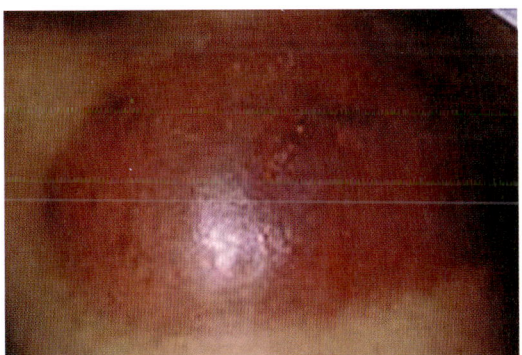

FIGURE 53.21. Phlegmonal abscess.

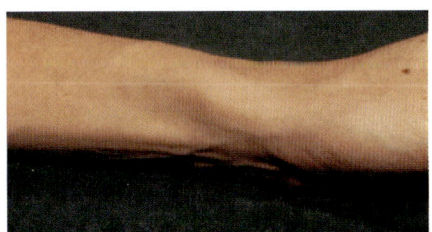

FIGURE 53.23. De Quervains tenosynovitis.

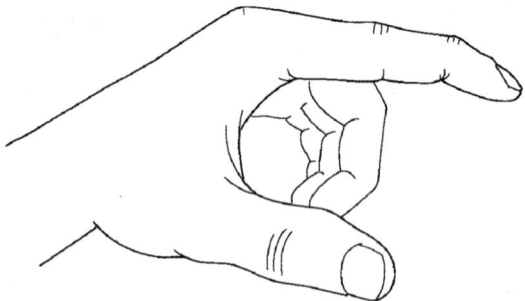

FIGURE 53.24.   Drop finger.

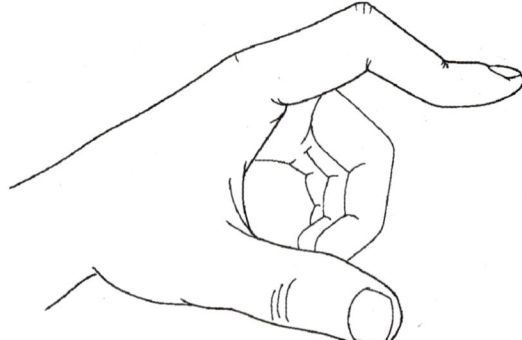

FIGURE 53.26.   Bouttonière defect.

Extensor/Dorsal DIP Joint Injuries

Pain on the dorsal aspect of a DIP joint combined with an extension deficit would imply the presence of a drop finger (extensor rupture) or avulsion fracture. A closed drop finger lesion should be treated conservatively with the joint in full extension using a small cast or prefabricated finger support for 6 weeks. Surgery is seldom indicated and seldom successful (Fig. 53.24).

Flexor/Volar DIP Joint Injuries

Pain on the volar aspect of a DIP joint with intact flexion of the PIP joint but absent flexion and forced hyperextension of the DIP joint would imply a lesion of the superficial digital flexor (Fig. 53.25).

Extensor/Dorsal PIP Joint Injuries

Pain on the dorsal aspect of a finger PIP joint combined with an extension deficit and forced flexion at the PIP joint, but with intact PIP extension and flexion would imply a boutonnière defect (Fig. 53.26).

Flexor/Volar PIP Joint Injuries

Pain on the volar aspect of a finger PIP joint and MCP joint may be associated with forced hyperextension

of the PIP joint; association with absent flexion at both the PIP and DIP joint would imply a complete rupture of the flexor apparatus. Intact DIP joint flexion but absent PIP joint flexion would imply damage to the deep flexor tendon. Surgery is indicated with all flexor ruptures and PIP joint exstensor ruptures (Fig. 53.27). Surgical repair of damaged tendons is best left to experts and should be performed in a sterile environment. It is also often necessary to explore the tendon injury by further opening the wound, so referral to a specialist center is recommended.

Collateral Ligament Injuries

Collateral ligament injuries can also occur at the PIP and DIP joints and are often associated with tiny avulsion fractures. Ligament stability is tested by performing varus and valgus tests. Ligamental defects are best treated with immobilization, either by taping the affected finger to its neighbor or by using "Buddy Loops" for 6 weeks. For the collateral ligament of the first MCP joint, see below.

Avulsion Fractures

These are not uncommon around the PIP or DIP joints, as valgus or varus stress of the collateral

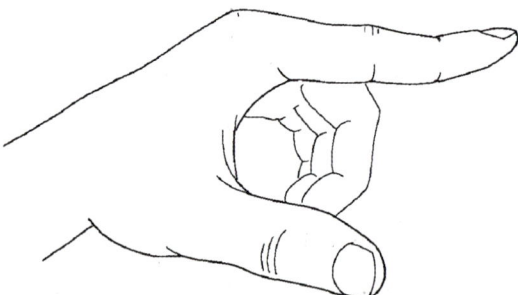

FIGURE 53.25.   Flexor rupture at DIP joint.

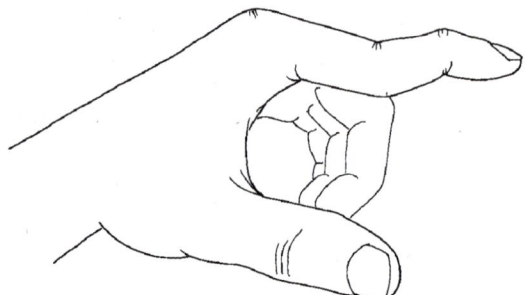

FIGURE 53.27.   Flexor rupture at PIP joint.

ligaments (which are often stronger than bone) may lead to a fracture rather than a ligamental injury. As a rule, these fractures can be treated conservatively by taping the injured finger to its neighbor. This dynamic form of immobilization seems to work better than a rigid cast, which often leads to the injured joint being stiff. If the fracture affects the joint and the avulsed segment affects more than one-third of the articular surface in width, then surgery is usually indicated.

53.5 ULNAR COLLATERAL LIGAMENT INJURIES OF THE FIRST MCP JOINT

Ulnar collateral ligament (UCL) sprain, also known as skier's or gamekeeper's thumb, occurs after a stretching or falling on an abducted thumb—the classical example being when a skier's pole becomes snagged. The athlete complains of a painful, swollen, stiff thumb with discomfort and often swelling at the first MCP joint, particularly on the ulnar aspect of the joint. Gently applied abduction stress may cause significant radial deviation of the thumb (Fig. 53.28).

Diagnosis

Test for laxity in the UCL by stressing the ligament: While stabilizing the first metacarpal with one hand, gently apply abduction stress to the extended joint using your other hand. Mobility should be compared with the healthy side. If there is a tear in the UCL, then abduction stress will cause increased radial deviation of the thumb. The test may also be carried out with the thumb flexed. Complete disruption of the UCL leads to pronounced radial deviation, and there may be as much as a 20-degree or greater difference in angulation when comparing both thumbs. Occasionally, the ligament becomes interposed between the metacarpal and the proximal phalanx, a so-called Stener lesion.

Treatment

In my part of the world, complete tears are referred to operation, although in some countries, complete ruptures are treated conservatively with a cast for 3 weeks. Partial tears are treated with a cast or splint for a minimum of 3 weeks followed by 3 weeks with dynamic splinting. These casts must be changed often to ensure that the cast is well molded at all times, particularly when the swelling resolves.

Taping before competition can support a previously injured UCL.

Return to Play

Full activity can be commenced when pain free and full ROM has been achieved. Thumb and joint strength should also be adequate for the sporting activity. One should allow for a period of 10 to 12 weeks after injury or surgery before commencing active sport. Routine activities that do not challenge the UCL can be initiated after 6 to 8 weeks.

53.6 HAND FRACTURES

Hand fractures can be divided into

- Carpal fractures
- Metacarpal fractures
- Finger fractures

Firstly, beware swellings in the dorsum of the hand. One obviously suspects a fracture if there is a

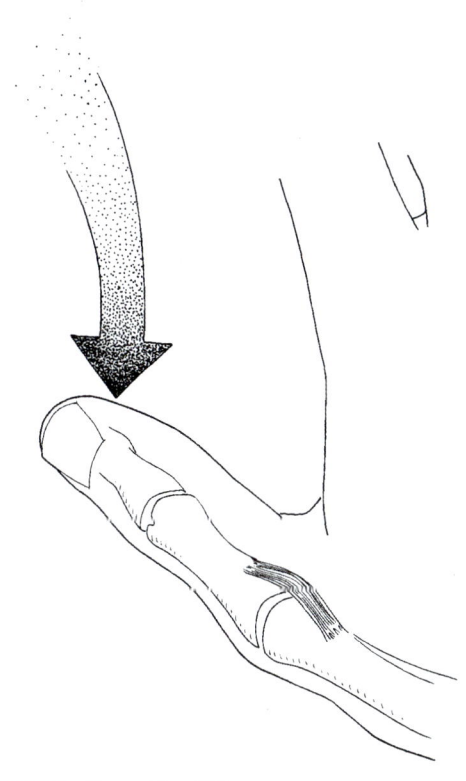

FIGURE 53.28. Normal first UCL.

swelling over bone. If the x-ray is negative but clinical findings implying a fracture are present, there is a temptation to put on a cast, just in case. This is accepted practice in many countries, as x-ray diagnosis is not always black and white (excuse the pun). If one goes for the safety-first regime, this may have serious consequences for one type of injury: carpal subluxations due to intercarpal ligament ruptures. If these are not correctly examined for, diagnosed, and treated, there is the danger of permanent dysfunction in the hand, either due to incorrectly plastering a dislocated bone or not plastering a fracture. I have seen this lesion and complication in several boxers.

Lunate Dislocations

These are uncommon lesions but must be examined for. The lunate is in the first carpal row on a line with the third metacarpal—if you palpate the radioulnar joint dorsally, the lunate is usually directly distal to this. Tenderness and swelling may imply a fracture and/or dislocation. Palpation may reveal swelling but also a recess when the lunate is dislocated toward the palmar surface.

If suspicion is aroused, apply ice and compress the injury site, refer to radiology, and request special x-rays of the lunate, or a CT scan.

Treatment usually requires surgery, unless the dislocation is moderate.

Scaphoid Fracture

The easiest fracture to miss is a fracture of the scaphoid bone. Classically, one palpates the anatomical snuffbox, but this is almost always tender with most wrist injuries. To examine the scaphoid, it is not enough to just press into the snuffbox at a 90-degree angle to the skin, because you are often only applying pressure to the styloid process of the radius and the wrist capsule. To elicit scaphoid tenderness, point your index finger in the direction of the third, fourth, and fifth MCP joints; you are now palpating the scaphoid. Tenderness here may indicate a scaphoid fracture rather than a distal radius injury. Whilst keeping the index finger in the snuffbox and pointing toward the MCP joints, and simultaneously placing one's thumb over the palmar aspect of the hand at the proximal end of the thenar eminence one can apply bidigital compression on the scaphoid—tenderness may indicate a scaphoid fracture (Fig. 53.29).

Why is this an issue? If you request an x-ray of the wrist, you will more than likely miss a scaph-

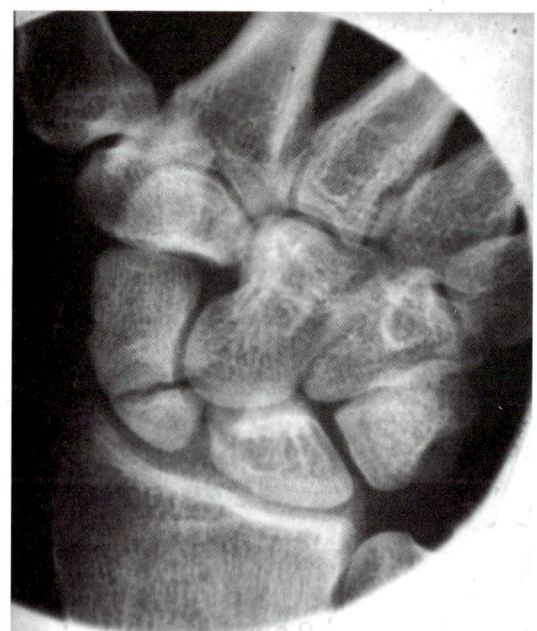

FIGURE 53.29. Scaphoid fracture.

oid fracture. Even if you correctly request a scaphoid series of x-rays, you can still miss a fracture as a high percentage of scaphoid fractures are not found on primary x-ray. If the patient has digital and bidigital tenderness, I apply a plaster cast for 1 week. If tenderness is still present after a week, then refer to CT or MRI. Athletes who are traveling tend to have poor follow-up, and scaphoid fractures can go undiagnosed. Complications can occur—potential malunion, avascular necrosis, etc.

One might avoid this scenario by ordering a CT scan of the scaphoid as the primary investigative procedure, but this is an expensive and not easily accessible examination in many parts of the world available and difficult to obtain in other parts of the world.

Diagnosis of Other Carpal Fractures

Usually, deep palpation and rotation of the wrist causes pain in fractured carpal bones. Fractures are usually, but not always, found on plain x-ray, though, like scaphoid fractures, CT is sometimes necessary.

Metacarpal Fractures

The most commonly seen metacarpal fracture is that of the fifth metacarpal. It is usually associated with fighting (not necessarily boxing). Sure, boxers injure and break the fifth metacarpal, but they also break other metacarpals and carpal bones as well. The fifth is more often seen in street fighting or wall punchers. Angulated or rotated fractures may require surgery or reduction. Apply ice and compression and send the athlete for a radiological evaluation. Always attempt to evaluate the presence or extent of finger rotation with metacarpal fractures.

Finger Fractures

These are not unusual, particularly after falls or when hit on the finger by a baseball or another opponent when blocking a throw (handball, American football), etc. It is not always easy to differentiate between a pure dislocation and fracture/dislocation clinically, so x-rays should be requested. If the waiting time for investigation is long—let us say 2 hours or more—then a closed reduction may be attempted to prevent long-term damage at the joint/fracture site. The main problem with finger fractures is that of rotation.

Tape or Buddy Loop the potentially broken finger to a neighboring finger and refer the patient to x-ray.

Finger rotation can be extremely difficult to evaluate but must always be examined for clinically and radiologically if suspected. A fracture can appear to be correctly aligned on an x-ray, but the finger may be rotated clinically.

I learned an old trick that can be useful in evaluating finger rotation associated with finger, or often, metacarpal fractures.

Gently flex each finger, one at a time, from the DIP toward the thenar eminence. The fractured finger will obviously stop before the others. Draw a line with a pen from the middle of the DIP joint down through the middle of the finger to the fingertip and continue the line over to the thenar eminence. Do this for all fingers. In most patients these lines meet over the proximal scaphoid in a 1-cm diameter circle. Compare both sides; does the fractured finger vary very much from its ipsilateral partners or from the contralateral side? This

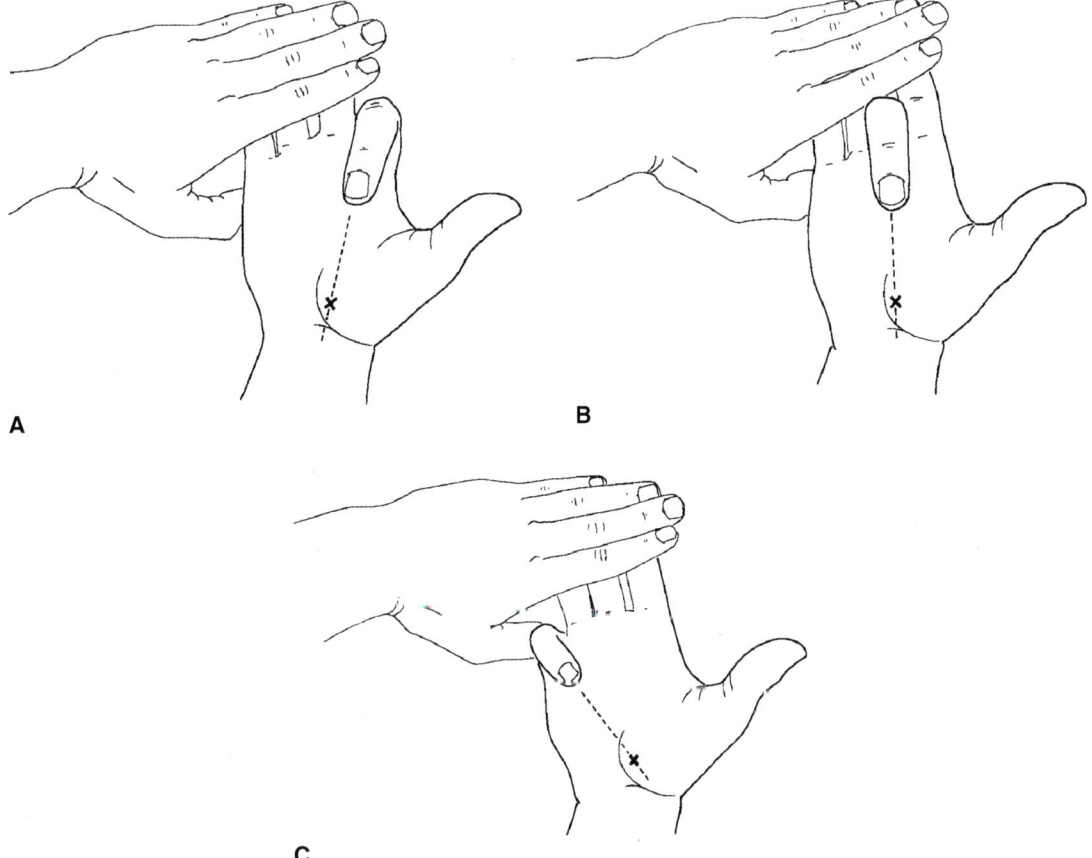

A

B

C

FIGURE 53.30. Normal flexion of second, third, and fifth fingers.

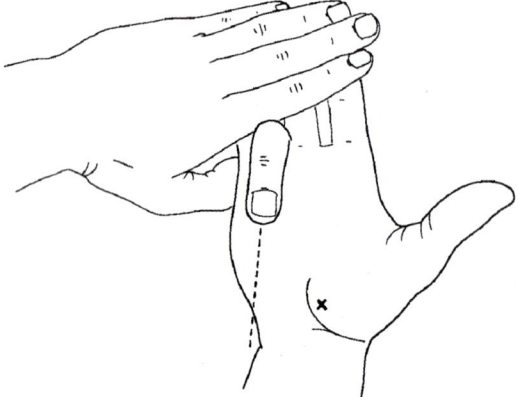

FIGURE 53.31. Abnormal rotation of fourth finger under flexion.

comparison may not always be accurate as many patients have crooked fingers, in particular slim girls or people with deformities from before. The test is worth trying, though. You will be fooled if the patient tries to flex all fingers at the same time. Flex them one by one and rotational defects become more visible. Finger rotation is important because it may affect the athlete's ability to grip (Figs. 53.30 and 53.31).

Open fractures or open dislocations require antibiotic treatment, intravenously on occasions.

Recommended Reading

1. Boyd R, Libetta C. Towards evidence-based emergency medicine: best BETs from the Manchester Royal Infirmary. Reimplantation of the nail root in fingertip crush injuries in children. *Emerg Med J.* 2002;19(2):141.
2. Brown RE. Acute nail bed injuries. *Hand Clin.* 2002;18(4):561–575.
3. Chang J, Vernadakis AJ, McClellan WT. Fingertip injuries. *Clin Occup Environ Med.* 2006;5(2):413–422, ix.
4. Jellinek NJ. Nail surgery: practical tips and treatment options. *Dermatol Ther.* 2007;20(1):68–74.

CHAPTER 54

Pelvic and Hip Injuries

Contributed by Roger Hackney, Chapel Allerton Hospital, Leeds; President, British Orthopedic Sports Trauma Association; former medical officer for UK athletics; three-time Olympic steeplechaser; and Peter Giannoudis, Professor, University of Leeds, Leeds General Infirmary Hospital, Leeds; President, British Trauma Society; President, European Society of Pelvis and Acetabulum; Greek Olympic marathon runner

Reviewer: Dr. Katharina Grimm, Head of Medical Office, FIFA

Pelvic and hip injuries comprise approximately 5% of all injuries sustained by athletes, with some athletic activities having higher incidences such as soccer, running, American football, horse riding, and hockey.

54.1 PRIMARY ASSESSMENT IN HIGH-IMPACT TRAUMA

Severe acute injuries to the pelvis, especially those that result in significant fracture, are a result of high-energy trauma. The most common causes in sport are from collisions in motor sports or falling from a horse. The attending physician must ensure that the area where the injury occurs is safe for the athlete, the medical team, other competitors, and spectators. There must be a mechanism in place for immediately stopping the race or game and summoning urgent help as required. Early resuscitation and evacuation of a severely injured athlete can be life saving.

The initial assessment of these injuries always should begin with a primary survey, which is performed at the spot before moving the injured. It is helpful to adopt the ATLS approach of evaluation as follows: Airway, Breathing, Circulation, Disability, Exposure and Environment (ABCDE).

The purpose of the ABCDE is to identify early life- and limb-threatening injuries that require immediate attention. By using the ABCDE approach, hemodynamic instability from an occult fracture should be identified readily. For instance, considerable volumes of blood may be lost into third spaces in the body following pelvic or femur fractures. Up to 3,000 mL of blood may be lost into the pelvic cavity alone, resulting in hemodynamic instability after a pelvic fracture. The injured area may require splinting, depending on the severity and type of injury with a pelvic binder or a pelvic sheet. Binding the legs together with a crepe bandage would reduce unnecessary movements of the pelvic ring and contribute to pain relief. While joint dislocations occur most commonly at the shoulders, elbows, and knees, hip dislocations should not be overlooked. Neurovascular injuries may occur following pelvic ring disruption or subsequent compartment syndrome. A compartment syndrome in the lower extremities may occur from bleeding and ischemia distal to the dislocation despite palpable pulses. For these reasons, a careful neurovascular examination must be performed. A limb with arterial compromise has a window of 6 hours from injury before irreversible tissue damage occurs.

It is of paramount importance to "clear" each step of the ABCDE algorithm before moving the injured athlete in any way. A secondary survey is carried out nearby in a protected space in order to identify other significant limb or organ injuries. A careful head-to-toe examination must be performed. In general terms, any major pelvic injury with possible fracture or ligamentous disruption should be referred to the hospital for assessment and early treatment in a timely fashion.

54.2 LACERATIONS AND PENETRATING INJURIES AROUND THE PELVIC GIRDLE

Wounds can be deep or superficial. They can also be associated with an underlying fracture of the pelvis, making the management of this type of injury an emergency.

Consideration of the mechanism of injury will assist in the assessment of soft-tissue damage and contamination since the velocity of the impact, the presence of any crush component, and the location where the injury occurred will aid the appreciation of the damaged area. The amount of energy absorbed by the pelvic ring creates a shock wave within the soft tissues that is responsible for any underlying bony comminution and for a variable degree of disruption and stripping of soft tissues, as well as creating a momentary vacuum that tends to suck foreign material into the depths of the wound. Specific environmental exposure should be taken into account. Injuries heavily contaminated by soil (equestrian sports, motocross, mountain biking, etc.) are associated with *Clostridium perfringens*, and wounds exposed to the environment of a lake or a river (waterskiing, canoeing, kayaking, etc.) carry the risk of infection by *Pseudomonas aeruginosa* or *Aeromonas hydrophila*. Tetanus status should be recorded and appropriate action should be taken in case of absent tetanus immunization or the last booster being more than 10 years ago.

Superficial wounds can be treated with irrigation, cleansing, and secure dressings to allow the athlete to continue competing. Suture materials can be used for repair of a simple laceration. Only if the EP is sure that no vital structures are involved should suturing at the competition site occur. Wound inspection and cleaning must be repeated once participation in sport has ended.

Deep wounds can be associated with profuse bleeding and/or neurological compromise, especially around the gluteal region. In these cases, the ATLS principles should be applied to optimize the initial management of the athlete. Major vessels at risk of injury include the superior/inferior gluteal artery, the obturator artery, the iliac vessels, and the femoral artery (Fig. 54.1), especially as a result of penetrating trauma in the inguinal region. In cases of an associated pelvic fracture with extensive soft-tissue disruption, bleeding can also occur from the fractures' edges and the low-pressure venous plexus of the pelvic ring. Neurological structures at risk of damage include the sciatic, femoral, and gluteal nerves as well as the sacral plexus in the presence of sacral fractures.

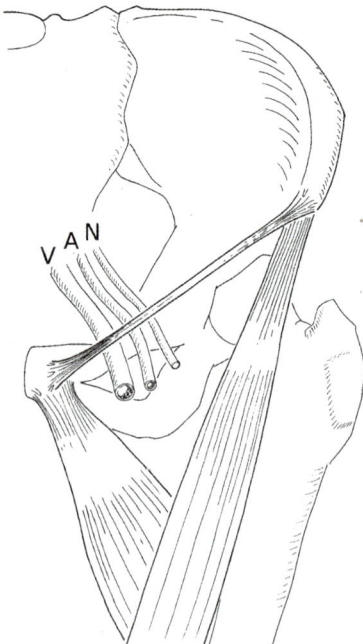

FIGURE 54.1. Femoral triangle with vessels.

Several intrapelvic organs are also at risk of injury such as the urinary bladder, the urethra, and the bowel. Detailed evaluation of the site of injury and correlation of the underlying anatomical structures are vital to make promptly the right diagnosis. Inspection of the urethral opening for blood and, if possible, careful rectal examination should be attempted to assess sphincter tone and, if applicable, position of the prostate. Passing of urine should be observed. The presence of leakage of urine in a lower abdominal wound or feces from a perineal wound should raise the suspicion of urinary bladder and/or bowel injury, respectively. Any active bleeding should be managed with direct pressure using sterile dressings. The depth of the wound should be assessed promptly. Open wounds should have pictures taken prior to being covered with a moist, sterile dressing. Any suspected fractures (i.e., of the pelvic ring) should be splinted with a pelvic binder and with a crepe bandage, immobilizing the two legs together. Assuming the injured athlete is hemodynamically stable, complex lacerations ideally should be managed in the more sterile environment of a clinic or of an emergency department. The decision to transfer the patient should be taken promptly by informing the local receiving clinic or hospital without any delay. Intravenous access and fluid administration should be initiated at the scene of the accident and at the same time if possible blood should be drawn to facilitate cross-match on arrival at the hospital. Accurate documentation of the vital signs and neurovascular status before transportation would help the clinicians at the receiving hospital to assess any changes in the athlete's condition. An accurate record of any drugs and fluid administered should accompany the patient.

54.3 HIP CONTUSION

Direct trauma to a muscle may result in a hematoma, as in the quadriceps muscle giving the "charley horse" or "corked thigh." Pain and loss of function from a severe blow are usually sufficient to preclude further participation. When the athlete wishes to continue he or she should be discouraged from continuing, the rationale being that further bleeding may lead to either a compartment syndrome or myositis ossificans (Figs. 54.2 and 54.3). Compartment syndrome has been described in both the thigh and the buttock. Severe pain out of proportion to the extent of the injury and restriction of range of motion should result in referral for urgent compartment pressure studies at an appropriate institution. Early referral is also desirable as the treatment of choice remains surgical decompression. Myositis ossificans is a potentially career-ending complication of a deep hematoma of the thigh. The prognosis is usually good if the knee can be flexed to 90 degrees after 24 hours.

54.4 MUSCULAR INJURIES

As a general principle, an acute muscle tear should result in the athlete ceasing competition. Muscle tears around the pelvis are common in contact

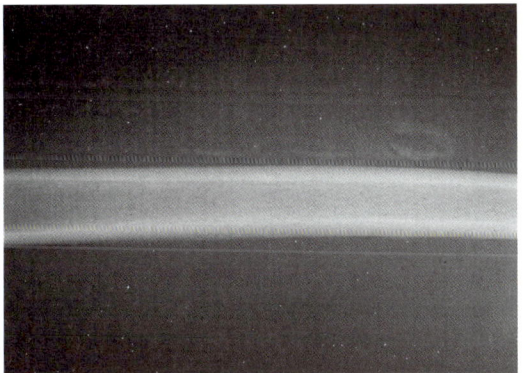

FIGURE 54.2. Quadriceps myositis ossificans (Courtesy of Graham Holloway, Orthopedic Surgeon, Swindon).

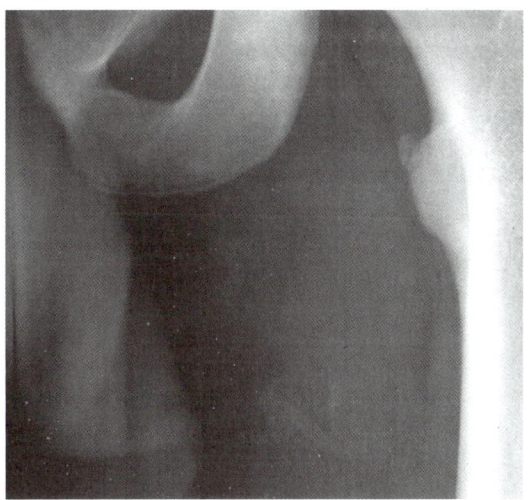

FIGURE 54.3. Myositis ossificans of the adductor muscle group.

twisting sports such as soccer. This can either be as an acute event or as an acute exacerbation of a chronic condition. The muscle group most commonly affected is the adductor muscle group. Diagnosis is usually simple: a history of a sudden, localized pain associated with swelling and loss of function. Traditional management with ice, compression, and elevation can be commenced immediately. Only rarely do muscle tears require hospitalization.

Long-standing adductor muscle or groin pain preventing further participation is frequently found in soccer, American football, rugby, and basketball. Many diagnostic terms have been created for different symptom combinations including adductor and groin pain such as sports hernia, adductor muscle tendinopathy, and osteitis pubis. Symptoms include pain referred along the adductor muscles, pain in the inguinal region reproduced by coughing or sneezing, and a loss of the ability to twist/turn or sprint. Examination reveals adductor muscle spasm, pain on resisted adduction of the hips, and tenderness over the pubic symphysis spreading out toward the inguinal region. In men, a painful cough impulse is most prominent on examining the inguinal canal by invaginating the scrotum. This test is diagnostic for an inguinal hernia. The affected player should be withdrawn from competitive sport and placed on a core stability rehabilitation program. An acute tear will require the player to be removed from the field of play. Diagnosis is made by clinical means: pain, swelling, and loss of function followed by bruising (Fig. 54.4). The extent of the injury can be assessed by ultrasound scan.

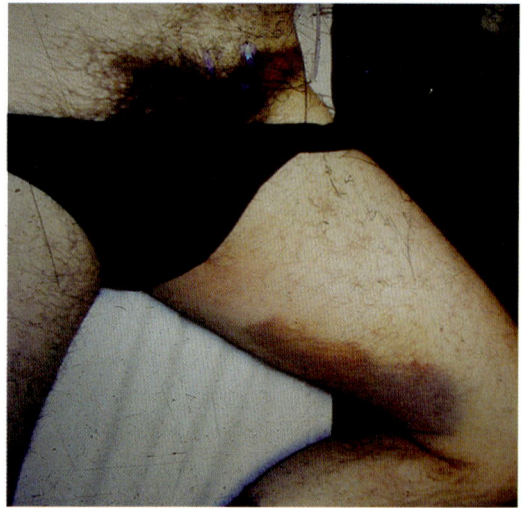

FIGURE 54.4. Extensive bruising tracking along the adductor fascia following acute tear of the inguinal wall (Courtesy of Andrew Grainger, consultant radiologist, Chapel Allerton Hospital, Leeds).

The rectus femoris muscle is prone to rupture at the site of the midthigh, the so-called thigh strain. This will be seen as a sudden swelling over the anterior midthigh. Treatment is conservative, and consists largely of stretching. Pain may persist until the rupture is completed.

Hamstring tears are characterized by a sudden tearing sensation in the muscle belly. This relatively common injury is managed with rest and a rehabilitation program to improve both flexibility and strength, paying attention to the strength ratio between the hamstring and quadriceps muscles. The diagnosis is made by ultrasound or, alternatively, by MRI, which is more sensitive. The origin of the muscle may be avulsed, resulting in a more complex problem. Plain radiographs may demonstrate an avulsed fragment of ischial tuberosity. A significant displacement should be managed by surgical repair.

Avulsion fractures may occur at any site of muscle attachment but are more common in adolescents at the site of an epiphysis. The most common site is the ischial tuberosity, where the long head of biceps femoris originates. The diagnosis is confirmed by plain radiograph. These injuries almost invariably unite spontaneously with full return to function but may take some weeks to do so. The psoas muscle is rarely injured acutely, but avulsion of the attachment at the lesser tuberosity has been reported as resulting in occlusion of the femoral artery. This requires urgent hospitalization.

54.5 PELVIC RING FRACTURES

As mentioned above, sport-related fractures or fracture dislocations of the pelvic ring result from high-energy trauma, mainly in high-impact sports, such as cycling and horse riding (Fig. 54.5). Their emergency management is described in this section.

Fractures of the ilium and the sacrum may occur with a backward fall resulting in a direct blow. Based on the direction of the force applied during the course of the accident, pelvic fractures may be classified according to the Young-Burgess classification system into anteroposterior

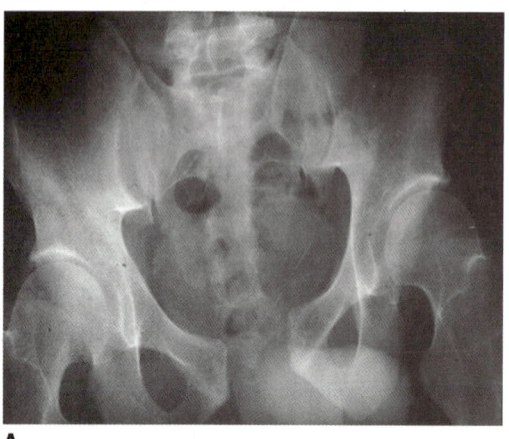
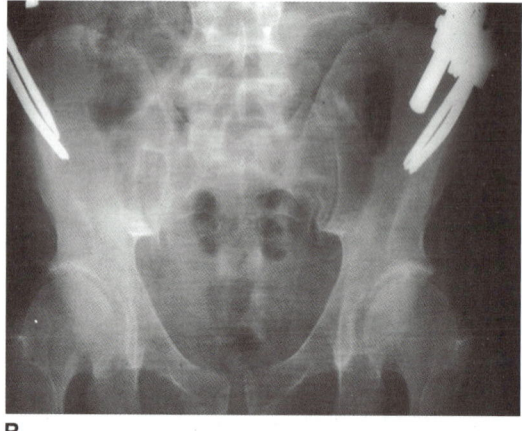

A   **B**

FIGURE 54.5. **A:** Radiograph, AP pelvis, illustrating an APC II injury (pubis symphysis diastasis, rotationally unstable) of a 28-year-old male who fell whilst horse riding. **B:** Radiograph, AP pelvis, revealing temporary stabilization of the disrupted pelvic ring initially with an external fixator.

compression (APC), lateral compression (LC), and vertical shear (VS) types, with further classifying of APC and LC according to their severity into I to III. In such injures, initial management involves the temporary stabilization of the pelvic ring with a binder, initiation of resuscitation, and prompt transfer of the injured athlete to the closest medical facility. Determining the relative stability of the fracture and the need for reduction and fixation requires an orthopedic specialist.

54.6 HIP DISLOCATION

Hip dislocations with or without associated acetabulum fractures may occur in contact sports, such as football, hockey, rugby, as well as horse riding.

The hip joint is inherently extremely stable and a great force is required to produce these injuries. While hip dislocations can be anterior, posterior, or central, posterior dislocations account for the majority of the injuries encountered in sports (Fig. 54.6).

The mechanism of posterior hip dislocation is an axial force exerted onto a flexed knee. Hip flexion and abduction increases the risk of an associated acetabular fracture. In general terms, hip dislocations are orthopedic emergencies. Neurological evaluation of the limb is of paramount importance to exclude sciatic nerve damage. Attempted maneuvers for reduction at the scene are not recommended. The dislocated limb should be immobilized. Prompt transfer to the local medical facility is desirable for early reduction of the dislocation

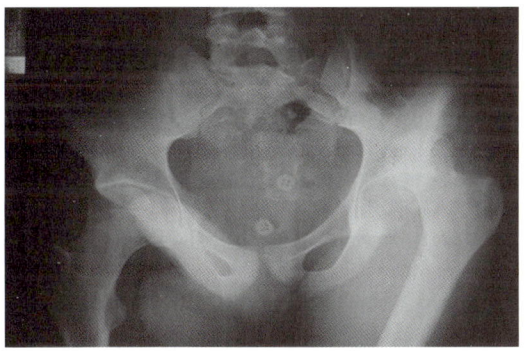

A

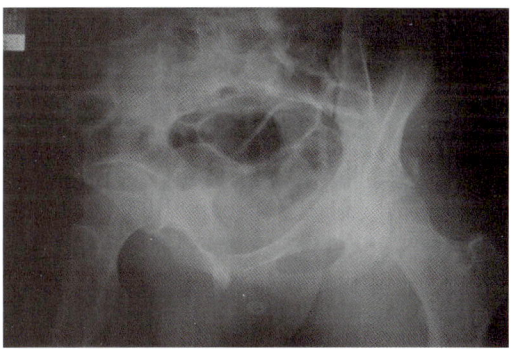

B

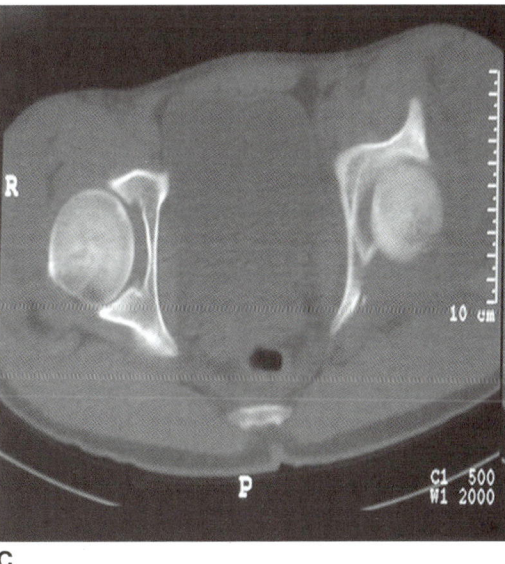

C

FIGURE 54.6. **A:** Radiograph, AP pelvis, showing a posterior fracture dislocation of the left acetabulum in a 24-year-old rugby player. **B:** Obturator oblique radiograph of left hip, revealing reduction of the dislocation, following manipulation under general anesthesia, and the posterior wall fracture. **C:** CT scan of the pelvis indicating the posterior wall fracture (*arrow*).

under general anesthesia. Plain radiographs should be taken prior to attempting reduction in order to evaluate the presence and the extent of a fracture of the acetabulum and the direction of the dislocation. CT scan should also be routinely obtained to exclude intra-articular loose fragments and injuries to the femoral head. Open reduction internal fixation is usually recommended in cases of fracture dislocations where the posterior wall segment covers >30% of the articular surface. In cases where there is less posterior wall involvement, the authors recommend examination of the injured hip under anesthesia for assessment of stability and the need for surgical reconstruction. Avascular necrosis, sciatic nerve injury, degenerative joint disease, and chondrolysis include the expected complications associated with hip dislocations.

A tear of the acetabulum labrum can lead to either recurrent hip instability or irreducible dislocation. It can also be the source of a painful catching type of pain. Differential diagnosis for this condition includes snapping of the iliopsoas tendon over the iliopectineal eminence and of the iliotibial band over the greater trochanter. The diagnosis can be made either with MRI arthrography or direct visualization of the hip with arthroscopy, allowing simultaneous treatment of the tear.

54.7 OVERUSE INJURIES

Pubic symphysis strain represents a degenerative condition of the pubic symphysis and surrounding muscle insertions, leading to chronic pain. It is frequently called osteitis pubis, though there is no evidence of an inflammatory process; it might be caused by repetitive microtrauma or shearing forces to the pubic symphysis. In a study performed in Canada in runners, this condition comprised 6.3% of the 222 overuse injuries found. The athlete's pain increases with running, kicking, or pushing off to change direction. However, the most specific test is the elicitation of tenderness over the pubic symphysis with a direct-pressure spring test. This pubic spring test has proven to be fairly specific and is very simple to perform as follows: Palpate the athlete's pubic bone directly over the pubic symphysis. The athlete is often tender to touch at that point. Slide your fingertips a few centimeters laterally to each side. Apply direct pressure on the pubic rami. With this pressure, the patient feels pain in the symphysis. Ipsilateral pressure may be applied to see if either side produces more pain or lateral pain. If the pain is not reproduced

over the pubic symphysis, other diagnoses must be considered.

Stress fractures in athletes are common, especially in endurance and repetitive type of sports such as long-distance running, soccer, American football, and gymnastics.

The classic symptom of a stress fracture is progressive activity-related pain that is relieved with rest. If activity is continued, pain usually increases and eventually becomes constant. The most common site of stress fractures in the pelvis is the inferior pubic ramus and is thought to be due to repetitive hip adductor contraction. Stress fractures of the pubic bone are more common in athletes, particularly in long-distance runners, as compared to the normal population. Symptoms include pain in the inguinal, perineal, or adductor region. Pain is relieved with rest and exacerbated by activity. Hip range of motion is often normal, but the athlete is unable to stand unsupported on the affected extremity. Gait is frequently antalgic. Tenderness to palpation occurs over the rami. If undisplaced, these fractures are easily overlooked on initial radiographs; radionucleotide bone scan or CT scan may provide a definite diagnosis. Treatment consists of protected weight bearing for 4 to 6 weeks followed by a gradual return to activity. Return to unrestricted activity usually takes 3 to 5 months.

Of major concern is the possibility of a stress fracture of the femoral neck. This may occur as an acute event in endurance running events. The typical story is pain occurring around mile 20 of a marathon race; the athlete continues to run but collapses a few miles later with a complete stress fracture of the femoral neck.

A more subtle onset occurring in distance runners may be observed after a recent change in training in terms of mileage or activity that often precedes symptoms. The athlete may present with groin, hip, thigh, knee, or nocturnal groin pain. An antalgic gait may also be present. Pain occurs at the end of range of hip motion, especially with internal rotation and flexion.

Any endurance runner with significant groin pain should be stopped from competing and mobilized exclusively non–weight bearing on crutches until appropriate investigations have been performed. Plain radiographs may reveal a localized periosteal reaction. However, in up to 50% of the cases, radiographs are normal and, if a stress fracture is suspected, further imaging in the form of a radionucleotide bone scan is required. The combination of radiograph and bone scan

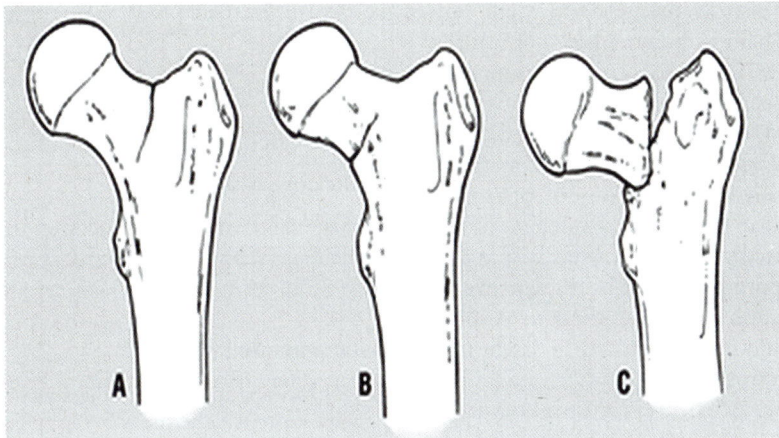

FIGURE 54.7. Femoral neck classification. **(A)** Tension; **(B)** Compression; **(C)** Displaced.

allows a correct diagnosis in 90% of cases. Lately, MRI scanning is more frequently used as the investigation of choice, having higher specificity than the radionucleotide bone scan, allowing better localization and grading of injury severity, and differentiating stress fracture from other bone and soft-tissue conditions such as avascular necrosis of the femoral head. Stress fractures of the femoral neck are high risk because of the potential morbidity associated with them due to disruption of the blood supply to the femoral head. Prognosis is based on the location, with fractures traditionally being classified as either a tension, compression, or a displaced fracture (Fig. 54.7).

Compression fractures occur at the inferomedial aspect of the femoral neck and are considered to be mechanically stable. If initial radiological investigation (plain pelvic x-ray and/or MRI) does not show displacement, non–weight-bearing locomotion with crutches, bed rest, and frequent repeat radiographs are advisable until the athlete is pain free. Serial radiographs should be taken, especially during the first 3 to 4 weeks in order to exclude fracture progression and potential displacement requiring immediate surgical stabilization. When radiographs reveal features consistent with sound healing, progressive weight bearing and activity can be permitted. Recurrence of pain warrants rest for 2 to 3 days, then resumption of activity at the last level tolerated.

Distraction or tension fractures occur in the superolateral aspect of the femoral neck, an area subjected to biomechanical tension. Propagation of the fracture line occurs perpendicular to the femoral neck. Tension-type fractures have a high risk of displacement and should always be referred to an orthopedic specialist for management. Standard treatment consists of internal fixation and non–weight bearing for 6 weeks, followed by 6 weeks of partial weight bearing.

A displaced femoral neck stress fracture is an orthopedic emergency. It necessitates immediate surgical reduction and fixation. Complications of fracture displacement include avascular necrosis, deformity, delayed union, and nonunion. Athletes may have to end their careers as a result of these complications.

Apart from intracapsular hip fractures to the femoral neck, there are instances where extracapsular hip fractures of the trochanter region may occur, particularly in athletes during high-impact sports. These injuries present with excruciating pain localized in the affected groin and with shortening and external rotation of the lower leg. Prompt diagnosis is essential to ensure early transfer to a hospital and surgical stabilization of the fracture.

Endurance runners may also rarely develop other stress fractures of the pelvic ring. Repetitive hip adductor contraction is thought to produce stress fractures of the pubic ramus. Symptoms include pain in the inguinal, perineal, or adductor region. Pain is relieved with rest and exacerbated by activity. Hip range of motion is often normal, but the athlete is unable to stand unsupported on the affected extremity. Gait is frequently antalgic. Tenderness to palpation occurs over the rami. A bone scan or an MRI is usually the investigation of choice. Treatment consists of protected weight bearing for 4 to 6 weeks followed by a gradual return to activity. Return to unrestricted activity usually takes 3 to 5 months.

Sacral stress fractures present with vague buttock or low back pain without a history of trauma. Examination reveals tenderness to palpation along the sacrum and sacroiliac joints. Plain radiographs rarely reveal the fracture. The investigation of choice is either a bone scan or an MRI. Treatment consists of rest with gradual resumption of activity. The event physician should be suspicious of this injury among running athletes, especially young women, who report sacral and buttock pain that does not adequately respond to treatment. Bone metabolism should be investigated to assess possible osteopenia or osteoporosis.

There are instances where either intracapsular or extracapsular hip fractures may occur during high-impact sports in athletes. These injuries present with excruciating pain localized in the affected groin and with shortening and external rotation of the lower leg. Prompt diagnosis is essential for early transfer to a hospital and surgical stabilization of the fracture.

54.8 FEMORAL TRIANGLE INJURIES

The structures in the anterior groin include the femoral artery, vein, and nerve. A laceration of the main artery to the lower limb is a life-threatening event. Immediate control of bleeding with direct pressure over the wound should be achieved. Other signs of serious bleeding include the following:

- Abnormal pulses
- Expanding hematoma
- A bruit or thrill over a major vessel
- Pallor
- Empty veins
- Decreased capillary refill
- Relative coolness

Management of severe bleeding is as per ATLS guidelines (see above).

Recommended Reading

Choi H, McCartney M, Best TM. Treatment of osteitis pubis and osteomyelitis of the pubic symphysis in athletes: a systematic review. *Br J Sports Med.* 2011;45(1):57–64.

Gustilo RB, Merkow RL, Templeman D. The management of open fractures. *J Bone Joint Surg [Am].* 1990;72-A: 299–304.

Moeller JL. Pelvic and hip apophyseal avulsion injuries in young athletes. *Curr Sports Med Rep.* 2003;2(2):110–115.

Scopp JM, Moorman CT. Acute athletic trauma to the hip and pelvis. *Orthop Clin N Am.* 2002;33:555–563.

Taunton JE, Ryan MB, Clement DB, et al. A retrospective case-control analysis of 2002 running injuries. *Br J Sports Med.* 2002;36(2):95–101.

Taunton JE, Ryan MB, Clement DB, et al. A prospective study of running injuries: the Vancouver Sun Run "In Training" clinics. *Br J Sports Med.* 2003;37(3):239–244.

Young JWR, Burgess AR. *Radiographic management of pelvic ring fractures: systemic radiographic diagnosis.* Baltimore: Urban & Schwarzenberg; 1987.

Acute Thigh Injuries

Contributed by Lars Engebretsen, Professor in University of Oslo, Head of Medical Science IOC and previously Team Physician Norwegian National Soccer Team, Rosenborg Football Team, Norwegian Olympic Team and Roald Bahr, Chair FIVB (Volleyball) MC, IOC Medical Committee, Professor in Norwegian School of Sports Sciences Oslo, Norway

Reviewer: Arild Aamodt, Professor in NTNU and Head of Orthopedic Department, St. Olavs University Hospital, Trondheim, Norway

OCCURRENCE

Muscle injuries are common in contact sports such as soccer, handball, rugby, and ice hockey. Studies show that up to 30% of all soccer injuries are thigh injuries. Muscles are injured by direct contact or in straining injuries where the muscle–tendon apparatus is suddenly stretched beyond its tolerance limit, tearing fibers and causing bleeding and pain. Other thigh structures, including nerves, vessels, and bone, may also be injured but are more often associated with high-energy trauma, such as falls in ski jumping and downhill skiing.

DIFFERENTIAL DIAGNOSES

Table 55.1 provides an overview of the differential diagnoses. Hamstring muscle strains are common and problematic, but contusions also occur frequently in contact sports like soccer. Hamstring avulsions in children, though rare, are painful and result in a long-term absence from sports activity.

DIAGNOSTIC THINKING

Thigh injuries can usually be treated by the event physician (EP) and seldom require surgical intervention. The EP must be able to identify the presence of a hematoma and distinguish between *intra*muscular and *inter*muscular lesions. Similarly, the EP must be able to diagnose and differentiate

between hamstring strains and ruptures (partial and total) and hamstring avulsions. Field side diagnosis is always difficult but early correct management (PRICE treatment) can facilitate examination by reducing swelling and pain. If pain and swelling do not allow for a satisfactory examination, the patient should be seen again after 48 hours. At that time, it is often significantly easier to make a definite diagnosis. Occasionally, a contusion may be associated with a fracture or an acute anterior thigh compartment syndrome, which obviously requires hospitalization for further examination.

CASE HISTORY

If a contusion is present, the patient usually states that he or she received a direct blow to the anterior aspect of the thigh. This causes immediate pain. If the patient's thigh is deformed after the injury, due to either dislocation or massive swelling, a fracture must be suspected, immobilized, the patient stabilized, and transferred to hospital. An acute compartment syndrome can develop after forceful direct trauma to the anterior thigh. The pain gradually becomes more intense as the pressure increases and the thigh becomes board-like on palpation. In such cases, intracompartmental pressure of 80 mm Hg or greater has been measured. Unlike in the lower leg (surgery becomes mandatory when pressure rises to 30 to 40 mm Hg), compartment syndrome in the thigh rarely causes nerve damage. Opening or surgical decompressing

TABLE 55.1	Overview of Current Differential Diagnoses of Acute Thigh Injuries	
Most Common	**Less Common**	**Must Not Be Overlooked**
Thigh contusion	Avulsion or total ruptures of the hamstrings and quadriceps	Acute compartment syndrome
Partial hamstring rupture		Fractured femur
Hamstring cramps		

of the compartment is still a rare event and is usually associated with high-energy trauma, such as a fall from a great height or motor vehicle accidents.

Ruptures are normally located at the muscle–tendon junction. When a rupture occurs, the patient has sudden, local, knife-like pain usually on the posterior aspect of the thigh. The diagnostic challenge is to differentiate between partial and total ruptures, avulsion fractures, and injuries in the tendinous substance. Again this can be difficult in the primary setting and magnetic resonance imaging (MRI) is needed to facilitate correct diagnosis. It can also be difficult to distinguish between partial ruptures and cramps. Some athletes, especially sprinters and contact sports athletes, have sudden anterior or posterior thigh muscle cramps of unknown origin.

CLINICAL EXAMINATION

Inspection: If a significant injury has occurred, the thigh will be swollen. Measuring the circumference of the thigh with a tape measure and comparing it with the healthy side can quantify the degree of swelling. A major contusion is always associated with some form of skin damage, leaving no doubt as to the seriousness energy forces involved. If the patient has a muscle or tendon rupture, a depression and bruising may be visible at the site of the injury and ecchymosis will gradually appear distal to the rupture site. This distal bruising is common with intermuscular injuries but usually absent with intramuscular injury, though contact point discoloration may be present.

Palpation: The anterior and posterior aspects of the thigh are palpated for tendon or muscle tearing. The thigh will be board-like if a compartment syndrome is present.

Functional tests: Testing the degree of reduced knee flexion can help distinguish between an *intra*muscular and an *inter*muscular injury, thus facilitating return-to-play predictions. If the compartments are intact, bleeding (usually in the vastus intermedius or rectus) is limited by the fascia. Therefore, an intramuscular hematoma leads to increased intramuscular volume and pressure, reducing the range of motion (ROM) in the muscle. This in turn reduces flexion in the knee joint. It is often easier to conduct functional tests and assessment 2 to 3 days after the injury occurs. Less than 90-degree flexion in the knee joint after a thigh contusion indicates intramuscular bleeding and a prolonged period of convalescence. Rehabilitation time is shorter for an intermuscular hematoma as there is less ROM restriction than with an intramuscular bleed. Functional muscle tests are also performed to distinguish between partial and total tendon–muscle ruptures. Both the quadriceps and the hamstring apparatus can be tested isometrically and dynamically to evaluate the degree of the injury.

SUPPLEMENTAL EXAMINATIONS

A plain x-ray will exclude a fracture and calcium deposits will gradually become visible after intramuscular bleeding if the patient develops myositis ossificans. MRI is accurate in determining muscle ruptures, particularly in the hamstrings and quadriceps. If compartment syndrome is suspected, then intracompartmental pressure measurements must be taken by a specialist.

55.1 Thigh Contusion

Contusions are the most common acute thigh injury in sport, and usually involve the quadriceps muscles. In a large Swedish study, 14% of all soccer injuries caused thigh contusions. The prognosis depends on the presence or absence of intramuscular or intermuscular bleeding. The muscles are rich in blood vessels and circulation is often maximal when the injury occurs. Therefore, injury causes significant bleeding, which may increase intracompartmental pressure that may lead to initial compartment syndromes and even myositis ossificans later on if the hematoma becomes organized and eventually calcifies.

Symptoms and signs: The patient experiences acute pain, eventually significant swelling and impaired function. If the patient has an intermuscular injury, ecchymosis is usually visible subcutaneously distal to the site of the injury after a couple of days.

Diagnosis: The diagnosis is based on the case history. The practitioner should be aware that a compartment syndrome may develop. If the knee cannot be flexed to more than 90 degrees, the injury is usually intramuscular.

Treatment by physician: PRICE treatment and NSAIDs are recommended. If an anterior thigh contusion is present, PRICE treatment should be administered with the hip and knee in flexed positions. This position increases counterpressure on the injured muscle and may reduce bleeding, which in turn facilitates early active mobilization after 2 or 3 days. If the patient has a major injury, it may be wise to wait 4 to 5 days before beginning active exercises.

Treatment by physical therapist: The physical therapist should start with circulation exercises, such as bicycling, as soon as possible. Stretching exercises are introduced early on but should always be conducted within the limits of pain. Massage may also be used to improve circulation, but not during the acute phase (the first 2 to 3 days).

Prognosis: Healing often takes as long as 6 to 12 weeks after an intramuscular bleed. Intermuscular bleeding can heal within a couple of weeks. If the injury is minor, strength will return to normal within a week. About 50% of muscle strength is regained within 24 hours. After 7 days, 90% of muscle strength has usually returned.

55.2 Hamstring Ruptures and Strains

Hamstring ruptures are common in soccer players, sprinters, and other athletes. The injury is usually due to a tear in the muscle–tendon junction in the semimembranosus, semitendinosus, or biceps femoris muscle. These muscles have long muscle–tendon junctions and an injury may occur at any location.

It is likely that reduced ROM makes an athlete more vulnerable to hamstring injury, particularly if the athlete has sustained a similar injury in the past. It is also assumed that weakness on the posterior aspect of the thigh compared to the anterior aspect (reduced hamstring/quadriceps ratio) increases the risk of hamstring injury. A preceding period of low back pain without nerve damage but with mild root signs is not uncommon. Low back

pain may cause the hamstring muscles to tighten and cramping may occur, making the thigh muscles more vulnerable to injury. The hamstring muscles are rich in blood vessels and circulation is often maximal when the injury occurs. However, hamstring injury rarely causes sufficient bleeding to increase intracompartmental pressure to the level where compartment syndromes occur. Myositis ossificans is also rare.

Symptoms and signs: A hamstring rupture causes immediate intense pain, like being struck in the back of the thigh, and the athlete has to cease activity. Strength is significantly reduced. The athlete can no longer run at maximal speed.

Diagnosis: Functional tests reveal reduced isometric and dynamic strength. Sometimes a torn tendon or muscle can be palpated. MRI will confirm the diagnosis and differentiate between partial and total tendon rupture or avulsion.

Treatment by physician: Initiate PRICE treatment and standard muscle rehabilitation training. If an acute ischial tuberosity tendon rupture has occurred, it can be surgically repaired with good results. The surgery should be performed within 2 weeks of the injury.

Treatment by physical therapist: The patient begins circulation exercises 2 days after the injury. The therapist should wait 4 to 5 days before beginning exercise therapy. This is followed by more intense exercise therapy, transverse massage, and possibly electrotherapy. The training progression should be carefully monitored, preferably in cooperation with the coach.

Prognosis: The prognosis is generally good; optimally, the athlete can return to training after a couple of weeks, but the injury often results in a prolonged absence from sports requiring explosive muscle use. There is an increased risk of recurrence if the athlete returns to sport activity too soon.

55.3 Acute Compartment Syndrome

Acute compartment syndrome is uncommon; nevertheless, it can be seen in sports such as soccer and ice hockey. It is most commonly found in the quadriceps as a forceful contusion; in this vessel-rich area, it may cause considerable bleeding and thus raised pressure. In high-energy femoral fractures, blood loss may be more than 2 L. Normal pressure in a muscle compartment is less than 20 mm Hg; however, pressure in the rectus femoris muscle compartment may increase to between 80 and 100 mm Hg. If there is no femur fracture present, pressure will often decrease after a short period of time making fasciotomy unnecessary. However, the situation must be monitored and increased pressure usually causes intense pain for some days after the injury.

Symptoms and signs: Symptoms are pain and muscle stiffness with findings of a hard, board-like muscle on palpation and painful knee flexion or extension.

Diagnosis: The patient can be monitored by measuring the circumference of the thigh and by comparing it with the opposite side. If the thigh circumference increases gradually, compartment syndrome may develop and the patient must be closely monitored clinically. Hospitals that frequently admit multitrauma patients will monitor the patient using pressure monitoring. Ultrasound or MRI may distinguish between diffuse muscle swelling and hematoma/muscle rupture.

Treatment by physician: Early PRICE treatment may reduce the risk of compartment syndrome development. Qualified personnel must monitor the patient if compartment syndrome is suspected.

Prognosis: The prognosis is good, but occasionally myositis ossificans develops, resulting in a long absence from sport.

55.4 Acute Nontraumatic Thigh Pain

Thigh pain is not common in athletes. Some athletes may experience acute pain in the thigh due to underlying chronic conditions such as

- Muscle fibrosis or scarring after previous trauma (hamstring strain or thigh contusion)

- Myositis ossificans after a previous muscle contusion—probably the commonest cause in soccer. The hematoma is usually absorbed after a few weeks but occasionally calcifies. At the start of the calcification process, the area is still swollen and often very tender (warm phase). Pain and swelling result in long-term reduced knee joint ROM. The calcification eventually stabilizes (cold phase).

- Stress fractures in the pubic rami (both superior and inferior) and femoral shaft and neck have been reported in female cross-country skiers. NB: the female triad.

- Osteogenic sarcoma may be located in the distal femur.

- Vascular anomalies may also occur, often where the popliteal artery passes between the lateral and medial gastrocnemius tendons at the knee.

- Referred pain due to back or hip problems

- Chronic compartment pain has been described in long-distance runners during periods of hard training. In Norway, the syndrome has also been seen in bicyclists and skaters.

- Sequelae after previous hamstring ruptures—not unusual in sprinters, soccer players, and others involved in intense, hard, eccentric muscle work. Scarred muscle tissue may limit ROM and cause pain and even sciatica due to local pressure.

- Nerve entrapment, for example, pain with sudden atrophy of the vastus lateralis

CASE HISTORY

The case history must include a history of acute trauma, in particular thigh trauma (myositis ossificans). It is important to know if the back, pelvis, or thigh have been exposed to unusually intense or prolonged exercise (not unusual in top class athletes) and the EP must consider the presence of stress fractures and/or compartment pathology.

CLINICAL EXAMINATION

Examination may reveal muscle atrophy (e.g., nerve entrapment at the vastus lateralis), swelling (myositis ossificans or tumors), or sequelae from a hamstring or extensor tendon rupture. Palpation may help confirm these findings. Individual muscle group function tests may help localize the injury. Neurologic status must be included in the examination as thigh pain often originates from the back. Although thigh pain due to circulatory disorders in young athletes is rare and difficult to assess clinically, lower extremity pulses should be checked.

SUPPLEMENTAL EXAMINATIONS

Radiographic examination: Frontal and lateral x-rays of the thigh and pelvis (including the hips) must always be taken to exclude stress fractures, myositis ossificans, or tumors. Remember of course that stress fractures are often not seen on x-ray.

Other examinations: A follow-up with an MRI (useful in diagnosis of stress fractures, myositis ossificans, muscle ruptures, and tumors) is often indicated. Ultrasound examinations may demonstrate ruptures in the extensor apparatus but depend on the skills of the operator. Scintigraphy is highly sensitive for stress fractures and tumors but is a nonspecific examination and if positive should be followed up with an MRI.

Recommended Reading

Davis KW. Imaging of the hamstrings. *Semin Musculoskelet Radiol*. 2008;12(1):28–41.

Heiderscheit BC, Sherry MA, Silder A, et al. Hamstring strain injuries: recommendations for diagnosis, rehabilitation, and injury prevention. *J Orthop Sports Phys Ther*. 2010;40(2):67–81.

Järvinen TA, Järvinen TL, Kääriäinen M, et al. Muscle injuries: optimising recovery. *Best Pract Res Clin Rheumatol*. 2007;21(2):317–331.

Järvinen TA, Kääriäinen M, Järvinen M, et al. Muscle strain injuries. *Curr Opin Rheumatol*. 2000;12(2):155–161.

Linklater JM, Hamilton B, Carmichael J, Orchard J, Wood DG. Hamstring injuries: anatomy, imaging, and intervention. *Semin Musculoskelet Radiol*. 2010;14(2):131–161.

Mason DL, Dickens V, Vail A. Rehabilitation for hamstring injuries. *Cochrane Database Syst Rev*. 2007;(1): CD004575.

Ojike NI, Roberts CS, Giannoudis PV. Compartment syndrome of the thigh: a systematic review. *Injury*. 2010;41(2): 133–136.

CHAPTER 56

Acute Knee Injuries

Lars Engebretsen, Scientific Director IOC, Prof. University of Oslo, and previously Team Physician Norwegian National Soccer Team, Rosenborg Football Team, Norwegian Olympic Team and Roald Bahr, Chair FIVB (Volleyball) MC, IOC Medical Committee, Prof. Norwegian School of Sports Sciences, Oslo, Norway

Reviewer: Arild Aamodt, Prof. Orthopedics, NTNU; Head of Orthopedic Department, St. Olavs University Hospital, Trondheim, Norway

Acute knee injuries constitute almost 5% of all acute injuries treated in physicians' offices, emergency rooms, and outpatient clinics. However, only 10% of these knee injuries are severe soft-tissue injuries, with meniscal ruptures and anterior cruciate ligament (ACL) ruptures being the most common. Half of all meniscal and ligament injuries in the knee are sport injuries. The annual incidence of ACL injuries and meniscal injuries is 2 to 5/10,000 and 1/1,000, respectively.

Acute knee injuries may be very severe. The largest annual insurance payments in Scandinavia are made for this category of sports injury. In Norway, there has been special focus on handball as the major cause of most cruciate ligament injuries, but soccer players and skiers also sustain numerous severe knee injuries. Three of four ACL injuries are sport related. Of all insurance losses from Norwegian handball, more than 10% were due to cruciate ligament injuries, most of which were sustained by women. The incidence of cruciate ligament injuries among Norwegian female elite handball players is 4% to 8%. Hence, every team loses one to two players per year to this injury.

Diagnostic Thinking

Knee injuries that cause blood to enter the joint must be evaluated by an orthopedic surgeon and are usually treated surgically, whereas injuries without hemarthrosis generally do not require acute surgery and can be evaluated and treated at the primary-care level. Therefore, it is important to detect injuries that cause hemarthrosis (see Table 56.1).

Intra-articular bleeding will usually occur within 12 hours of an injury, so if a patient presents with a swollen knee in this period, it may be assumed that the knee contains blood. If in doubt as to the presence of hemarthrosis, one can aspirate the joint; however, this procedure must be performed in a sterile manner. The likelihood of an ACL rupture being present is more than 85% if the patient is female, has hemarthrosis, and was playing team handball when the injury occurred.

A peripheral bucket-handle meniscal injury can be repaired if the patient is operated within a couple of weeks. An osteochondral injury can also be repaired during this acute phase; lateral lesions in particular are much easier to repair during this first 2-week period. Injuries that require urgent treatment are fractures, a fracture/dislocation, or a major knee injury (such as a dislocation) with possible vascular and nerve injury. It is worth noting that, in the Scandinavian countries, surgery is not performed on an ACL injury until 4 to 8 weeks have elapsed, unless there are other concomitant injuries that require emergency surgery.

The goal of the clinical examination during the acute phase is to determine whether a reparable meniscus, cartilage injury, or fracture exists. A routine x-ray will usually reveal a regular fracture, whereas clinical evaluation and magnetic resonance imaging (MRI) will reveal a meniscal or an osteochondral injury. ACL injuries and patellar dislocations may be demonstrated clinically without MRI. If the patient has a dislocated knee, the clinical examination will reveal so much instability

TABLE 56.1 Overview of Current Differential Diagnoses of Acute Knee Injuries

Most Common	Less Common	Must not be Overlooked
Injuries that usually cause hemarthrosis		
ACL rupture	LCL rupture	Knee dislocation
Peripheral meniscus rupture	Cruciate ligament avulsion in children	Rupture in the extensor apparatus
Fracture of the tibial plateau	Fractures: Osteochondral	
Dislocated patella	Femoral condyle, Patella	
Injuries that usually do not cause hemarthrosis		
Central meniscus rupture	Cartilage injury	Epiphyseal injuries—children
MCL rupture	PCL rupture	Total rupture LCL apparatus

that there will be no doubt as to the severity of the injury. These patients must be transported to an orthopedic department for immediate care.

Case History

Information about the injury mechanism often suggests a diagnosis even before the patient is examined. A thorough case history is extremely important and should include information from trainers, coaches, or team mates, whenever possible. Performing a feinting, sidestep movement or landing on a nearly extended and slightly valgus/varus knee is typical of a basketball or handball ACL injury.

This ACL injury is often accompanied by a partial lateral meniscal injury (in 70% of cases) and a so-called bone bruise (where the subchondral bone becomes compressed and injured) in the lateral femoral condyle and tibial plateau in more than 80% of cases). Hyperextension trauma is not uncommon in soccer. The ACL gets torn when an opponent falls over the athlete's knee and presses it backward. Trauma to the lateral side of the knee often injures the medial structures and may, in addition, cause an injury to the ACL.

TABLE 56.2 Overview of Current Differential Diagnoses of Knee Pain

Most Common	Less Common	Must not be Overlooked
Patellofemoral pain syndrome	Osteochondral injuries	Unstable osteochondritis dissecans
Patellar tendinopathy	Osteochondritis dissecans	Posterior and combined instability
Quadriceps tendinopathy	Popliteus tendonitis	
Meniscus injuries	Biceps tendonitis	Tumor
Knee instability	Iliotibial tract tendonitis	
	Bursitis	
	Medial plica syndrome	
	Osgood–Schlatter disease	
	Sinding–Larsen disease	
	Knee osteoarthritis	

Recreational skiers are usually injured when the tip of their ski gets stuck in the snow, causing valgus external rotational trauma to the knee. This results primarily in tearing of the MCL, followed by the medial meniscus, and occasionally by the ACL as well. In addition, these patients often have bone bruises. The ACL may also tear, even at low speed, if a downhill skier falls backward, putting all his weight on the outer ski. This causes the ski to cut inward, causing internal rotational trauma to the knee. In the same situation, the ski can also cut outward, causing external rotational trauma, which will also injure the ACL.

Top professional skiers can also sustain ACL injuries after a typical combination of factors—after a jump, the athlete lands with his weight behind his centre of gravity, and with concentric use of the quadriceps with the knee in slight varus or valgus position, the back of the ski hits the ground. Again the history or TV observation will help one to make a correct diagnosis. Alternatively, this same mechanism also causes medial bone contusion in men or tibial plateau fractures in women (instead of an ACL injury).

Posterior cruciate ligament (PCL) injuries usually occur as a result of a direct blow to the anterior tibia. Of all PCL injuries, 50% result from traffic accidents (e.g., when the knee hits the dashboard) and the other half are sport related (e.g., by falling to the floor in handball or crashing into the sideboard in ice hockey). Approximately 50% of PCL injuries are isolated, whereas the other 50% of patients have injuries to the LCL and the popliteus tendon.

Patellar dislocations usually occur after a direct blow to the medial patellar margin, with the knee slightly flexed (e.g., hitting the knee of a slalom gate). Valgus trauma in handball may also cause the patella to dislocate (often with spontaneously relocation). Patients with patellar dislocations will have hemarthrosis and will complain of pain along the medial patellar retinaculum.

56.1 CLINICAL EXAMINATION

Inspection

With the patient's knee at rest on a pillow at 15- to 20-degree flexion, inspect both knees from the foot of the examination table. Intra-articular fluid is usually obvious due to knee swelling. If at least three of the four main ligaments (ACL, PCL, MCL, and/or the LCL) are torn, the knee is dislocated.

This is a major injury and when the knee is examined, there is often no doubt as to the injury severity. However, several hours may pass from the time of injury to the time of examination; swelling and intense pain may make satisfactory examination difficult. One may see that the patella is laterally dislocated or possibly in an alta (high) or baja (low) position, indicating a rupture of the patellar or the quadriceps tendon, respectively.

Palpation

The patellar tendon, the patellar retinaculum, and the quadriceps tendon are palpated for pain or discontinuity. Medial ligaments cannot be felt directly, but painful attachment points at the femoral condyle and on the medial tibia are typical for MCL injury. The LCLs and the biceps tendon can however be easily palpated and both sides should be compared. If major lateral injuries have occurred, the LCL and the biceps tendon are often less easily recognized. The joint spaces can be palpated and a meniscus injury will usually cause tenderness when palpated.

Movement

Normal range of motion (ROM) in the knee joint is from 0- to 10-degree extension to 140-degree flexion and more. In an acute knee injury, both flexion and extension will often be reduced and one must also test for locking. The challenge is in determining whether locking is real or due to so-called pseudolocking. With real locking, fragments are to be found wedged between the femur and the tibia, thus preventing normal movement, for example, a ruptured meniscus (as with a bucket-handle tear) or displaced pieces of the ACL or cartilage. When the equally frequent pseudolocking occurs, there are no structures physically blocking mechanical movement—limitations in ROM are initiated by intense pain.

Neuromuscular Function

Bilateral examination and comparison of the dorsal pedal and posterior tibial pulses are obligatory. Strength and sensibility should also be checked; the musculature innervated by the Peroneus nerve is frequently weakened particularly after varus trauma or after a dislocated knee. In such cases, the patient will have reduced strength when dorsiflexing the big toe or the entire foot and possibly a loss of sensibility between the first and second toes.

Special Tests: If the patient has an acute knee injury, a series of special tests exist to evaluate the integrity of the cruciate ligaments, the collateral ligaments, and the menisci. To ensure objectivity, one must always compare the injured knee with the healthy side.

Varus or Valgus Stress Test 30 Degrees

This test (see Fig. 56.1) is used to determine the presence of a collateral ligament injury. The knee is held at 30-degree flexion and loaded in varus or valgus so that the collateral ligaments are stretched. Using a finger, the practitioner palpates the stretched joint space and attempts to evaluate the amount of ligamentous laxity, that is, by estimating how much the joint space increases due to valgus/varus loading. MCL and LCL injuries are graded according to how wide a joint space opening can be created: grade I < 5 mm difference between sides; grade II 5 to 10 mm difference; and grade III > 10 mm difference between sides. This test may also be positive for physeal injuries in children and tibial plateau fractures in adults.

Lachman Test 30 Degrees

The test (see Fig. 56.2) is used to evaluate the ACL. With the patient lying supine, flex the knee to approximately 30-degree flexion. Some examiners also externally rotate the knee. Placing one hand behind the tibia with the thumb on the tibial tuberosity and the other hand around the front of the patient's thigh, one attempts to pull (draw) the

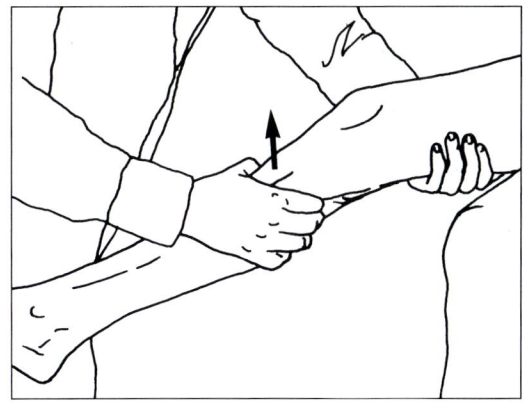

FIGURE 56.2. Lachman test for the anterior cruciate ligament. (MediClip image © 2003 Lippincott Williams & Wilkins. All rights reserved.)

tibia anteriorly on the tibia. An intact ACL should prevent this forward translation and the movement will have a firm endpoint. If compared to the healthy knee, anterior translation of the tibia is more pronounced and is associated with a soft endpoint—a positive test is defined and an ACL injury may be present.

Posterior Drawer Test 90 Degrees

The test (see Fig. 56.3) is used to evaluate the PCL. With the knee flexed at 90 degrees and the examiner sitting on the patient's foot, the tibia is pushed straight backward. If the PCL is torn, the tibia will slip backward in relation to the femur.

Sag Test

The test (see Fig. 56.4) is used to evaluate the PCL. The patient is placed in a supine position with the hip and knee flexed. When a PCL injury exists, the tibia will sag backward compared with the healthy side.

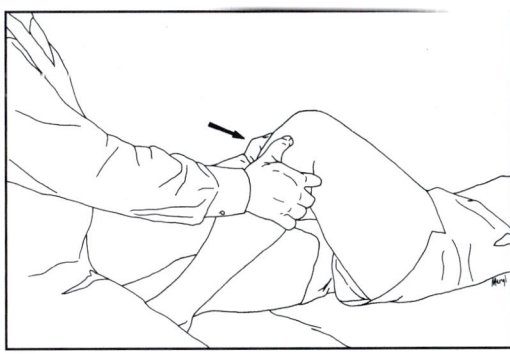

FIGURE 56.3. Posterior drawer test. (MediClip image © 2003 Lippincott Williams & Wilkins. All rights reserved.)

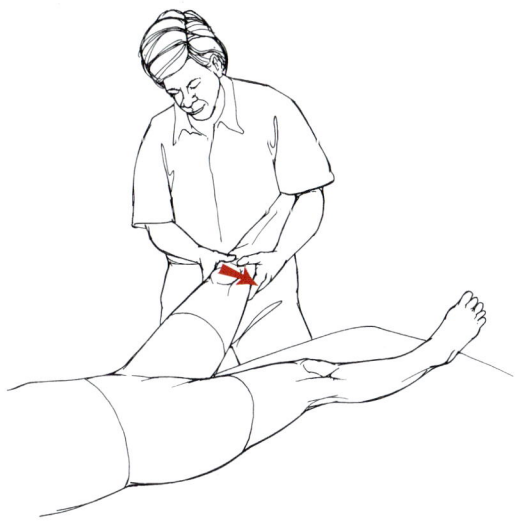

FIGURE 56.1. Valgus stress test.

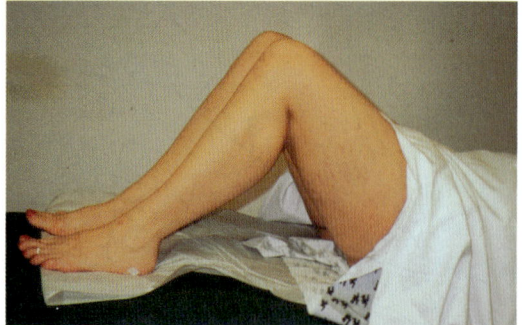

FIGURE 56.4. Sag test. (From Berg D, Worzala K. *Atlas of Adult Physical Diagnosis*. Philadelphia, PA: Lippincott Williams & Wilkins, 2006, with permission.)

Posterolateral Lachman 30 Degrees

The test (see Fig. 56.5) is used to examine for potential injuries to structures in the posterolateral corner—the LCL, the popliteus tendon, and the popliteofibular ligament. Think of a reversed Lachman, with the knee flexed at about 30 degrees, push the tibia posteriorly in an externally rotated position.

Recurvatum Test

This test (see Fig. 56.6) is also used to evaluate a potential posterolateral ligament injury. With the patient supine, both feet are lifted up from the surface. If a major injury to the posterolateral ligament and other posterior structures has occurred, the injured knee becomes hyperextended.

McMurray Meniscus Test

This test (see Fig. 56.7) is used to evaluate the lateral and medial menisci. The knee is flexed to

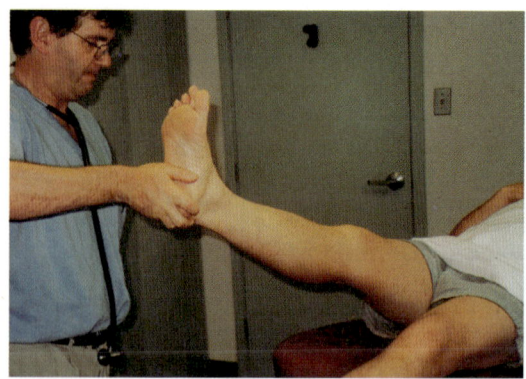

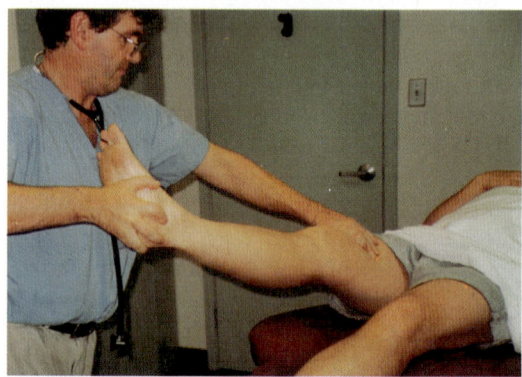

FIGURE 56.6. Technique for recurvatum test (Godfrey's) for posterior cruciate ligament sprains/rupture. (From Berg D, Worzala K. *Atlas of Adult Physical Diagnosis*. Philadelphia, PA: Lippincott Williams & Wilkins, 2006.)

90 degrees, after which it is gradually and passively extended. To test the medial meniscus, the EP holds a finger in the medial joint space while the tibia is externally rotated and slight valgus pressure is applied to the joint. The lateral meniscus is tested by applying pressure to the lateral joint space with simultaneous internal rotation

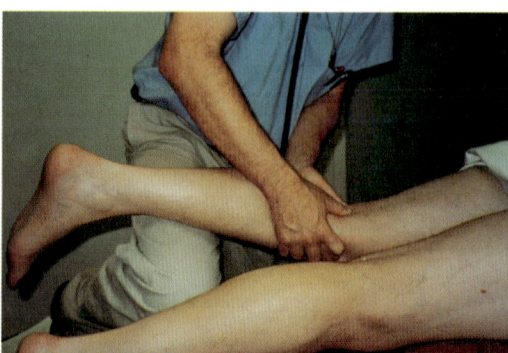

FIGURE 56.5. Posterolateral Lachman test. (From Berg D, Worzala K. *Atlas of Adult Physical Diagnosis*. Philadelphia, PA: Lippincott Williams & Wilkins, 2006.)

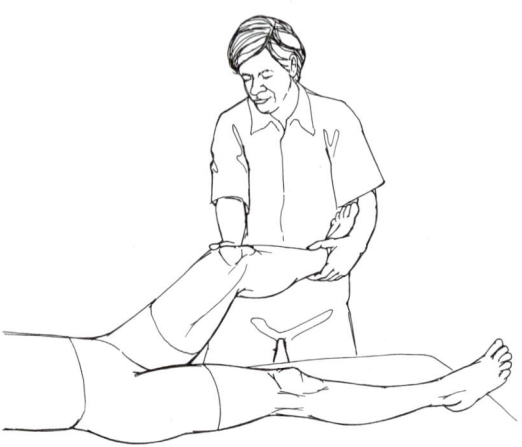

FIGURE 56.7. McMurray's test to assess the medial meniscus.

and varus stress. The test is positive if the patient feels pain in the joint space. If a medial meniscus injury has occurred, a click can sometimes also be palpated by the fingertip—this also represents a positive test.

Supplemental Examinations

Routine x-rays should always be ordered for acute knee injuries, but if special tests are needed, it is probably best to leave this to a specialist.

Radiographic Examination

Fractures can be located with frontal and lateral x-rays. If a tibial plateau fracture is suspected, oblique x-rays can also be ordered. If an ACL injury is suspected, look for avulsion of the intercondylar eminence.

Other Examinations

If an epiphyseal injury is suspected, routine x-rays should be taken. If these are negative and there is pain on palpation of the growth zone, fluoroscopy during stress testing should be considered. MRI is accurate for demonstrating cruciate ligament, meniscal, and collateral ligament injuries. Note that when the extremities are examined by MRI, the entire extensor apparatus is not routinely included, so quadriceps ruptures may be overlooked. Ruptures in the extensor apparatus may be revealed on ultrasound, but again, the usefulness of this method depends a great deal on the skill of the operator.

56.2 MEDIAL OR LATERAL COLLATERAL LIGAMENT RUPTURE

Approximately 40% of all severe knee injuries involve the MCL. The most typical injury mechanism is when an opponent falls over the patient's slightly flexed knee, pressing it into valgus. These injuries are often isolated and are primarily limited to the origins or insertions of the MCLs. LCL injuries are less common but more complicated as the lateral side consists of a series of ligaments and tendons. An injury to the LCL often involves the iliotibial tract, the biceps apparatus, the popliteus apparatus, or the lateral gastrocnemius tendon as well. MCL injury usually involves only the MCL. LCL injuries are generally caused by an external trauma to the medial side of the knee or by a hyperextension trauma. Ligament injuries are traditionally divided into grades I to III, based on the grade of the opening in the joint space during stress tests (see above) and are often combined with injuries to the cruciate ligaments and the menisci.

Symptoms and Signs

The patient has intense pain medially or laterally. There may not always be swelling in the joint, but reduced flexion and extension is typical in the acute phase. Hemarthrosis is usually present with LCL injuries.

Diagnosis

The valgus test is positive (usually grade I) if the patient has a MCL injury. A positive varus test indicates a major LCL injury. The EP should compare findings with the healthy side. If the LCL cannot be palpated, there is usually a major injury involving the popliteus tendon, the biceps, and other structures on the lateral side. If a major varus injury has occurred, a recurvatum test is also often positive. A total ligament rupture often causes less pain than a lesser injury. The EP should always take a routine x-ray to exclude a fracture.

Treatment by Physician

Acute treatment of grade I injuries is based on the PRICE principle. Many patients benefit from special orthotic devices that contain ice water and apply compression. NSAIDs will reduce pain and swelling and are useful in the first 3 to 5 days. Rehabilitation should then begin, with the goal of repairing strength, motion, and neuromuscular function. MCL grades II and III injuries are treated for 6 weeks with full flexibility orthoses. An orthopedic surgeon must evaluate LCL grades II and III, often with the assistance of MRI. Grade III LCL injuries are often treated surgically. Unless the ACL is reconstructed, combined ACL + grade II/III MCL/LCL injuries lead to a highly unstable knee. In some cases, the ACL will be reconstructed while the collateral ligaments are treated with a brace. In other cases, the LCL will also be repaired simultaneously with the ACL reconstruction. Collateral ligaments should never be surgically treated on their own if the ACL is also torn.

Treatment by Physical Therapist

Exercises may begin as soon as pain allows, usually after 2 to 4 days. The patient should avoid exercises with valgus stress. When swimming, breaststroke should be avoided.

Prognosis

Grades I and II collateral ligament injuries often normalize after 6 to 12 weeks. Grade III injuries depend on accompanying injuries and therefore usually take significantly longer time to heal. With the exception of major lateral injuries, the athlete can usually return to sport activity after rehabilitation without major problems.

56.3 ANTERIOR CRUCIATE LIGAMENT RUPTURE

Women are injured three to five times more often than men. A cruciate ligament injury is usually total, but as the ACL consists of two parts, cases in which only the posterolateral or the anteromedial section of the ligament is torn do occur. Of the patients with ACL, about 75% sustain meniscal injuries at the same time, 80% have bone contusion, and 10% have accompanying cartilaginous injuries that require treatment. Some also have accompanying injuries to the MCL or LCL.

Symptoms and Signs

ACL injuries usually cause rapid swelling (hemarthrosis within 12 hours) and are very painful. The patient often states that the knee gave way when attempting to bear weight immediately after the injury occurred. It is often difficult to complete an adequate examination immediately after the injury occurs. The usual tests can be performed as described after a few days (usually a week). Lachman test is positive if the end point is soft. It is unnecessary, and generally impossible, to do pivot shift tests during the acute phase.

Diagnosis

Diagnosis is based on a positive Lachman test, which is a highly accurate test when performed by a trained specialist (>90% accuracy compared to arthroscopic findings). Greatly limited movement in the joint may be due to a bucket-handle meniscal tear or osteochondral injury and an MRI should be ordered. The practitioner should take x-rays to exclude a fracture or avulsion of the intercondylar eminence. Diagnostic arthroscopy alone should not be necessary for this injury; the diagnosis is made clinically.

Treatment by Physician

For acute injuries, the PRICE principle is recommended. The patient often needs crutches and NSAIDs reduce swelling and pain. If it is not possible to make a definite diagnosis during the acute phase, the EP or primary-care physician should check the patient after 5 to 7 days. Only patients with fractured or dislocated knees need to be admitted to the hospital within the first few hours.

56.4 MENISCAL INJURIES

The meniscus is the knee's shock absorber. The meniscal ligaments also help to stabilize the knee joint. Meniscus injuries may occur in isolation or in combination with ligament injuries. About 75% of patients with ACL injuries sustain a simultaneous meniscal injury. A medial meniscal injury increases loading on the cartilage in the medial joint compartment and increases the risk of arthrosis. A lateral meniscal injury is more serious than a medial one, as the lateral meniscus is of greater significance to joint stability, so injury increases the risk of future instability and arthrosis. The risk of developing arthrosis depends on the extent of meniscal injury. Figure 56.8 shows the most common types of injuries. The most important determinant factors are whether the injury is located peripherally in the so-called red zone (where there is a good blood supply) and can therefore be repaired, or centrally in the avascular white zone where the injured portion must be removed.

Symptoms and Signs

Meniscal injuries that cause hemarthrosis are peripheral and usually reparable. Unfortunately, peripheral injuries are less common than radial and horizontal ruptures, which usually cause less bleeding but do cause pain and eventually edema due to accompanying local synovitis. A peripheral rift may cause a bucket-handle rupture, which will often cause locking in extension and is well suited to repair.

Diagnosis

Diagnosis is based on pain in the joint space and a positive McMurray test. If hemarthrosis exists, joint movement is often reduced. In contrast to a blood-filled joint where reduced ROM is determined by pain, a bucket-handle meniscal tear often causes locking due to an elastic resistance to extension. MRI is accurate in demonstrating meniscal injuries but is not always necessary for making the diagnosis. MRI examination can subdivide a meniscal injury into four types: grade I—slightly increased signal; grade II—increased signal in the

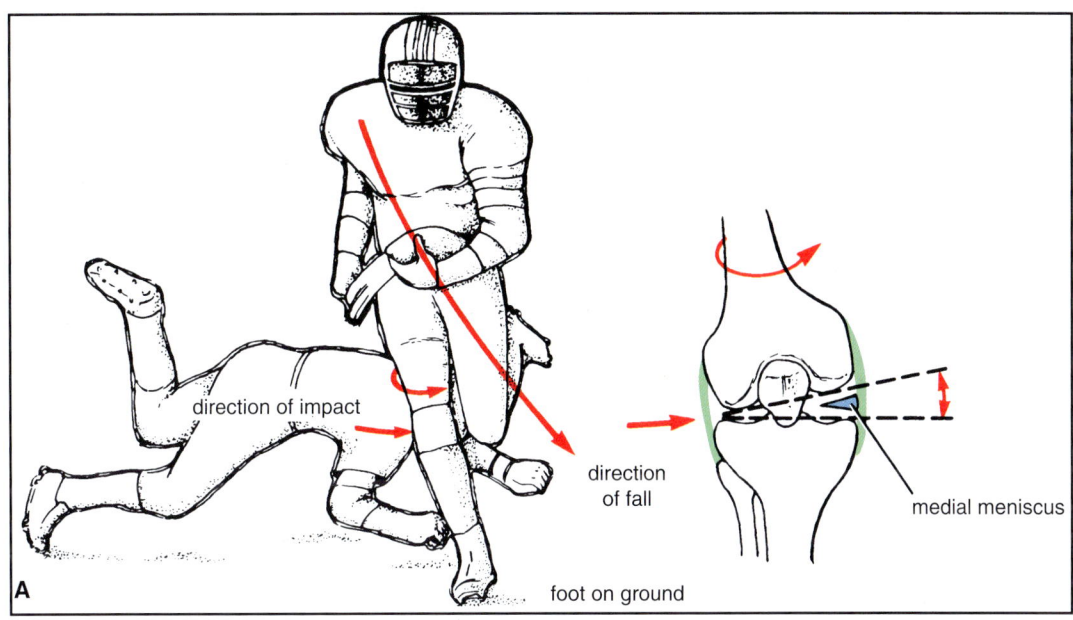

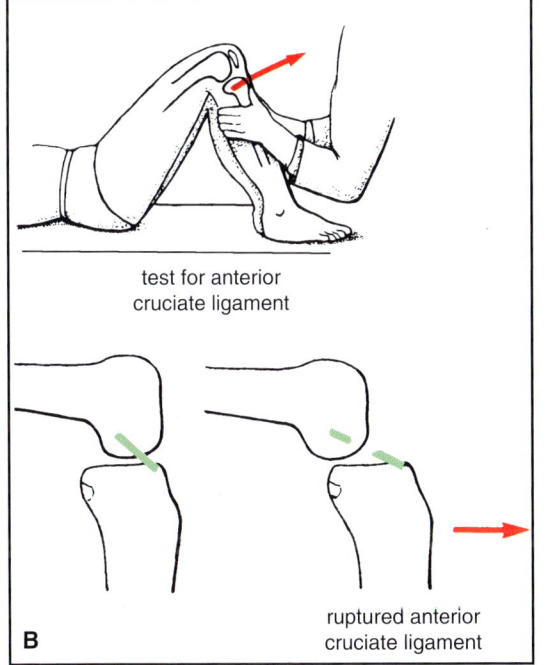 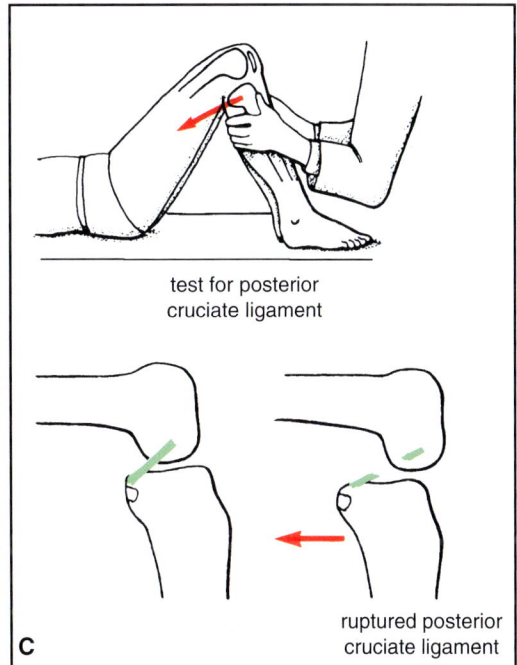

FIGURE 56.8. **A.** Mechanism involved in damage to the medial meniscus of the knee joint from playing football. Note that the right knee joint is semiflexed and that medial rotation of the femur on the tibia occurs. The impact causes forced abduction of the tibia on the femur, and the medial meniscus is pulled into an abnormal position. The cartilaginous meniscus is then ground between the femur and the tibia. **B.** Test for integrity of the anterior cruciate ligament. **C.** Test for integrity of the posterior cruciate ligament. (From Snell. *Clinical Anatomy.* 7th ed. Lippincott Williams & Wilkins, 2003.)

entire meniscal substance without penetrating the surface; and grades III and IV—superficial ruptures with a dislocated meniscus. In children and adolescents, grades I and II can heal spontaneously, whereas grades III and IV usually require surgery.

Treatment by Physician

It is preferable to perform arthroscopic repair of a peripheral rupture within the first 2 weeks after injury. If there is a minor rupture, an arthroscopic partial resection is performed. Small ruptures that do not go through the entire meniscus may heal without surgery.

Prognosis

Prognosis is generally good. A sutured meniscal injury requires a period of at least 4 to 6 months' rest before the athlete returns to sport activity in which the knee is subjected to torsional loading. The athlete may return to sport activity within 4 weeks of a minor resection. The long-term prognosis is not known. A total resection of the medial meniscus puts the patient at high risk for radiographic arthrosis 10 years later on, whereas a partial resection appears to cause only a moderately increased risk of arthrosis.

56.5 DISLOCATED PATELLA

After cruciate ligament and meniscal injuries, the commonest cause of hemarthrosis is patellar dislocation (see Fig. 56.9). Normal patella function is necessary to achieve good extensor strength. Some athletes have poor patellar stability and the patella may be dislocated laterally either spontaneously or due to a medial blow as from a slalom gate.

Symptoms and Signs

While a patellar or quadriceps tendon rupture causes significant local swelling, a dislocated patella always causes hemarthrosis. The patella

Patellar dislocation

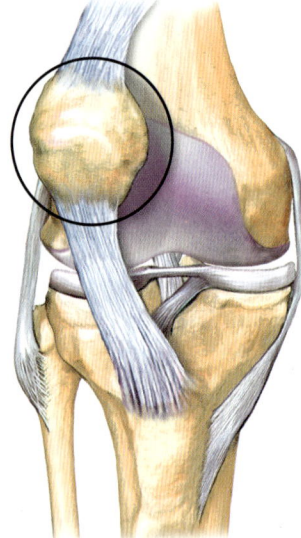

FIGURE 56.9.   Traumatic knee injuries: patellar dislocation.

almost always dislocates laterally and usually causes the knee to lock in flexion. If the patella is reduced before the physician arrives, the diagnosis may be more difficult to make. This may occur spontaneously and almost immediately, without the patient realizing what has happened. However, palpation along the medial patellar edge and in the ligaments will always cause pain in an otherwise stable knee joint.

Diagnosis

Diagnosis is based on reduced ROM, particularly flexion and on pain along the medial patellar edge. There is pain and apprehension when attempting to lateralize the patella.

Patients usually have significant hemarthrosis. The practitioner should always take x-rays, as a dislocation may result in avulsion or an osteochondral fracture from the patella or lateral femoral condyle.

Treatment by Physician

The patella must always be reduced. If at the Fieldside, reduction may be attempted immediately after the injury, otherwise patients often need anesthesia. Extending the knee and pushing the patella anteriorly and medially reduces the dislocation. After reduction, the patella is stabilized with a cast brace, orthosis, elastic bandage, or tape for some weeks. There is good evidence that after early surgical repair of the patellar retinaculum, recurrence is rare. Nonsurgical treatment of younger active patients, such as with a cast or orthosis for 6 to 8 weeks, results in redislocation in more than 50% of patients. If there is an avulsion fracture, then the need for surgery increases.

Treatment by Physical Therapist

Exercise therapy is recommended.

Prognosis

The prognosis is very good. The athlete almost always returns to sporting activity after 3 or 4 months.

56.6 FEMORAL CONDYLE/TIBIAL PLATEAU FRACTURE

Traffic accidents and falls are a more usual cause of this injury than sporting accidents. However, tibial plateau fractures are relatively common in girl skiers. The same injury mechanisms that cause cruciate ligament and collateral ligament injuries may also result in fractures, most frequently of the tibial

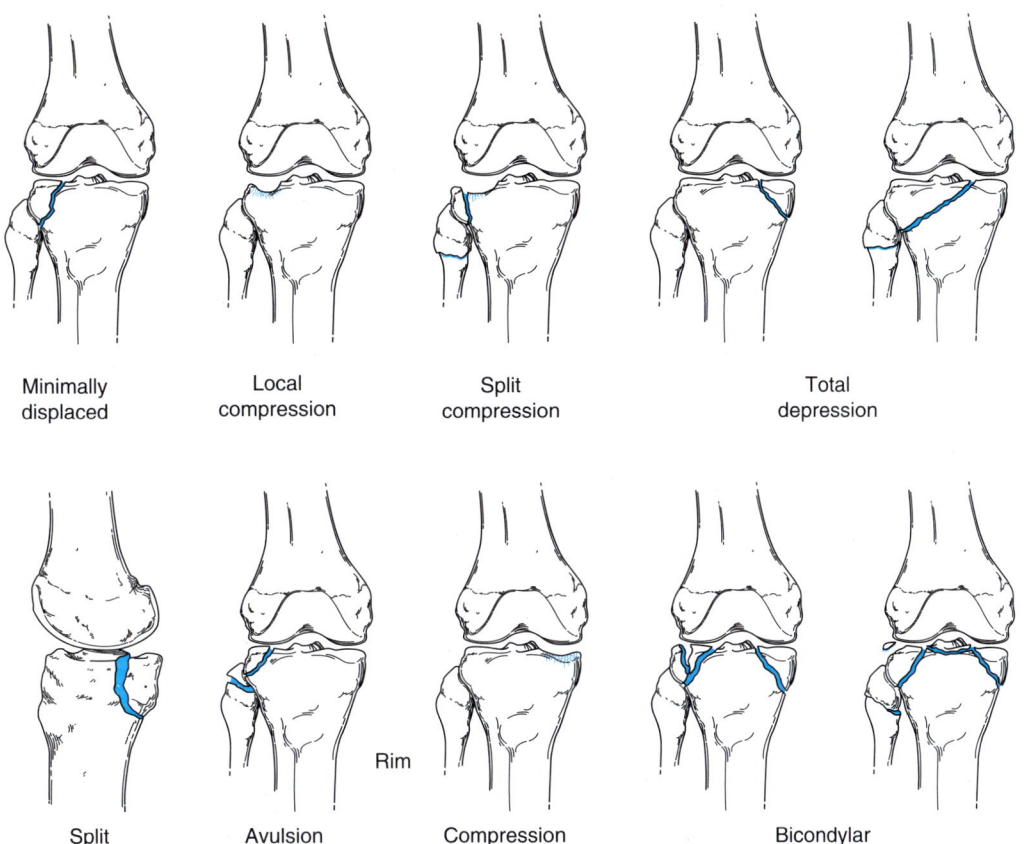

Minimally displaced

Local compression

Split compression

Total depression

Split

Avulsion

Rim

Compression

Bicondylar

FIGURE 56.10. Hohl's revised classification of tibial plateau fractures: minimally displaced (22%), local compression (28%), split compression (18%), total depression (13%), split (3%), rim avulsion or compression (5%), and bicondylar (11%). (From Bucholz RW, Heckman JD. *Rockwood & Green's Fractures in Adults*. 5th ed. Lippincott Williams & Wilkins, 2001.)

plateau (see Fig. 56.10) and less commonly of the femur or patella. These fractures are more often seen in older recreational skiers than in younger athletes. A tibial plateau fracture may cause a step in the joint surface and blood enters into the joint from the bone marrow. If this step is more than 2 to 3 mm, the patient must undergo surgery to avoid arthrosis and instability in the joint later on.

Symptoms and Signs

The patient will have pain from loading and hemarthrosis. Tibial plateau fractures must be suspected when the patient has sustained a high-energy trauma, especially in elderly patients and patients with osteoporosis.

Diagnosis

X-rays will usually be sufficient, but occasionally the depression of the tibial plateau is so minor that only an MRI image can demonstrate the lesion.

Oblique views may also be helpful. The EP should watch for epiphyseal injuries in children. They may be difficult to diagnose radiologically, so the physician should always take comparative contralateral x-rays when the patient is 15 years or younger.

Treatment by Physician

Patients should be referred to x-ray and, if a fracture is found, to an orthopedic surgeon for evaluation. Many of these injuries require surgery.

Prognosis

Prognosis depends entirely on the nature of the fracture, which may vary from major plateau compression in ski jumpers to minimal depression fractures in recreational slalom skiers. The normal healing period for minor injuries is 6 to 12 weeks, but the athlete must reckon with 3 months away from sporting activity.

56.7 POSTERIOR CRUCIATE LIGAMENT RUPTURES

Only 10% of cruciate ligament injuries affect the PCL (see Fig. 56.11). In more than half of these cases, combined injuries are involved. Sporting accidents are responsible for 50% of all PCL injuries; the remainder are caused by traffic accidents. The most common PCL injury mechanism is when the upper portion of the tibia is hit against a static object such as a hockey sideboard or by an opponent falling directly on the tibia pressing it posteriorly. A direct blow from the front may push the tibia backward in relation to the femur, causing an isolated PCL injury. The blow often comes from an anteromedial or anterolateral direction to the tibia.

Symptoms and Signs

The patient often tells that (s)he sustained a direct blow to the tibial tuberosity as described above. Generally, the patient experiences intense pain after the injury. Patients with PCL injuries do not necessarily have hemarthrosis with early swelling, but swelling eventually occurs in some patients.

Diagnosis

The diagnosis is made clinically, based on a positive posterior drawer test and a positive Sag test. Patients often sustain combined injuries and must be carefully examined for other knee injuries. The patient should also have an MRI examination for this reason.

Treatment by Physician

A patient with an isolated PCL injury is treated with active rehabilitation and does not need to be referred to an orthopedic surgeon. Patients with combined injuries, especially those with major

lateral injuries or dislocated knees, should be surgically treated, preferably within 2 weeks of being injured. As is the case for ACL injuries, orthoses do not have any documented effect on these injuries.

Treatment by Physical Therapist

Patients often require several months of training, which includes strength training and neuromuscular training. It is particularly important to train the quadriceps muscle after a PCL injury as this may limit slipping of the femur in relation to the tibia.

Prognosis

Isolated PCL injuries seldom cause symptoms during sports activity. However, the knee may gradually become less stable, due to stretching of the secondary stabilizers. Some of these patients will eventually require surgery.

56.8 KNEE DISLOCATION

Knee dislocations (see Fig. 56.12), though rare, are important to detect due to the prevalence of vascular and nerve injuries. In sport, this injury results after a major fall, for example, in ski jumping or from a motorcycle, but dislocations may also occur in soccer and handball. A dislocated knee is defined as damage to at least three of the knee's four main ligaments—the MCL, LCL, PCL, and ACL.

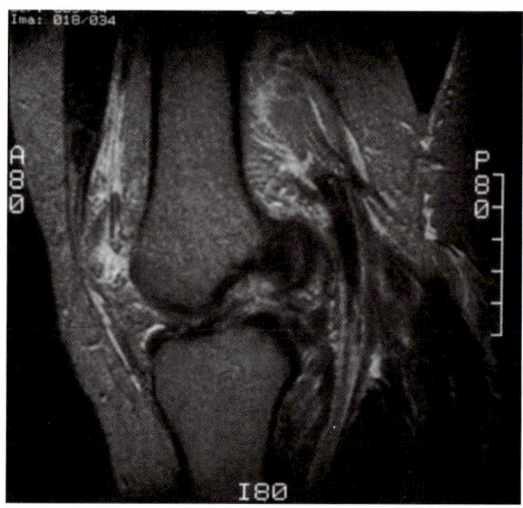

FIGURE 56.12. Midsubstance anterior cruciate ligament (ACL) and posterior cruciate ligament (PCL) tears on magnetic resonance imaging in a low-velocity knee dislocation. (From Bucholz RW, Heckman JD. *Rockwood & Green's Fractures in Adults.* 5th ed. Lippincott Williams & Wilkins, 2001.)

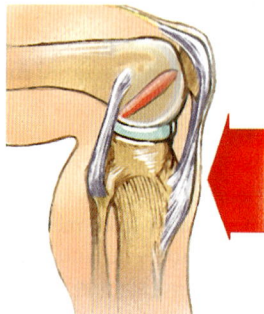

FIGURE 56.11. Knee injury mechanism for PCL injury.

Symptoms and Signs

The patient usually has intense pain. About one of three patients show signs of peroneal nerve injury. The EP should always check for a dorsal pedal pulse as 10% of these patients have a vascular injury. If the artery is torn at knee level, circulation must be restored within a few hours. If more than 8 hours have elapsed, then the amputation rate is as high as 80%.

Diagnosis

The diagnosis is based on the knee being unstable in at least three directions. In a conscious patient, there is no doubt about the presence of a major injury. Lachman test and posterior drawer test are positive, in addition to the varus or valgus test at 30-degree knee flexion.

Treatment by Physician

In rare cases, reduction on site when the injury occurs may be difficult. The knee should be stabilized with an orthosis, brace, or vacuum splint. An x-ray should be taken immediately to assess the injury. At the hospital, the patient will undergo an MRI and accurate neurologic and vascular diagnostic tests to evaluate the scale of the injury. If vessels are injured, the patient should have vascular surgery immediately, injured ligaments will be attended to a few weeks later. If no vascular injury has occurred, the cruciate ligaments will be reconstructed and the collateral ligaments will be repaired a week later.

Prognosis

This is such a severe injury that only a few patients return to sporting activity.

56.9 QUADRICEPS/PATELLAR TENDON RUPTURE

Total rupture of the patella or quadriceps tendon occurs rarely. The injury mechanism is generally a fall on a flexed knee. Patient drug use, such as the use of corticosteroids in rheumatic patients, may contribute to weakening of the tendon. This type of injury has also been related to anabolic steroid abuse.

Symptoms and Signs

The main symptoms are pain and weakened or absent knee extension. If the patient's extensor apparatus is ruptured, (s)he will be unable to keep the extremity extended when it is lifted from the table. Patients also sustain partial injuries that allow extension of the knee but there will be pain and probably reduced strength on resistance testing.

Diagnosis

MRI or ultrasound examinations are helpful in making the diagnosis.

Treatment by physician

Extensor apparatus ruptures require surgery within 2 weeks.

Prognosis

The prognosis is good, but the athlete often loses some flexion ability during the first year after injury.

56.10 CHONDRAL AND OSTEOCHONDRAL INJURIES

In up to 90% of major knee injuries, crushing of the subchondral bone occurs, damaging both the bone and the bone marrow under the cartilage. Eventually, the cartilage over the bone is also affected. Despite this, cartilage may appear normal. About every tenth patient referred for knee arthroscopy has a cartilaginous injury and about half of these may benefit from surgery that preserves cartilage. Osteochondritis dissecans (OCD) occurs in patients with no history of knee trauma.

Symptoms and Signs

Patients always have a history of torsional trauma, which is often followed by activity-dependent joint swelling, periodic pain, and occasional locking.

Diagnosis

It is difficult to make a clinical diagnosis unless locking occurs. Therefore, arthroscopy is often indicated if the patient has recurring edema or locking. An x-ray may reveal OCD. An MRI may reveal other cartilage disorders. The physician should be aware that smaller MRI apparatuses, designed for examining the extremities, are poorly suited to cartilage diagnostics.

Treatment by Physician

Usually, a loose fragment of cartilage will be removed during arthroscopy. Occasionally, the cartilage may be fixed with pins. A number of possible treatments are available, such as microfracture technique, mosaic plasty, and cartilage transplantation, but the long-term results of these treatment forms are not known.

Prognosis

Short-term prognosis is good. In the long term, lesions of more than 2 cm^2 increase the frequency of osteoarthritis and may significantly reduce knee function after 10 years.

56.11 PATELLAR FRACTURE

Patellar fractures occur due to direct trauma to the patella, such as a bicycle fall or a blow from a puck, or if the athlete's knee padding is inadequate. In sport, transverse fractures are the most common, but longitudinal fractures also occur.

Symptoms and Signs

The patient experiences immediate intense pain and rapid swelling and is unable to stand upright. The fracture cleft can often be palpated.

Diagnosis

X-ray of the patella confirms the diagnosis.

Treatment by Physician

Surgery using pins and steel wire are used, the goal being to stabilize the fracture without leaving a step in the articular surface. The patient may bear load after a few days provided the knee is immobilized in extension using an orthosis weight.

Treatment by Physical Therapist

Physical therapy focuses on mobilization after 1 to 2 weeks, with emphasis on ROM and isometric strength training after 2 weeks.

Prognosis

Prognosis is good in the short term, in the sense that a patellar fracture almost always heals within 6 to 8 weeks. The problem is often a long-term reduction in flexion, particularly from cartilage injuries where symptoms usually do not appear until about 3 to 12 months later, when the patient begins full loading.

56.12 SPECIAL INJURIES IN CHILDREN

Children have growth zones in both the femur and the tibia and an apophysis at the tibial tuberosity. This makes the knee a particularly vulnerable area. Even if the injury may clinically resemble a ligament injury in adults, an x-ray will often demonstrate an epiphyseal or an avulsion injury. The ACL is particularly vulnerable to avulsions, whereas collateral ligament injuries are often confused with detachment of the epiphysis. Acute pain in the tibial tuberosity is often confused with Schlatter's disease, but instead there may be varying grades of patellar tendon avulsion from the tuberosity (Ogden grades I to IV). Instead of a ruptured patellar tendon or quadriceps tendon, a child may have what is known as a sleeve fracture, in which the patellar tendon with its insertion to the patella is torn off like a glove. It is important to remember that knee injuries in children should usually be immobilized, whereas adults often require early active rehabilitation already after a couple of days. Meniscal injuries in children differ from those in adults in that some children have rifts in a discoid meniscus (a large meniscus that covers the entire surface of the tibia). Others have partial injuries; still others have meniscus cysts. Unlike adults, the entire child meniscus is vascularized, so that conditions for healing are good. Therefore, the possibilities for repairing meniscal injuries in children, with both conservative and surgical treatment, are good. Hence, it is crucial to detect these injuries early.

Symptoms and Signs

Cruciate ligament injuries in children are rare, but they do occur. Avulsions are the most common injury. In both cases, the child has acute swelling in the knee, much pain, and limited extension and flexion. An acute meniscal injury will usually cause the joint to swell. In contrast, grade I epiphyseal injuries of the femur or tibia (which cause instability on valgus or varus testing) or avulsion of the tibial tuberosity only cause local swelling and local tenderness.

Diagnosis

Lachman test is positive if the patient has a cruciate ligament injury, whereas varus and valgus tests are positive if the patient has an epiphyseal injury. Avulsion of the tuberosity causes pain when the extensor apparatus is used; sleeve fractures make it impossible for the patient to keep the knee in an extended position. X-rays are necessary when looking for an epiphyseal injury and should be compared with the healthy side. MRI may be helpful in determining if locking is due to a meniscal injury and if cruciate ligament injury is due to an avulsion or substance tear.

Treatment by Physician

The initial treatment of knee injuries is the same for children and adults (the PRICE principle). But while time is usually not a major issue in the treatment of adult injuries (with the exception of knee dislocations), knee injuries in children require immediate treatment. A qualified professional must diagnose an extension deficit in a child within a few days. An ACL avulsion injury can be reinserted during the first 2 weeks. There is currently no surgical alternative for substance ruptures. This patient group will be treated with an orthosis until the patients have reached adulthood when ligaments can be surgically reconstructed. Orthoses can be used for all twisting activity and will prevent dislocations and new major injuries in the presurgical period. Epiphyseal separation from the tibia or femur that causes varus or valgus instability must be treated by immobilization for 4 to 5 weeks. Grade I and II avulsions from the tibial tubercle can be treated by immobilization for 4 to 5 weeks, whereas grade IV (total separation) must be evaluated for surgery. Sleeve fractures from the patella require surgical treatment.

Prognosis

Follow-up studies of children who undergo surgery for cruciate ligament avulsion show very good results with respect to stability and function. Epiphyseal injuries increase the risk of growth disturbances, but this rarely occurs if the patient has the most common grade I injury. The prognosis is also very good for cartilage and meniscus injuries in children, and they seldom cause symptoms in later life.

56.13 LACERATIONS AROUND THE KNEE

(For a general description of the treatment of lacerations see Chapter 17).

Usually, if the athlete has a cut, then he/she should leave the field of play for wound inspection.

First evaluate the wound—is there arterial bleeding? The likelihood of there being serious arterial bleeding in a nonfractured thigh or calf is extremely rare. However, in some sports, for example, ice skating, short track skating, and ice hockey, there is a danger of deep lacerations and the potential for large artery damage due to deep cuts from sharp skating blades.

Here, compression is the answer. Suturing large artery lacerations in the field is nigh impossible and one risks worsening the injury. Compression with a sterile glove and a thin compress is the only viable option. Do not use too many bandages as this only reduces the amount of pressure that can be applied and soaks up more blood.

Ensuring circulation by giving intravenous fluid is essential. If you are the only medical person present, then get assistance from another player or coach and get them to compress the bleeding artery at the site of the cut—then put in at least one IV cannula, hang up two infusion bags with saline or plasma expanders, check that the airways are free (insert a tongue suppressor if necessary), give oxygen via a mask, and then change positions with your assistant. Get someone nearby to ring the helicopter or ambulance, let them hold the phone while you speak to the emergency central—informing them of the seriousness of the injury, keeping your hand compressing the wound at all times. Ask for immediate helicopter or ambulance assistance. Be prepared for a rapid clinical deterioration. If the ambulance does not have a competent physician or paramedic on board, then I would advise the Event Physician to travel with the patient to hospital in these exceptional circumstances. If the sports event has to be stopped because the Event Physician has left the arena, then so be it. A life is more important than a game!

Minor arterial bleeds are much less dramatic, but blood loss can be significant if ignored. Once again, compression is the key. Observe the patient throughout the period of treatment. If you choose to ligate the small artery with a suture, then do this in the medical room. Remove the patient from the field of play, clean the wound thoroughly, seriously consider giving the patient a tetanus vaccine (check your national guidelines here) and suture if you are competent and if the situation demands it. If you do not feel competent to suture the wound, transfer the athlete to hospital or suitable clinic, compressing until there is haemostasis. One may then apply an elasticated stretch bandage to compress the wound.

Major venous bleeds are rare in the thigh—again you need to have a deep gash. The leg veins are more exposed, but again serious bleeds from cuts are rare. Compression is often enough to give adequate haemostasis. Suture if necessary. Again, wound hygiene and an antitetanus booster vaccine should be considered.

If the wound is over the knee joint or ankle joint, then inspect the wound for muscle and ligament injury (look for ruptures of the patellar ligament in particular, as there is little fat protection)—check muscle and ligament function distal to the wound. If intact function, evaluate the wound for bleeding, if none, then close the wound after thorough cleaning. Again, apply an elasticated stretch bandage to compress the wound afterward.

Never close the wound if you suspect or are unsure of an underlying muscle, ligament, major nerve, or capsule injury. If in doubt, cover the wound with a wet saline bandage; transfer the patient to a hospital for further evaluation.

56.14 CONTUSIONS

Treating bruises with ice packs or cold packs is still the treatment of choice. I usually apply ice for 15 to 20 minutes with mild compression, then recommend compression bandaging for 2 hours before repeating the icing/bandaging process every 2 hours. When compressing the wound with ice, use mild pressure (15–20 mm)—do not press too hard. Remember there may be a fracture beneath the bruised tissue! Contusions are often associated with muscular tears, so check for muscular dysfunction distal to the bruise. The RICE concept is the standard form of treatment —Rest, Icing, Compression, and Elevation.

56.15 OTTAWA KNEE RULES

A knee x-ray is only required for knee injury patients with any of these findings:

- Age 55 or over

- Isolated tenderness of the patella (no bone tenderness of the knee other than the patella)

- Tenderness at the head of the fibula

- Inability to flex to 90 degrees

- Inability to weight bear both immediately and in the casualty department (four steps—unable to transfer weight twice onto each lower limb regardless of limping)

CHAPTER 57

Acute Leg Pain in the Absence of Trauma

Contributed by J. Preston Wiley, Professor, University of Calgary; International Rugby Board; President, American College of Sports Medicine/Canadian Academy of Sports Medicine, Canada; and David McDonagh, FIBT and FIMS

Reviewer: Andrew Thomson, Netherlands Bobsleigh Team and FIBT, den Haag, Holland

Diagnosing leg pain requires a three-pronged approach. Firstly, by taking a good history, one can find out if this is a first-time event or, as often is the case, a recurring problem, indicating a chronic overuse injury or vascular or neurologic claudication. Secondly, the patient can indicate where the pain is localized (having him or her point to the painful area is a useful technique). There are typical conditions for each region of the leg: anterior, medial, lateral, or posterior regions. Thirdly, one must determine if the pain is of muscle, nerve, bone, or vascular pathology.

Pain on activity that disappears with rest may imply the presence of a compartment syndrome, claudication, or stress fracture. Claudication pain is almost always reproducible with the same level of loading, compartment pain may vary, and stress fracture pain often worsens in intensity over time and becomes constant. Always inquire about back pain and stiffness, as referred pain from lumbar pathology is always in the differential diagnosis. A compartment syndrome is usually associated with a tight and sometimes swollen compartment. Pain due to a deep vein thrombosis (DVT) is almost always located in the posterior aspect of the calf, and the patient often points to the area between the proximal one-third and proximal one-half of the calf.

The only condition that is potentially life threatening is a DVT, and this requires immediate investigation and treatment. Failure to diagnose an acute Achilles tendon rupture may lead to chronic long-term problems. This condition should be identified by the event physician (EP)

and referred urgently to an orthopedic surgeon. The other conditions need further investigation as well, but this is not the EPs task. The EP must exclude serious illness and then decide if the athlete can participate in the event. This decision usually is based on the level of pain, mobility and functionality, and further risk of injury. Advise the patient to seek further medical help in determining the cause of the leg pain.

57.1 DEEP VEIN THROMBOSIS

DVT of the leg is notoriously difficult to diagnose or, to put it more correctly, notoriously difficult to exclude. The potential for partial tears in the gastrocnemius and soleus muscles is present in most sports and much more likely to occur than a DVT in a young athlete. Yet DVTs do occur in the sporting population, and women on the oral contraceptive pill are at higher risk. There are no definitive clinical tests. Homans' sign, long considered an important sign for leg DVT, is no longer considered a reliable test but is still used. Accuracy estimates vary from 8% to 56% of cases of proven DVT.

Clinical Presentation

DVT can cause leg pain symptoms but can be asymptomatic. Common signs and symptoms include the following:

- Acute or chronic cramp-like pain in the calf with possible radiation to the ankles and feet.

- Swelling/pitting edema in the affected leg; this can include swelling down to the ankles and feet.

- Redness and warmth over the affected area.

- Palpation tenderness over the thrombosis, on the posterior aspect of the calf.

- Homan's sign: The athlete's knee is placed in the flexed position. The examiner should forcibly and abruptly dorsiflex the patient's ankle and observe for pain in the calf and popliteal region—a positive sign. Most authors now agree that Homans' sign is limited use in the diagnosis of DVT (as noted above).

Conclusion

DVTs are often notoriously difficult to diagnose. If a DVT is suspected, emergent referral to a tertiary medical facility is required for definitive testing and treatment. Ultrasound with or without a D-dimer test are the most commonly used assessment tools. Venography is less commonly done now but is still an option. It can be extremely difficult to differentiate clinically between a partial calf muscle tear and a DVT.

Treatment

Once a suspicion of DVT arises, then rapid transport to a hospital is recommended due to the risk of pulmonary embolism (PE). Having made a definite diagnosis of DVT or PE, treatment is traditionally with anticoagulants.

Predisposing Factors

Many factors have been recognized such as prolonged periods of immobility (e.g., after surgery, after or during prolonged fracture casting), long flights on an airplane, contraceptive pill use, smoking, and inherited or acquired medical conditions (e.g., protein C deficiency, protein S deficiency, antithrombin III deficiency, factor V Leiden mutation, lupus anticoagulant or anticardiolipin antibodies). Virchow's triad of venous stasis, endothelial injury, and hypercoagulability states can help to identify general risk factors for venous thrombosis.

Endurance athletes are exposed to many of these factors during prolonged strenuous exercise, with microtrauma and increased endothelial injury, dehydration, and hemoconcentration.

Effort thrombosis of upper limb vasculature results from microtrauma to the axillosubclavian vein, leading to activation of the coagulation cascade and subsequent DVT formation, and although not very common, must be diagnosed in those with upper limb symptoms and signs in athletes with overhead sports.

57.2 CLAUDICATION—VASCULAR AND NEUROLOGIC

Intermittent claudication symptoms in the leg are rare in young, healthy athletes, though they can occur and must be recognized. The classical symptoms are the same as in older patients:

- Pain with activity—almost always in the calf.

- Pain occurs consistently with the same amount of activity.

- Pain is deep and achey—almost never sharp.

It can be difficult to differentiate between the pain caused by claudication, chronic compartment syndrome, and a stress fracture.

Vascular Claudication

There are many potential causes of vascular insufficiency of the limb in young persons: premature accelerated atherosclerosis, arteritis, thromboangiitis obliterans, adventitial cystic disease, microemboli, collagen vascular diseases, coagulopathies, etc. The commonest cause of vascular leg pain in athletes is popliteal artery entrapment syndrome (PAES), which usually affects young men between the ages of 20 and 40 years.

One must always palpate the popliteal, dorsalis pedis, and posterior tibial arteries—comparing side to side. Occasionally, a difference in pulse strength comparing both sides can be detected. The presence of distal pulses does not rule out arterial injury. PAES is found in young muscular sportsmen and may be due to a number of anatomic anomalies. Assessment of the pulse and further investigation must assess flow with the ankle fully plantar and dorsiflexed. Any suspicion of vascular claudication requires further investigation. The EP should inform the athlete of the need to contact the team physician for further investigation.

Neurologic Claudication

Neurologic claudication is almost always a result of lumbar or sacral nerve root compromise. The back examination can be surprisingly normal in this scenario. EP referral to the athlete's team physician is warranted to assess for such conditions as spinal stenosis, spondylolisthesis, or degenerative disc disease.

57.3 COMMON PERONEAL NERVE INJURY

A branch of the sciatic nerve, the common peroneal nerve curves around the head of the fibula, before branching into the deep and superficial branches. Damage is caused by injury to the lateral aspect of the knee during sports activities and also during knee surgery. A fracture to the head of the fibula is a common traumatic cause of nerve injury (the classic "bumper injury"). Prolonged icing of the lateral knee may cause temporary injury (neuropraxia) due to the nerve's superficial position as it rounds the fibular neck.

Injury to the common peroneal nerve will affect both branches, the superficial and deep peroneal nerves (Figs. 57.1 and 57.2).

- Deep peroneal nerve: This nerve courses anteriorly around the fibula neck into and supplying the anterior compartment muscles of the leg and also sends a sensory branch to the space between the first and second toes.

- Superficial peroneal nerve: This nerve supplies the lateral compartment muscles of the leg and sends off sensory branches to the distal anterior leg and anterolateral aspects of the ankle and proximal foot.

Clinical findings depend on the level of nerve injury, but may include

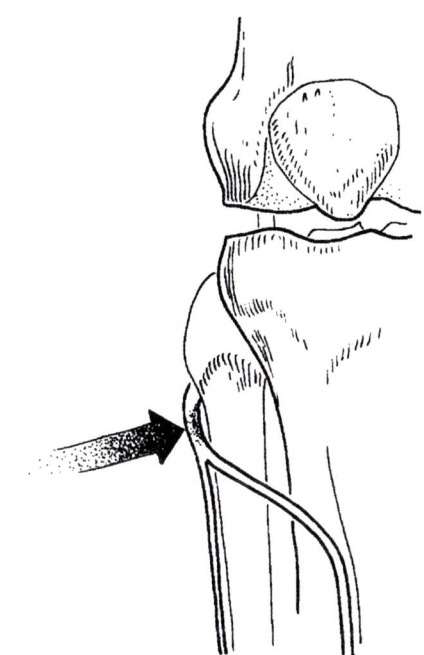

FIGURE 57.2. External compression injury to the common peroneal nerve.

- Decreased sensation, numbness, tingling, or paresthesia of the anterolateral leg, ankle, and proximal foot

- Weakness of ankle dorsiflexion or eversion

- Gait abnormalities

- Foot drop

For the EP, findings are more often associated with a fracture; however, symptoms may occur from a hematoma or after a kick to the lateral knee. Neurologic impairment should prompt the EP to refer the athlete for further immediate assessment.

57.4 LEG COMPARTMENTS

The leg is classically considered to have four compartments (Fig. 57.3):

- *Anterior compartment* containing the ankle dorsiflexors and toe extensors—tibialis anterior, extensor hallucis longus, extensor digitorum longus, fibularis tertius. The compartment is supplied by the deep peroneal nerve and anterior tibial artery.

- *Superficial posterior compartment* containing the ankle plantar flexors—gastrocnemius, soleus, plantaris. The compartment is supplied by the tibial nerve and perforators of the posterior tibial artery.

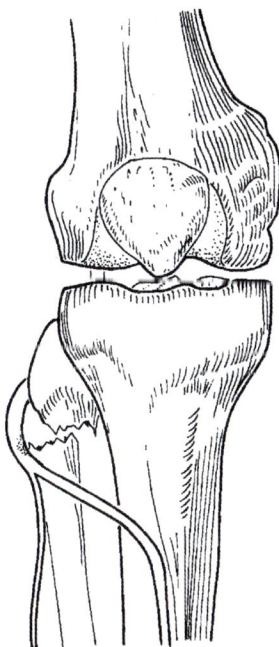

FIGURE 57.1. Head of fibula fracture with injury to the common peroneal nerve.

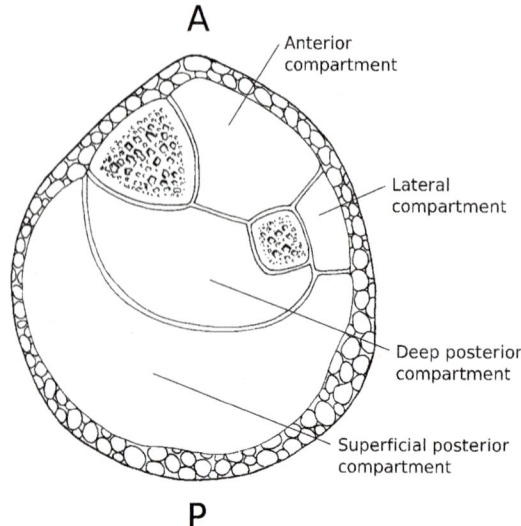

A

Anterior compartment

Lateral compartment

Deep posterior compartment

Superficial posterior compartment

P

FIGURE 57.3. Leg compartments.

- *Deep posterior compartment* containing the invertors of the foot and toe flexors—flexor hallucis longus, flexor digitorum longus, tibialis posterior. The compartment is supplied by the tibial nerve and the posterior tibial and fibular (peroneal) arteries.

- *Lateral compartment* containing the foot evertors—fibularis (peroneus) longus, fibularis (peroneus) brevis. These muscles also are involved in plantar flexion. The compartment is supplied by the superficial peroneal nerve and perforating branches of the fibular (peroneal) artery.

Acute Compartment Syndrome

Acute compartment syndrome (ACS) is usually caused by trauma, as with a closed leg fracture or extremity contusion. It has also been reported that intense physical exercise can cause an ACS; however, this is a very uncommon occurrence. Several hours may pass after an injury before ACS symptoms develop. Within the muscle compartment, swelling and/or bleeding creates pressure on capillaries and nerves. When the pressure in the compartment exceeds the blood pressure within the capillaries, the capillaries collapse. This disrupts the blood flow to muscle and nerve cells. Without a steady supply of oxygen and nutrients, nerve and muscle cells begin to die. Unless the pressure is relieved quickly, this can cause permanent tissue damage and necrosis.

An acute compartment disorder is a medical emergency requiring prompt diagnosis and treatment. The athlete will complain of pain that seems out of proportion to the injury. Pulses distal to the compartment are usually normal. Stretching the compartment muscles usually intensifies the pain as will strength testing. While the clinical history and findings may give a clue to the cause of the leg pain, intracompartmental pressure measurement confirms the diagnosis and the athlete should be referred for emergency fasciotomy.

Compartment symptoms can arise in an immobilized extremity, such as in the leg after the application of a fracture cast. A patient who complains of intense and worsening pain 2 to 3 hours after a fracture needs urgent reassessment. If the injured limb continues to swell after a rigid cast has been applied, an acute compartment syndrome may arise.

Chronic Exertional Compartment Syndrome

Athletes may present with acute leg pain that may be due to a chronic disorder, such as chronic exertional compartment syndrome (CECS). The pain for CECS is characterized by pain and swelling that come on with exercise (also called exercise-induced compartment syndrome). The pain disappears with rest. Discomfort occurs in the specific leg compartment(s) that is involved and may be accompanied by numbness distal to the injury site or by difficulty in moving the foot. Symptoms usually disappear when activity stops, though aching may persist for 20 to 30 minutes. There may be a tendency for the "second day phenomenon," where pain comes on sooner and is more intense with the same activity on the second day.

CECS is defined as a clinical condition in which increased pressure within a closed anatomical space (a specific anatomic compartment) compromises the circulation and function of the tissues within that space. CECS is a reversible condition upon rest. Prolonged pain should alert the EP to think of ACS, prompting emergent referral to a tertiary medical facility.

Diagnosis

- Specific anatomic location (one of the leg's four compartments)

- Exercise-induced pain with palpable tenderness and tightness over the affected compartment muscles (except for the deep posterior compartment, where tenderness along the medial tibial border will be found)

- Possible muscle weakness on strength testing specific to the muscles involved

- Possible numbness distally

Treatment

For the EP, treatment basically involves the athlete being observed until the pain disappears. The athlete should be referred to the team physician for further assessment. No treatment has ever shown to be effective for CECS (apart from avoidance of provoking exercise) except for fasciotomy. If pain is not relieved by rest, ACS or other pathology needs to be considered and emergent referral to an orthopedic surgeon is appropriate for further assessment.

57.5 STRESS FRACTURE

Typically, a stress fracture will initially ache only after activity, then during and after activity, then all the time. Eventually, there may be swelling over the fracture, along with tenderness. The area of pain is usually quite focal and athletes can point with a finger to the injured area. The pain is often worse on loading. Palpation and percussion may illicit pain. Hopping on the affected leg may cause pain and absence of pain can be useful in making return-to-play decisions.

Stress fractures are one of the commonest lower extremity injuries in runners; the most common site is the tibia, followed by the fibula, metatarsals, and tarsals.

- Stress fractures are caused by a number of factors that include the repetitive application of force, muscle fatigue, and biomechanical factors. Stress fractures initially are merely microcracks within the trabeculae and cortex. Thus, plain x-rays initially are negative. Imaging using a bone scan or MRI may be required to make the diagnosis. In uncommon cases, the bone may go onto nonunion (e.g., midshaft anterior cortex tibia stress fracture or talar navicular stress fracture) or complete fracture (related to persistent exercise or a sudden load).

- Like any fracture, it is important to determine if there is any deficiency in bone architecture. This may occur in amenorrheic females (female athlete triad), elder female athletes (postmenopausal osteoporosis), and transplant recipients, to name a few.

Predisposing factors include

- High-impact repetitive sports such as running, track and field, basketball, tennis, or gymnastics

- Female athletes with abnormal or absent periods (osteoporosis or osteopenia)

- Anorexia/bulimia

- Osteoporosis or other bone pathology (inherited conditions, postmenopause, transplant recipients, those treated with chemotherapy)

- Sudden lifestyle changes—for example, from a sedentary lifestyle to an active training regimen

- Hypothyroidism

If, as an EP, you suspect a stress fracture, then you should advise the athlete to discontinue sporting activity, and either arrange appropriate physician follow-up or arrange an x-ray of the leg. This may not show a fracture but may show other underlying bone pathology, such as tumor, osteomyelitis, etc. Negative x-rays do not exclude a stress fracture and the athlete may need further investigation with either a bone scan or an MRI. If the patient is from out of town, then after receiving the negative x-ray results, you must inform the athlete of the need for further investigation and advise him or her to rest the leg until these tests have been initiated and completed.

On-site treatment is based on the RICE principle. NSAIDs may help against pain or swelling in the acute phase. In more severe cases, one may have to either immobilize the affected bone with a splint or cast or make the limb non–weight bearing using crutches, but this is usually done by other physicians further down the treatment chain. It is important for athletes to stop activity to prevent progression to a complete fracture.

57.6 PERIOSTITIS, SHIN SPLINTS, MEDIAL TIBIAL STRESS SYNDROME, TIBIAL STRESS INJURIES

As with Achilles tendinopathies, there are an array of confusing terms regarding exercise-induced medial leg pain. The term *shin splint* should never be used as it is a term that has been used in too many circumstances to have any meaning. Many alternative terms have been proposed over the years for medial leg pain such as tibial stress syndrome, medial tibial stress syndrome, medial tibial syndrome, posterior tibialis syndrome, soleus syndrome, and tibial periostitis. In 1982, Mubarak introduced the term *medial tibial stress syndrome* (MTSS), and this now seems to be the term of choice favored by sport medicine clinicians, though the use of *periostitis* is also very common. This terminology came into being to describe the bone scan findings of diffuse patchy uptake in the distribution of the soleus attachment on the tibia. This finding can also be seen on MRI but can never be seen on x-ray. Mubarak specifically stated what MTSS was, but also specifically stated what it was not—it was not CECS and it was not a tibial stress fracture (TSF). We have discussed compartment syndromes and stress fractures above.

MTSS is a common condition in all sports requiring running activity. It is an overuse injury that gradually develops over a period of weeks or months. Individuals typically complain of pain in the middle and distal aspects of the posterior medial tibial border. Pain often presents on the initiation of an activity, usually running, disappears for a while, and then often returns hours after the race has been completed, even the day after the event. If ignored, and if the athlete continues to train, pain may progress and become constant, even at rest. Periostitis does not lead to stress fractures, but it is possible to have both MTSS (periostitis) and a stress fracture. This is important to know as treatment for one condition may not necessarily help both conditions.

Clinical Findings

Tenderness over the posteromedial margin of the middle to distal third of the tibia is the classical finding—the area of tenderness is usually at least the distal third of the leg. Tenderness due to a stress fracture is usually more localized. MTSS tenderness may be intense and may also involve adjacent soft tissue with soft-tissue swelling and even induration. Passive stretching of the soleus muscle and hop tests may reproduce symptoms.

Treatment

Emergency treatment is limited to RICE principles and NSAIDs; however, if the athlete has classic MTSS symptoms, he or she should be warned against training in the near future and informed of the need to contact a specialist and of the need for radiological investigation to exclude stress fractures, tumors, osteomyelitis, etc. It is important that, if the athlete wishes to compete despite the pain, MTSS is differentiated from a stress fracture. There has been no association of occult fracture associated with MTSS/periostitis, *but* there has been with stress fractures. The latter diagnosis clearly puts the athlete at risk of significant injury.

57.7 ACHILLES TENDON RUPTURES

Achilles tendon ruptures are more common in older athletes, usually over 30 years age. In the younger athlete, musculotendinous junction

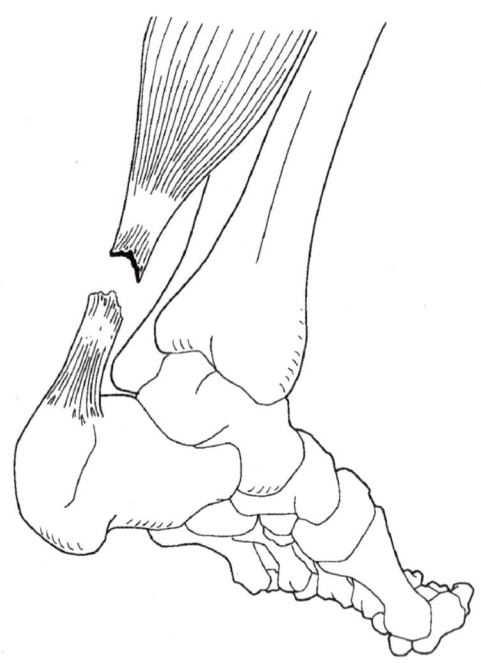

FIGURE 57.4. Achilles tendon rupture.

ruptures are commonest, but more distal tendinous ruptures can also occur. Injury often occurs in sports that require sudden pivoting, jumping, and running. The patient may notice immediate discomfort and pain after a forceful push-off with an extended knee at the start of a sprint race, or the patient may have stumbled during a soccer tackle or ski trip and broken the fall with a forced dorsiflexion of the ankle, thus overstretching the Achilles tendon. The same mechanism is seen in tennis, badminton, and many other sports. Tears can also occur after falls from height. Patients may or may not have antecedent pain (Figs. 57.4 and 57.5).

Clinical Findings

Sudden and severe pain may be felt at the back of the ankle or lower calf. The athlete often reports a snapping sound, followed by swelling and stiffness and finally bruising. Weakness becomes apparent with walking or tiptoeing. A gap may be seen and felt in the tendon or at the musculotendinous junction. Plantar flexion of the foot is weakened but may still be present due to the activity of the tibialis posterior, peroneal, and long toe flexor muscles.

a. Thompson's test: The classical test for Achilles tendon functionality. With the patient lying prone and with both feet extending over the end of examining table, squeeze the calf muscles on the affected side. If the Achilles tendon is intact,

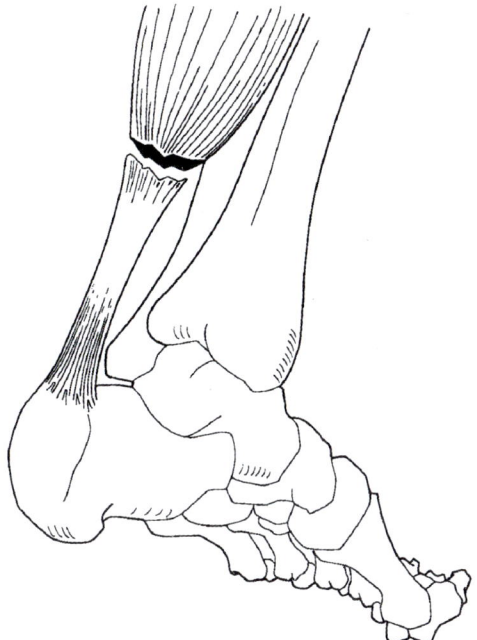

FIGURE 57.5. Musculotendinous Achilles rupture.

then the foot will plantarflex; if the tendon is ruptured, the foot will not. This test is less accurate a week after the injury.

b. Prone plantar flexion strength test: With the patient in the same position and both feet hanging over the end of the table, ask the patient to plantarflex both feet while the examiner applies resistance to the soles of both feet. There is usually a marked difference in strength, the patient complains of pain at the injury site, and the tendinous tear or gap may become more visible and may be more easily palpated. This test may confuse the examiner into thinking that there is a partial injury/tear as the other plantar flexors (tibialis posterior, toe flexors, and peroneal muscles) are still functional and will give plantar flexion. The inability to single toe raise on the affected side should lead the examiner to suspect a complete rupture.

c. Hyperdorsiflexion sign: With the patient in the same position, flex both knees to 90 degrees, then passively dorsiflex both feet maximally and compare sides.

d. Perhaps the most useful observation is to assess the attitude of the foot in relation to the leg (resting foot angle) with the athlete prone and feet over the end of the bed. The ruptured side will usually be more dorsiflexed than the normal side.

Predisposing Factors

These include, among others, previous partial injury to the tendon, tendonitis, tendinosis, soleus muscle atrophy, local steroid injections, and systemic conditions such as hyperparathyroidism or gout.

Treatment

If suspected, then sporting activity should be discontinued. Ice and a compressive bandage should be applied. If possible, immobilize the foot in the plantar flexed position. The patient should be referred to an orthopedic specialist for definitive care, which may be either nonoperative or operative. If late at night, the patient can wait until the morning before contacting the hospital, though one must have eliminated a DVT as the cause of pain.

57.8 ACHILLES TENDINOPATHY

This common condition of the midportion of the Achilles tendon is often seen in runners and athletes who do a lot of running training, such as boxers, footballers, etc. This problem has been known by many names in the past (e.g., Achilles peritendinitis, Achilles tenosynovitis, Achilles peritendinopathy, and Achilles tendinitis/tendonitis). However, as there is little or no inflammation, the preferred term is now Achilles tendinopathy, and where there is ultrastructure change suggestive of degenerative change, the term tendinosis can be used.

Traditionally, Achilles tendinopathy occurs 2 to 5 cm proximal to the insertion on the calcaneus. Pain is often worse in the morning or after exercise. There is often localized tenderness, thickening, or swelling, and crepitus may occasionally be felt over the tendon. Strength deficit is unusual unless pain restricts effort.

For the EP, there is not a lot one can do. Usual symptomatic treatment with ice and physiotherapy, and local treatment with the use of mild analgesics can be tried. Some therapists will try to tape to prevent excessive planter flexion, but these are all experimental interventions. For quick power sports such as sprinting activity, there may be a slight increase in risk of rupture. Local corticosteroid injections are usually discouraged as there is a risk of further weakening an already degenerated tendon and potentially increasing the risk of rupture. Inquiry as to potential underlying rheumatologic disorders, such as Reiter's syndrome, is appropriate. Use of fluoroquinolone antibiotics should be stopped as this class of athletes have been associated with the development of tendon disorders.

There are many options for treating this condition, but none, to date, are guaranteed. There is good evidence for an eccentric rehabilitation program, but other options such as orthotics, foot wear change, use of a nitroglycerin patch, extracorporeal shock wave therapy, laser therapy, and others have all been used with varying degrees of success. The treatment is prolonged so that referral to a physician to monitor the treatment is appropriate.

Insertional Achilles tendinopathy or enthesopathy occurs at the Achilles tendon insertion onto the calcaneus. The pain and tenderness usually associated with swelling is right at the insertion. The cause of this condition is unknown. In some cases, a prominent superior calcaneal tuberosity (Haglund's deformity) is present, which may be due to a combination of bony impingement on the bursa and tendon with chronic overuse.

As with noninsertional tendon disorders, there is often a gradual pain onset, particularly after exercise, and especially after running uphill. The difference between the two conditions is one of location. Differentiating between midsubstance and insertional Achilles tendinopathy has little consequence for initial treatment; however, it may have important consequences for subsequent rehabilitation and possible surgical treatment.

57.9 HAGLUND'S HEEL

Chronic irritation of the back of the heel, usually caused by pressure from the heels of stiff running shoes, may lead to the development of a bony growth on the posterior superior aspect of the calcaneus near the insertion of the Achilles tendon.

With this bony prominence on the one side and the rigid Achilles tendon on the other, the bursa becomes impinged and bursitis develops. Similarly, soft tissue near the Achilles tendon can become irritated leading to a painful condition that is exacerbated by pressure and use of the Achilles. Haglund's deformity is more common in women, in those with high-arched feet or rearfoot valgus, and in patients with "tight" Achilles tendons (which can be genetic or a tendon that has been exposed to repetitive microtrauma).

Clinically, the athlete presents with a painful, sometimes red and inflamed heel in the area around the Achilles tendon attachment. There may be a bony prominence or signs of chronic skin friction. The lesion may be bilateral. The lesion can often be bilateral and is confirmed on x-ray.

Treatment

Acute irritations can be treated with NSAIDs, painkillers, topical anesthetics, and ice. Pads can be attached over the irritated area to diminish friction; similarly, insoles can help change the angle of the calcaneus and reduce irritation. Shoes can be modified. Gastrocnemius/soleus/Achilles stretching exercises may help in the less-acute phases. The athlete should avoid running uphill or on hard surfaces, if possible. Cycling may also cause discomfort (Fig. 57.6).

57.10 ANATOMIC DIAGNOSES

By localizing the source of pain in the leg, here is a quick reference based on anatomic structure to some of the likely differential diagnoses (Table 57.1).

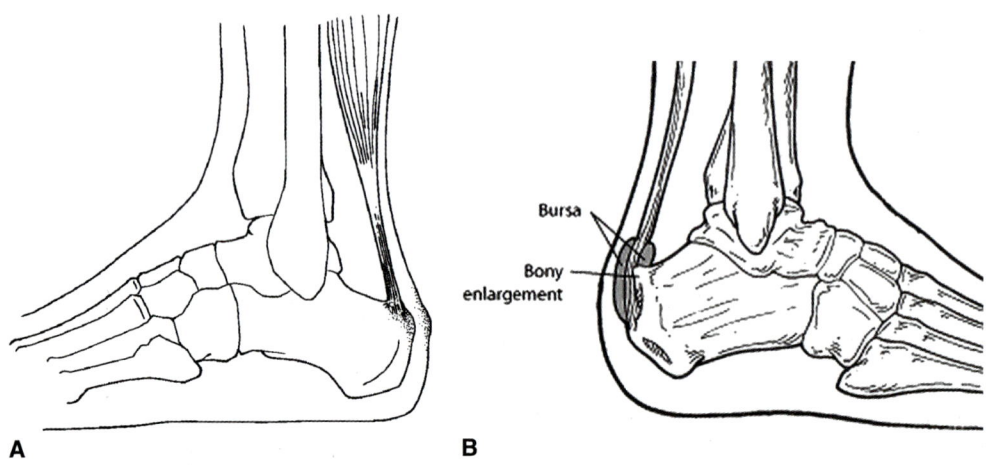

FIGURE 57.6. **A.** Normal foot. **B.** Haglund's heel with bone impingement on the bursa.

TABLE 57.1 Differential Diagnosis of Leg Pain Based on Anatomical Location

Anatomic Location	Structure	Differential Diagnosis
Anterior	Bone	Anterior cortex midshaft tibial stress fracture
	Muscle	Chronic compartment syndrome (anterior)
	Nerve	Lumbar referred (L4 or L5)
		Common/deep peroneal nerve injury
Lateral	Bone	Fibula stress fracture
	Muscle	Chronic compartment syndrome (lateral)
	Nerve	Lumbar referred
		Common/superficial peroneal nerve injury
		Superficial peroneal nerve entrapment
Medial	Bone	Tibia (stress fracture or periostitis)
	Muscle	Tibialis posterior tendinopathy/tenosynovitis
		Chronic compartment syndrome (deep posterior)
	Nerve	Tarsal tunnel syndrome
Posterior	Muscle	Chronic compartment syndrome (superficial)
	Nerve	Lumbar referred (S1 or neural claudication as seen in spinal stenosis)
	Vessel	Deep vein thrombosis
		Atherosclerotic disease (vascular claudication)
		Popliteal artery entrapment

Recommended Reading

Alfredson H. Chronic midportion Achilles tendinpathy: an update on research and treatment. *Clin Sports Med.* 2003;22(4):727–741.

Bernardi E, Camporese G, Buller HR, et al. Serial 2-point ultrasonography plus D-dimer vs whole-leg color-coded doppler ultrasonography for diagnosing suspected symptomatic deep vein thrombosis: a randomized controlled trial. *JAMA.* 2008;200(14):1652–1659.

Blackman PG. A review of chronic exertional compartment syndrome in the lower leg. *Med Sci Sports Exerc.* 2000;32(3 suppl):S4–S10.

Chad DA. Lumbar spinal stenosis. *Neurol Clin.* 2007;25:407–418.

Fredericson M, Jennings F, Beaulieu C, et al. Stress fractures in athletes. *Top Magn Reson Imaging.* 2006;17(5):309–325.

Gourgiotis S, Villias C, Germanos S, et al. Acute limb compartment syndrome: a review. *J Surg Educ.* 2007;64(3):178–186.

Howard JL, Mohtadi NGH, Wiley JP. Evaluation of outcomes in patients following surgical treatment of chronic exertional compartment syndrome in the leg. *Clin J Sport Med.* 2000;10(3):176–184.

Khan RJK, Fick D, Brammar TJ, et al. Surgical interventions for treating acute Achilles tendon ruptures (review). *Cochrane Database of Systematic Reviews.* 2004;(4)3:CD003674.

Paavola M, Kannus P, Järvinen TAH, et al. Achilles tendinopathy. *JBJS.* 2002;84-A(11):2062–2076.

Rompe JD, Furia JP, Maffulli N. Mid-portion Achilles tendinopathy: current options for treatment. *Disabil Rehabil.* 2008;30(20–22):1666–1676.

Schepsis AA, Jones II, Haas AL. Achilles tendon disorders in athletes. *Am J Sports Med.* 30(2):287–305.

Shadgan B, Menon M, O'Brien PJ, et al. Diagnostic techniques in acute compartment syndrome of the leg. *J Orthop Trauma.* 2008;22(8):581–587.

Spitz DJ, Newberg AH. Imaging of stress fractures in athletes. *Radiol Clin North Am.* 2002;40(2):313–331.

Stager A, Clement D. Popliteal artery entrapment syndrome. *Sports Med.* 1999;28(1):61–70.

Taunton JE, Ryan MB, Clement DB, et al. A retrospective case-control analysis of 2002 running injuries. *Br J Sports Med.* 2002;36(2):95–101.

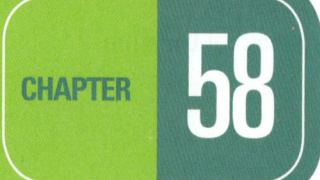

CHAPTER 58

Muscle Cramps and Strains in Runners

Contributed by Martin Schwellnus, Professor, University of Cape Town, FIFA Medical Centre of Excellence, and IOC Research Centre, Cape Town, South Africa

Reviewer: David McDonagh

Acute exercise-associated muscle cramping (EAMC) has been defined as a "painful spasmodic involuntary contraction of skeletal muscle that occurs during or immediately after muscular exercise." Muscle cramps can be a manifestation of some underlying medical disease, but the majority of these medical diseases are rare and most athletes with cramping suffer from EAMC. Epidemiological studies indicate that about 30% to 50% of all endurance athletes will experience cramping at some stage in their careers. The causes, diagnosis, and treatment of acute EAMC are still not well understood but will be briefly discussed.

58.1 WHAT CAUSES CRAMPS DURING EXERCISE?

Anecdotal observations, first reported more than 100 years ago, have led to the common belief that cramps in athletes are caused by shortages of "electrolytes" (sodium, chloride, magnesium), "dehydration," heat, or a combination of these factors. In general, there is a lack of scientific support for these theories, and most recent prospective cohort studies have shown no association between either serum electrolyte disturbance or dehydration and the development of EAMC.[3] In contrast, there is a growing body of evidence from animal studies, human laboratory studies, and epidemiological studies that EAMC is associated with muscle fatigue when athletes exercise at a higher intensity or for a prolonged duration, particularly in hot, humid environments. There is evidence that muscle fatigue results in abnormal control of the nerves that cause muscle contraction, which then results in EAMC. This is supported by

the common observations that EAMC is localized to working muscles, and is relieved by static stretching that invokes reflex muscle relaxation.

58.2 WHO IS AT RISK OF DEVELOPING CRAMPING DURING EXERCISE?

The risk factors for acute EAMC have recently been reviewed using evidence-based medicine criteria. Risk factors for EAMC for which there is good evidence (level I) include a past history of EAMC and increased exercise intensity (race pace and subjective assessment of intensity). Risk factors for which there is some, but weaker, evidence (level 11 or III) are exercising in hot or humid environmental conditions, increased exercise duration, irregular stretching habits, shorter daily stretching time, a positive family history of EAMC, longer history of running, increased body mass index, and increased age. Other risk factors that are not associated with EAMC (level IV evidence) are dehydration, serum electrolyte disturbances, and increased sweat loss and sweat sodium concentration.

Furthermore, muscles most prone to cramping are those that span across two joints (hamstring muscles, one of the front thigh muscles, some of the calf muscles, and foot muscles). These are also the muscles that are often contracted in a shortened position during exercise.

58.3 DIAGNOSIS OF ACUTE EAMC

The clinical features of acute EAMC are skeletal muscle fatigue followed by twitching of the muscle ("cramp prone state"). This progresses to spasmodic spontaneous contractions and eventual frank muscle cramping with pain. Relief from the "cramp prone state" occurs if the activity is stopped or if the muscle is stretched passively. Once activity is ceased, episodes of cramping are usually followed by periods of relief from cramping. Cramping can be precipitated by contraction of the muscle in a shortened position (inner range).

The clinical examination of an athlete with EAMC typically shows obvious distress, pain, a hard contracted muscle and visible fasciculation (twitching) over the muscle belly. In most instances, the athlete is conscious, responds normally to stimuli, and is able to conduct a conversation. Vital signs and a general examination usually reveal no abnormalities. In particular, most runners with acute cramping are not dehydrated or hyperthermic.

An athlete who has generalized severe cramping or is confused, semicomatosed, or comatosed should be treated as a medical emergency that requires immediate hospitalization where full investigation is required.

58.4 MANAGEMENT OF EAMC

The immediate treatment for acute cramping is passive stretching of the affected muscle groups and then holding the muscle in stretched position until fasciculation (twitching) ceases. Supportive treatment is by keeping the athlete at a comfortable temperature and by providing oral fluids, if required. Athletes with recurrent acute EAMC should be investigated fully to exclude other medical conditions.

58.5 PREVENTION OF EAMC

The key to the prevention of cramps is to protect the muscle from developing premature fatigue during exercise by being well trained, to reduce exercise intensity particularly if exercise is performed in hot and humid environmental conditions, to perfor regular stretching, to ensure adequate nutritional intake (carbohydrates), and to perform activity at a lower intensity and for a shorter duration.

Recommended Reading

Parisi L, Pierelli F, Amabile G, et al. Muscular cramps: proposals for a new classification. *Acta Neurol Scand.* 2003;107(3):176–186.

Schwellnus MP, Derman EW, Noakes TD. Aetiology of skeletal muscle "cramps" during exercise: a novel hypothesis. *J Sports Sci.* 1997;15(3):277–285.

Schwellnus MP, Drew N, Collins M. Muscle cramping in athletes—risk factors, clinical assessment, and management. *Clin Sports Med.* 2008;27(1):183–194.

Wilder RP. Preface: The runner. *Clin Sports Med.* 2010;29(3): xv–xvi.

CHAPTER 59 Acute Rhabdomyolysis

Contributed by Wayne Derman, Professor; and Dr. Dale Rae, University of Cape Town, FIFA Medical Centre of Excellence, and IOC Research Centre, Cape Town, South Africa

Reviewer: David McDonagh

Rhabdomyolysis is defined as the destruction and disintegration of skeletal muscle with leakage of intracellular enzymes including myoglobin and creatine kinase (CK) into the circulation. This can be a potentially serious condition, with resultant electrolyte abnormalities, acute renal failure (ARF) and disseminated intravascular coagulation (DIC), which can be life threatening. While rhabdomyolysis can occur through a variety of causes including crush injuries, trauma, drugs, toxins, infections, muscle enzyme deficiencies, and endocrine abnormalities, exertional rhabdomyolyis refers to the above-mentioned syndrome that occurs in association with physical exercise and has been documented in many different sports. Mild forms of exertional rhabdomyolysis are thought to be more common than previously appreciated, but severe exertional rhabdomyolysis can be devastating.

59.1 PATHOPHYSIOLOGY

Although there are many possible causes of rhabdomyolysis, there are two common events that occur in all etiologies. The first is direct injury to the sarcolemma, and the second is failure of energy supply within the muscle cell. Both events lead to a rise in intracellular calcium. Activation of calcium-dependent neutral proteases and phospholipases results in destruction of myofibrillar, cytoskeletal, and membrane proteins, and lysosomal digestion of fiber contents occurs. Excessive release of myoglobin into circulation, which is filtered by the kidney, is toxic to the renal tubule and can cause ARF.

59.2 RISK FACTORS

Risk factors include deconditioned athletes or participation in high-intensity unaccustomed exercise, high ambient temperature or humidity, and inadequate fluid intake. Furthermore, athletes who have certain medical conditions—including myopathy, dystrophinopathies, sickle cell trait, previous/recent history of viral illness, heat illness/exhaustion, renal insufficiency, or previous episodes of exertional rhabdomyolysis—are at risk of exertional rhabdomyolysis. The use of certain drugs, supplements, and medications could also predispose to exertional rhabdomyolysis. These include cocaine, alcohol, ephedrine, amphetamine, barbiturates, aspirin or other analgesics, clofibrate, gemfibrozil, statin agents, phenothiazines, and phencyclidine.

59.3 DIAGNOSIS

Symptoms of exertional rhabdomyolysis include a recent history of an acute vigorous bout of exercise followed by skeletal muscle pain, swelling, and the passing of red-brown (Coca-Cola–like) urine or little/no urine at all. Patients can also complain of nausea, abdominal, or lower back pain. A careful history should evaluate the presence of risk factors. Clinical signs might include excessive tenderness on palpation of the swollen muscle group and athletes with suspected exertional rhabdomyolysis should be observed for the development of features of compartment syndrome.

Biochemical findings in cases of acute rhabdomyolysis include the presence of hemo/myoglobin in the urine (without the presence of red blood cells), elevation of serum CK (can be up to 1 million U per L) or aldolase, hyperkalemia, hypocalcemia, hyperphosphatemia, hyperuricemia, a high creatinine:BUN ratio, hypoalbuminuria, and the accompanying features of ARF or DIC.

Screening by using a urine dipstick test for orthotolidine and CK is a useful combination for the condition.

59.4 MANAGEMENT

Management includes vigorous fluid replacement and strict patient monitoring of urine output and fluid overload. The patient should be cooled if there is associated heat illness. The use of furosemide and alkalinization of the urine is controversial. Hyperkalemia can be treated with glucose and insulin and an exchange resin such as sodium polystyrene sulfonate.[6]

It is important to monitor the patient's metabolic status, urea and electrolytes, calcium, phosphate, and CK concentrations as well as the prothrombin time, partial thromboplastin time, and platelet counts. Depending on the severity of the condition, dialysis or hemofiltration may be required. Patients with suspected compartment syndrome should be referred for surgical opinion regarding the need for fasciotomy.

59.5 PREVENTION

Athletes should be encouraged to follow the general principles of exercise training, namely, the application of gradual increasing training loads and not to undertake excessive unaccustomed exercise. Furthermore, adherence to international guidelines regarding participation of exercise in the heat and fluid replacement is important.

It is also important that the emergency or team physician has a high index of suspicion of this condition, particularly in athletes with risk factors.

Recommended Reading

Clarkson PM. Exertional rhabdomyolysis and acute renal failure in marathon runners. *Sports Med.* 2007;37:361–363.

Figarella-Branger D, Baeta Machado AM, Putzu GA, et al. Exertional rhabdomyolysis and exercise intolerance revealing dystrophinopathies. *Acta Neuropathol.* 1997;94:48–53.

Galvez R, Stacy J, Howley A. Exertional rhabdomyolysis in seven division-1 swimming athletes. *Clin J Sport Med.* 2008;18:366–368.

Line RL, Rust GS. Acute exertional rhabdomyolysis. *Am Fam Physician.* 1995;52:502–506.

Makaryus JN, Catanzaro JN, Katona KC. Exertional rhabdomyolysis and renal failure in patients with sickle cell trait: is it time to change our approach? *Hematology.* 2007;12:349–352.

Sandhu RS, Como JJ, Scalea TS, et al. Renal failure and exercise-induced rhabdomyolysis in patients taking performance-enhancing compounds. *J Trauma.* 2002;53: 761–763.

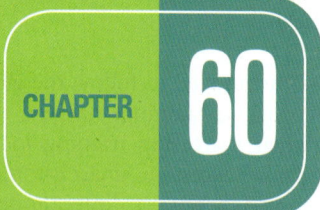

CHAPTER 60

Ankle Sprains

Contributed by Jack Taunton, CMO, Vancouver 2010 Winter Olympic Games; Professor, University of British Columbia; and Dory Boyer, Deputy CMO, Vancouver 2010 Olympic Winter Games

Reviewer: Ketil Holen, University Hospital, Trondheim; Team Physician, Rosenborg Football Club, Norway

60.1 ANKLE SPRAIN EPIDEMIOLOGY: INCIDENCE AND MECHANISM OF INJURY

Ankle sprains are the most common injury among recreational and competitive athletes, representing 11.8% of all injuries and the greatest time lost from practice and games. They are associated with a recurrence rate reported to be as high as 70% to 80%. Most ankle injuries in males result from participation in sports like basketball, American football, soccer, volleyball, and cross-country running. In females, ankle sprains are associated with the practice of cross-training, basketball, badminton, volleyball, handball, and gymnastics. Some 85% to 90% of all ankle sprains involve the lateral ligament complex and result from excessive plantar flexion and inversion of the ankle. The first structure to be injured is the anterior talofibular (ATF) ligament and then, with increasing inversion force, the calcaneofibular ligament and the posterior talofibular ligament (Fig. 60.1). Inversion injuries to the lateral ankle ligaments are associated with subtalar ligament injury in 70% to 80% of cases.

Eversion injuries to the medial collateral ligament are rare. These injures are known to result in longer rehabilitation with more pain and chronic instability. Injuries to the inferior tibiofibular complex (syndesmosis injuries), seen in approximately 10% of all sprains, also have a slower rehabilitation process. These sprains are most commonly seen with hypereversion and occasionally hyperinversion injuries.

Noncontact ankle sprains are now thought to be the result of poor foot position just before or during foot strike. With insufficient recruitment of muscles to support the foot in this position at foot strike, the ankle is forced into inversion. This theory suggests that poor joint position sense is a primary cause of ankle inversion sprains.

Other injuries closely associated with the ankle include distal tibial stress fractures, tibialis posterior tendinopathy, and peroneal tendinopathy.

60.2 ANKLE JOINT EXAMINATION

Physical examination of the acute ankle sprain should include inspection, palpation, evaluation of range of motion, muscle strength assessment, and tests of joint laxity. The severity of the sprain is represented by the immediate amount of swelling, pain, and disability. Local tenderness about the three lateral ligaments is the most common finding. With a severe inversion, tenderness over the talus can suggest an associated osteochondral injury to the talus. With an eversion sprain, tenderness is found on the medial ligament complex and the distal medial malleolus. Tenderness over the syndesmosis with the inferior tibiofibular complex can be enhanced by compression of the tibia and proximal third of the tibia and fibula (the squeeze test).

Associated findings can include tenderness over the peroneal tendons posterior to the lateral malleolus when an injury includes subluxation or dislocation of these tendons. Strength testing during resisted eversion can often demonstrate subluxation or dislocation of the tendon.

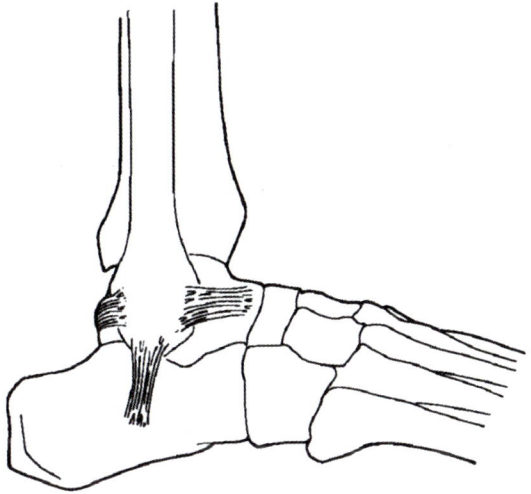

FIGURE 60.1.   Ankle ligaments.

Examination of the peroneus brevis close to the insertion in the base of the fifth metatarsal can reveal an avulsion injury. More proximal tenderness at the base of the fifth metatarsal tubercle can be seen with a Jones fracture. Tenderness with compression of the calcaneus could represent a fracture of the anterior process of the calcaneus (beak fracture) or of the anterior calcaneal articular facet. Tenderness over the lateral talus, as seen in snowboarders, can represent a fracture of the lateral talar process. Resisting eversion can reveal weakness of the tibialis posterior muscle.

Laxity assessment of the ATF ligament is done with the anterior drawer test. A positive test done in plantar flexion indicates damage to the ATF with anterior displacement of 4 mm or more, and complete disruption can be suggested by the absence of a firm endpoint. If the anterior drawer is positive in the neutral position, involvement of the calcaneofibular and posterior talofibular ligaments should be suspected. A positive talar tilt test, done by holding the calcaneus and inverting or everting the hind foot, suggests the involvement of the calcaneal fibular and subtalar ligaments. Both ankles should be tested to compare findings.

Always check for continuity of the Achilles tendon in your exam and check for tenderness and stability of the midfoot and tarsal–metatarsal forefoot region. Significant hop pain points to a more severe injury and is often associated with a fracture and requires imaging.

60.3 ANKLE SPRAIN GRADING

Ankle sprains are often graded from I to III.

- Grade I sprains—primarily to the ATF ligament—some swelling, mild tenderness, and only slight pain on inversion stress. Loss of function is minimal. On clinical exam, the anterior drawer test is negative or equal to the opposite side and talar tilt is normal. If ultrasound is done, there is only minor ligament damage.

- Grade II sprains—involve both the ATF and the calcaneofibular ligament. There is moderate swelling and moderate loss of function with difficulty bearing weight. Hopping may be possible but causes considerable pain. Inversion stress results in significant pain and both ligaments are very tender to palpation. No pain on tibiofibular squeeze. Increased anterior drawer test and mild talar tilt are noted. The best opportunity to assess the athlete is in the field of play before swelling increases and before the range of motion is restricted by swelling and reflex muscle spasm. Alternatively, one may have to wait some days when pain and swelling have decreased, but by then the event may be over.

- Grade III sprains—involve the posterior talofibular ligament in addition to the ATF and CF ligaments. With this injury, walking and hopping are very difficult and, with complete lateral ligament complex involvement, there is a significantly positive anterior drawer test with soft end feel, positive talar tilt, marked swelling and tenderness, and significant functional impairment. Talar tilt test is positive although the clinical value has been debated.

60.4 ANKLE SPRAIN TREATMENT

Grades I and II sprains are managed with PRICES, taping and/or bracing, and active physiotherapy.

Grade III sprains will usually be treated with a below-knee functional walking cast for 5 to 6 weeks followed by active physiotherapy.

For the elite athlete with significant instability, surgical repair is often the best choice because it reduces the risk of recurrent ankle sprains. After surgery, a functional walking boot is used and a rehabilitation program is implemented, similar to grades I and II sprains with range of motion, strength, and proprioceptive drills, leading to protected mobilization with sport-specific drills.

60.5 ANKLE IMAGING

Of the estimated six million ankle x-rays done in North America each year, only 15% are positive for significant fractures. The Ottawa rules established by Stiell et al. have improved this situation considerably. An x-ray should be done if there is pain in the malleolar zone, associated with an inability to bear weight for four steps both immediately and on assessment in the emergency department. In addition, x-rays are required if there is tenderness along the distal 6 cm of the posterior edge of the fibula or tip of the lateral malleolus and/or bony tenderness along the distal 6 cm of the posterior edge of the tibia or tip of the medial malleolus. Tenderness over the base of the fifth metatarsal also requires an x-ray.

Persistent pain about the talus, navicular, or calcaneus bones following a severe ankle injury may be due to occult fractures not seen on plain initial x-rays and may require imaging with bone scans, CT scans, or MRI.

Examples of this are osteochondral fractures of the talus or lateral process fractures most commonly seen in snowboarders. High-resolution ultrasound is very useful for investigation of tendon injury and subluxation plus injury to the ligaments, especially the lateral complex and bursal swelling.

60.6 ANKLE SPRAIN—IMMEDIATE MANAGEMENT TO REHABILITATION

After the assessment in the field, the decision must be made as to whether the athlete can continue to play. If there is significant pain when hopping, then the athlete needs further investigation. The aim is to reduce swelling and pain and to initiate early protected range of motion. This can be achieved by PRICES. Ice packs or a Cryo/Cuff can be used at this stage. Stabilization with taping or with an orthotic device is appropriate, along with the use of crutches for initial non–weight bearing. Referral to physiotherapy is important at this stage with the initiation of range of motion exercises followed by strength drills and static exercises, progressing to dynamic balance.

Fraser's acute stage (first 48 hours) management is to control swelling, edema, and hemorrhage in order to reduce synovial reaction that slows recovery of the range of motion. This is achieved by compression with open-basket taping or tensor wrap with foam horseshoes around the malleoli, plus elevation with periodic ankle pumping with a Cryo/Cuff. Swelling, edema, and hemorrhage can also be controlled with icing, using ice bags directly applied to the skin in a cycle of 15 minutes on and 45 minutes off for the first 3 hours, then 15 minutes every 3 hours.

To further unload compressive forces on the joint, Fraser stresses modified activity with partial weight-bearing crutch walking. Early mobilization is the key to preventing joint stiffness and promoting an earlier return to sport. Early mobilization of the ankle and subtalar joint (eversion movement first) followed by gentle ROM exercises (featherweight-bearing squat motion, gentle stair subtalar joint oscillations, and open chain active ROM focusing on dorsiflexion and eversion) is recommended.

In the subacute stage of 2 to 21 days, swelling is more synovial and edematous, so open-basket tape or tensor wrap with the foam horseshoe is continued as swelling will increase as day to day activity is increased. For patients with persisting pain in the anterolateral region after established stability and normal ROM, anterolateral synovial impingement (ALSI) is a common problem. This requires MRI arthrography and very often arthroscopic synovectomy. Similarly, chondral injuries may cause persisting symptoms.

60.7 ANKLE SPRAIN RETURN-TO-PLAY CRITERIA

See Chapter 73.9.

60.8 ANKLE SPRAIN PREVENTION

Prevention measures for ankle sprains have been researched and include proprioceptive and balance training, strength exercises, taping, bracing, and shoe modifications.

Recommended Reading

Stiell IG, McKnight RD, Greenberg GH, et al. Implementation of the Ottawa ankle rules. *JAMA*. 1994;271(11): 827–832.

CHAPTER 61

Ottawa Ankle and Foot Rules

Contributed by David McDonagh, Chair, FIBT Medical Commission

Reviewer: Ketil Holen, University Hospital, Trondheim; Team Physician, Rosenborg Football Club, Norway

The Ottawa ankle rules were developed at the department of emergency medicine in Ottawa, by Stiel et al. Before the introduction of the rules, most patients with ankle injuries were x-rayed. However, the vast majority of x-rays revealed no fracture, and this proved to be costly and time-consuming, not to mention a possible health risk. Several studies have confirmed the sensitivity of these rules. Bachmann et al., conducted a meta-analysis on 32 studies, reporting on 15,581 patients. They concluded that the incidence of false negatives (i.e., fractures) was extremely low (as low as 0.3%) and that the false negative results may just as well be due to physician skill variations as due to faults with the Ottawa rules. The rules are now widely accepted and used around the world and are an important tool in the event physician's kit.

61.1 ANKLE ASSESSMENT

Test the ability to walk four steps (immediately after the injury or at the emergency department) and note localized tenderness of the posterior edge or tip of either malleolus (four spots). If there is

tenderness or inability to walk four steps, then an ankle x-ray is also indicated if there is

- Bone tenderness at A
- Bone tenderness at B
- Inability to bear weight both immediately and in the casualty department

61.2 MIDFOOT ASSESSMENT

A foot x-ray is required if there is any pain in the midfoot zone and any of these findings (Figs. 61.1 and 61.2):

- Bone tenderness at C
- Bone tenderness at D
- Inability to bear weight both immediately and in the casualty department.

Recommended Reading

Bachmann LM, Kolb E, Koller MT, et al. Accuracy of Ottawa ankle rules to exclude fractures of the ankle and midfoot. *BMJ.* 2003;326:405–406.

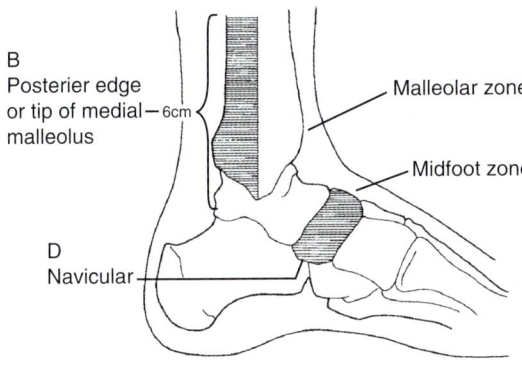

FIGURE 61.1. Medial view.

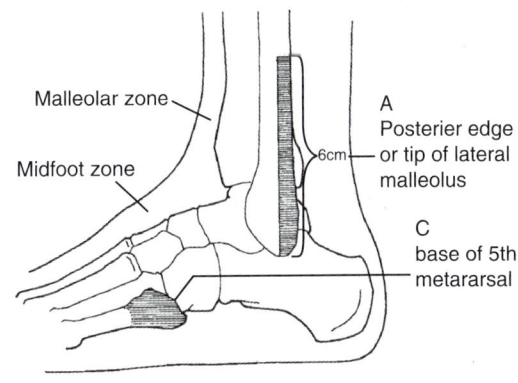

FIGURE 61.2. Lateral view.

Foot Injuries

Contributed by Jack Taunton, CMO, and Dory Boyer, Deputy CMO, Vancouver 2010 Olympic Winter Games, University of British Columbia, Vancouver, Canada

Reviewer: Ketil Holen, University Hospital, Trondheim; Team Physician, Rosenborg Football Club, Norway

For simplicity, foot injuries in the field of play will be divided into forefoot injury, midfoot injury, and rearfoot injury.

62.1 FOREFOOT INJURIES

Houghton stated that the most significant causes of forefoot pain include turf toe, sesamoiditis, metatarsal stress fractures, Morton's neuroma, and Freiberg's avascular necrosis.

Turf toe is seen in soccer, football, and basketball players with a forced dorsiflexion of the first metatarsal phalangeal joint and a sprain of the plantar capsular ligament. The joint is painful and swollen with restricted motion of the joint. Management consists of icing, NSAID medication, a stiff sole or rocker bar on the shoe to restrict further dorsiflexion of the joint, taping, and then graduated range of motion exercises and intrinsic foot exercises. Return-to-play is generally 2 weeks for a grade II sprain and 6 weeks for a grade III sprain. Repeated sprain might lead to a chronic condition that occasionally needs surgery.

Sesamoid injury is seen in running and jumping sports with repetitive impact and can result in a complex of pathology from inflammation and stress fracture to fracture. If the athlete has a congenital bipartite sesamoid, the fibrous union can be seen with forced dorsiflexion and impact. Investigation includes plain x-rays. Bone scan and follow-up CT scan are often required to make the diagnosis. Return-to-play is delayed with a fracture due to prolonged healing time. Orthotic modification with sesamoid cutout can often unload the sesamoid and permit a pain-free walk–run program.

Metatarsal stress fractures are commonly seen in the aerobic running phase of training. Bone density must be considered, and variants in foot morphology of the excessively pronated foot leading to second metatarsal stress fractures and fourth and fifth metatarsal stress fractures in the varus pes cavus foot. The athlete presents with a pain progression profile—initial pain after running, to slowly progressing pain while running, and finally pain on hopping and walking. Initial x-rays are normal and the diagnosis is confirmed by a CT scan or MRI.

Jones stress fracture of the proximal fifth metatarsal is notorious for nonunion due to avascular necrosis and for requiring internal fixation. Some may be treated with electromagnetic bone stimulation and non–weight bearing while maintaining fitness through pool running with healing time of 8 to 10 weeks. The typical stress fracture heals in 4 to 6 weeks, and a walk–run program is started when the athlete is pain-free to hop. Orthotic foot control and appropriate footwear are important with a motion control shoe for the pronated foot and curved lasted shock-absorption sole for the more rigid cavus foot. Alternatively, surgical treatment with an intramedullary screw may be more appropriate.

Morton's Neuroma

Burning forefoot pain and paresthesia typically between the third and fourth interspaces in a tight boot (figure skates, ski boots, tight running shoes) bring the diagnosis of Morton's neuroma. The interdigital nerve can get compressed with an entrapment that can lead to swelling and scarring of the nerve. On exam, tenderness is localized and can be increased with metatarsal head compression, which can occur with a click, and a Tinel's sign over the interspace can

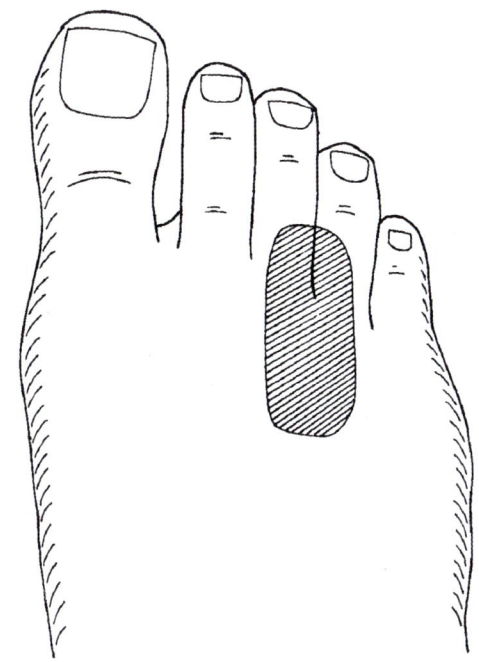

FIGURE 62.1. Morton's neuroma.

be produced. Management involves a wider shoe or boot, orthotic with metatarsal pad to open the interdigital space, local cortisone injection in the acute phase, and if it persists, surgical excision. In rehabilitation, intrinsic muscle strength, arch curls, and balance drills are very important (Fig. 62.1).

Freiberg's avascular necrosis

In the adolescent runner or jumper, pain over the second or third metatarsal head can represent Freiberg's avascular necrosis. This can be confirmed on x-ray although x-rays can be normal in the early stages, and a bone scan and follow-up CT scan or MRI can confirm the diagnosis. The natural history of this process is 2 to 3 years, and the foot should be protected with orthotics and metatarsal pads to unload the involved metatarsal head to prevent deformity. In the early phases, activity must be modified to cycling and pool running.

62.2 MIDFOOT INJURIES

The most commonly underdiagnosed causes of midfoot pain are the navicular stress fracture and tendinopathies of tibialis posterior and of peroneus longus and brevis. Both tendinopathies can be assessed with high-resolution Doppler ultrasound, and if partial tears are identified, a Ritchie brace for protection and extensive physiotherapy may be used together with an appropriate orthotic to stabilize the foot postbracing.

Navicular stress fracture is a challenge due to poor vascularization, like the scaphoid, leading to nonunion. The central one-third of the navicular becomes impinged during foot strike and is further compromised with excessive foot pronation. It is typically seen in jumpers, runners, sprinters, and basketball players presenting with a vague midfoot pain increasing with accelerated training. Torg identified tenderness at the *N* spot on the proximal dorsal surface with an 81% sensitivity for stress fracture. Plain x-rays have low yield with sensitivity of approximately 33% but good specificity.

Bone scan, although nonspecific, has a high sensitivity with diagnosis confirmed on CT scan or MRI with high sensitivity and high specificity but higher cost. You will see stages of a navicular stress injury—first with normal x-rays, positive bone scan, and negative CT scan—a stress reaction proceeding on a continuum as bone stress continues to a true stress fracture with positive CT scan. The current standard of care as outlined by Koehle is 6 weeks of non–weight-bearing immobilization followed by a 6-week functional rehabilitation program. Khan et al. (1994) reported an 86% success rate with this program. For failures with nonunion or fragmented fracture, then surgery is required. Electromagnetic bone stimulation 8 hours per day can be used if there is delayed healing at 6 weeks. Also, pulsed ultrasound for just 30 minutes daily can be used, but the effect of this and the electromagnetic treatment is still under debate.

62.3 REARFOOT INJURIES

Rob Lloyd-Smith gave an excellent summary of rearfoot pain in the athlete. For brevity, I will confine my discussion to plantar fasciitis, calcaneal stress fracture, and tarsal tunnel syndrome.

Plantar fasciitis is a common chronic condition seen in runners, walkers, and jumpers, plus individuals who stand for prolonged periods. It is a degeneration of the collagen usually at the origin from the medial calcaneal tubercle and is often associated with microtears. It presents with morning heel pain and pain with prolonged standing and push off in jumping and running. The athlete often has limited dorsiflexion and has, more often, pronated feet, but some of the most challenging cases are seen with the cavus foot. If it presents bilaterally, you must consider a seronegative arthropathy such as Reiter's, psoriasis, inflammatory bowel or bladder, and/or sacroiliitis (ankylosing spondylitis). Imaging with high-resolution Doppler ultrasound can confirm the presence of microtears, neovascularization, and increased thickening. Ultrasound-guided hyperosmolar dextrose injections

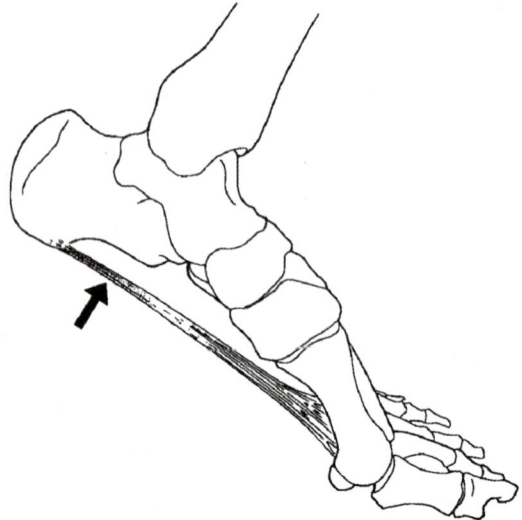

FIGURE 62.2. Plantar fasciitis.

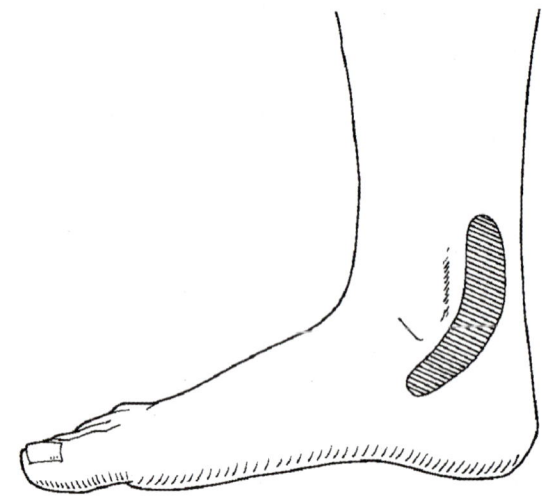

FIGURE 62.3. Tarsal tunnel syndrome.

(sclerotherapy) have a 75% to 85% success rate at 1 year. Similar success rates can be seen with Achilles and patellar tendinopathy.

Treatment traditionally consists of a night splint or Strassburg sock, stretching, low-dye arch taping, icing, physiotherapy, graduated eccentric heel drops, and appropriate orthotics and shoes. For chronic cases, extracorporeal shock wave therapy has been studied. Corticosteroid injections have been used in the past but postinjection ruptures can occur (Fig. 62.2).

Calcaneal stress fracture is similar to other stress fractures and is seen more frequently in female athletes. Lloyd-Smith reports on a female bimodal distribution with the 18- to 30-year-old females being long-distance runners and the next peak in over 60-year-old female walkers and golfers. Pain is initially vague then becomes more localized as stress continues. Clinically, there is pain to hop and pain on calcaneal compression. The diagnosis can be confirmed with a positive bone scan as initial x-rays are often nondiagnostic. Follow-up CT scan or MRI will show the extent of the stress fracture. Bone density assessment for associated osteopenia or osteoporosis is recommended. The standard treatment is activity modification, and ambulation is usually comfortable in a below-knee walking cast. Fitness can be maintained by pool running or cycling. Once pain-free to hop, the athlete can progress on a walk–run program, working with a physiotherapist addressing strength, flexibility, and balance exercises.

Tarsal tunnel syndrome is an underdiagnosed complex compression neuropathy of the posterior tibial nerve as it travels under the flexor retinacu-lum of the medial ankle. The compression can result in both motor and sensory involvement often in a pronated foot that can be rigid with an associated tarsal coalition. The pronated foot causes nerve tension as the heel rolls into valgus and the forefoot abducts. Pain is reported to be a burning numbness or tingling that can radiate proximally or distally. On exam, a positive Tinel's sign may be elicited with tenderness over the tarsal tunnel but can be confused with tenderness at the origin of the plantar fascia from the medial calcaneal tubercle. Investigation with ultrasound may reveal thickening of the nerve or adjacent tendons (i.e., tibialis posterior, flexor digitorum longus, flexor hallucis longus) or ganglion, varicosity, or lipoma as the source of the compression. X-ray may show an impinging osteophyte. EMG and nerve conduction tests are often normal with sensory studies being the most sensitive. In this condition, also consider other causes of compression neuropathy—diabetes, B_{12}, and thyroid deficiencies.

Treatment consists of orthotic foot control to reduce foot valgus, better heel counter, motion control shoes, arch and gastrocnemius stretching, ankle and foot strengthening plus balance drills. For pain control and night relief, Gabapentin and Pregabalin and a corticosteroid injection under ultrasound guidance may give some relief. Surgery is always stated to be a last resort with success rates varying from 44% to 95% reported (Fig. 62.3).

Recommended Reading

Bucholz RW, Heckman JD, Court-Brown CM, et al. *Rockwood and Green's Fractures in Adults* (7th Ed.). Philadelphia, PA: Lippincott Williams & Wilkins, 2009.
Canale ST, Beaty J. *Campbell's Operative Orthopaedics* (11th Ed.). Philadelphia, PA: Mosby, 2007.

CHAPTER 63

Foot Conditions

Contributed by David McDonagh, Chair, FIBT Medical Commission

Reviewer: Ketil Holen, University Hospital, Trondheim; Team Physician, Rosenborg Football Club, Norway

63.1 JOGGER'S TOE/TENNIS TOE

Trauma-induced subungual or periungual hemorrhage is common among athletes. When toes slide forward repetitively, the nails collide with the front of the shoes, and may lead to hematoma formation, onycholysis, and subungual hyperkeratosis. A black–blue discoloration is frequently observed under the distal nail plate, sparing the proximal nail. Specific mechanical stresses in various sports may lead to different nails being affected. Similar hemorrhages can occur in workers who wear steel-toed shoes or boots. The differential diagnosis includes subungual melanocytic nevus or malignant melanoma, and biopsy of the nail bed may be warranted, especially if the discoloration is unilateral or extends to the nail fold (known as Hutchinson sign).

Management

Properly fitted shoes and orthotic devices may help prevent the forefoot from slamming into the toe box. If a patient presents with an acute subungual hemorrhage, drainage with a needle or a heated paper clip through the nail plate can quickly reduce local pressure and discomfort.

63.2 FOOT BLISTERS

Shearing forces during exercise, compounded by perspiration, can separate the layers of the epidermis and lead to friction blisters, which are often quite painful and debilitating. New or poorly fitted footwear is a frequent culprit.

Management

Properly fitting shoes and socks worn without folds and creases, as well as frequent sock changes in order to avoid moisture accumulation, are cornerstones of blister prevention. Socks made of synthetic materials (e.g., acrylic) may help to collect moisture and keep it away from the skin. Antiperspirant agents containing aluminum chloride applied to the bottom of the feet before athletic activity may be effective in reducing foot blisters. In a double-blind trial in which military cadets applied either an antiperspirant containing 20% aluminum chloride or a placebo to their feet for at least 3 nights before a long hike, the rate of foot blisters in the group using the antiperspirant was only 21%, compared with 48% in the placebo group ($p < 0.01$). However, the cadets who used the antiperspirant were also significantly more likely to experience foot irritation (57% vs. 6%, $p < 0.01$). Toe padding may also prevent blistering. Once blisters form, it is generally recommended that small ones (diameter < 1 cm) be left intact and large ones drained using an aseptic technique. The blister roofs should be left in place as a protective covering in order to accelerate healing. Moleskin tape, which is available over the counter, can be used in the form of a "blister doughnut" that is applied over the area.

63.3 PLANTAR WARTS—VERRUCAS

Warts are viral tumors caused by the *Human papillomavirus* (HPV) of which at least 70 or more subtypes have been defined. Plantar warts (verrucas) may be single or multiple inwardly growing "myrmecia" on the sole of the foot. They have a hard crusty surface, are usually tender, and are painful when squeezed. Multiple clusters of mosaic warts may arise on the sole of the foot and can be spread by direct contact or autoinoculation. The presence of multiple warts may, occasionally, indicate that that the patient has an immunosuppression disorder.

Treatment

There is no quick and easy treatment for foot warts, so there is not a lot the event physician can offer there and then. Applying pressure pads may relieve the pain somewhat during competition and is worth trying if the athlete has a lot of pain; similarly, the application of Xylocaine cream may have some limited effect but is messy, and bandages do not sit very well. Injecting the sites with anesthetic is not recommended (I have never done this) as the injection is extremely painful and there is a risk of spreading the viral infection deeper into the foot. Occlusion treatment is rarely effective in adult patients. The use of chemicals may be indicated but is a time consuming and not always very effective form of therapy. So-called wart paints may contain salicylic acid or cytotoxic agents such as Podophyllin. Do not use Podophyllin on pregnant women.

Cryotherapy can be helpful but is not usually readily available at a sports event. Patients often experience pain and tenderness after treatment, so therapy before an event does not usually facilitate participation. Scraping down the wart and then covering with duct tape may alleviate the pressure somewhat, but again, it is difficult to predict the effect of therapy.

One can conclude by saying that if an athlete presents with a verruca, there is not a lot the EP can do there and then (Figs. 63.1–63.2).

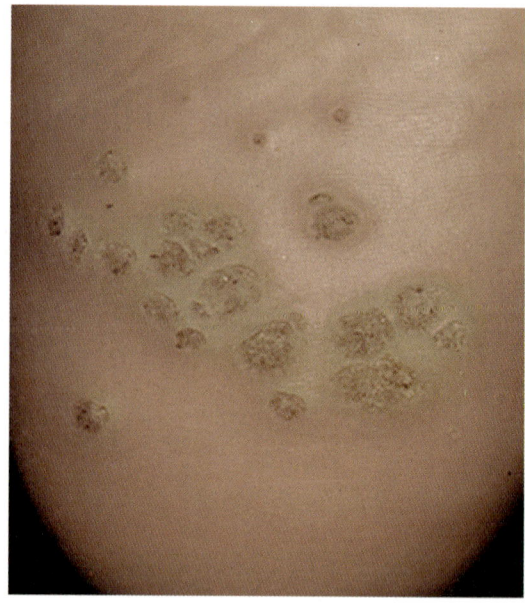

FIGURE 63.2. Plantar warts.

63.4 TINEA PEDIS

Tinea pedis is caused by a dermatophyte fungal infection, most frequently *Trichophyton rubrum*, *T. interdigitale*, or *Epidermophyton floccosum*.

These dermatophytes usually present in the warm sweaty areas of the feet and the groin (tinea cruris) and are most commonly seen in young adult male athletes. Fungal spores can survive for months or years in showers, changing rooms, and swimming pools. Walking barefoot in these areas or towel sharing is not recommended. Similarly, athletes who sweat profusely or wear tight occlusive footwear, or those who wear the same socks or shoes for long periods are more likely to get infected.

Tinea pedis can present in many forms, among others:

- Athlete's foot, where there is often soggy scaling and irritable skin between the toes, often the fourth and fifth toes

- Blister clusters on the sides of the feet or insteps

- Moccasin feet, where there is extensive dry hyperkeratotic skin changes on the sole of the foot

- Chronic patchy dry scaling hyperkeratotic lesions on the sole of the foot

The diagnosis of tinea pedis should be confirmed by scraping off a skin sample and sending it to microscopy and skin culture. Treatment is usually based on a combination of correcting the predisposing factors and by the topical application of antifungal creams, often for several weeks.

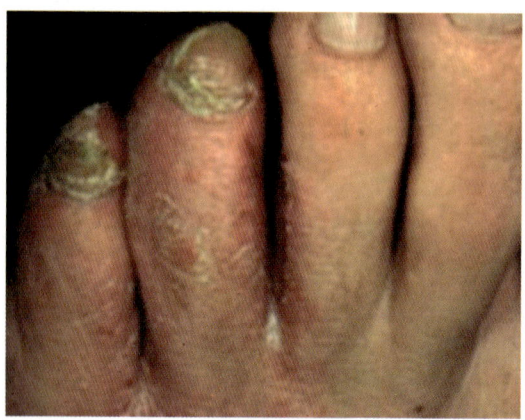

FIGURE 63.1. Athlete's foot.

Failure to respond may be due to incorrect diagnosis (psoriasis or dermatitis), fungal resistance, incorrect choice of antifungal cream, reinfection from other parts of the body, or reexposure from other family/team members.

63.5 CALLUSES AND CORNS

Calluses and corns are areas of thickened skin most often found on the feet or hands. Calluses are localized areas of painless thickened skin. Corns, or clavi, may be dry or damp, may be inflamed, and are usually painful. Both are caused by repetitive microtraumas to the skin, resulting in an increase in keratinocytes. Both may present in any sport that involves running or holding a bat or racquet. Calluses are usually not a problem for the EP, but corns may become debilitating for runners. I usually try to shave the corn with a rounded #15 blade, carefully cutting/scraping away the thickened skin until the skin becomes pink. Do not try to cut into pink tissue as this almost always ends up in a cut, which is painful and usually prevents running. Sometimes the clavus has a darkened area at the tip of the cone. Some practitioners use a file, but I find a blade to be better. Do not use a straight #11 blade as these seem to cause more small cuts. Once removed, the affected areas should be padded or toes separated using a soft material. Correctly sized protective gloves or shoes should be utilized. For special cases, individualized orthotics may be made (Fig. 63.3).

63.6 INGROWN TOENAILS

Many teenagers and young men, and hence athletes, have problems with ingrowing toenails. This condition usually affects the big toe but not exclusively so. The condition is believed to be caused by repetitive pressure or trauma to the periungual skin (soccer players kicking a ball), tight shoes and boots, profuse foot sweating, and, possibly, poor foot hygiene. There may well be a genetic component as some nails appear to be broader than the underlying nail bed.

The condition arises when the periungual skin is perforated by the nail plate and results in an inflammatory and infectious process at the trauma site. In the early phase, there may be slight swelling of the nail folds, but as the process continues, the inflammation becomes chronic due to a combination of friction, compression, infection, and scarring. Hypertrophic tissue grows at the point of contact between the nail and periungual skin; this tissue appears to have poor vascularization, which may explain the frequency of infection and the poor effect of oral antibiotics. Unfortunate patients can become infected with *Staphylococcus aureus* bacteria and develop chronic, difficult-to-treat infections. When these changes have become chronic, they will not, in my experience, improve unless the nail and the hypertrophic tissue are removed.

If an athlete presents with an ugly, purulent, swollen, red, painful toe, immediate palliative treatment is seldom possible. These patients need surgery—usually a combination of partial nail avulsion, removal of hypertrophic tissue, and partial nail matrix excision or phenolization. For milder cases, a partial nail avulsion and the use of steroid creams can occasionally allow an athlete to participate in sport the next day, but this is only a stopgap solution to be used only in extreme circumstances. In mild cases, warm soapy foot baths may help against a moderate edema with slightly infected skin. As mentioned earlier, oral antibiotics are often a waste of time.

Recommended Reading

Clayton YM. Clinical and mycological diagnostic aspects of onychomycoses and dermatomycoses. *Clin Exp Dermatol.* 1992;17(Suppl 1):37–40.

Focht DR 3rd, Spicer C, Fairchok MP. The efficacy of duct tape vs cryotherapy in the treatment of verruca vulgaris (the common wart). *Arch Pediatr Adolesc Med.* 2002;156(10):971–974.

Knapik JJ, Reynolds K, Barson J. Influence of an antiperspirant on foot blister incidence during cross-country hiking. *J Am Acad Dermatol.* 1998;39(2 Pt 1):202–206.

Knapik JJ, Reynolds K, Barson J. Risk factors for foot blisters during road marching: tobacco use, ethnicity, foot type, previous illness, and other factors. *Mil Med.* 1999;164(2):92–97.

van Brederode RL, Engel ED. Combined cryotherapy/70% salicylic acid treatment for plantar verrucae. *J Foot Ankle Surg.* 2001;40(1):36–41.

Zuber TJ. Ingrown toenail removal. *Am Fam Physician.* 2002;65(12):2547–2552, 2554.

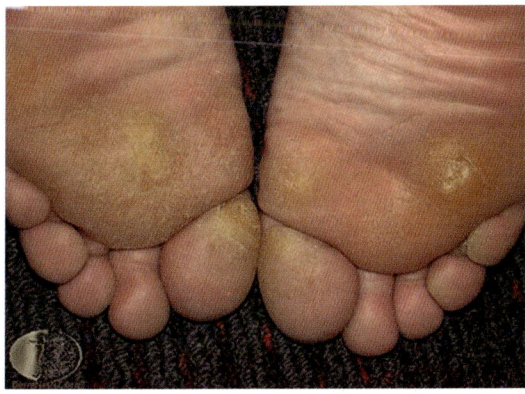

FIGURE 63.3. Calluses.

CHAPTER 64

Dermatological Infections

Contributed by David McDonagh, Secretary, AIBA Medical Commission

Reviewer: Kristin Ryggen, Dermatology Department, St. Olavs University Hospital, Trondheim, Norway

This chapter is not meant to be an atlas of dermatology, just a short overview of common skin infections that can be seen at a sports event.

One of the commonest sporting conditions is that of an infected wound, usually a couple of days after a cut, scrape, or scratch. As a rule, if the infection appears superficial, then it is probably due to a *Streptococcus* infection. Deep infections, involving the full dermis and subdermis, are often caused by staphylococci, many of which are penicillin resistant. Many sores are a mixture of both, but do not forget herpes simplex or *Borrelia* infections.

64.1 STREPTOCOCCAL INFECTIONS

Streptococcus pyogenes (group A) is the commonest pathogen in humans and in adults may present as a pharyngitis (strep throat) or cellulitis. On occasions, streptococci can be more invasive and toxigenic and can cause life-threatening conditions such as necrotizing cellulitis/fasciitis/myositis and streptococcal toxic shock syndrome. Immune-mediated poststreptococcal infection sequelae may occasionally occur, such as acute rheumatic fever and acute glomerulonephritis.

In children, streptococci may also present as scarlet fever or impetigo, though these conditions are rarely seen at a sports event, due to the age of the infants and the unlikelihood of parents allowing children to participate when ill.

Strep Throat

Strep throat is caused by group A *Streptococcus* bacteria and is the most common bacterial infection of the throat and is spread by droplets or secretions between athletes living in close contact with each other. Symptoms usually have their debut 2 to 5 days after exposure and usually begin with a fever and sore throat with varying degrees of malaise, nausea, loss of appetite, difficulty swallowing, headache, muscle and joint stiffness, etc. On examination, there may be redness of the throat, white patches on the tonsils or pharynx, and tender or swollen neck lymph nodes. A throat swab can be taken, but again time limitations make this an unlikely procedure for an event physician. Rapid immunoassay tests are quicker but false negatives do occur in up to 10% of cases depending on the kit being used. False positives are rare. Most sore throats (viral) get better on their own, but strep throats should be treated with antibiotics—penicillin is still very effective. Ibuprofen may alleviate symptoms somewhat, as well as gargling with salt water (5 mL of salt in 1 L of warm water) before an event. Avoid swallowing this water.

Streptococcal Skin Infections

As a rule, these are mostly superficial infections of sores; however, they may have a surrounding cellulitis or erysipelas. Clean the sore with tap water (unless contaminated; if so, use salt water), and rub away surface bacteria and foreign bodies. If the sore looks infected, it is common to start oral antibiotic treatment. It is not usual to take a bacterial culture. If there is surrounding cellulitis, often a darker color nearer the wound and lighter in the periphery, mark these areas with a pen and write the time and date on the border (e.g., "2300, 07/07"). This may appear overexaggerated but can be a very useful indicator as to how fast the infection is spreading. In my part of the world, northern Europe, this clinical picture usually responds to oral penicillin (660 mg × 4, or 1 g × 4 if very red or covering a larger area). Lymphangitis is not uncommon and seldom serious; sepsis is not common despite its high incidence in old wives' tales.

Cellulitis

Cellulitis is a spreading bacterial infection of the skin and the tissues immediately beneath the skin. Cellulitis may be caused by many different bacteria but streptococcal infections are commonest. Staphylococci can also cause cellulitis, especially after bites by humans or animals or in "dirty" environments. Cellulitis can also occur in skin that is not visibly injured.

Clinical Findings: Cellulitis most commonly develops on the legs and arms. The initial findings are of redness, swelling, pain, and tenderness over the affected area, which will also be warm on palpation. The borders of the affected area are usually less distinct than those found in erysipelas. Some patients have only mild symptoms but others may complain of fever and chills. There may be an associated local lymphadenitis and lymphangitis, which may even lead to bacteremia, though this is rare in healthy athletes. In athletes, mild cases may be treated by oral antibiotics such as penicillin; however, some physicians choose cephalexin, which is usually effective against both streptococci and staphylococci. Symptoms of cellulitis usually disappear after a few days of antibiotic therapy but often get worse before the antibiotics take effect. Antibiotics should be continued for 7 to 10 days, and a final check should be made by the athlete's physician before discontinuing treatment.

Erysipelas

Less common than cellulitis, it usually presents with a red, swollen, raised, warm, hardened, and painful rash (often described as having the same consistency as an orange peel). Nearby lymph nodes may be swollen and lymphangitis may be present. Lymph nodes may be swollen, and lymphedema may occur. An erysipelas lesion can be distinguished from cellulitis as it usually has sharper and more rapidly advancing borders. The borders do not blend as much into the nearby normal skin as seen in cellulitis. Lesions tend to occur in the extremities but may also affect the face around the eyes, ears, and cheeks. Raised antistreptolysin O titer levels occur only after 7 to 10 days, so this is of little use for the event physician. Patients may also have high fever, chills, fatigue, malaise, headaches, vomiting, and general illness within 48 hours of the initial infection.

Oral antibiotics, such as penicillin, are usually effective, but must be taken for several weeks and not the usual 7-day treatment. For severe infections, with bullae or extensive lesions, intravenous penicillin is needed.

Lymphangitis is inflammation of one or more lymphatic vessels, usually caused by a streptococcal infection from a wound or scrape in an arm or a leg. Often, there is peripheral cellulitis followed by bacterial spreading to the lymph vessels producing red, warm, tender stripes from the infected area toward the axilla or groin. Lymph nodes in the groin or axilla may become enlarged and feel tender. There may be associated fever, chills, tachycardia, even headache, malaise, and drowsiness. Sepsis can occur. Oral penicillin is usually effective.

Lymphadenitis almost always results from an infection in the skin, ear, nose, or throat but can also occur in infectious mononucleosis, cytomegalovirus infection, streptococcal infection, tuberculosis, or even syphilis. Lymph node affectation may be local or spread. Infected lymph nodes enlarge and are usually tender and painful. The patient may have a fever. Enlarged lymph nodes that are not red, painful, and tender may indicate other serious disorders (e.g., lymphoma or tuberculosis).

Treatment depends on the infecting organism. Oral antibiotics are usually sufficient for bacterial infections. Once the infection has been treated, lymph nodes usually return slowly to their normal size. They may remain enlarged for a period, but tenderness usually disappears within a week. Peritonsillar abscesses will not improve with antibiotics and need to be drained.

Necrotizing skin infections, including both necrotizing cellulitis and necrotizing fasciitis, are severe and dramatic forms of cellulitis that result in tissue necrosis. Some necrotizing skin infections spread on the outer layers of skin only and are termed necrotizing cellulitis. Other infections also spread inward through the layer of fat to muscle fascia and along the surface of the fascia. Most studies would imply a polymicrobial cause, though infection with a single pathogen is reported in about 15% of cases. *Streptococcus* is the most common causative organism, in particular the toxic shock strains of group A β-hemolytic streptococci.

A whole array of other bacteria have been found in these necrotic lesions, though it is uncertain if these bacteria are causal or opportunistic. They include gram-positive and gram-negative aerobic bacteria, anaerobic bacteria (including the *Clostridium* species), fungi, and other species.

Some necrotizing skin infections begin at puncture wounds or lacerations, particularly if these are "dirty" wounds. Some infections begin postsurgically; some bacteria may escape from the intestine and spread to the skin.

Clinical Findings

These are usually defined as being early or late. I have only seen two cases in my almost 30 years as an MD. Both had similar clinical presentations; none presented in a sporting environment. Both were almost sent home by the triage nurse at the emergency department, as the patients complained of great pain in insignificant wounds—the first, a wasp bite; the second, a tiny scratch. In both cases, the clinical findings were almost minimal. Both complained of uncharacteristic pain. This type of patient can easily be ignored, initially. The first patient had a wasp bite with no visible wound, just redness and swelling at the bite site. In the space of 30 minutes, his pain increased and he had developed an 8-mm-diameter ulcer in the skin.

Early findings are very nonspecific, and these include pain, cellulitis, swelling, fever, and later, tachycardia, sore induration, and numbness around the sore. Later findings are severe pain, skin discoloration (purple or black), blistering, hemorrhagic bullae, crepitus (gas), open sores, discharge, severe sepsis or systemic inflammatory response syndrome, and multiorgan failure.

Symptoms often begin as with cellulitis.

Treatment

Once suspected, immediate transfer to a hospital is advised and early IV antibiotics should be administered, even if this disturbs later blood culture results.

64.2 STAPHYLOCOCCAL SKIN INFECTIONS

A common cause of dermatological infections, staphylococci can be divided into two groups:

- *Albans*—usually not a problem, but can cause infections
- *Aureus*—even if present, they are not always the cause of an infection. A survey of cuts in our

department showed that of 100 "contaminated wounds" (i.e., cuts and scrapes), 45 patients had *Staphylococcus aureus* present in their wounds, but of these, only 40% developed an inflammation/infection.

Staphylococcus infections seem to be commoner in health personnel and in health workers with paronychias. Some people have *Staphylococcus* bacteria colonization of the nose without being symptomatic and are considered nasal carriers. On occasion, these nasal bacteria may cause repeated infection in the patient and can be a source of contagion.

Clinical Findings

As a rule, staphylococcal infections begin as superficial infections (often in inflamed tissue after trauma, insect bite, irritated hair follicle, itchy skin) with cellulitis, but may spread downward into the skin and subdermis as opposed to the classical streptococcal pattern. There are many clinical varieties of staphylococcus infections including furuncles, carbuncles, and abscesses. People with HIV or AIDS or other immune disorders are more at risk of infection.

Hidradenitis suppurativa is an inflammation and blocking of the apocrine sweat glands in the axillary, pubic, perianal, and genital areas. They may also occur under the breasts and result in painful accumulations of pus under the skin. For mild cases, oral tetracyclines may be attempted, though there is a strong risk of reinflammation. An antibiotic prescription is about as much as an EP can offer. Severe cases often need surgery.

Folliculitis is an infection of a hair follicle, often caused by *S. aureus* bacteria. They may be superficial or deep and may develop into abscesses. They are usually painful and the athlete seldom has any other illness symptoms. Squeezing these lesions is not recommended. Most cases are one-off events; however, if these lesions are multiple, recurring, or extremely painful, then treatment, as for impetigo (below), is indicated.

"Hot-tub folliculitis" is a specific type of folliculitis that can begin anytime 6 hours to 5 days after bathing in unclean or poorly chlorinated water. It occurs mostly in the torso and buttocks and is caused by the bacterium *Pseudomonas aeruginosa*. The condition usually goes away after a week without any treatment. Adequate chlorination of the tub is necessary to prevent further recurrences.

Furuncles are abscesses that involve a hair follicle and the surrounding tissue. They are usually small and relatively superficial (Fig. 64.1).

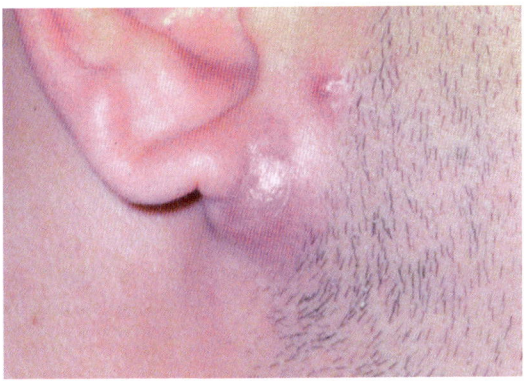

FIGURE 64.1. Furuncle. (Reprinted from Berg D, Worzala K. *Atlas of Adult Physical Diagnosis*. Philadelphia, PA: Lippincott Williams & Wilkins; 2006, with permission.)

Carbuncles are multiple furuncles that are connected to each other below the skin surface. Furuncles and carbuncles should not be incised locally; they often require surgery and antibiotics (often IV) such as Diclocil for several weeks (Fig. 64.2).

Impetigo is a skin infection usually caused by *S. aureus*, *Streptococcus pyogenes*, or both, characterized by the formation of scabs, often yellow-crusted, and, sometimes, small blisters filled with yellow fluid. It is usually a disease of childhood and is not commonly seen in sport. It commonly affects the face, arms, and legs and is more itchy than painful and may cause extensive scratching. It is a very contagious condition, particularly in children. The infected area should be washed gently with soap and water, or with other antimicrobial agents such as dibromopropamidine isethionate (Brulidine) several times daily. If large areas are involved or the

athlete appears ill, antibiotics should be considered. People who are nasal carriers are treated with topical antibiotics applied to the nasal passages.

Staphylococcal scalded skin syndrome (SSSS) is a rare infection in which a superficial skin infection deteriorates dramatically due to staphylococci toxin release. This is usually pediatric condition, in children under 5 years of age, with fever, pain, and erythema that spreads quickly and is associated with epidermal scaling (Nikolsky's sign), looking almost like second degree skin burns. Pain is usually the dominant symptom. Outbursts of toxic staphylococcal infections have also occurred in female athletes using tampons.

Methicillin-resistant Staphylococcus aureus *(MRSA)* is, per definition, resistant to the antibacterial activity of methicillin and other related penicillins. Most strains of *S. aureus* are ß-lactamase producing and thus degrade penicillin. Methicillin was developed in the 1960s and was not degraded by ß-lactamase—initially. Methicillin was later replaced by better antibiotics, such as flucloxacillin; however, certain strains of *S. aureus* emerged that were resistant to these newer antibiotics. These new strains were called MRSA.

Fortunately, other antibiotics can still be used to treat MRSA infections, but most of these drugs must be administered intravenously and are not available in tablet form.

64.3 ABSCESSES

An abscess is a localized collection of pus surrounded by infected tissue, usually caused by superficial bacteria that spread downward into subcutaneous tissue and other structures.

Causes

- Organisms infiltrate through the skin, usually via a penetrating wound or sore
- There may be tissue contamination from nearby infected tissue
- Dissemination via lymphatic or blood-borne transport from distant sites
- Migration of normal flora into a sterile area

Predisposing Factors

- Reduced immune response
- Diabetes

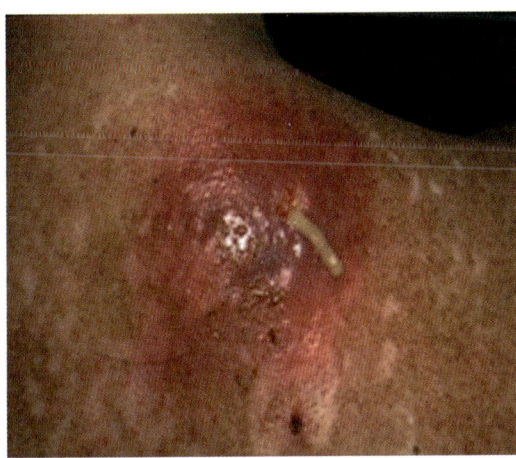

FIGURE 64.2. Carbuncle.

- Foreign bodies
- Obstruction of normal organ drainage
- Tissue ischemia
- Tissue necrosis
- Fluid collection in tissue—hematoma, transudate, injected substances

Pathogenesis

- Cellulitis
- Leukocyte invasion
- Increase in size due to pus invasion or pressure necrosis

Children

If there is a history of recurrent abscesses, or abscess complications—such as bacteremia or sepsis, then one must always suspect underlying pathology such as immune suppression, neutropenia, leukocytopenia, chronic granulomatoses, etc.

Clinical Findings

- Tender, painful, red, warm swelling, with or without an elevated pustule
- Sick patient often with high fever
- If the abscess is mature but has no central pustule, you may find that the skin over the top of the abscess is flaccid, lifeless, and easy to rupture, even on palpation

Complications

- Bacteremia
- Rupture into other structures
- Bleeding
- Reduced organ function
- Anorexia
- Osteomyelitis
- Lung abscess

Common Abscesses Seen in Sport and the General Population

- Fingers and toes—paronychia
- Sacral abscesses
- Back of the neck
- Groin region—hidrosadenitis

Common Pitfalls

- Breast abscesses should be referred to a hospital due to the pain involved in drainage
- Abscesses with a diameter of more than 4 cm (this figure varies around the world) should be referred to a hospital
- Never empty an abscess if there are multiple tops; there is usually no central pus reservoir
- Beware of furuncles and carbuncles—even if these lesions have silly names and sound like Tolkien Shire dwellers, they are often serious and painful conditions and should not be incised by inexperienced hands. Refer these lesions to a hospital

Treatment

Spontaneous rupture is a pretty safe way of avoiding an incision; the problem is that the patient will have more pain, may have more fever, and be more ill. Failure to incise may cause the abscess to spread. While abscesses normally take 3 to 5 days to mature, some may rupture spontaneously before the athlete returns for surgical drainage. *C'est la vie*, but it can be a bit messy.

Antibiotics may help prevent a deep staphylococcus infection from becoming an abscess.

Antibiotics can also help the abscess maturation in the lead-up to an incision.

Surgical technique is important. It is all about knowing which lesions to incise; timing (making an incision at the right time in abscess maturation); where to make your incision; not damaging healthy or inflamed tissue and following Langer's lines if possible; making a big enough and deep enough incision; removing dead tissue and all the pus and avoid leaving pockets. Make one clean incision if you can.

Beware

Beware so-called tracking abscesses, abscesses that have fistulated from a deep source, or abscesses that are not primarily cutaneous or subcutaneous (e.g., thenar abscesses): Drainage is often not enough; the palm has often to be surgically opened and debrided. Beware perianal abscesses; they may indicate intra-abdominal pathology.

Abscess Anesthesia

Topical numbing/freezing anesthetic spray—my favorite for superficial abscesses—works quickly and lasts just a few seconds, giving just enough time to make the incision but often helps little against the pain caused by squeezing out the pus.

Single nerve-block anesthesia can be effective, but you have to wait 10 to 15 minutes for the anesthetic to take effect.

Local anesthesia is to be avoided as a rule (unless you have no other options), mostly due to the fact that it is extremely painful, it does not work very well, and you may inadvertently puncture the abscess making it difficult to make a clean incision.

Advice

- Never lean over an abscess while making an incision: You may get the pus straight in your face or eyes.

- Use a face mask to protect your face and maybe reduce the smell.

- If the smell is overbearing or sickening, dip two cotton buds in salt water, stick one up each of your nostrils and then put on a face mask. You may sound a little nasal, but it is better than vomiting.

- Have plenty of clean paper towels to squeeze and absorb the pus.

- If you cannot get any pus out, your incision may have been too superficial, the incision may have been misdirected, you may have incised too early, there may be deeper pockets of pus, or your diagnosis was wrong.

- When finishing up, place a drain in the wound crater, preferably in the distal, caudal (nearest the ground) end, so that pus can flow by gravitational forces along the drain out of the wound into an absorbing bandage. Do not pack the wound crater with bandages, either initially after incision or while applying new dressings. If the wound opening is packed with dressings, then pus will not drain away and wound healing will be delayed.

- Bandages and drains should be changed at least daily the first 2 to 3 days. Most skin abscesses dry out after 2–to 3 days and the drain will simply fall out as the wound crater diminishes.

64.4 BORRELIA

According to the European Union Concerted Action on Lyme Borreliosis (EUCALB, http://meduni09.edis.at/eucalb/cms/index.php?option=com_content&task=view&id=15&Itemid=38) up to 60% of patients with early localized Lyme borreliosis may present with an erythema migrans (EM), which usually erupts within 2 to 30 days after a tick bite. The lesion can vary in both size (up to 30 in.—75 cm in diameter) and color (faint or pink/red) and typically "clears from the central area." The patient may also have flu-like symptoms such as fever, fatigue, myalgia, arthralgia, headache, or a stiff neck. These symptoms can vary from continent to continent, country to country. The dermatological lesion is usually self-limiting and will resolve without treatment, but most experts recommend the administration of antibiotics to prevent possible disease progression (penicillin, tetracyclines, cephalosporins, etc.—the choice varies in different countries).

It is beyond the scope of this manual to go into any more detail, but the EP should be aware of the classical EM presentation and suspicion should be alerted if the patient presents with the classical bull's-eye lesion, especially if the patient has come from an endemic area populated by larger animals such as deer, sheep, cows, or horses. Not all patients know, or remember, if they have been bitten by a tick (Fig. 64.3).

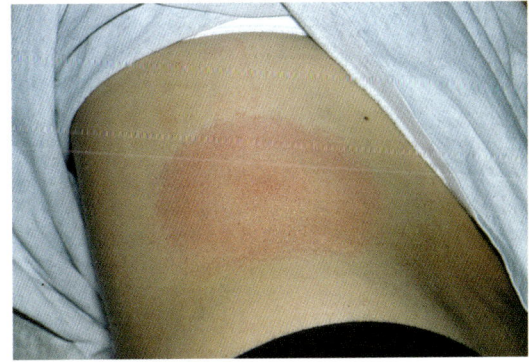

FIGURE 64.3. Erythema migrans. (Reprinted from Goodheart HP. *Goodheart's Photoguide of Common Skin Disorders.* 2nd ed. Philadelphia, PA: Lippincott Williams & Wilkins; 2003, with permission.)

64.5 SPORTS-INDUCED ACNE (ACNE MECHANICA)

This lesion looks similar to acne vulgaris; however, it usually occurs in areas covered by protective gear in contact sports. American football players, rugby and ice hockey players, and equestrian riders can have follicular papules pustules, and nodules where the skin comes in contact with helmet strap on the forehead, around the ears, or under the chin. Caddies may experience acne mechanica over their golf-bag–carrying shoulder. Allergic contact dermatitis caused by substances found in sports equipment (e.g., rubber chemicals such as thiurams, mercaptobenzothiazole, and carbamates) needs to be considered in the differential diagnosis of acne mechanica. The former appears more eczematous and pruritic and can be confirmed by specialized patch testing.

Treatment

Try to remove (alleviate) the cause of irritation and treat with tetracycline antibiotics or benzoyl peroxide creams.

64.6 VIRAL SKIN INFECTIONS

There are three viral skin conditions common in sport: verrucas, molluscum contagiosum, and herpes simplex.

Warts are known to be transmitted by direct contact, particularly in showers and changing rooms. Swimmers seem to be particularly susceptible to plantar verruca. The use of sandals while showering may limit transmission. Painful warts can be difficult to treat and often an event physician has little to offer athletes with plantar warts other than padding and support. One can cut away some of the wart in an emergency situation, but this does not usually help.

Molluscum contagiosum can also be transferred by contact, in particular wrestling. The lesions are typical discrete, "pearl-like," skin-colored papules and can be removed surgically. One should exercise care with early surgery as this may lead to scarring in young athletes. However, wrestlers may demand removal as multiple mollusca may result in the athlete failing a skin inspection by a referee.

Herpes simplex infections have been extensively documented in wrestlers and judo and have been given the name herpes gladiatorum (Fig. 64.4),

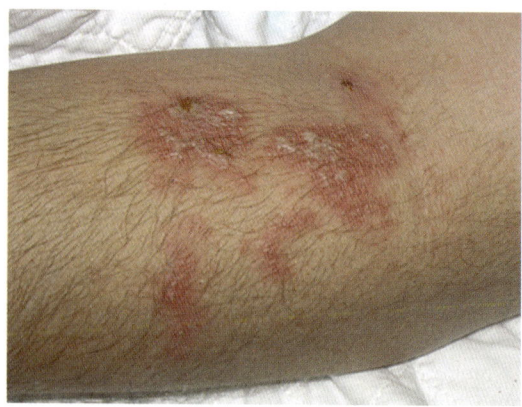

FIGURE 64.4. Herpes gladiatorum.

but are also seen in rugby. An extremely aggressive variant of type 1 virus, BgK1, is prevalent amongst Sumo wrestlers in Japan where even deaths have been reported due to systemic complications. Clinically, lesions present as vesicles on an erythematous plaque. Vesicle rupture may result in erosions. Transmission is primarily through skin-to-skin contact, so infected wrestlers should be promptly removed from competing to inhibit involuntary spreading of the virus. Oral antiviral tablets need some days to work, so early detection is important if an athlete is to compete. In my experience, antiviral creams do not seem to help very much on skin lesions, though they do seem to be effective when combined with oral antivrals when treating herpes opthalmicus.

64.7 FUNGAL SKIN INFECTIONS

The event physician may be asked to treat tinea cruris fungal groin infections. These are usually caused by anthropophilic dermatophytes, in particular *Epidermophyton floccosum* and *Trichophyton rubrum*. The condition is more common in men than in women and is contagious, often being spread by sharing damp towels or by direct contact. Good general hygiene is important in prevention and daily washing, though not scrubbing, is recommended. Athletes should avoid wearing wet or dirty clothing that have not been washed since the last training session. It is quite common for athletes with groin infections to have "athlete's foot" as well.

It is important to treat both the toes and the groin, as all body foci must be treated to prevent future relapse.

These lesions are usually easily recognizable for a sports physician. They present as a large, scaly,

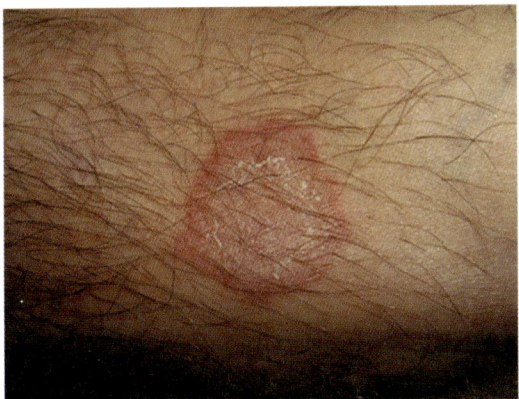

Recommended Reading

Abraham N, Double M, Carson P. Open versus closed surgical treatment of abscesses: a controlled clinical trial. *Aust N Z J Surg.* 1997;67(4):173–176.

Ban F, Asano S, Ozawa S, et al. Analysis of herpes simplex virus type 1 restriction fragment length polymorphism variants associated with herpes gladiatorum and Kaposi's varicelliform eruption in sumo wrestlers. *J Gen Virol.* 2008;89(Pt 10):2410–2415.

Barnes SM, Milsom PL. Abscesses: an open and shut case. *Arch Emerg Med.* 1988;5(4):200–205.

Bergfeld WF, Taylor JS. Trauma, sports, and the skin. *Am J Ind Med.* 1985;8(4–5):403–413.

Freeman MJ, Bergfeld WF. Skin diseases of football and wrestling participants. *Cutis.* 1977;20(3):333–341.

de Tullio D, Rossi C, Bolzon S, et al. Necrotizing fasciitis: a surgical emergency. *Updates Surg.* 2010;62(2):83–87.

Simms MH, Curran F, Johnson RA, et al. Treatment of acute abscesses in the casualty department. *Br Med J Clin Res Ed.* 1985;284(6332):1827–1829.

Sorensen C, Hjortrup A, Moesgaard F, Lykkegaard-Nielsen M. Linear incision and curettage vs. deroofing and drainage in subcutaneous abscess. A randomized clinical trial. *Acta Chir Scand.* 1987;153(11–12):659–660.

Stewart MPM, Laing MR, Krukowski ZH. Treatment of acute abscesses by incision, curettage and primary suture without antibiotics: a controlled clinical trial. *Br J Surg.* 1985;72(1):66–67.

Verit A, Verit FF. FOURNIER'S gangrene: the development of a classical pathology. *BJU Int.* 2007;100(6):1218–1220.

FIGURE 64.5. Tinea gladiatorum.

red–brown patch on the groin; they may be bilateral and may spread to the scrotum. These patches tend to itch. On palpation, they often have a different consistency than normal skin.

Treatment is relatively easy: A local topical antifungal cream (e.g., clotrimazole) is usually effective. Oral treatment is seldom necessary. It is important that the athlete makes certain lifestyle changes if hygienic issues are apparent.

Tinea Gladiatorum

Tinea gladiatorum refers to the contagious fungal lesions that occur in wrestlers, *T. tonsurans* being the most prevalent. The incidence reported varies. Treatment as above (Fig. 64.5).

CHAPTER 65

HIV/AIDS and Tropical Infections

Contributed by David McDonagh and James Sekajugo, Uganda Health Ministry, Kampala, Uganda

Reviewer: Jan Kristian Damås, Infectious Diseases Department, St. Olavs Hospital, Trondheim, Norway

The majority of tropical diseases are easily preventable through enforcement of proper personal and environmental hygiene measures. However, if not avoided or prevented, they can cause serious illness, which will disrupt training programs and result in suboptimal performance.

Febrile infections adversely influence the respiratory, cardiovascular, musculoskeletal, and thermoregulatory systems with decreased mental concentration. Players with undetected infections are consequently exposed to a higher risk of injury.

Prevention of these diseases from occurring in the first place is the best approach. When they occur, the event physician is expected to be able to detect them, advise the player on his or her suitability to play, appropriately manage the infection, and take the necessary precautions to prevent spread of the infection to other members of the team. As part of case management, it may be necessary to refer the affected player to a specialized disease treatment center and to notify the disease in question to the relevant health authorities where required.

Physicians dealing with athletes from diverse regions of the world need to sufficiently acquaint themselves with the disease signs and symptoms, the incubation period, the mode of transmission, and the geographical distribution of the common tropical diseases. This information will be key to identifying the disease in question and in taking the most appropriate course of action within the short time the EP may have with the athlete before, during, or after a competition.

Athlete health care teams in disease-endemic regions should teach athletes how to initiate the first line of defense against disease by observing personal, food, water, and environmental hygiene. It is important that they limit their exposure to rodents and bloodsucking insects, which are vectors of many tropical disease pathogens. They should take vaccinations when and where they are required.

Traveling teams should seek information and expert advice on the endemic tropical diseases and recent history of epidemics at their intended destination. For example, malaria and dengue fever are known to be endemic in some parts of the world; epidemics of meningococcal meningitis, cholera, and hemorrhagic fevers are reported wherever they occur. This information will enable the team or event physician to assess the potential health risks to his entourage and to prepare to counter them. It is, for example, important to be aware of drug-resistance patterns of malaria parasites at the intended destination and to select the most effective chemoprophylactic agent to administer to the team. Necessary vaccinations should be given; advice on food and water hygiene, and vector repellents should be reinforced. The team should be reminded to carry condoms and to use them whenever necessary. The team physician should travel with sufficient medical supplies for the specific treatment of expected infections even when chemoprophylaxis has been administered to the team before travel.

The event physician should have high index of suspicion when a player presents with any of the following features:

- A positive history of travel or contact with persons from an endemic area

- Fever, flu-like symptoms

- Skin rash

- Jaundice

- Lymphadenopathy

- Muscle and joint aches and pains, which could be mistaken as exercise related and ignored

These are some of the commonest presenting features of acute tropical disease infections. Investigations should immediately be ordered to make a proper diagnosis and to administer the correct treatment. The player's participation in any sports activity should be temporarily suspended until the nature of the disease has been established and until the infection has been controlled. Remember to control team members and coaching staff due to the risk of contagion.

65.1   HIV/AIDS

HIV/AIDS deserves special mention. HIV/AIDS is now a global epidemic that has hardest hit the most important source of manpower in Africa, the 15- to 49-year age group. The vast majority of infections are found in developing countries in sub-Saharan Africa and southeast Asia. Football is widely played in these regions, which are also an important source of players for professional football clubs in the developed world. It is, therefore, important to prevent new HIV infections in the sporting populations of these regions as part of measures to limit HIV infections in the global sports population.

Confidential voluntary counseling and testing (VCT) for HIV is encouraged for all members of the football community. HIV-negative athletes should be encouraged to remain negative by observing the known HIV infection prevention methods and practices. HIV infection is not a contraindication to participation in athletic activities. HIV-positive players must however know the risk they pose to their playmates and have a responsibility to avoid getting their body fluids into contact with others. Universal precautions and proper hygiene must be observed at all times when managing football injuries during training and competition.

In the case of accidental exposure to contaminated body fluids, test for the source and exposed players for the HIV antibodies (HIVAb). There is a high risk of HIV transmission if the body fluid in question is blood, the source person is HIV positive, and the exposed person has broken skin or mucous membrane. In such a case, HIV postexposure prophylaxis with HIV PEP is recommended

within 1 to 2 hours for 4 weeks. HIV PEP should not be considered if there is no potential of HIV transmission, for example, if the body fluid in question is noninfectious (e.g., saliva, sweat). It should be noted that only a small percentage (<3%) of occupational exposures to HIV result in HIV transmission. HIV PEP has side effects and there is limited data on its efficacy. It is advisable to carefully consider the toxicity of HIV PEP against its efficacy before administering it.

65.2   MOSQUITO-BORNE ILLNESSES

There are many diseases that can be transmitted by mosquitoes, the commonest being

- Dengue

- Malaria

- Japanese encephalitis

As mentioned above, early symptoms and signs may be vague with all these diseases. The clue is to take a good history and to keep in mind that athletes today travel extensively and may be exposed to diseases not commonly found locally. Always ask the athlete if he or she has traveled recently, where he or she has traveled to, whether he or she was bitten by anything, and whether the water he or she drank was clean. It is difficult to make a diagnosis without various lab tests; however, for the EP, it is important to be suspicious and enquire about these disorders, which are often overlooked or never thought of until someone asks the question, "Have you been abroad recently?" If you suspect a "tropical" disorder, refer the athlete to a specialist.

65.3   DENGUE

Dengue is transmitted to humans by *Aedes* mosquitoes and is endemic in the tropical regions of the Caribbean, the American continents, the South Pacific, Asia, and Africa (Fig. 65.1). More than a quarter of the world's population lives in areas where dengue infections can be acquired.

The *Aedes aegypti* mosquito is often found in cities and towns and is reported to prefer biting humans in the early and late afternoon, but can feed at anytime. Mosquitoes breed in or near water, so avoid having stagnant water in flower pots, buckets, cans, etc. There may be less of a risk in clean, modern hotels than in small, private homes and villas.

There are at least four serotypes, and exposure to more serotypes may increase the likelihood of

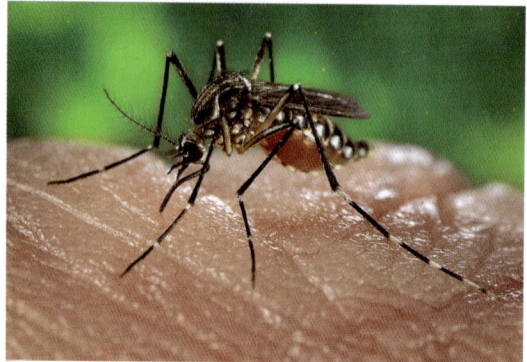

FIGURE 65.1. *Aedes* (dengue) mosquito, note the white stripes on the body. (Courtesy James Gathany.)

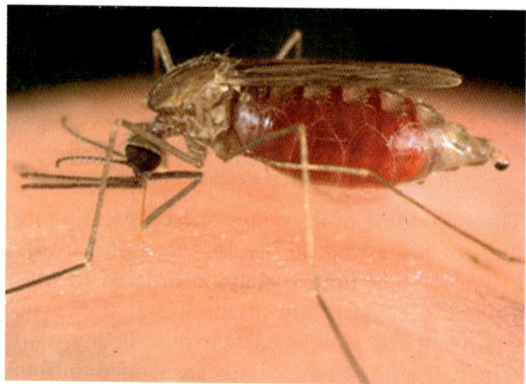

FIGURE 65.2. *Anopheles* (malaria) mosquito.

the potentially fatal dengue hemorrhagic fever (DHF). The virus has an incubation period of 3 to 14 days (or 4 to 7 days) in the majority of cases. The virus infection can be asymptomatic or cause illnesses ranging from mild fever to severe disease, including DHF with

- Fever
- Increased vascular permeability leading to hemorrhage with
- Raised hematocrit (20% over baseline values)
- Thrombocytopenia (<100,000 platelets/μL)
- Abdominal or pleural effusions
- Hypoproteinemia

Approximately 1% of dengue patients develop DHF. The patient often presents with fever, which usually resolves after 3 to 5 days. Patients may then develop increased vascular permeability leading to seepage into the pleural and abdominal cavities, hematuria, and hematemesis. Dengue shock syndrome can also occur with circulatory failure and has a reported fatality of 10%. Previous dengue infection may increase the risk of DHF.

Patients should rest and drink plenty of water initially and should avoid aspirin. Acetylsalicylic acid and other NSAIDs are often contraindicated due to their anticoagulant properties. Patients with acute dengue must be monitored for signs of DHF, so consider admission to a hospital, as early fluid therapy appears to reduce morbidity and mortality. Obviously, patients must be admitted if they develop abdominal or chest pain, prolonged vomiting, or altered mental status.

It is also possible for a player to have debut symptoms of malaria at a football event (e.g., if he or she has been at a precamp before the event).

65.4 MALARIA

Another mosquito-borne disease, this time carried by the *Anopheles* mosquito (Fig. 65.2), can inject one of four malaria parasites into humans, *Plasmodium vivax*, *P. ovale*, *P. malariae*, or *P. falciparum*. A fifth parasite, *P. knowlesi*, can also infect humans though it primarily affects other primates. Parasites enter red blood cells and multiply, finally causing the cell to rupture, with release of new parasites that enter new red blood cells. This can eventually lead to anemia. Some species, notably *P. falciparum*, invade liver cells, grow, and multiply, finally causing the hepatocyte to rupture with release of daughter parasite cells into the blood stream.

The *Anopheles* mosquito, and therefore the malaria disease, is most virulent in Africa—from the sub-Saharan countries in the north to the South African border in the south. Malaria is also found in Asia, roughly forming an isosceles triangle from Hanoi in the north to Indonesia in the south, all through southeastern Asia over to Damascus. In South America, basically the whole continent north of Rio de Janeiro, with the exception of the northeastern Brazilian coast as well as the northern Andes, are potential malaria areas. This belt spreads north into Central America and the eastern coast of Mexico.

Diagnosis of malaria can be difficult, due to its often diffuse presentation but also due to the fact that medical facilities may be somewhat limited in some of the countries where the disease is prevalent.

Early clinical presentation may include

- Fever
- Chills
- Sweating
- Headache

- Muscle pain
- Nausea and vomiting
- Fatigue
- Elevated temperature

A more severe form of malaria (caused by *P. falciparum*) may present with the following findings:

- Altered mental status
- Coma
- Neurological focal signs
- Severe anemia
- Dyspnea

The initial clinical presentation may be vague and varied, so diagnosis is confirmed by laboratory tests. These should be taken as early as possible so that treatment can be initiated. Malaria parasites can be identified in the lab by taking a blood smear, staining it (often with the Giemsa stain) and then identifying the parasites under a microscope. Rapid diagnostic tests (RDTs, immunochromatographic tests) are also available, and though these appear to be quite promising, they are not yet considered as being the "gold standard" and are mostly used as adjunct tests. A list of commercially available malaria RDTs can be found at http://www.wpro.who.int/rdt/.

65.5 JAPANESE ENCEPHALITIS

Another mosquito-borne infection, this time caused by the Japanese encephalitis flavivirus, affects the meninges and brain. It is most commonly seen in the vicinity of rice paddy fields in south and southeast Asia, particularly when these are flooded and there is an abundance of mosquitoes. The majority of infections are mild, presenting with fever and headache, but in some cases, patients can present with high fever, headache, neck stiffness, altered intellectual function, coma, seizures, and paralysis. To confirm the diagnosis, further lab tests need to be conducted.

Treatment is supportive.

Fortunately, an effective vaccine is available—one primary vaccination and two boosters—and these should be taken by athletes before traveling to these areas.

65.6 LEISHMANIASIS

This is a sand fly–borne infection. Leishmaniasis is found in approximately 90 countries around the world and, according to the CDC in the United

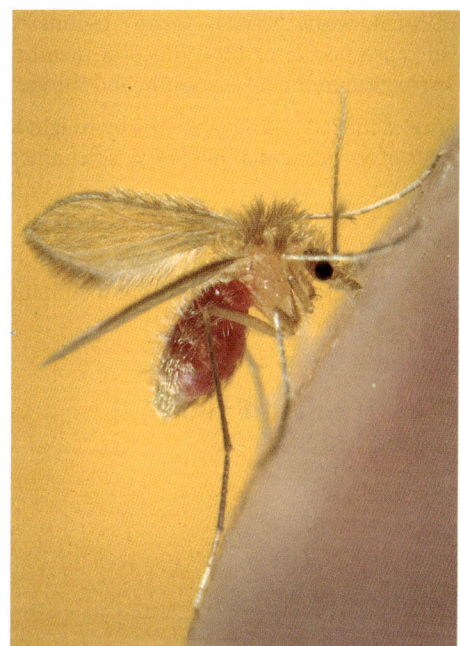

FIGURE 65.3.   Phlebotomine sand fly (leishmaniasis). (Courtesy James Gathany.)

States, over 90% of cutaneous leishmaniasis cases are found in Afghanistan, Algeria, Brazil, Iran, Iraq, Peru, Saudi Arabia, and Syria. More than 90% of visceral leishmaniasis cases occur in Bangladesh, Brazil, India, Nepal, and Sudan. Leishmaniasis is caused by the protozoa *Leishmania* and is transmitted after bites from the phlebotomine sand fly (Figs. 65.3 and 65.4).

Leishmaniasis may present with a variety of symptoms but has three classic forms:

- Cutaneous forms—produces skin ulcers on the face, arms, and legs

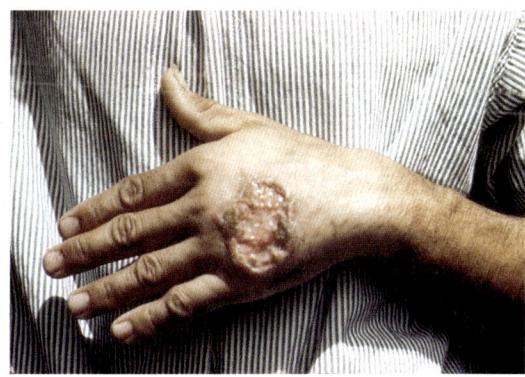

FIGURE 65.4.   Cutaneous leishmaniasis.

- Mucocutaneous forms—forms lesions that can cause partial or total mucosal membrane destruction in the nose, mouth, and throat

- Visceral forms—is characterized by weight loss, bouts of fever, anemia, and hepatosplenamegaly

Treatment

Treatment is usually with antimony-containing compounds.

65.7 WATER-BORNE TROPICAL DISEASES

These include

- Typhoid

- Hepatitis A

- Leptospirosis

65.8 TYPHOID

Food or water that has been contaminated by urine or feces containing the *Salmonella typhi* or *S. paratyphi* bacteria may cause this disorder. Recent episodes have only occurred in areas with contaminated water and poor sanitation. Shellfish from contaminated areas can also be a source of infection, as can foods contaminated by food handlers. Symptoms usually develop within 1 to 3 weeks after exposure and may be mild or severe in nature. Paratyphoid fever has similar symptoms to typhoid fever but generally runs a milder course. Symptoms may include high fever, gradually rising fever, cough, malaise, headache, constipation or diarrhea, hepatosplenomegaly,

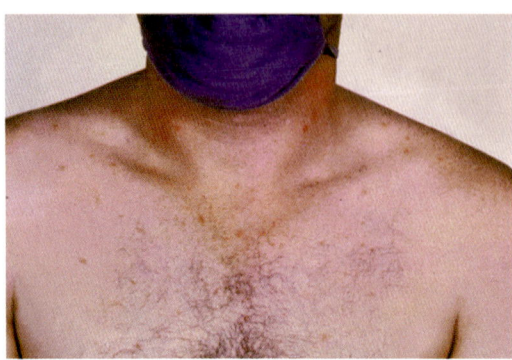

FIGURE 65.5. Rose-colored spots on the chest.

abdominal pain and tenderness, rose-colored spots on the chest, and in extreme cases, neurological focal signs, coma, renal impairment, and shock (Fig. 65.5). Later complications may develop such as myocarditis and osteomyelitis. Classically, temperature rises over 2 to 3 days, then remains elevated for another 10 to 14 days. If untreated, the patient deteriorates; diarrhea may become florid and bloody.

Patients can be contagious even after they have recovered after an infection (e.g., Typhoid Mary).

Diagnosis is based on a suspicion of contamination, clinical findings, and lab tests. These include stool and blood cultures, elevated WBC, and elevated transaminases. Widal test may be positive.

Treatment is dependant of the locality, as drug resistance is regrettably common. Chloramphenicol has been the drug of choice for many years .

65.9 HEPATITIS A

Though not necessarily a tropical disorder, it is found all over the world. Hepatitis A is most often seen in areas of inadequate and contaminated water supplies as well as in areas with poor hygiene and sanitation (Asia, Africa, Central and South America). The virus can be transmitted through the fecal contamination of water and food and again by food handlers, or fruits and vegetables washed with contaminated water.

The disease may present in a mild form with symptoms lasting only 1 or 2 weeks; however, the usual picture is of a 2- to 6-week illness. Some patients can be ill for up to 6 to 9 months.

Clinical Findings

- Abrupt onset of fever

- Malaise

- Tiredness and weakness

- Loss of appetite

- Nausea, vomiting

- Abdominal discomfort (due to hepatomegaly)

- Followed by jaundice with darkish urine

Blood tests for Hepatitis A antibody, transaminases, and electrolytes should be taken; it is normal to check for other forms of hepatitis as well. Treatment for hepatitis A is supportive. Effective hepatitis A vaccines are available.

65.10 LEPTOSPIROSIS

Leptospirosis is caused by infection with the spirally shaped bacteria *Leptospira*. Humans are usually infected when they come into contact with contaminated water (i.e., where contaminated animals have urinated in the water) usually through small skin cuts and abrasions or via the mucous membranes of the eyes, nose, and mouth. The disease is found worldwide but is more prevalent in the humid tropics. Canada and the United States have very low incidences. Statistics collection is poor in many countries and may thus give a false security when visiting certain countries. According to Pappas, the countries with the highest incidence are the Seychelles, Trinidad and Tobago, Barbados, Jamaica, Costa Rica, and Sri Lanka.

The clinical findings in the acute phase are varied and there are many presentations, from mild to severe. Mild cases can present with fever, chills, headache, myalgia, abdominal pain, vomiting, and diarrhea, whereas severe cases can present with Weil's syndrome (jaundice, renal failure, hemorrhage, and myocarditis with arrhythmias), meningitis/meningoencephalitis, or even pulmonary hemorrhage with respiratory failure.

Clinical diagnosis is difficult due to the various presentations and the ease with which a physician can suspect other prevalent disorders such as dengue and other hemorrhagic fevers. Blood tests are necessary to make a diagnosis.

65.11 TRAVELER'S DIARRHEA

Athletes may develop diarrhea when traveling, and this is usually due to exposure to water or food that has been contaminated by fecal and other bacteria, but also viruses and protozoa. As we all know, gastroenteritis can be highly "unexotic" and can also easily occur at home as well as abroad.

Symptoms usually develop 2 or 3 days after arrival, and this usually indicates a local contamination as being the cause. In locations where hygiene is good, it is more likely that the diarrhea has a viral origin rather than being due to some form of bacterial food or water poisoning—though bacteria contaminated food and water are found all over the world. Viruses may also be spread via food and water. Common signs and symptoms include

- Fever
- Nausea, vomiting
- Headache
- Frequent, sometimes painful, loose, watery, or bloody stools
- Abdominal bloating and cramping

The commonest bacterial causes are

- *E. coli* and subtypes (by far the commonest causative agents)
- *Shigella* species
- *Salmonella* species
- *Campylobacter jejuni*
- *Clostridium* species
- *Yersinia* species

When traveling, many teams bring their own food and beverages, and this may help against bacterial infections, but perishable products (which are common sources of contamination) such as raw leafy vegetables, fruits, seafood, and unpasteurized cheese are often purchased locally. Restaurants and street vendors are common sources of food poisoning. Tap water may also vary in quality around the world, and in some places it is even wise to brush teeth with bottled water and to keep the mouth closed when showering—lower the shower head to neck height. Contaminated ice cubes are also a potential risk. Protozoal diarrhea causes include *Giardia duodenalis*, *Entamoeba histolytica*, and *Cryptosporidium parvum*. Viral causes include noroviruses (including Norwalk), rotaviruses, and enteroviruses.

Escherichia coli

The WHO, in an unusually humoristic section on its website, classifies *E. coli* bacteria as the good, the bad, and the ugly. The good refers to the harmless *E. coli* gut bacteria; the bad being those *E. coli* (ETEC) that release enterotoxins and cause diarrhea and cramps; and the ugly being the potentially life-threatening enterohemorrhagic *E. coli* (EHEC) strains.

Enterohemorrhagic *Escherichia coli*: Most strains of *E. coli* are harmless; however, some strains may cause illness that progresses to a bloody diarrhea—EHEC of which the O157:H7 serotype is probably the best known. The EHEC strains produce enterotoxins called verotoxins (or Shiga-like toxins), which are similar to *Shigella dysenteriae* toxins, and can cause a hemorrhagic colitis and even a life-threatening hemolytic uremic syndrome (HUS) with acute renal failure, hemolytic anaemia, and thrombocytopenia. It appears to be more prevalent in younger teenagers and children.

Foods implicated in outbreaks include salami, hamburgers, unpasteurized dairy products, and unwashed fruits and vegetables.

Salmonella

Salmonellosis is usually contracted after ingesting contaminated meat, poultry, eggs, and milk, but also green vegetables, and can cause an enterocolitis. Athletes must avoid undercooked chicken or turkey as well as undercooked eggs. Certain pets also carry *Salmonella*, reptiles in particular. Symptoms develop quite quickly after ingestion—from around 8 to 48 hours. There are over 2,500 strains of *Salmonella* and, of these, the "egg-bug" *S. enteriditis* is one of the better known, having being responsible for tens of thousands of infections around the world. Although the strain may vary, the clinical picture is often similar and findings usually include

- Acute onset of fever
- Abdominal pain, cramps, tenderness
- Diarrhea (can contain blood if prolonged or profuse)
- Nausea and vomiting
- Myalgia

Symptoms can last for up to a week and the patient can often feel very sick. Keeping the patient hydrated is important, and it is important to replace lost electrolytes. Antibiotics are seldom indicated unless the infection is severe or systemic, and many experienced physicians believe that oral antibiotics only make the patient more ill. Diarrhea usually disappears after some days, though it may take time to restore normal bowel movements. Loperamide can be used but is often not very effective in the first 2 of 3 days, particularly if the infection is severe. Loperamide is not recommended if the patient has a fever or if the stools are bloody. The danger with these infections is that sepsis or severe dehydration may occur. Diagnosis is confirmed by stool or blood tests.

Giardia

The *Giardia* parasite can be found in feces contaminated food or water, including drinking water but also swimming pools, hot tubs, and spas. Symptoms of giardiasis usually begin 1 to 2 weeks after exposure and include nausea, vomiting, stomach discomfort and pains, flatulence, diarrhea, and reportedly greasy stools that tend to float. Symptoms may last for several weeks, though chronic cases are well known. Giardia is found all over the world but is more common in countries and areas where water is contaminated by animal feces. Laboratory diagnosis is necessary with stool analysis. Treatment includes supportive treatment and the use of medications such as metronidazole, quinacrine, and others.

Noroviruses

These infections usually occur in enclosed environments (e.g., where a group of athletes is living together) and are often very contagious. The virus may be spread through food, utensils, fluids (shared juice, milk cartons), or contaminated surfaces or objects when patients then place their hands in their mouths. Symptoms include nausea, vomiting, diarrhea, stomach cramps, fever, chills, headache, muscle aches, and tiredness. The illness usually begins suddenly and the athlete may feel sick for a couple of days. If possible, it is a good idea to isolate athletes immediately, preferably in a new location. Stool and nasopharyngeal swabs can be taken, but athletes may become sick before these results become available. Treatment is supportive.

Rotaviruses

Again, this virus spreads through person-to-person contact, contaminated objects, and airborne droplets. Symptoms usually appear approximately 2 to 3 days after infection and include fever, nausea, vomiting, abdominal pain, and diarrhea. There is no specific drug treatment. A rotavirus vaccine exists. Rehydration, as with all diarrhea disorders, is important.

Enteroviruses

This is a large group of viruses including the coxsackieviruses, echoviruses, and polioviruses. The nonpolio enteroviruses are some of the commonest viral infectious agents, probably second only to rhinoviruses. Infected patients usually present with sudden onset of fever, upper respiratory and gastrointestinal complaints, malaise, sore throat, nausea, vomiting, headache, myalgia, and diarrhea. Symptoms usually last for 3 to 7 days. The virus can be detected by taking swabs from the nasopharynx or stool. Again, hygiene procedures and isolation as well as supportive treatment are all that one can offer.

No nonpolio enterovirus vaccine is available.

Advice to the Event Physician

If possible, it is a good idea to isolate athletes immediately, preferably to a new location. Athletes should be removed from the suspected location; the location should be cleaned properly and ventilated, and strict hygiene procedures should be enforced.

Sports events are often completed before laboratory results become available and definitive medication is usually not indicated or available. The EP most offer supportive treatment and make general recommendations including cessation of eating and drinking for some hours to let the stomach settle, followed by active rehydration with water or sports drinks. A gradual return to eating with easily digestible foods is recommended when nausea and vomiting have disappeared. Avoidance of milk and dairy products, fatty food, or spicy food is recommended initially. Plenty of rest is always recommended.

Loperamide (Imodium) can be used if the diarrhea is troublesome, usually two tablets initially, followed by another tablet with each loose stool. The use of antiemetics and antipyretics can also be considered.

More severe cases should be referred to a hospital.

65.12 GEOGRAPHICAL OVERVIEW OF INFECTIOUS DISEASES

The U.S. Centers for Disease Control and Prevention (CDC) in Atlanta gives an excellent overview of the diseases one can be exposed to in different countries around the world.

For more information, look up http://wwwn.cdc.gov/travel/destinations/list.aspx.

65.13 RECOMMENDED VACCINES FOR TRAVELERS

Once again, the CDC offers excellent advice on what vaccines are recommended in various countries. For more information, see http://wwwn.cdc.gov/travel/destinations/list.aspx.

Recommended Web Sites

World Health Organization: http://www.who.int/en/
The Centers for Disease Control and Prevention (CDC): http://www.cdc.gov/

Recommended Reading

Cook GC, Zumla AI (eds.). *Manson's Tropical Diseases.* Philadelphia, PA: Saunders, 2008.

Guerrant RL, Walker DH, Weller PF. *Tropical Infectious Diseases: Principles, Pathogens & Practice* (2 Volume Set). Philadelphia, PA: Elsevier, 2005.

Mandell GL, Bennett JE, Dolin R. *Mandell, Douglas, and Bennett's Principles and Practice of Infectious Diseases* (7th Ed.). New York, NY: Churchill Livingstone, 2010.

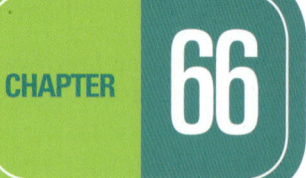

CHAPTER 66 Child and Adolescent Injuries

Contributed by Michel Binder, Member, FIG Medical Commission, France, and Michel Léglise, Vice-President, FIG; Chair, FIG Medical Commission; Coordinator, IOC Medical Commission working group Sports, Children and Adolescents, France

Reviewer: Talia Alenabi, Secretary General, Asian Federation of Sports Medicine, Tehran, Iran

There are five concepts that are essential in understanding the goals of sports medicine treatment:

- A child is in a constant state of physical and psychological growth as he or she moves toward adulthood: He or she has a vacillating free will that is influenced by those around him or her.

- Sport must remain a fun activity, chosen and loved by the child who practices it.

- A child is a mosaic of growth cartilage. Acute trauma or chronic microtraumas will often cause growth cartilage injury.

- Overtraining has a counterproductive effect and results in deteriorating performance levels or affects essential areas of the child's overall well-being, such as loss of motivation, pain, asthenia, relational disturbances, emotional disorders, sleep or eating disorders, troubles in keeping up with educational demands, etc. Therefore, a balance must be established between the needs of the child and the demands of sport.

- The execution of certain elements must be limited once distress has been identified.

66.1 GROWTH REFERENCE POINTS

Puberty (pubic pilosity) begins at 11 years bone age in girls and 13 years bone age in boys. Menstruation begins around 13 years bone age. Girls reach their adult height at 15 years bone age; boys, at 17 years bone age.

Certain primarily female sports (notably artistic gymnastics, figure skating, classical dance), when practiced intensively, may affect a child's growth rate: There may be a parallel deceleration of bone maturation (sometimes up to years' retarded growth as compared to real age) and a subsequent delay in growth to mature adult height, though the child's adult height will not be different from what it would have been had he or she not practiced sport. This deceleration of bone maturation explains delayed puberty and subsequent delayed muscular development, which has an impact on the muscular capacity of young athletes and which explains delayed growth cartilage pathologies.

It is important that the team physician does not oversee hormone deficiency disorders in these cases, so a full serological hormone evaluation must be made.

66.2 ROLE OF A PEDIATRIC SPORTS PHYSICIAN

The role of a physician is of primary importance; the pediatric sports physician must encourage, but in no way force, an athlete to develop his or her talents. The physician should also be able to evaluate an athlete's ability to be active even if he or she has a cardiac murmur, scoliosis, or some other form of disability that may or may not affect his or her sporting ability.

It is important to monitor young athletes, to detect signs of overexertion early on. A physician may need to curb, modify, and modulate the child athlete's sporting activity at an early stage in order to help the child stay in that particular sport.

The physician should educate the young athlete on the need to lead a healthy lifestyle with propter nutrition (four meals, complex sugars, water, calcium, etc.). The physician should also inform on the benefits of sport, the need to respect the rules of sport and fair play, the need to be able to control minimal pain; and finally, endeavor to induce a level of psychological stability (motivation, pleasure, mastery, pursuit of glory) in the young athlete. A physician should explain to an athlete's parents that their role differs from that of a coach and that parents must be aware of danger signs such as excess psychological pressure being applied by domineering coaches. The physician should offer information on doping matters and prevent creating a bond between the unnecessary intake of food supplements (e.g., vitamins) with sporting success and possibly subsequent dependency tendencies that may lead to doping at a later stage.

A physician must inform the young athlete of the importance of systematically inquiring of his or her doctor or pharmacist if a prescribed medication is on the WADA Prohibited List, in order to foster a sense of responsibility in relation to doping matters.

It is important to realize that acute trauma in a child may result in injuries to the epiphyseal or apophyseal growth cartilage (Fig. 66.1A,B); a child is a mosaic of growth cartilage.

Chronic overexertion with direct impact on apophyseal growth cartilage in a child may lead to osteochondrosis, whereas in an adult, it would lead to tendinitis (Fig. 66.1A,B).

66.3 ACUTE TRAUMA

Fractures in children have their own pathogenicity including frequency, anatomical relationship to diaphyseal or epiphyseal areas, etc. While many fractures will only cause moderate discomfort for a period of time, other fractures may cause serious initial damage and may be associated with injury to the growth plates and result in growth cartilage disorders.

The most frequently seen fractures are of the clavicle, the radius and ulna, metacarpals, the tibia, and the fibula. The sports most commonly associated with injuries in young athletes usually involve

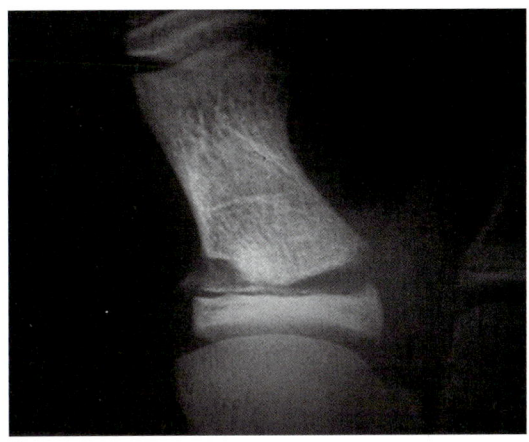

A

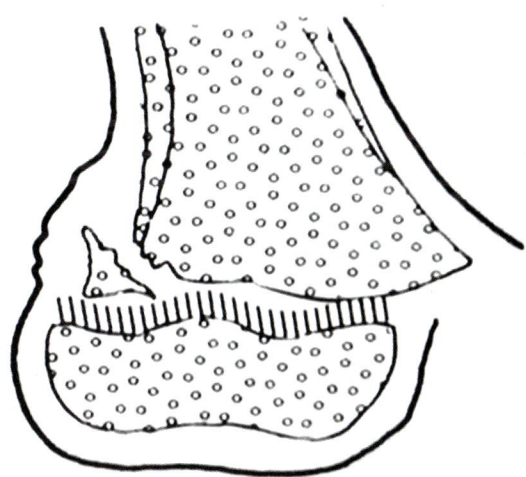

B

FIGURE 66.1. Separation of epiphysis, Salter-Harris type II. **A**: X-ray of base of the thumb. **B**: Schematic diagram.

running and jumping, but also contact and combat sports, where injuries are often associated with blows or falls.

Fractures

(Diaphysis—the shaft; metaphysis—the zone between the epiphysis and diaphysis; epiphysis—the end of a long bone that is separated from the main bone by the growth plate; apophysis—a bony outgrowth such as a process, tubercle, or tuberosity) (Fig. 66.2).

Diaphysis (Shaft) Fractures: If not grossly distorted, dislocated, or associated with soft-tissue injuries, diaphyseal fractures are usually less severe in that the growth cartilage is not affected. Moderate dislocations that would require reduction in an adult may not be necessary in a child due to their ability to remodel bone.

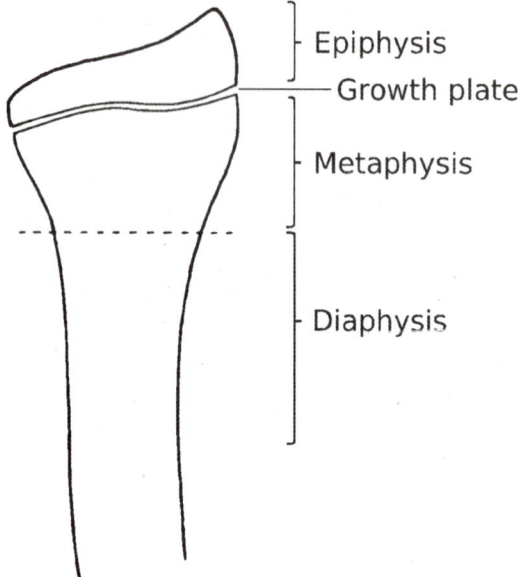

FIGURE 66.2.   Immature bones.

Metaphyseal Fractures: Fractures to the radial metaphysis are the most frequently seen fractures in children. Associated scaphoid fractures can also be present (and overlooked) and must be systematically eliminated. Typically, these fractures occur when trying to break a fall with an extended wrist (Fig. 66.3).

Epiphyseal Fractures, Dislocations: Epiphyseal fracture or dislocation usually occurs at the wrist, ankle, knee, humeral head, and elbow epiphyses (Fig. 64.4).

In children, cartilage is like a nail and ligaments are like strings attached to that nail. If you pull on the strings, the nail may give way. A muscle sprain sustained by a child athlete can often be associated

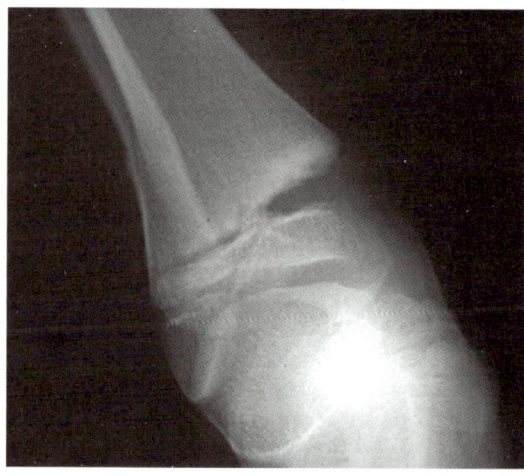

FIGURE 66.4.   Salter-Harris type I distal radius epiphyseal separation.

with an epiphyseal cartilage fracture and should be treated as such until proven otherwise.

Similarly, a muscle tear in children should be treated as an apophyseal cartilage fracture until proven otherwise. An epiphyseal fracture is serious in that it may impact on growth cartilage, with the possibility of premature growth plate ossification (epiphysiodesis), which may lead to shortening or angulation of the bone. Reduction or relocating of fractured or dislocated bone must be exact.

In most cases of displacement, surgical treatment is necessary.

Avulsion Fractures: Avulsion of the ischial tuberosity ossification nucleus, at the point of tendinous insertion, can, as we all know, also occur in adults (Fig. 66.5).

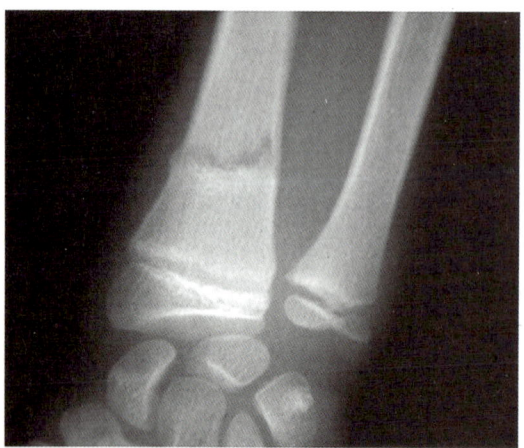

FIGURE 66.3.   Fracture to the radial metaphysis.

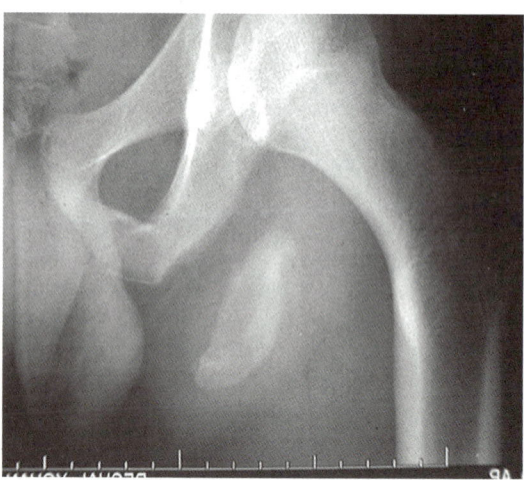

FIGURE 66.5.   Avulsion of the ischial tuberosity ossification nucleus.

Avulsion of the tibial tuberosity at the point of patellar ligament insertion is a more common injury; this avulsion fracture is a potentially disabling injury (surgical repair is not always possible or successful until the bone reaches maturation at the age of 15 years, after the patellar epiphyses have reached full ossification).

Other Injuries: In the child athlete's knee, lateral meniscal lesions are commonest and may result in constitutional discoidal dysplasia. The decision to operate on meniscal lesions in children is often individual but most agree that lesions in areas with good blood supply (red zone) should be sutured. Tearing of the anterior cruciate ligaments is rare.

The cervical spine is also at risk in certain contact or vaulting sports, notably rugby, with the swift engaging at the scrum, the banging of heads, scrum collapse, and head-to-head collisions being prevalent. All spinal traumas must be considered serious, even if an athlete is able to stand up after the incident. The same is true for any cranial trauma accompanied by loss of consciousness or altered intellectual activity. A cervical sprain is potentially unstable and should be considered a neurological risk. Athletes should desist from training immediately, until a complete medical examination can be performed.

Patellar dislocations occur in adolescents with existing patellofemoral dysplasia and may be the result of painful chronic patellar instability, or due to acute trauma.

As for wounds and bumps, they are countless.

It is imperative that an injured child terminates training immediately. Only after a full medical examination has been completed should a young athlete recommence training, and then, only if the athlete so desires and is not in pain.

Dental Fractures

Dental trauma requires rapid intervention; the quicker the athlete is treated, the greater the chance is of salvaging the tooth in working condition. If a tooth has been evulsed, it should be reimplanted within 20 minutes of the accident.

66.4   CHRONIC REPETITIVE TRAUMA

Tendinitis and muscular tearing are very rare in children, whose tendons are attached to unossified apophyseal cartilage. In cases of intense and repeated tensile stress or multiple percussions, the

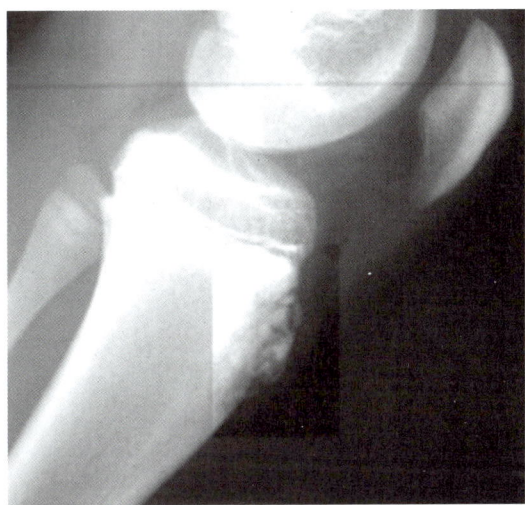

FIGURE 66.6.   Fragmented appearance of tibial apophysis of the knee.

tendon resists and growth cartilage begins to bulge and dissipate; the result is apophyseal osteochondrosis (Fig. 66.6).

Osteochondrosis

Osteochondrosis occurs as a result of chronic repetitive microtrauma in children, often after

- Tensile stress on the apophyseal cartilage (apophyseal osteochondrosis is to children what tendinitis is to adults)

- Compression of the articular endochondral cartilage (articular osteochondrosis)

Osteochondrosis is a common condition in sportingly active children and adolescents between the ages of 7 and 16 and is caused by overexertion, incorrect training, or training on improper surfaces. The condition results in pain and functional disability, especially in the lower limbs (takeoff and landing, acceleration, kicking, abrupt changes in direction), but also in the upper limbs (throws, flips).

In gymnastics, symptoms appear while the athlete is in action and subside with rest. Palpation of the affected ossification nucleus is painful and swelling is often found. Alternate contraction and overstretching of the adjoining muscle is painful; the patient identifies this pain. Usually, no effusion in the adjacent joint is noted. Clinical signs are often sufficiently characteristic; however, the radiological findings of the ossification nucleus can be extremely varied, even showing a shattered or fragmented, irregular appearance. Supplementary

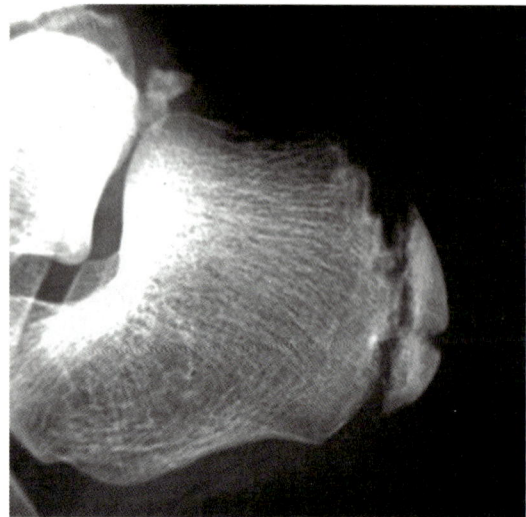

FIGURE 66.7. Sever's disease.

radiological examination should be considered even if the clinical findings are normal, in order to eliminate the possibility of a skeletal tumor, osteomyelitis, or other inflammatory condition.

Obesity contributes to the onset of these conditions, as do precocious intensive training, repetitive movements, exclusive resistance training, insufficient warm-up, poorly designed training exercises, or overly intensive training (duck walk, squats, jumps, hopping on one or two feet, push-ups).

The most common sites are at the posterior calcaneus, at the point of insertion of the Achilles tendon (Sever's disease)—presenting between the age of 7 and early puberty—and the anterior tibial tuberosity, at the point of insertion of the patellar tendon (Osgood-Schlatter's disease), most common in 9 to 15 year olds (Figs. 66.7, 66.8A and 66.8B).

Other areas can be affected depending on types of activity:

- Anterior superior iliac spine
- Midpoint of the kneecap
- Epicondylar or epitrochlear nuclei of the elbow
- Femoral condyles
- Patellar facets
- Talus
- Tarsal navicular bone
- Second metatarsal
- Femoral condyle (Fig. 66.9A–C)

Accessory ossification nuclei may also be affected:

- Accessory tarsal scaphoid
- The base of the fifth metatarsal
- Sesamoid bone at the distal end of the first metatarsal

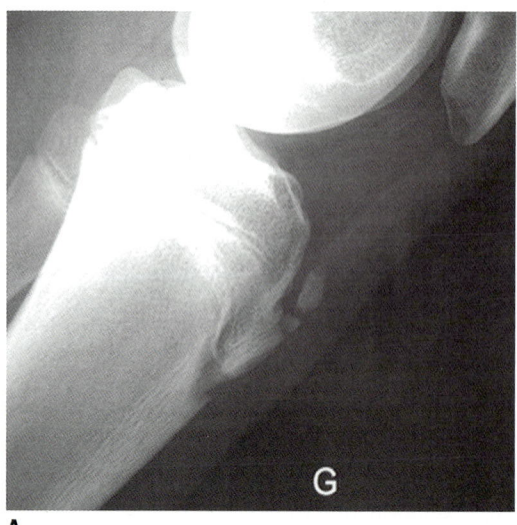

A

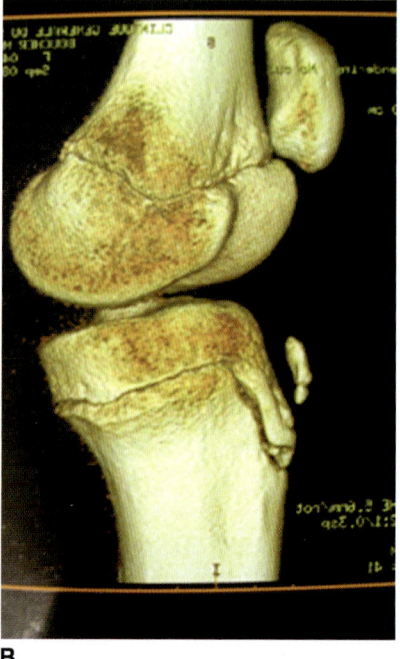

B

FIGURE 66.8. Osgood-Schlatter disease. **A**: X-ray. **B**: 3-D scan.

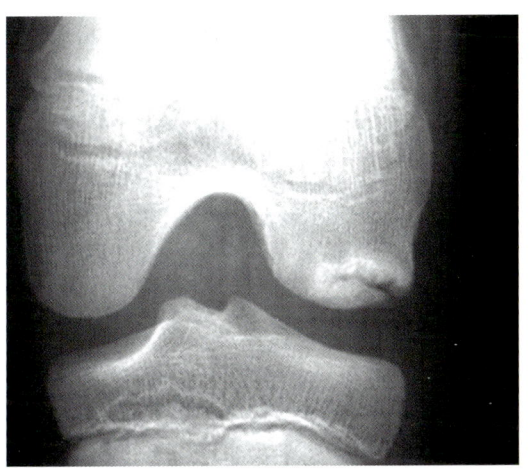

A

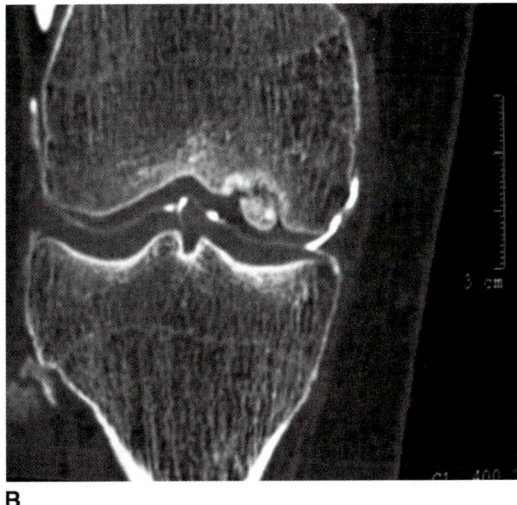

B

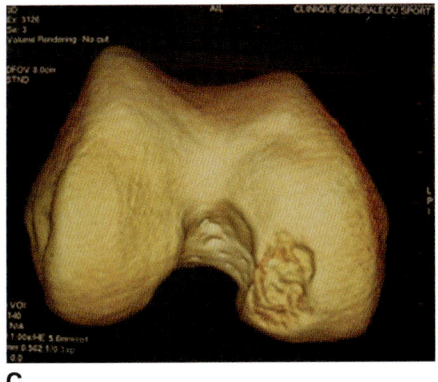

C

FIGURE 66.9. Internal condyle osteochondritis. (**A**) X-ray, (**B**) MRI, (**C**) 3-D scan.

Scheuermann's Disease

Also called juvenile osteochondrosis of the spine (or juvenile vertebral epiphysitis—[Fig. 66.10]), this condition is caused by repetitive intervertebral stress such as lifting or jumping; the disease is characterized by the advent of dorsal or dorsal lumbar pain after a heavy strain or after holding a prolonged static position. Complications may include permanent kyphosis of the upper spine.

Treatment of Osteochondrosis

Treatment is quite simple to explain; practical enforcement (patient compliance) is quite another issue. No formal sports restrictions should be placed on the child athlete; rather, let the level of pain decide the appropriateness of any given activity. Rest is often necessary but must be justified and relative. There is no use prohibiting a child from practicing a sport if he or she is running up the stairs, playing at school breaks, roller skating with his or her friends, or carrying a heavy backpack. Thus, treatment includes informing physical education teachers, coaches, and parents, as well as heightening awareness in the child. Immobilization is justified in unmanageable hyperalgia only, and for a duration of 3 weeks.

Surgery may be required where there are complications and repercussions (residual intratendinous osseous sequestration, surplus bone excision). Back braces may become necessary as the kyphosis (Scheuermann's disease) progresses.

Spondylolisthesis

Lumbar pain in athletes is the consequence of excessive strain that combines vertebral compression and rotational motions with an exaggerated lumbar curve. Stress of this kind may lead to a fracture when there is an acute trauma to the isthmus of the fifth lumbar vertebra, caught in a pincer movement between the vertebrae above and below.

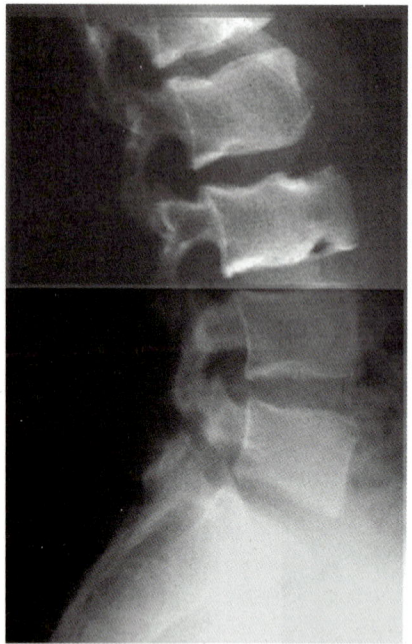

FIGURE 66.10.   Scheuermann's disease.

This is isthmus lysis. The posterior process of the vertebra having been broken, the vertebra slips forward (much like a slippery bar of soap), resulting in spondylolisthesis.

Six percent of the nonsporting general population present with this type of lysis. Its onset occurs progressively, starting at the age of 2 to 5 years when a child begins to walk and explore his or her sense of equilibrium at the expense of a lumbar curve compressing the fifth lumbar vertebra. Pain may become aggravated during adolescence when inappropriate or overly intense lumbar stress is applied.

While an acute traumatic fracture justifies immobilization using an orthopedic brace for a 2- to 3-month period, painful decompensation of a preexisting isthmus lysis is not a contraindication to the practice of sport, however intense, providing the activity does not trigger too much pain.

Early and rigorous pain management is effective in the treatment of pathologies involving overexertion of this kind; the child and his caregivers must remain vigilant. From an unpleasant sensation to the violent externalization of pain, discomfort is expressed in a way that reflects the child's age. The child's perception of pain differs depending on the maturity of nociception, the way he or she communicates, and how he or she expresses emotion in a relational context.

A child will need to learn to identify pain and communicate it to receptive caregivers, who will explain its cause clearly and in simple terms. The child respects the condition by easing up, and by modifying or terminating an activity after pain onset. A great many conditions involving overexertion could be avoided if only a child would learn to effectively manage pain.

Treatment may also involve alterations to a training program or of technical elements, modifications to equipment, adequate physical preparation, a progressive training routine, and sufficient warm-up.

66.5   CONCLUSION

Responsibility for a juvenile athlete falls to coaches, educators, parents, and doctors; it is a task that requires diligence and sensitivity. These adults will need to be on the lookout for signs of overexertion or of poor training techniques, which may translate into a general imbalance in the life of a young athlete: everything from a lack of motivation, counterperformance, asthenia, and social and emotional disturbances, to insomnia, eating disorders, and even difficulty in school.

CHAPTER 67

The Paralympic Athlete

Contributed by Peter Van de Vliet, International Paralympic Committee, Bonn, Germany; and Faculty, Kinesiology and Recreation Management, University of Manitoba, Canada

While sport contributes significantly to one's quality of life, it has even greater importance for the disabled athlete as it offers not only the possibility of physical rehabilitation but also helps introduce/reintroduce athletes with a disability into society. Furthermore, sport teaches independence.

Sport for people with a physical disability was introduced after World War II, to assist the large number of injured ex-servicemen, ex-servicewomen, and civilians with medical and psychological needs. Nowadays, people with a disability participate in high performance as well as in competitive and recreational sports. Public awareness has increased. More and more individuals with a disability are finding interest in sport. The Beijing 2008 Paralympic Summer Games sports program comprised 20 sports, while five sports were included in the Vancouver 2010 Paralympic Winter Games. Sport has now become a viable option for individuals with a disability.

The International Paralympic Committee (IPC) is the global governing body of the Paralympic Movement. The IPC organizes both Summer and Winter Paralympic Games and serves as the International Federation for nine sports, for which it supervises and coordinates World Championships and other competitions, from the developmental to the elite level. The IPC represents more than 160 countries, IFs, regional organizations, and four particular international sports organizations for the disabled (i.e., International Wheelchair and Amputee Sports Federation, International Blind Sports Association, Cerebral Palsy International Sport and Recreation Association, and the International Sports Federation for Persons with Intellectual Disability). The IPC is committed to enabling Paralympic athletes to achieve sporting excellence and to developing sport opportunities for all persons with a disability from the beginner to elite level. In addition, the IPC aims to promote the Paralympic values, which include courage, determination, inspiration, and equality.

67.1 PARALYMPICS—KNOW YOUR AUDIENCE

With participation in sport comes an associated risk of injury. Despite the growing awareness and popularity of Paralympic sport, there continues to be a relative paucity of understanding the injury patterns and risk factors for injury among elite athletes. The few studies that have been published comparing sport participation by both able-bodied and disabled individuals suggest that athletes with a disability do not have a significant greater overall risk of injury than their able-bodied counterparts, although the functional consequences of injury to an athlete with an underlying impairment can be considerably greater than for an able-bodied athlete. For example, a comparatively "routine" shoulder overuse injury that might be a mere "nuisance" for an able-bodied athlete may compromise the ability of a C6-lesion tetraplegic athlete (an athlete with a high neck lesion, impacting the function of both lower and upper limbs) to remain independently mobile, to say nothing of dramatically interfering with his or her participation in sport.

An understanding of common disabilities and injuries will assist athletes, their coaches, therapists, and trainers, as well as all event (medical) staff in identifying possible medical problems and activities that may lead to injuries or medical complications. This enables all involved to take the steps necessary to ensure safe and effective training techniques and maximize competitive performance on the one hand and optimize event-related medical services on the other hand.

Traditionally, there are six different athlete groups represented in the Paralympic Movement:

- Athletes with amputation
- Athletes with spinal cord injuries
- Athletes with cerebral palsy (CP)
- Athletes with intellectual impairment
- Athletes with visual impairment
- *Les autres* (a group of athletes not covered by any of the previous ones)

Athletes are categorized in the different sports ("classified") according to their ability to perform certain movements and tasks in that particular sport so that their sport performance is comparable to other athletes with similar ability. The objective of classification is to allow competitive success to be determined by strategies, skills, and talent of athletes and teams and not solely due to the function determined by the athletes' physical, sensorial, or intellectual ability, similar to the concept of weight classes or separate events for men and women.

Amputee athletes suffer from congenital or acquired amputations (traumatic, bone cancer, bone infection, diabetes, etc.). Occasionally, amputee athletes experience phantom sensations, painful cramping feelings and hypersensitivity. Amputee athletes may compete with or without orthotic or prosthetic devices, depending on the sport in which they participate.

The group of "spinal cord" athletes typically includes athletes with spinal cord injury, spina bifida, and postpolio paralysis. The neurological level of injury corresponds with the lowest level of the spinal cord that exhibits intact motor and sensory function. Associated conditions can include spasms and spasticity, urinary tract infections, thermoregulation disorders, skin breakdown, pressure sores and decubitus ulcers, autonomic hyperreflexia, osteoporosis and heterotopic ossification, and joint contractures.

Athletes with spina bifida or myelomeningocele experience muscle weakness, sensory loss, and bowel and bladder dysfunction similar to a spinal cord injury. Particular attention should be given to orthopedic complications of the spine and legs and the enhanced risk of hydrocephalus development. Poliomyelitis is an infectious impairment caused by a virus that destroys motor nerve cells and causes permanent muscle weakness and paralysis. Unlike spinal cord injury and spina bifida, postpolio paralysis results in problems with movement but not with sensation or autonomic nervous system function. Depending on the extent of paralysis, athletes may experience joint contractures and osteoporosis. Asymmetrical muscle function often results in the development of muscle tightness and restriction around limb joints, and spine curvatures.

CP includes a wide range of conditions involving a problem with control of voluntary movement or coordination. CP usually results from a complication in the pre-, peri-, or postnatal period that leads to an injury to the areas of the brain that control movement, speech, muscle tone, and coordination. Associated conditions often include seizure disorders and perceptual speech and swallowing disorders.

Les autres (French for "the others") is an umbrella term for athletes with a wide range of conditions resulting from various neurological, neuromuscular, or musculoskeletal disorders, but who do not fit into the traditional profiles as described above. Typical examples are achondroplasia, muscular dystrophy, multiple sclerosis, mutilated hands or feet, congenital deformities, etc. In the majority of sports, *les autres* athletes compete together with athletes with other physical impairments in accordance with their functional ability.

To be eligible for Paralympic sports, athletes with intellectual impairment must have a significantly subaverage general intellectual functioning (defined as IQ < 75) and concurrent limitations in adaptive skills, acquired before the age of 18. Additionally, they show reduced "sports intelligence," or limitations in the conative domain (conation refers to the mental processes that activate and/or direct behavior and action, such as processing speed, visual–spatial intelligence, memory) that impact directly on sport participation. Intellectually disabled (ID) athletes may be challenged with associated conditions such as seizures, significant loss of strength, joint hypermobility, and eventually, reduced self-care.

Visual impairment is the consequence of a functional loss of vision, rather than an eye disorder itself. Eye disorders that can lead to visual impairments result from disease, trauma, or congenital or degenerative conditions that cannot be corrected by conventional means. This functional loss of vision is typically defined as manifesting with visual acuity defects, significant central or peripheral field defect, or reduced peak contrast sensitivity. Associated conditions may include loss of body balance and reduced orientation.

67.2 MANAGEMENT OF COMMON MEDICAL PROBLEMS

Generally, the same safety and medical considerations apply to both Paralympic and able-bodied athletes. Precautions should be taken to prevent accidents from occurring and to make the sporting environment a safe and positive one. Safety precautions should not be so extreme so as to take away the "sense of achievement" that is inherent to sports participation. One of the greatest handicaps that people with a disability, in general, have had to confront has been to deal with the overbearing concerns of caregivers and society in general. Although these types of concerns have been well intended, they have often stifled the independence and hampered the freedom of disabled athletes.

As with able-bodied athletes, Paralympic athletes should be "cleared" for sport and checked that they do not have medical complications that may limit or prohibit involvement in (competitive) sport. Team physicians should have a medical history report available on all athletes at an event. Athletes themselves have the responsibility to pass on appropriate medical (and technical) information to coaches, event organizers, and the like upon request.

An awareness of the risks of common medical problems experienced by Paralympic athletes is essential to prevent the development and progression of the unfortunate condition(s), and important for care staff to identify the possible medical problems the athletes might face. Issues such as the extent of muscle and joint involvement, muscle tone and coordination, sensory loss, heat/cold intolerance, susceptibility to fractures, dangers of exacerbation, or the likelihood of progression of disease symptoms are all important considerations.

Though it is expected that Paralympic athletes should practice routine preventive measures to achieve and maintain optimal health to achieve maximal performance, research has shown that Paralympic athletes often do not seek medical consultation for problems they consider inherent to their impairment. Consequently, they too often try to "work through" an illness or disease. Unfortunately, this "self-management" sometimes prevents from proper assessment of the problem

and appropriate medical care at an early stage in its development.

67.3 COMMON MEDICAL PROBLEMS AND INJURIES

The medical care of Paralympic athletes should be related to the sport-specific risks and demands, as well as to the nature of the impairment. Though relatively few studies are available, alpine skiing, wheelchair track and road racing, paracycling, and wheelchair basketball are among the highest-risk sports. In addition, medical problems and injuries are positively correlated with frequency and intensity of training and competition.

Analysis of medical encounters reported at major events shows that athletes present to medical stations more often for the same medical problems as the general population than they do for medical problems usually related specifically to their impairment.

The following are most common injuries occurring in Paralympic athletes.

Soft-tissue Injuries

Soft-tissue injuries typically result from repetitive stress on joints and muscles. Shoulder and elbow joints are particularly vulnerable to repetitive motions, as well as contact surfaces between amputee stump and socket. Particular attention should be given to carpal tunnel syndrome. The repetitive trauma of wheelchair propulsion creates additional forces on the nerves that run from the forearm to the palm of the hand. The carpal tunnel compresses these nerves. This results in pain, tingling, and loss of strength and/or hand sensation.

Muscles are often strained when in a stretched position and contracting with great force against strong resistance, which commonly occurs in sport performance. Weaker, smaller muscles (e.g., shoulder rotator cuff) are particularly prone to such strain in disabled athletes. The result is an impingement syndrome or painful condition caused by continued compression of a tendon that then inflames. Since soft-tissue injuries are related to direct and repetitive trauma, it is essential to schedule adequate rest and recovery between practice times and competitions.

In addition to soft-tissue problems, cartilage degeneration, periarticular fibrous tissue tears, and loss of bone circulation may occur over time. Extensive forces imposed by weight bearing and continuous overhead activity decrease circulation to the structures of, in particular, the shoulder (e.g., wheelchair users) and hip (e.g., lower limb amputees) joints. Surgical decompression is sometimes the only alternative left to relieve chronic shoulder pain resulting from repetitive strains.

Paralympic athletes often report scrapes, cuts, bruises, blisters, and floor and wheel burns. They are particularly at risk for accidental injury from incidental contact with the wheelchair, prosthesis, or ground after a fall. Occasionally, friction burns occur due to an inappropriate fitting into the device (wheelchair too wide, prosthesis to small). If a prosthesis is not fitted correctly and it rubs on the stump, or if the stump sock moves against the stump, then friction occurs. This can cause blistering of the stump and result in several days' loss of training and competition. Particular attention should be given to the problems occurring when the skin is wet (e.g., swimming, rowing, sailing). Athletes sensitive to abrasions and lacerations often wear protective long sleeves or gloves, or strap themselves into their chairs to minimize injuries during falls (i.e., wheelchair rugby players).

Sensory Disorders and Skin Breakdown

Sensory disorders and skin breakdown often occur in spinal cord injury, spina bifida, and other nervous system–related impairments combined with excessive friction related to repetitive movements. The result is pressure sores due to shearing of the superficial tissue over bone, in particular, in tissue areas over bony prominences (especially on the buttocks and hips). The blood supply to the skin and underlying tissues is cut off. Athletes vulnerable to pressure sores should very regularly (visually) inspect insensitive skin. Persistent redness, hardening of the skin, or a raised area are first signs of a pressure sore and should immediately result in relief of all pressure from sitting, restrictive clothes, or prosthesis fitting until the redness resolves and normal skin color returns. If not treated appropriately, skin breakdown (decubitus ulcer) may progress to serious deep infection in muscle and bone. Caretakers should be sensitive to any red, hardened or raised area that has been subjected to sustained pressure. If pressure is not relieved immediately, the area can progress to an open sore (ulcerate) and result in a serious infection involving skin, muscle, and bone. Customized seating may alleviate pressure, but horizontal rest, mostly lying on the stomach or side, is recommended.

Temperature-regulation Disorders

Thermal injuries are common in all Paralympic athletes. Paralysis affects the body's ability to perspire below the site of the lesion, especially among athletes with high-lesion levels. Similarly, due to the loss of a limb, the ratio of surface area to body volume in amputee athletes is different. Consequently, both paralyzed as well as amputee athletes may suffer from overheating.

Muscle paralysis induces impaired circulation. In addition, blood flow is relatively low to the skin and deep tissues. A sensory deficit also often causes lack of pain sensation that normally serves as a warming mechanism. As a result, it is easier to sustain both burns and cold injuries (frostbite). Additionally, the same circulatory problems slow down and complicate the healing of the wounds afterwards.

Athletes with higher lesions often also have problems with core body–temperature regulation due to the loss of normal blood-flow regulation via the central nervous system. This may be compounded by their inability to sweat or shiver below the level of spinal cord injury. Typically, these athletes wet their own t-shirts or moisture themselves with plant sprinklers. Fans also are a common aid along the field of play (e.g., wheelchair rugby).

While sunscreen may be used, athletes with more severe dysfunction may have difficulties to apply their own protective cream or clothing. And, although sunscreen helps protect against sunburn, it can also make the athlete susceptible to heat intolerance; sunscreen may inhibit and impair cooling, especially in athletes who do not sweat normally.

High temperatures and humidity intensify heat intolerance. Initial symptoms include muscle cramps, whereas more severe heat illness results in heat exhaustion, with similar symptoms to able-bodied athletes.

Underestimated as an important cause of thermoregulatory disorders is dehydration. Athletes, in particular CP athletes, easily become dehydrated because the athletes start breathing rapidly and lose water from perspiration. Athletes with high support needs are less able to take fluids during sports participation without assistance due to their severe mobility problems. In addition, those who have communication or cognitive disorders may not readily report symptoms of cold intolerance. Some athletes may also restrict water intake because of bladder problems (see below).

Bladder Dysfunction and Urinary Tract Infections

Athletes with neurological disorders often have neurogenic bladders, due to inadequate or incomplete bladder emptying, indwelling catheters, or intermittent catheterization, and consequently have increased vulnerability to bladder infections, kidney stones, and urinary tract obstruction. Bladder infections often cause pain and increased muscle spasticity, as well as blood pressure disturbances (see below). In a worst-case scenario (i.e., with continued physical activity or sport participation), bladder infection may extend to kidney and bloodstream infections, causing severe illness or death. Many athletes take preventive medication. In case of an acute infection, antibiotic treatment should be initiated, and the athlete should refrain from any activity before body temperature normalizes. Although infections can be treated, they are best prevented by simple measures. By far, the simplest one is to ensure adequate fluid intake to regularly flush out the bladder. Additionally, athletes require clean areas in order to avoid contamination during handling and use of catheters, connecting tubes, and bags.

Blood Pressure and Blood-flow Problems

Some muscle and joint diseases have associated problems in blood flow. This can be caused by artery spasm of the hands of feet and may be induced by lower temperatures. Athletes with paralyzed muscles may lack blood return due to the inability of muscular pumping action. Edema in the paralyzed limbs is likely to occur, in particular when the blood flow is obstructed from wearing tight clothing or using straps around the legs or trunk. Circulation problems also occur when athletes rapidly change position, in particular from lying to sitting or standing position. In particular, wheelchair-bound athletes may lack the rapid response from the heart and blood vessels to position or movement changes. Those athletes often experience orthostatic hypotension, due to the inability of the sympathetic nervous system to accommodate a rapidly shifting blood volume.

Disabled athletes may also experience low blood pressure in hot or humid environments, especially when they are already dehydrated (see Chapter 69). Athletes are very vulnerable to this hypotension in long-lasting opening and closing ceremonies or when they watch peer Games while exposed to full sunshine.

A particular case of high blood pressure likely to occur in Paralympic athletes is that of autonomic dysreflexia. This is a reflex syndrome that is unique to individuals with spinal cord injury at lesion levels above T6. This reflex can occur spontaneously and results in a sympathetic discharge that elevates the arterial blood pressure and associated cardiovascular responses, which can enhance physical performance. The stimulus usually occurs in an area without sensation and triggers a series of reflexes resulting in abnormally high blood pressure, sweating, goose pimples, and/or flushing of the face and neck combined with headache. Paralympic athletes with spinal cord injury who compete in wheelchair sports may voluntarily induce autonomic dysreflexia prior to or during the event in order to enhance their performance. Research has demonstrated that this practice, which is commonly referred to as "boosting" in athletic circles, improves middle distance wheelchair racing performance by approximately 10% in elite athletes with quadriplegia. However, autonomic dysreflexia is a medical emergency. Failure to resolve the problem may result in stroke due to elevated blood pressure. Since the situation is triggered by a stimulus from a bladder or bowel obstruction, immediate action to empty the bladder or evacuate the bowels is to be undertaken, together with moving the athlete to a sitting position to reduce blood pressure.

Osteoporosis and Fractures

Although fractures are uncommon and occur in only a few sports (e.g., alpine skiing), paralyzed athletes have often osteoporotic bones that can fracture even with minor trauma. Since many athletes lack the sensation that accompanies a bone fracture, any evidence of an abnormal body position, swelling, redness, bruising, or grinding sensations should be further examined through imaging, having been initially immobilized. Fractures may also occur due to falls as a consequence of reduced balance. This can be the result of loss of sensation (e.g., incomplete lesions), coordination problems (e.g., CP athletes), loss of proprioception (e.g., prosthesis running), or unforeseen obstacles (e.g., visually impaired athletes).

Other

In the case of tetraplegic athletes, the diaphragm muscle is generally the only respiratory muscle that remains functional. The respiratory function of the muscles of the chest wall is usually paralyzed below the level of the injury. This loss of function affects the ability to cough and thereby clear the respiratory passage. Consequently, respiratory infections are more likely to occur, particularly when the sports activities are performed under less favorable environmental conditions.

CP athletes are more likely to have convulsive disorders than their able-bodied peers. Not only is fatigue a major inductor, CP athletes, similar to athletes with intellectual disability, may suffer epileptic attacks when they become overly distressed. Team physicians should have this convulsive tendency documented on the individual athlete's medical files and event physicians should monitor athletes with epilepsy in the cool-down period as seizures are more likely to occur in this period rather than during the activity itself.

There is some evidence to suggest that there may be an increase in intraocular pressure during explosive activities (i.e., powerlifting, rowing, judo, shot put), in particular in athletes with preexisting glaucoma.

67.4 COORDINATING MEDICAL SERVICES AT EVENTS

Despite the best planning, accidents do occur. It is, therefore, important that organizers solicit experienced medical personnel and carefully determine emergency contingencies. Prior to the event, medical staff should be informed about common disability-related problems, about the medical services, facilities, and policies that will be available, and of course, about expected medical procedures. Nearby hospitals with comprehensive emergency services should be identified and contracted, and consultation with a specialized rehabilitation care center is advisable. Prosthetists, orthotists, and wheelchair repair specialists should be approached regarding their ability to provide services and assistance. Accessible medical services will largely facilitate the work for all involved. Health care professionals should hold malpractice and professional liability insurance coverage and be licensed to practice in

the region where the competition is being held. Additionally, the organizers should have an adequate liability insurance to cover participants. It is important to note, at this stage, that this insurance policy should not exclude exacerbations of previously existing injuries or impairments.

It is recommended that the emergency medical teams have experience in the extrication of athletes from adaptive equipment (i.e., monoski shells, ice sledges, racing chairs, hand cycles), or at least familiarize themselves with the equipment that is available.

Due to the variety of Paralympic sports, event medical services need to be tailored to reflect the needs and demands of each particular sport or discipline. The following criteria should be considered: who participates (impairment groups: wheelchair users vs. amputees vs. visually impaired athletes), which (adaptive) equipment will be used, where does the activity take place (outdoor vs. sports hall vs. water), and what are the environmental conditions (winter vs. summer; altitude vs. air quality). It is recommended that key medical staff attend Paralympic sports events before the commencement of their own event.

Finally, disabled athletes must comply with antidoping regulations published by WADA. All medical personnel must familiarize themselves with these rules to properly advise and treat the athletes.

Recommended Reading

Australian Sports Commission. *Coaching Athletes with Disabilities: An Australian Resource.* www.ausport.gov.au/publications/catalogue/index.asp.; 2005.

Curtis KA. Health smarts: strategies and solutions for wheelchair athletes. *Sports 'n Spokes.* 1996;22:25–31.

Ferrara MS, Davis RW. Injuries to elite wheelchair athletes. *Paraplegia.* 1990;28:335–341.

Laskowski ER, Murtaugh PA. Snow skiing injuries in physically disabled skiers. *Am J Sports Med.* 1992;20:553–557.

Webborn N, Willick S, Reeser JC. Injuries among disabled athletes during the 2002 Winter Paralympic Games. *Med Sci Sports Exerc.* 2006;38:811–815.

Williams R. *First Aid: A Guide for Adapted Sports Coaches.* Atlanta, GA: The American Association of Adapted Sports Programs; 2006.

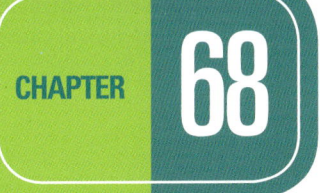

CHAPTER 68

The Hypothermic Patient

Contributed by Inggard Lereim, Vice Chairman, FIS Medical Committee, and Professor, NTNU, Trondheim, Norway; and Peter Jenoure, University of Basel, Switzerland

Reviewer: David McDonagh

Many winter and some summer sports take place in weather conditions that can lead to hypothermia. Obviously, the condition becomes more serious if it occurs during competition, where there are demands for increased metabolism and body function. Hypothermia can also be considered as a failure of the body's biological regulatory system (homeostasis), which is normally able to maintain the core body temperature to a near-constant level and can easily occur when the organism is exposed to such cold that its internal mechanisms become unable to replenish the heat lost to the surroundings.

This may be due to low temperature or the wind-chill effect. The temperature lowering effects of wind have previously been ignored by organizers of winter competitions; as a result, severe cases of hypothermia have been reported. Obviously, hypothermia is more often seen in outdoor winter sports, and an important part of an event physician's duty is to ensure that adequate preventative measures are in place.

Organizers of outdoor summer sports events should not neglect this risk; there are many examples of hypothermia cases described in cycling during mountain stages when unforeseen snow appears, in high-altitude trails (Tour du Mont Blanc), and in long-distance swimming, to mention a few examples. Sport activities with a risk of hypothermia are alpine skiing, cross-country skiing, ski jumping, freestyle skiing, kayaking, cycling, swimming in open water, altitude trails, cyclo-cross, and triathlon.

68.1 PREVENTION

Appropriate clothing is probably the best way to prevent hypothermia. Wearing cotton in cool weather is a common error as cotton retains water,

and water rapidly conducts heat away from the body. Even in dry weather, cotton clothing can become damp from perspiration and chilly after the wearer stops exercising. Synthetic and wool fabrics provide far better insulation when wet and dry quicker. Some synthetic fabrics are designed to help remove perspiration from the body. In air, up to 40% of body heat is lost through the head, so probably the most preventative measure one can take is to cover the head.

Heat loss on land is very difficult to predict due to multiple variables such as clothing type, the amount of clothing, amount of insulating body fat on the athlete, environmental humidity, personal sweating after exertion, the circumstances surrounding the hypothermic episode, etc. Heat is lost much quicker in water, hence the need for appropriate clothing in cold-weather activities such as kayaking. Water temperatures that would be quite acceptable as outdoor air temperatures can quickly lead to hypothermia. For example, water immersion at a temperature of 10°C can be expected to lead to death in approximately 1 hour, and water temperatures hovering at freezing can lead to death in as little as 15 minutes.

Alcohol consumption prior to cold exposure may increase one's risk of becoming hypothermic. Alcohol acts as a vasodilator, increasing blood flow to the body's extremities, thereby increasing heat loss. Ironically, this may cause the victim to feel warm while he or she is rapidly losing heat to the surrounding environment.

Twenty to fifty percent of hypothermal deaths are associated with a phenomenon known as paradoxical undressing. This typically occurs during moderate to severe hypothermia as the victim becomes disoriented, confused, and combative.

The hypothermic victim may begin discarding the clothing he or she has been wearing, which, in turn, increases the rate of temperature loss. There have been several published case studies of victims throwing off their clothes before help reached them. Rescuers who are trained in mountain survival techniques have been taught to expect this effect. One explanation for the effect is a cold-induced malfunction of the hypothalamus, the part of the brain that regulates body temperature. Another explanation is that the muscles contracting peripheral blood vessels become exhausted (known as a loss of vasomotor tone) and then relax, leading to a sudden surge of blood (and heat) to the extremities, fooling the victim into feeling warm.

68.2 CLINICAL STAGES

In mild hypothermia, body temperature drops by 1°C to 2°C below the normal temperature; in moderate hypothermia, by between 2°C and 4°C; and finally, in severe hypothermia, the core temperature drops below approximately 32°C. Severe hypothermia should not be encountered in an organized sports event; however, milder forms are more frequently seen.

Core Temperature: Symptoms and Signs

- Mild hypothermia (36°C to 35°C): Shivering, sensation of cold

- Moderate hypothermia (34°C to 32°C): Violent shivering, sluggish thinking, poor coordination with loss of hand control, confusion, mood changes, pale skin with reddish or pink areas

- Severe hypothermia
  - 35°C: Shivering is intense.
  - 33°C: Shivering decreases.
  - 32°C to 30°C: Shivering replaced by muscular rigidity, confusion, semiconsciousness, dilated pupils; later, bullae may develop.
  - 30°C to 29°C Stupor, rigidity, slow pulse, and respiration. The peripheral portion of the limbs, head, and unprotected parts of the body will have obvious signs of local lesions such as bullae, wounds, or necrotic areas (depending on the lapse of time).
  - 28°C to 26°C: Unconsciousness, arrhythmias, an imperceptible pulse and blood pressure, shallow respiration. Cardiac monitoring is necessary, if possible, by an EEG to detect if

ventricular fibrillation is present, which, if not treated rapidly and adequately, will cause death.

68.3 TREATMENT

Few authors have reported survival when a core body temperature of 19°C was recorded.

- Mild hypothermia: The patient is brought into a sheltered, warm room, given warm drinks, dried, changed into warm clothes, and covered with blankets, thus gradually warming the undercooled athlete. If necessary, close body contact with a companion can be considered. It is of the utmost importance that the body core is warmed up to prevent cold blood being forced toward the heart, which may cause death. For this reason, it is very important to make sure that the first aid providers do not rub the patient's body but try to transfer their own body heat to the patient. Place the patient in a horizontal position, first wrapping the patient in plastic to prevent further heat loss before lying him or her down on a woolen blanket. Check the airway, give oxygen, and establish an IV access. Protect the patient from wind. Take off cold and wet clothes only when indoors in a warm environment.

- Moderate hypothermia: A patient with moderate hypothermia between 34°C and 30°C must be resuscitated by a warm bath initially at a temperature of 26°C, increasing to 42°C over a period of 7 to 8 minutes. The patient should be encouraged to drink warm fluids, and if possible warm, moisturized air should be inhaled. Moderate and severe cases of hypothermia require immediate evacuation and treatment in a hospital. Moderate and severe hypothermia may be exacerbated by after drop (i.e., the core body temperature continues to fall even when the patient has been removed from the cold to a warmer area). Good results can be achieved when the patient breathes warm air and oxygen. It appears to be more effective in decreasing the effect of after drop than rewarming in a bath from 26°C to 40°C. Warming can also be accomplished by more invasive techniques such as warm fluid infusions or even lavage (washing) of the bladder, stomach, chest, and abdominal cavities with warmed fluids for severely hypothermic patients. These patients have an increased risk of cardiac arrhythmias and care must be taken to minimize jostling and other disturbances until they have been sufficiently warmed, as these arrhythmias are very difficult to treat while the victim is still cold.

- Severe hypothermia: A patient with severe hypothermia, with fixed, dilated pupils; impalpable pulses; nonrecordable blood pressure; and a core temperature below 30°C should be taken to a hospital as soon as possible, preferably by helicopter. Cardiac monitoring should be established as soon as possible because of the dangers of cardiac arrest. Rapid, central rewarming with humidified oxygen and warm air using a ventilating bag should be started. Cardiac massage and defibrillation are not necessary if the core temperature is below 30°C and unless ventricular fibrillation occurs. The patient should be treated as gently as possible to avoid precipitating ventricular fibrillation.

A thermometer that can record down to −18°C should be available. Intraesophageal and rectal electronic thermometers are more accurate and reliable.

An important tenet of treatment is that a person is not dead until he or she is warm and dead. Remarkable accounts of recovery after prolonged cardiac arrest have been reported in patients with hypothermia. This is probably due to the fact that the low temperature prevents some of the cellular damage that occurs when blood flow and oxygen are lost for an extended period of time.

68.4 PRACTICAL CONSEQUENCES FOR THE EVENT PHYSICIAN

At events where there is even the slightest risk of hypothermia, the main duty of the event physician is to initiate all possible measures to reduce this danger. Close cooperation with local weather services can be useful. Knowledge of the hypothermic condition is widely spread through the medical and paramedical professions, so education of first aid personnel is important.

It also important to warn the athletes if the competition is to be held in extremely cold conditions: Advise proper clothing and raise awareness of hypothermia symptoms, etc. As mentioned above, prevention is the key.

In some sports, such as cross-country skiing, the regulations stipulate a temperature minimum below which a competition cannot take place. In borderline situations, the jury will often go ahead with an event and the event physician will not be consulted. However, if the event physician has a seat on the jury, he or she has much greater influence over decisions made.

Recommended Reading

Keatinge WR, Khartchenko M, Lando N, et al. Hypothermia during sports swimming in water below 11 degrees C. *Br J Sports Med*. 2001;35(5):352–353.

Wilkerson JA, Giesbrecht GG. *Hypothermia frostbite and other cold injuries: prevention, recognition, rescue, and treatment*. Seattle, WA: Mountaineers Books, 2006.

CHAPTER 69

Hyperthermia and Heat-Related Conditions

Contributed by Andreas Niess, Professor, University of Tübingen, Germany

Reviewer: Dr. James Macdonald, University of California, Santa Cruz, United States

Augmented ambient temperatures reflect a major challenge for training or competing athletes, especially during endurance exercise. Besides detrimental effects on endurance performance, warm or hot conditions can induce environmental heat stress, which may even lead to life-threatening events.

Endurance athletes, as well as athletes in ball sports, sprinters, or strength athletes can suffer from hot conditions. In these athletes, muscle cramps are the main reasons for interrupting or stopping competition. Additionally, heat-associated problems affect not only exercising athletes but also officials and spectators who are coaching or watching the event.

69.1 PHYSIOLOGY OF THERMOREGULATION DURING EXERCISE

During exercise, most of the heat produced is gained from working muscle. In working muscle, only 25% of the energy produced is transformed into mechanical work, while the remaining 75% results in heat production. For every liter of oxygen consumed by working skeletal muscle per minute, 270 W of heat energy is produced. Most of this heat is delivered by the venous vessels to the body core. An increase in body core temperature leads to the stimulation of heat receptors, which activate the hypothalamic thermoregulatory center. In turn, this area in the brain initiates distribution of the heated blood to the body's surface via augmented cardiac output and active sympathetic cutaneous vasodilatation.

A sufficient transfer of heat from the body's surface to the ambient environment depends on evaporative heat loss, conduction, convection, and radiation. However, the latter three mechanisms of cooling are impaired if ambient temperatures are high. Under such conditions, evaporation of perspiration is the only remaining mechanism for heat loss. As heat loss through sweat vaporization depends on the existing environmental water vapor pressure, increased humidity will compromise evaporative heat transfer from the body at a given ambient temperature. If heat production by working skeletal muscle exceeds the capacity of the thermoregulatory system, uncompensatory heat stress occurs. Under such conditions, exercise performance is strongly compromised, heat exhaustion may occur, and the risk of heat illness becomes high.

The WBGT is a useful index of environmental heat stress. In addition to the existing temperature, the calculation of the WBGT factors in the humidity and radiant heat into a determination of the actual influence of heat stress on the body. Values for WBGT above 27.8°C are considered to be a very high risk for heat illness.

A number of mechanisms are known or assumed to negatively affect exercise performance under elevated ambient temperatures. These include an increased blood flow to the cutaneous capillaries, dehydration via sweat loss with a subsequent decrease in plasma volume, and as a result of this, a decline of blood flow to the exercising muscles. Growing evidence exists that, beyond peripheral factors, increased brain temperature as a result of reduced heat removal seems to reduce the activity of central motor centers. To what extent increased reliance on carbohydrate utilization, disturbances in mitochondrial respiration, actin–myosin interactions, or decreased enzyme functions contribute to muscle fatigue during exercise in the heat await further confirmation.

TABLE 69.1	**Factors That Negatively Affect Thermoregulatory Function and Risk Factors for Heat Illness**

- Dehydration
- Low physical fitness
- Obesity
- Sleep deprivation
- Medication (antidepressants, diuretics, antihistamines, antihypertensives, alpha-1 blockers, attention deficit hyperactivity disorder drugs, some stimulants)
- Alcohol or caffeine intake
- Sunburn
- Skin diseases
- Sweat gland dysfunction
- Prepubescent age or age > 40 y
- Prior history of heat illness
- Upper respiratory infection, gastroenteritis

Adaptation to elevated ambient temperatures has been shown to be a relatively rapid process. Daily repeated exercise sessions in the heat are sufficient to prolong time to fatigue and attenuate the rise of the core temperature. Such acclimatization can normally be induced by exercising under elevated ambient temperatures for 8 to 14 days. There is some evidence that approximately 75% of the acclimatization process occurs during the first 5 days. The most important mechanism responsible for heat adaptation is improved perspiration.

In this context, a better evaporative heat loss is the result of a

- Greater sweat volume
- Lower sweat sodium content
- Decrease in the sudomotor (sweat gland stimulation) threshold

Moreover, an expansion of plasma volume and better vascular regulation improve blood transfer to the skin and therefore contribute to heat dissipation.

69.2 HEAT ILLNESS AND HYPONATREMIA

Heat illnesses include

- Exertional heatstroke (EHS)
- Heat syncope
- Exertional heat exhaustion
- Exertional heat cramps

Heat exhaustion and EHS usually occur under hot conditions, especially if there is high humidity. If the WBGT exceeds 28°C, there is a highly increased risk of heat illness. However, EHS and heat exhaustion can also occur under normal temperatures if exercise is intense or prolonged, or if the body's innate thermoregulatory capacity is in some way inhibited (e.g., wearing many layers of clothing or taking certain medicines such as some antihypertensives).

The onset of heat exhaustion and exertional heat cramps does not necessarily require excessive hyperthermia, while EHS is defined by hyperthermia with a body core temperature >40°C. Whether it occurs during exercise or at rest, EHS poses a serious health risk, the successful treatment of which mainly depends on early recognition and onset of cooling intervention.

Hyponatremia is not a typical form of heat illness but can also occur more frequently if prolonged exercise is performed in heat. Hyponatremia is usually induced via excessive fluid ingestion during endurance exercise. Symptoms and treatment of the different forms of heat illness are summarized in Table 69.2.

69.3 RECOMMENDATIONS FOR PREVENTION OF HEAT ILLNESS

The following recommendations can be used to help prevent heat illness and to manage exercise in the heat.

TABLE 69.2	Exercise-Associated Hyponatremia and Forms of Heat Illness: Predisposing Factors, Symptoms, Prevention, and On-Site Treatment		
	Predisposing Factors	**Symptoms/Clinical Manifestation**	**On-Site Treatment**
Exertional heat cramps	Muscle fatigue, dehydration, large sodium loss Long duration, high-intensity events in the heat	Painful cramps, mostly in exercising muscle groups Intestinal cramps may also occur	Rest, prolonged stretching, oral ingestion of sodium (0.5–1.0 g/L or 1/4–1/8 teaspoon sodium to 300–500 mL water). In refractory, painful muscle cramps, intravenous treatment with benzodiazepines can be considered. In these cases, continuing exercise is not possible (NB: doping regulations). Prevention: Maintaining fluid and salt balance; if much sweat is perspired, daily salt intake should be increased to 5–10 g.
Heat syncope	Prolonged standing in the heat Sudden rise from lying or seated position	Loss of consciousness	Move the athlete to a cool room, place in a supine position with feet raised, monitor vital signs; recovery usually occurs quickly once supine. Replacing fluid deficit by oral ingestion is usually sufficient. Prevention: Be aware of pre- or near-syncopal symptoms; these can indicate inadequate hydration.
Heat exhaustion	Existing risk factors for heat illness (e.g., high body mass index, low fitness, low acclimation state) Unaccustomed exercise intensity, dehydration	Inability to continue exercise, fatigue, core temperature <40.5°C, wet and mostly cool skin, nausea, hypotension, tachycardia, vomiting, mild confusion, headache, disturbed coordination	Move the person to a cool room, place in a supine position with feet elevated, remove clothing, monitor vital signs, including rectal temperature.[a] Oral fluid administration in conscious persons, swallowing well. In other cases, intravenous fluid administration (0.9% sodium). If no improvement occurs, further evaluation and transportation to an emergency facility is necessary.

(Continued)

TABLE 69.2	**Exercise-Associated Hyponatremia and Forms of Heat Illness: Predisposing Factors, Symptoms, Prevention, and On-Site Treatment (*Continued*)**

	Predisposing Factors	**Symptoms/Clinical Manifestation**	**On-Site Treatment**
Exertional heat stroke (EHS)	Existing risk factors for heat illness (e.g., high body mass index, low fitness, low acclimation state) Unaccustomed exercise intensity, dehydration	Core temperature >40°C, tachycardia, hyperventilation (with pCO_2 often <20 mm Hg), hypotension, delirium, convulsion or coma Multiorgan dysfunction syndrome	Immediate recognition is paramount to survival. Move the patient to a cooler room, remove clothing, cool immediately (cold water immersion, application of cold packs to neck, axilla, groin; fanning of the undressed body while wetting the skin surface). Monitor vital signs, including rectal temperature.[a] Intravenous fluid administration (0.9% sodium). Rapid transfer to an emergency facility.
Exercise associated hyponatremia (EAH)	Excessive drinking behavior Extremely hot environment conditions Exercise duration > 4 h	Plasma sodium concentration < 135 mmol/L Nausea, vomiting, headache, disorientation, confusion, agitation, respiratory distress, seizures, coma	*Asymptomatic EAH:* Restrict oral fluid intake until onset of renal excretion. *Symptomatic EAH:* Monitor vital signs, ensure intravenous access. For experienced medical staff, persons with EAH exhibiting confusion, respiratory insufficiency, nausea, or vomiting can be treated with intravenous administration of 100 mL of sodium 3% over a period of 10 min (NB: doping regulations). Rapid transfer to an emergency facility.

[a]Oral, ear, skin, temporal, and axillary measurements should not be used to assess body temperature in suspected heat illness.

Individual Risk Assessment

For individual risk assessment, persons exercising/competing in the heat should be asked for

- Prior history of heat illness
- Current medications
- Training state
- Acclimation state
- Individual practice of fluid intake
- Clothing and protective gear
- Further risk factors of heat illness (see Table 69.1)

Acclimatization

A minimum of 5 to 10 days should be allowed, depending on age, planned activity, environmental conditions, training status, and individual experiences in hot climates and exercising in the heat. Also, at least four to seven exercise sessions with a minimum of 60 to 90 minutes duration should be planned in this period. A gradual increase in exercise intensity and duration is recommended.

If more intense training is necessary during the first days of acclimatization, then sessions should be scheduled during the early morning or late evening to avoid extreme heat stress.

Remember, young athletes may take longer to acclimatize. There is no specific adaptation to intense humidity. Therefore, acclimatization to hot and humid environments can be planned in locations with hot but dry weather conditions.

Hydration

A hydration strategy should be planned prior to exposure to warm or hot ambient conditions.

The daily drinking volume has to be adapted to existing conditions. To avoid dehydration during stays in warm or hot ambient temperatures, standardized measurements of naked body weight (e.g., in the morning after urinating) should be performed. Prior assessment of baseline body weight is helpful and euhydration can be assumed if fluctuations of morning body weight remain below 1%.

Note that fluid requirement may further increase once acclimation occurs.

Adequate sodium intake via consumption of sodium-rich foods, salted snacks, or sodium-containing drinks can help to sustain the sodium–fluid balance.

Euhydration before starting training or competition is mandatory. Sufficient fluid intake during the day and the evening before is recommended, especially if a certain extent of exercise-induced dehydration was present the preceding day. Preexercise hydration is based on the ingestion of approximately 500 mL fluid in the last 30 to 120 minutes prior to exercise.

During exercise, dehydration exceeding a loss of 2% of body weight should be avoided. On the other hand, the risk of hyponatremia increases if excessive drinking during prolonged exercise leads to weight gain. For repeated fluid replacement, 150 to 200 mL every 15 to 20 minutes and not more than 800 mL per hour during endurance exercise or ball sports is recommended. However, the large individual variability of fluid loss during exercise in heat may necessitate an individual adjustment of drinking volume. For this purpose, prior assessment of individual fluid loss during exercise under warm or hot temperatures by measuring body weight changes is a helpful tool.

If the duration of exercise exceeds 1 to 2 hours, beverages consumed before and during exercise should contain 0.5 to 1.0 g per L of sodium. If intense (duration > 60 min) or prolonged exercise (>90 min) is performed, an addition of 5% to 8% carbohydrates (50 to 80 g per L) can be beneficial for exercise performance. A mixture of different sugars (maltodextrine, glucose, fructose, sucrose)

has been shown to further enhance oxidation rates of ingested carbohydrates.

Hyperhydration agents provide equivocal benefits and have several disadvantages.

After exercise, full replacement of fluid and electrolyte losses is necessary for complete recovery. Under these conditions, the addition of sodium is also important for retaining ingested fluids. To achieve rapid rehydration, especially if the recovery period is short and/or the fluid loss is large, for every kilogram of body weight lost, a volume of 1,500 mL fluid should be ingested.

Otherwise, a more moderate approach to electrolyte and fluid supply is recommended by ingestion of normal electrolyte-containing food combined with water.

Fluid administration via intravenous infusion provides no advantages, unless it is medically indicated. In this context, one should be aware that intravenous infusions for nonmedical reasons are now prohibited by the WADA.

Clothing/UV Protection

Heat storage by wearing inappropriate clothing should be prevented. White or light-colored and loose-fitting textiles are recommended. Textiles should be highly permeable for heat and allow for evaporation of sweat near the skin.

In some sports, protective clothing is necessary or required by the rules of the sport. Note: Helmets, protective pads, and gloves disturb heat dissipation and can induce uncompensable heat stress.

Avoid prolonged exposure to direct UV radiation. Even if only technical or tactical training is performed, protection from direct sun exposure has to be considered. If direct exposure to solar radiation cannot be prevented, UV protection is strongly recommended.

Note: An existing sunburn can disturb thermoregulation and is a known risk factor for heat illness.

Recommended Reading

ACSM Team Physicians. Selected issues in injury and illness prevention and the team physician: a consensus statement. *Med Sci Sports Exerc.* 2007;39(11): 2058–2068.

Almond CSD, Shin AY, Fortescue EB, et al. Hyponatremia among runners in the Boston marathon. *N Engl J Med.* 2005;352:1550–1556.

Armstrong LE, Casa DJ, Millard-Stafford M, et al. ACSM position stand: exertional heat illness during training and competition. *Med Sci Sports Exerc.* 2007;39: 556–572.

Armstrong LE, Epstein Y, Greenleaf JE, et al. ACSM position stand: heat and cold illness during distance running. *Med Sci Sports Exerc.* 1996;28:i–x.

Bouchama A, Knochel JP. Heat stroke. *N Engl J Med.* 2002;346:1978–1988.

Cheung SS, McLellan TM, Tenaglia S. The thermophysiology of uncompensable heat stress. *Sports Med.* 2000;29:329–359.

Coris EE, Ramirez AM, Van Durme DJ. Heat illness in athletes. *Sports Med.* 2004;34:9–16.

Hargreaves M, Febbraio M. Limits to exercise performance in the heat. *Int J Sports Med.* 1998;19:S115–S116.

Hew-Butler T, Almond C, Ayus JC, et al. Consensus statement of the 1st international exercise-associated hyponatremia consensus development conference, Cape Town, South Africa, 2005. *Clin J Sport Med.* 2005;15:208–213.

Larsen T, Kumar S, Grimmer K, Potter A, et al. A systematic review of guidelines for the prevention of heat illness in community-based sports participants and officials. *J Sci Med Sports.* 2007;10:11–26.

Naughton GA, Carlson JS. Reducing the risk of heat-related decrements to physical activity in young people. *J Sci Med Sports.* 2007;11:58–65.

Nielsen B. Heat acclimation—mechanisms of adaptation to exercise in the heat. *Int J Sports Med.* 1998;19:S154–S156.

Nybo L. Hyperthermia and fatigue. *J Appl Physiol.* 2008;104:871–878.

Sawka MN, Noakes TD. Does dehydration impair exercise performance? *Med Sci Sports Exerc.* 2007;39:1209–1217.

Wendt D, van Loon LJ, Lichtenbelt WD. Thermoregulation during exercise in the heat: strategies maintaining health and performance. *Sports Med.* 2007;37:669–682.

CHAPTER 70

Inevent and Postevent Nutrition

Contributed by Jan Hoff, Professor, Sports Exercise Department, Norwegian University of Science and Technology, Trondheim, Norway

Reviewer: Julia Alleyne, Canadian Skating Team, University of Toronto, Canada

For many non–sports physicians, the whole topic of nutrition and hydration can appear very complicated and confusing. To aid the event physician who may be asked to give advice to athletes, here are some basic facts.

70.1 PREEVENT NUTRITIONAL ADVICE

Preevent hydration, if needed, should start several hours before competition to allow time for fluid absorption and for urine excretion to return to normal. Sports drinks with carbohydrates also help fill up the body's carbohydrate stores. Extra salt (snacks) can help stimulate thirst.

A preevent meal 1 to 4 hours before competition should be carbohydrate rich and the food should have a slower carbohydrate release than sports drinks, hence the use of cereals, bread, pancakes, rice, or pasta. Sports bars and sports drinks are more often used in the hours just before the competition.

70.2 INEVENT NUTRITIONAL ADVICE

During an event lasting more than an hour, both water and carbohydrates (6% to 8%) should be supplied.

Salty sweaters need added salt and should choose a sport drink that contains added salt, or they should mix in salt themselves.

Drinking 0.4 to 1.0 L sports drink per hour "ad lib" or with regular 10- to 20-minute intervals, containing 0.15 to 0.25 L per portion, should be individually determined and based on previous experience and measurements of weight loss.

Adding caffeine to the sport drink during the latter part of the competition might enhance performance.

Practicing drinking during exercise is important. Athletes need to develop this skill in order to ensure high-quality training and to train the body to react positively to inevent drinking.

70.3 POSTEVENT NUTRITIONAL ADVICE

After exercise, it is important to fully replace used water, carbohydrates, and electrolytes.

The absorption rate is faster the first 30 minutes after exercise and this time zone should be utilized.

The volume of sports drinks or sweetened drinks/water combinations that should be consumed should be more than the amount of fluid lost in the event. For every kilogram of weight loss, 1.5 L of fluid should be consumed: Fluid intake should be 150% of weight reduction.

Consuming salt snacks postexercise might enhance thirst and ease rehydration.

20 g protein in a protein drink or a protein bar immediately after training or competition might enhance the training effect.

70.4 SUPPLEMENTS

Macronutrients and water are primarily used for producing energy during training and competition. Macronutrients mostly contain carbohydrates, but also protein and, to a far lesser degree, fat. A few other substrates are important, not so much for performance enhancement, but more to avoid performance reduction due to energy loss and dietary deficiencies (e.g., sodium, vitamins, and minerals).

Remember, ATP and phosphocreatine (PCr) stored in the muscles provide energy for the first 6 or 7 seconds, and the anaerobic energy system might provide further short-term energy with lactate production; however, the continuous demand for energy is primarily dependent upon aerobic energy production to restore the short-term energy sources. The most important substances in inevent and postevent nutrition are carbohydrates and water.

70.5 CARBOHYDRATES

Carbohydrates are the easiest available energy source and supply most of the energy needed for sports activity. A 70-kg person stores about half a kilogram of carbohydrates. Most carbohydrates are stored as muscle glycogen, but a smaller amount—<100 g—is also stored in the liver. The amount of carbohydrate stored in the muscle is based on the level of training, usually measured in terms of maximal aerobic capacity (VO_{2max}), which determines the athlete's capacity to produce energy through oxidative metabolism (i.e., the higher the VO_{2max}, the greater the carbohydrate stores).

This can be illustrated by the fact that all athletes, regardless of their VO_{2max} status, have sufficient carbohydrates to perform 1 to 1.5 hours of hard work. Energy production rates are usually far higher in top marathon runners ($VO_{2max} > 85$ mL $\times$ kg^{-1} $\times$ min^{-1}) as compared to less well-trained soccer players ($VO_{2max} > 65$ mL $\times$ kg^{-1} $\times$ min^{-1}). To run a marathon requires pretty much the same amount of energy no matter if you are a top athlete or a less trained individual; however, time factors will be very different. A high-aerobic capacity soccer player may run 13 to 14 km during a match and thus needs approximately 30% to 40% more energy than the low-aerobic capacity soccer player (<10 km), and this energy comes almost entirely from carbohydrates.

A marathon run requires around 12,000 kJ (similar to ~750 g carbohydrate), although 5% to 20% of the energy is provided by fat oxidation. The percentage of VO_{2max} also determines the percentage of fat used for energy production. The longer the competition time, the lower the percentage of VO_{2max} that can be sustained. Repeated sprints, as in ball games, quickly empty the local carbohydrate stores. Improved oxidative metabolism has been shown to double the number of sprints during a soccer match. Athletes competing for more than an hour need refueling of carbohydrates. Excess carbohydrate feeding will be transformed to and stored as body fat. There do not seem to be any significant differences between men and women in their ability to utilize or store carbohydrates. Females at all levels have a 10 mL $\times$ kg^{-1} $\times$ min^{-1} lower VO_{2max} than men and have consequently lower carbohydrate stores.

Reduced carbohydrate stores do not influence performance during prolonged exercise until they are almost empty when the athlete may experience sudden exhaustion and acute hypoglycemia and may often have to terminate the competition. Most athletes during prolonged exercise now use sports drinks to prevent emptying their carbohydrate stores. The commonest cause of in-competition hypoglycemia is probably the lack of adequate carbohydrate replacement after previous training sessions where the athlete competes with reduced carbohydrate stores. The condition is easily and quickly corrected with carbohydrate feeding, preferably by using standard sports drinks containing 6% to 8% carbohydrates.

There is no evidence that carbohydrate feeding in the last hour before competition has any negative effect on performance, although a few athletes do report rapid onset of fatigue and show symptoms of hypoglycemia. These athletes are however easily detected and the timing of carbohydrate feeding before competition has to be individually determined.

Glycogen Loading

In untrained subjects, a period of high-fat/low-carbohydrate feeding and emptying of carbohydrate stores followed by a high-carbohydrate diet will prolong the time before hypoglycemia sets in by as much as 20%. Carbohydrate stores are however increased as part of the training adaptation to endurance capacity. Thus, in trained subjects, the effect of carbohydrate feeding is far lower and also not practical, as the reduced carbohydrate period leads to reduced training effects. The fact that carbohydrates can be supplied during most events has also reduced the need for carbohydrate feeding.

Dental Hygiene

Excessive use of sports drinks may cause dental problems, so pure water is often used for training that is <1 hour of continuous work or for training that does not have the potential to empty carbohydrate stores.

Symptoms of Hypoglycemia

- Confusion, abnormal behavior, or both, such as the inability to complete routine tasks
- Visual disturbances, such as double vision and blurred vision
- Seizures, though uncommon
- Loss of consciousness, though uncommon

Diabetes/Medical Conditions and Hypoglycemia

With diabetes, the effects of insulin on the body are drastically diminished, either because the pancreas does not produce enough insulin (type 1 diabetes) or because the body's cells are less responsive to insulin (type 2 diabetes). As a result, glucose tends to build up in the bloodstream and may reach dangerously high levels.

Intake of too much insulin relative to the amount of circulatory glucose can cause blood sugar levels to fall even resulting in hypoglycemia. Hypoglycemia may also occur after the intake of diabetes medication if insufficient glucose is ingested or if exercise is more intensive than normal. Diabetic athletes are usually experienced with these problems and are usually well regulated.

Hypoglycemia is also associated with eating disorders, medications connected to treatment of kidney failure, or with quinine, which is used to treat leg cramps and also used in the prevention and treatment of malaria.

70.6 WATER

Rigorous exercise causes body temperature to rise; the body responds by initiating heat loss through increased skin blood flow and increased sweat secretion. Of all the energy used by the body, only 25% or less is transferred to mechanical work; most of the energy represents heat production. The body's need for heat loss is primarily determined by

- The metabolic rate
- The external temperature
- Humidity and wind
- Clothing

Also, body size and body composition may affect the need for heat loss.

Fifty to sixty percent of the body mass is water. Daily water turnover without training or competition is 2 to 4 L in a temperate climate of which 0.3 to 0.4 L is lost via respiration, 0.6 to 0.8 L via skin evaporation, and the rest as urine and in the feces. One gram of carbohydrate binds approximately 3 g of water that is released as metabolic water when oxidized. Generally, metabolic water production equals the amount of water lost through respiration. Sweat losses can be substantial during hard work and can be as much as 5 L for a 70-kg male during a marathon in warm conditions, which represents 7% of body weight. Sweat rates are individual and vary for different sports but are usually in the region of 0.5 to 2 $L \times h^{-1}$. The thirst mechanism is rather insensitive and does not provide sufficient drive to induce adequate drinking. The body is less able to cope with restrictions in water intake than for food.

Performance Reduction with Water Loss

A reduced body mass of 1% to 2% due to dehydration substantially reduces aerobic power and performance, by maybe as much as 10%. The greater the dehydration level, the greater the physiological strain and the greater the inhibited aerobic performance level. This reduction in performance is less in cold environments. Dehydration of more than 2% of body mass seems to affect mental or cognitive performance negatively. Dehydration by 3% to 5% of body weight does not seem to influence muscle strength or anaerobic performance. However, a reduction in performance is shown when performing intermittent work, such as in playing soccer.

Detecting Hydration Status

Acute changes in body mass are regularly due to loss of water. Changes in body mass, both suddenly and over time, could be detected by determining body weight before and after exercise, nude and dry. A body mass diary should be kept, based upon morning body mass after urinating, which has been shown to be a stable measurement parameter (<1%) for athletes. Urine color has been shown to provide a reasonable "in-the-field" estimate.

More advanced controls of hydration status require the testing of urine and blood, though these tests are more invasive and time consuming. They include urinary volume, color, protein content, specific gravity, osmolality; or blood hematocrit, hemoglobin, plasma osmolality, sodium concentration, plasma testosterone, adrenaline, noradrenaline, cortisol, and atrial natriuretic peptide.

Rehydration

The purpose of drinking during training and competition is to keep one's hydration status stable and to prevent a decrease in exercise performance. Sweating rates are very individual and may differ from 0.4 to 1.8 $L \times h^{-1}$. It is therefore recommended that athletes monitor their body weight through a standard competition or training, to determine the water loss that should be compensated. A suggested fluid intake for a marathon runner is to drink 0.4 to 0.8 $L \times h^{-1}$ ad libitum, while more fluid will definitely be required by a faster, heavier athlete competing in a warm environment. Portions of 0.15 L every 10 to 15 minutes during a race are commonly used. There are individual reactions to drinking during a race, and it is thus important that inevent drinking skills are developed.

In some sports, such as soccer, rehydration during each 45-minute half is difficult and might thus reduce performance. However, the rehydration is equally difficult for the opponent and might keep a relative balance between the teams and athletes. A rehydration strategy at half time is of vital importance for continued performance.

After exercise, the goal is to fully replace any fluid deficits. If the recovery period is short (<12 hours), aggressive rehydration programs should be applied. If there is enough time for rehydration, the athlete is still recommended to drink 1.5 L of fluid for every kilogram of body mass lost in the competition because drinking leads to excess urine production. The fluid absorption rate is—three to four times higher directly after activity compared with resting conditions before, and though the rate falls, it stays elevated for 39 minutes after training or competition. Intravenous fluids do not seem to have any advantage over hydration strategies.

Health

When training or competing in hot environments, dehydration is the commonest cause of illness, although overhydration may lead to hyponatremia, an even more severe health problem that is discussed in the "salt/electrolytes" section below.

Dehydration increases the risk of heat exhaustion and heat stroke (20% of heat stroke hospitalizations in soldiers are commonly associated with dehydration). Dehydration combined with vomiting further increases the risk of heat stroke. Also, cardiac autonomic instability and altered intracranial volume have been associated with dehydration. Dehydration can increase the risk of acute renal failure secondary to exertional rhabdomyolosis. Rhabdomyolosis (rapid breakdown of skeletal muscle and release of potentially nephrotoxic substances) is most often observed with dehydration combined with inexperienced overexertion, and is primarily defined by a serum CK value >10 times normal.

70.7 SALT/ELECTROLYTES

There is a wide variation in salt intake and recommendations around the world. There are also substantial differences in sweat loss as well as salt content in sweat between individuals. The group of athletes that needs attention in this respect is the "salty sweaters," commonly and simplistically defined as those athletes whose training shirts or body leave salty stains when drying up. Acclimatization to heat reduces the salt content and increases the sweat rate to cope with the higher temperatures. Sodium and chloride are commonly lost with salty sweaters, whereas other electrolytes such as potassium and magnesium seem to be preserved to a higher degree. In hot conditions with high sweat rates, the salty sweaters should use sports drinks containing salt/sodium chloride. If a nonsalty sport drink is distributed, add a teaspoon of salt per liter of sports drink for these salty sweaters.

Health

Sodium deficits are associated with, but are not the only cause of, muscle cramps. Salty sweaters seem however to be more prone to muscle cramps.

Exercise-associated hyponatremia is a rapid drop of plasma sodium and has on occasions been fatal. In long-lasting races, symptomatic hyponatremia is more likely to occur in smaller, less-lean athletes who run slowly, sweat less, and drink excessive water and other hypotonic drinks before, during, and after the race.

70.8 CAFFEINE

Caffeine is included in several beverages and, if consumed in relatively modest doses, does not increase urine output or induce dehydration. Caffeine is a central stimulator that has been removed from the doping list, as its effect on performance seems to be modest (as are the potential side effects). Positive effects on performance have however been shown, but not in a dose–response manner, so that a modest dose (<6 mg $\times$ kg^{-1}) seems to have the same effect as higher doses. Many endurance athletes seem to prefer the use of caffeine-enriched sports drinks in the latter part of longer races.

70.9   PROTEIN

A 70-kg male with normal body composition contains approximately 17 kg of proteins. Proteins are the body's building blocks and are the main content of muscles, skin, and other organs. The human body contains more than 10,000 different proteins. There are eight essential amino acids that are necessary to form the protein mass of the body. Protein from milk, meat, fish, and eggs contains all the essential amino acids, whereas proteins from grains, soy, and vegetables do not. A nonsports person uses approximately 1 g of protein per kilogram of body mass a day to maintain body composition. The body turns over the total amount of body protein every 250 days. With heavy training and competition, protein turnover increases by 2 to 3 fold, dependent upon the type of training. Morphological adaptations to training are primarily protein synthesis, dependent upon available amounts of protein. As most athletes eat more food than the average population, they usually ingest enough protein unless they are totally addicted to junk food. Unlike the other nutrients carbohydrates and fat, the body does not have separate stores for protein. Excess protein is synthesized to and stored as fat. Recent research has shown that if proteins containing essential amino acids are consumed directly after exercise, then training responses can be enhanced significantly as opposed to waiting two hours before taking a meal. The reason seems to be that the protein synthesis triggered by training might be reduced if enough protein or amino acids are not available. There is no evidence to suggest that the ingestion of separate amino acid supplements enhances sports performance.

Protein seems not to be an important nutrient during competition or training but might help directly after training or competition to assist the protein synthesis.

There do not seem to be any health issues directly linked to moderate protein feeding of 1 to 3 g per kilogram of body mass per day.

70.10   FAT

Fat provides energy stores, and even slimmer athletes regularly have fat stores that are sufficient for competitions and training. Sports training and competition are regularly performed at a high intensity and thus are more carbohydrate than fat dependent. Endurance athletes also regularly have higher VO$_{2max}$ than the rest of the population; the ability to use fat as an energy source is dependent upon the percentage VO$_{2max}$ the activity represents. In everyday nontraining activities, athletes thus burn more fat than the average population. It is a common misunderstanding that low-intensity training burns the most fat, as recent studies and physiological deduction have shown that increased VO$_{2max}$ is the decisive component, for which training with higher aerobic intensities are more efficient. Fat is regularly a part of an athlete's diet with approximately 15%.

There is no evidence that fat plays a role in inevent or postevent nutrition. Fat is not linked to inevent or postevent health issues.

70.11   CREATINE

Creatine is a nutrient, an amino acid that is usually found in normal diets. One kilogram of fresh steak contains 5 g of creatine. Its use as an ergogenic aid is widespread. Creatine is stored in muscle as PCr and helps the regeneration of ATP in the muscle. PCr stored in the muscle can supply energy for up to a 6- to 8- second all-out event such as a maximal sprint and is regenerated after <1 minute's rest. A possible performance enhancement effect has not been clearly shown. Increased PCr stores in the muscle could theoretically improve performance in repetitive sprints with breaks of <1 minute. However, increased PCr stores seem to occur after training with repeated sprints. Performance enhancement is thus most likely observed with repeated sprints in subjects untrained in that specific respect. Secondly, increased PCr stored in the body binds water and increases body weight, typically 1 to 2 kg in a 3- to 5-day creatine loading, and more over time. In sports where body mass has to be carried, the increased mass will reduce acceleration and subsequently require higher energy demands that may counteract any improvement in repeated sprints. A possible performance enhancement seems thus to be limited to situations where the body weight is not fully carried, at least not uphill, such as in cycling and rowing. In sports where body weight is the driving force—such as bobsleigh, luge, downhill skiing, or certain contact sports (rugby or American football) or throwing sports (discus, shot put)—the story might be different. There are no indications that creatine feeding induces health problems.

Recommended Reading

American College of Sports Medicine, American Dietetic Association, Dietitians of Canada. Nutrition and athletic performance. *Med Sci Sports Exerc.* 2000;32(12):2130–2145.

Hoff J, Helgerud J. Endurance and strength training for soccer players: physiological considerations. *Sports Med.* 2004;34(3):165–180.

Maughan RJ. Fluid and carbohydrate intake during exercise. In: Burke LM, Deakin V, eds. *Clinical Sports Nutrition.* 2nd ed. Sydney: McGraw Hill; 2000:369–395.

Maughan RJ, Burke LM. *Handbook of Sports Medicine and Science; Sports Nutrition.* Oxford: Blackwell Publishing; 2002.

Maughan RJ, Shirreffs SM. Nutrition and hydration concerns of the female football player. *Br J Sports Med.* 2007;41(Suppl 1):i60–i63.

Sawka MN, Burke LM, Eichner ER, et al. American College of Sports Medicine position stand: exercise and fluid replacement. *Med Sci Sports Exerc.* 2007;39(2):377–390.

Siegel AJ, Januzzi J, Sluss P et al. Cardiac biomarkers, electrolytes, and other analytes in collapsed marathon runners. *Am J Clin Pathol.* 2008;129:948–951.

Stofan JR, Zachwieja JJ, Horswill CA, et al. Sweat and sodium losses in NCAA football players: a precursor to heat cramps? *Int J Sport Nutr Exerc Metab.* 2005;15(6):641–652.

Rehrer NJ, Burke LM. Sweat losses during various sports. *Aust J Nutr Diet.* 1996;53(Suppl 4):S13–S16.

CHAPTER 71 — Diabetic Emergencies

Contributed by Kathryn E. Ackerman, Harvard Medical School, Childrens Hospital, Boston, USA

Reviewers: Dr. Margo Hudson and Dr. Katharina Grimm, FIFA

Diabetes mellitus (DM) is a chronic endocrine disorder characterized by hyperglycemia caused by either decreased insulin secretion, decreased insulin action, or both. While the health benefits of physical activity are numerous, diabetic athletes should be evaluated before beginning an exercise program. The physician must exclude conditions that predispose to injury (severe autonomic or peripheral neuropathy, preproliferative or proliferative retinopathy, and macular edema) or cardiovascular disease (uncontrolled hypertension). The physician must also advise against certain types of exercise (e.g., those requiring valsalva maneuvers, such as powerlifting, or exercises performed at high altitudes).

71.1 TYPES OF DM

Type 1 DM accounts for 10% to 15% of all cases of diabetes. It is characterized by the destruction of beta cells, leading to deficient insulin production but normal insulin sensitivity. Type 2 DM accounts for the vast majority of the other 85% to 90% of cases.

It is characterized by variable abnormalities in insulin secretion and insulin sensitivity. Both types of diabetes, in the uncontrolled state, will have increased hepatic glucose output and decreased glucose uptake in muscle and adipose tissue. However, in general, only patients with type 1 DM are at risk of severe lipolysis leading to diabetic ketoacidosis (DKA).

Other secondary causes of DM have been recognized and new categories of DM are being added as we learn more about genetic and environmental predisposing factors. But for the team physician considering treatment modalities, it is most important to know if the athlete's disease is more similar to type 1 or type 2.

Also, knowing the athlete's general diabetes control is important in anticipating his or her response to athletic activity and medical treatment. Thus, in this chapter, variations of DM will only be referred to under the global categories of "type 1" and "type 2."

71.2 TYPES OF DM TREATMENT

The primary goal of diabetes management is to keep blood glucose as close to the normal range as possible, without causing hypoglycemia. Various baseline therapies exist. For some individuals with type 2 DM, this may include a form of insulin. For type 1 DM, insulin is always indicated. Types of insulin are listed in Table 71.1. Preferences and availability differ worldwide; however, premixed combination insulins are falling out of favor and are suboptimal in athletes whose insulin needs will fluctuate dramatically throughout the day depending on activity level.

Oral hypoglycemic agents and noninsulin injectables are listed in Table 71.2. It is important to know if an athlete on oral agents is on a drug that has the ability to contribute to hypoglycemia, such as sulfonylureas and meglitinides.

71.3 HYPOGLYCEMIA

There are many factors that need to be considered in understanding the development of hypoglycemia during exercise. Factors include exercise intensity

TABLE 71.1 Types of Insulin

Human Insulin and Insulin Analogs	Time of Onset of Action	Peak of Action	Duration of Action
Rapid-acting			
Aspart, glulisine, lispro	10–15 min	1–2 h	3–5 h
Short-acting			
Regular	0.5–1 h	2–4	4–8 h
Intermediate-acting			
NPH	1–3 h	4–10 h	10–18 h
Long-acting			
Detemir	1 h	none	up to 24 h
Glargine	2–3 h	none	24+ h
Premixed insulin			
Aspart mix 70/30 (70% aspart protamine + 30% aspart)	10–20 min	1–4 h	10–16 h
Lispro mix 75/25 (75% lispro protamine + 25% lispro)	10–15 min	1–3 h	10–16 h
Lispro mix 50/50 (50% lispro protamine + 50% lispro)	10–15 min	1–3 h	10–16 h
70/30 (70% NPH + 30% regular)	0.5–1 h	2–10 h	10–18 h
50/50 (50% NPH + 50% regular)	0.5–1 h	2–10 h	10–18 h

and duration, blood glucose concentrations before initiating exercise, the time relation of exercise to meals, basal/bolus insulin doses, an individual's physical fitness level, his or her insulin sensitivity, and the adequacy of his or her counterregulatory responses to exercise.

In people without DM, insulin levels decrease during exercise, but in DM patients who take exogenous insulin, levels do not decrease with activity. Increased insulin impairs hepatic glucose production and can induce hypoglycemia 30 to 60 minutes after exercise begins. Counterregulatory hormones (e.g., glucagon, catecholamines, growth hormone, glucocorticoids) may be impaired in patients with neuropathy or frequent hypoglycemic episodes. In addition, exercise improves insulin sensitivity in skeletal muscle, leading to postexercise, late-onset hypoglycemia, often at night when the athlete is sleeping. In fact, in patients with type 1 DM, exercise increases the risk of severe hypoglycemia up to 31 hours after cessation of activity.

In general, signs and symptoms of hypoglycemia occur when blood glucose drops below 70 mg per dL (3.9 mmol per L), but this number varies among individuals. Sweating, tachycardia, palpitations, hunger, nervousness, trembling, headache, and dizziness are early autonomic symptoms. Unfortunately, these are often hard to differentiate from responses experienced during vigorous exercise. If the blood glucose level continues to fall, neuroglycopenic symptoms may be observed and include fatigue, blurry vision, impaired cognition, loss of coordination, aggression, confusion, seizures, and loss of consciousness. Each individual has his or her own specific response to hypoglycemia, and ideally the team physician should be familiar with these prior to the athlete's sport participation.

This poses particular problems for the EP who may know very little about the athlete's diabetic status. Table 71.3 shows an action plan for hypoglycemia and initiating or returning to play.

TABLE 71.2 Types of Oral Hypoglycemic Agents and Noninsulin Injectables

Drug	Mechanism of Action	Peak of Action	Duration of Action	Risk of Hypoglycemia
Sulfonylureas	Stimulate insulin release			Yes
Glimepiride		2–3 h	24 h	
Glipizide		1–3 h	12–24 h	
Glipizide GITS		6–12 h	24 h	
Glyburide		4 h	12–24 h	
Micronized glyburide		2 h	12–24 h	
Meglitinides	Stimulate insulin release			Yes
Nateglinide		20 min	4 h	
Repaglinide		1 h	4–6 h	
Biguanides	Decrease hepatic glucose production			No
Metformin		2–3 h	12–18 h	
Metformin extended release		4–8 h	24 h	
α-Glucosidase inhibitors	Slow gut carbohydrate absorption	N/A	2–3 h	No
Acarbose		N/A	2–3 h	
Miglitol		N/A	2–3 h	
Thiazolidinediones	Increase peripheral insulin sensitivity			No
Pioglitazone		N/A	days–weeks	
Rosiglitazone		N/A	days–weeks	
DPP-IV inhibitors	Increase glucose-dependent insulin release and suppress glucagon release			No
Sitagliptin		1–4 h	24+ h	
Incretin mimetics	Increase glucose-dependent insulin release and suppress glucagon release			No
Exenatide[a]		1–2 h	6–8	
Amylin analogs	Suppress glucagon release, delay gastric emptying, and promote satiety			No
Pramlintide[a]		20 min	3 h	

[a]Injectable medication.

TABLE 71.3 Action Plan for Hypoglycemia

Mild Hypoglycemia[a]	Severe Hypoglycemia[b]	Postexercise, Late-Onset Hypoglycemia
Check blood glucose	Check blood glucose if possible—exclude other causes of change in mental status	Check blood glucose
Based on blood glucose: • If glucose > 50 mg/dL, administer 15 g of fast-acting solid or liquid carbohydrate[c] • If glucose ≤ 50 mg/dL, administer 25–30 g of fast-acting solid or liquid carbohydrate[c]	Activate emergency medical system and mix and administer glucagon injection from glucagon kit[d] or administer 50% dextrose IV Assess response • If athlete does not respond to glucagon or 50% dextrose, transfer to medical facility • If athlete has regained consciousness and is able to swallow, have athlete eat complex carbohydrate[e]	Based on blood glucose: • If glucose > 50 mg/dL, administer 15 g of fast-acting solid or liquid carbohydrate[c] • If glucose ≤ 50 mg/dL, administer 25–30 g of fast-acting solid or liquid carbohydrate[c]
Recheck blood glucose in 15 min If glucose still low, administer another 15 g of fact-acting carbohydrate[c] and add 15 g of complex carbohydrate[e] to sustain effect Recheck blood glucose in 15 min • If glucose in normal range, athlete is *not* on a long-acting glucose lowering medication, and is feeling better, monitor for 15 to 30 min and then consider allowing return to play • If athlete is on a long-acting glucose-lowering drug, continue to monitor and do not allow return to play until after peak of medication has passed	Continue to monitor Do not allow same-day return to play and assess cause (eg, medication dosing) before allowing resumption of physical activity in future	Recheck blood glucose in 15 min If glucose still low, administer another 15 g of fact-acting carbohydrate[c] and add 15 g of complex carbohydrate[e] to sustain effect Continue to monitor blood sugar periodically; note time of postactivity hypoglycemia to plan snack or decrease in medication after future activity (e.g., if hypoglycemia during night, decrease bedtime insulin and consider bedtime snack)

[a]Athlete is conscious and can follow commands.
[b]Athlete is unconscious, unable to follow commands, and/or unable to swallow.
[c]Examples: glucose tablets or gel, hard candy, juice, honey
[d]Because glucagon may cause nausea and/or vomiting, make sure athlete is on his or her side to prevent aspiration.
[e]Examples: crackers, bagel.

TABLE 71.4	Action Plan for Hyperglycemia and Returning to Play Considerations	
Type of Individual with DM	**Fasting Blood Glucose (≥4 h after eating a meal)**	**Comments**
Adult or child with type 1 DM	≥250 mg/dL (13.9 mmol/L)	Check for ketones, and if positive, do not exercise. Treat DKA.[a]
	251–300 mg/dL (14–16.7 mmol/L)	Check for ketones, and if negative, OK to perform physical activity.[b]
	>300 mg/dL (16.7 mmol/L)	Check for ketones, and if negative, may exercise with extreme caution.[b]
Child with type 1 DM	≥250 mg/dL (13.9 mmol/L)	Check for ketones, and if positive, do not exercise. Treat DKA.[a]
	251–350 mg/dL (14–19.5 mmol/L)	Check for ketones, and if negative, OK to perform physical activity.[b]
	>350 mg/dL (19.5 mmol/L)	Do not exercise. Hydrate and adjust insulin/dietary regimen.[a]
Adult or child with type 2 DM	≤350 mg/dL (19.5 mmol/L)	May exercise.[b]
	>350 mg/dL (19.5 mmol/L)	Do not exercise. Hydrate and adjust medication/dietary regimen.[a]

[a]If the athlete experiences a change in mental status that does not improve within 15 min of treatment, he or she should be taken immediately to the hospital.
[b]Continue to monitor blood glucose during activity. If blood glucose ≥ renal glucose threshold of 180 mg/dL (10 mmol/L), have athlete increase consumption of non-carbohydrate beverage to avoid dehydration.

71.4 HYPERGLYCEMIA

Exercise may cause hyperglycemia in patients with DM. In athletes who are underinsulinized and/or have poor baseline control, exercise (particularly high-intensity exercise) leads to increases in blood glucose levels and may eventually lead to Diabetic Ketoacidosis (DKA). High-intensity exercise is associated with increases in catecholamines, free fatty acids, and ketones, all of which decrease muscle glucose utilization and increase blood glucose. In the well-controlled athlete, these changes may be transient (decreasing in 30 to 60 minutes), but poor insulin balance along with stress regarding sports performance may increase counterregulatory hormones and perpetuate the hyperglycemia (Table 71.4).

71.5 PREVENTION

Each athlete with DM should have a care plan for training as well as for matches/games/races. These should include the elements listed in Table 71.5

and should be familiar and available to the coach, team physician, and EP.

Fasting glucose should be checked, following guidelines in Table 71.4. The pre-exercise meal should be ingested 1 to 3 hours before the activity and should consist of low glycogenic index foods and include protein to ensure continuous, but not too rapid, glucose absorption. Immediately prior to the activity, the athlete should check blood sugar again, with an ideal goal of 120 to 180 mg per dL (6.7 to 10 mmol/L). The athlete should continue to monitor his or her blood glucose throughout the sporting activity, supplement with carbohydrates when needed, and continue to hydrate and reassess every 30 to 60 minutes depending on his or her baseline control and exercise level.

Often, as athletes become more experienced with their glucose control and training habits, these intervals may lengthen. Elite athletes often get to an awareness of their personal responses to exercise such that they know when to consume extra carbohydrates or check their blood sugar based on exercise duration and/or symptoms.

TABLE 71.5 Diabetes Care Plan

Blood glucose monitoring	• Working lactometer, lancets, test strips • Pre-exercise exclusion values • Recommendations for monitoring frequency
Medication list	• Insulin: type, dose, frequency; insulin adjustment plan based on activity and correction doses for hyperglycemia • Other meds used by athlete
Hypoglycemia guidelines	• Symptoms and typical blood glucose level of symptomatic hypoglycemia • Plan for hypoglycemia: glucose source, amount of glucose, and instructions for glucagon (glucagon injection kit should be readily available)
Hyperglycemia guidelines	• Symptoms and typical blood glucose level of symptomatic hyperglycemia • Plan for hyperglycemia correction • Ketone test strips if DM type 1
Emergency contact information	• Family member and physician contact information, as well as consent for medical treatment
Medical alert tag	• With athlete at all times

Those using insulin should inject in areas away from exercising muscles approximately 1 hour before activity, as exercise, massage, and heat can increase rate of absorption. If possible, the athlete should try to anticipate the intensity and duration of activity to better adjust insulin dosing and carbohydrate intake. See Table 71.6 for a guide.

INSULIN PUMPS

DM individuals using insulin pumps receive insulin through a continuous subcutaneous infusion. They may have basal insulin settings that are consistent throughout the day (e.g., 1.0 unit per hour for 24 hours) or vary (e.g., 0.5 unit per hour from midnight to 6 AM, 1.2 unit per hour from 6 AM to 12 PM, 1.0 unit per hour from 12 PM to 5 PM, 1.4 unit per hour from 5 PM to midnight). In addition, pump users have bolus insulin doses administered prior to meals. Insulin pump settings may be adjusted prior to activity based on trial and error similarly to injectable insulin guidelines in Table 71.6.

Depending on the activity and athlete preference, pump users may discontinue the pump during sport and switch to injectable insulin. If the pump is removed before physical activity, hyperglycemia is more of a risk and a long-acting injectable insulin should be

TABLE 71.6 Injectable Insulin Adjustment Guidelines[a]

Activity	Duration	Peaking Insulin Adjustment
Low, moderate, or high intensity	<30 min	No adjustment
Low intensity	30 to > 60 min	Decrease by 5%
Moderate intensity	30–60 min	Decrease by 10%
	>60 min	Decrease by 20%
High intensity	30–60 min	Decrease by 20%
	>60 min	Decrease by 30%

[a]Individual needs vary.

used appropriately. If the pump is continued during activity, pump malfunction or detachment (e.g., from contact or sweat) may lead to hyperglycemia, overinsulinization and subsequent hypoglycemia. Insulinpump athletes who experience hyperglycemia or hypoglycemia should always have their pumps examined at the beginning of the athlete assessment.

71.6 CONCLUSIONS

While general guidelines may be helpful for treatment of a diabetic athlete, individual treatment based on the athlete's diabetes information and care plan is more important. The athlete should keep a log of glucose levels, dosing with insulin and other medications, dietary intake, and exercise to better understand his or her individual dietary and medication needs with various activities. Such knowledge, with ongoing adjustments, will improve glucose control and help prevent hypo/hyperglycemia. In the event of hypoglycemia or hyperglycemia, the severity and cause of such an episode must be kept in mind when making return-to-play decisions.

ACKNOWLEDGMENT

Special thanks are due to Dr. Margo Hudson for her review and suggestions.

Recommended Reading

Albright A, Franz M, Hornsby G, et al. American College of Sports Medicine position stand. Exercise and type 2 diabetes. *Med Sci Sports Exerc*. 2000;32(7):1345–1360.

American College of Sports Medicine and American Diabetes Association joint position statement. Diabetes mellitus and exercise. *Med Sci Sports Exerc*. 997;29(12):I–vi.

American Diabetes Association Web site. http://www.diabetes.org. Accessed April 17, 2011.

Beazer RS. *Joslin's Diabetes Desk Book: A Guide for Primary Care Providers*. 2nd ed. Boston, MA: Joslin Diabetes Center; 2007.

Diabetes Exercise and Sports Association Web site. http://www.diabetes-exercise.org. Accessed April 17, 2011.

Modigliani G, Iazzetta N, Corigliano M, Strollo F. Blood glucose changes in diabetic children and adolescents engaged in most common sports activities. *Acta Biomed*. 2006;77(Suppl 1):26–33.

Inzucchi SE. *Diabetes Facts and Guidelines*. New Haven, CT: Yale Diabetes Center/Takeda; 2007.

Jimenez CC, Corcoran MH, Crawley JT, et al. National athletic trainers' association position statement: management of the athlete with type 1 diabetes mellitus. *J Athl Train*. 2007;42(4):536–545.

Sigal RJ, Kenny GP, Wasserman DH, et al. Physical activity/exercise and type 2 diabetes: a consensus statement from the American Diabetes Association. *Diabetes Care*. 2006;29(6):1433–1438.

CHAPTER 72 — Drowning and Immersion Accidents

Contributed by Suzanne Shepherd, Associate Professor of Emergency Medicine, Hospital of the University of Pennsylvania, Philadelphia, United States

Reviewer: David McDonagh

Drowning incidents at organized sports events are extremely rare. However, incidents can occur, and if the event physician is involved with water sports, he or she must be alert to predisposing causes, potential dangers, diagnostic paradigms, and treatment modalities. For open-water swimming events, the EP must evaluate existing rescue plans before an event, ensure that well-functioning warning systems are in place, ensure that communication systems function and that staff are trained in these systems, ensure that staff are positioned in such a manner that they have rapid access to the athlete, and finally that they have the necessary competence and equipment to treat all categories of submersion incidents.

Drowning has been defined as death secondary to asphyxia while immersed in a liquid, usually water, or within 24 hours of submersion.

At the 2002 World Congress on Drowning, held in Amsterdam, a group of experts suggested a new consensus definition for drowning in order to decrease the confusion over the number of terms and definitions (>20) referring to this process that have appeared in the literature. The group believed that a uniform definition would allow more accurate analysis and comparison of studies, allow researchers to draw more meaningful conclusions from pooled data, and improve the ease of surveillance and prevention activities.

The new definition states that drowning is a process resulting in primary respiratory impairment from submersion in a liquid medium. Implicit to this definition is that a liquid–air interface is present at the victim's airway. Outcome may include delayed morbidity or death, death, or life without morbidity. The terms *wet drowning*, *dry drowning*, *active* or *passive drowning*, *near drowning*, *secondary drowning*, and *silent drowning* would be discarded.

The classic image of a victim helplessly gasping and thrashing in the water rarely is reported. A more ominous scenario of a motionless individual floating in the water or quietly disappearing beneath the surface is more typical.

72.1 PATHOPHYSIOLOGY

The principal physiologic consequences of drowning are prolonged hypoxemia and acidosis.

After initial gasping and possible aspiration, immersion stimulates hyperventilation, followed by voluntary apnea and a variable degree and duration of laryngospasm. This leads to hypoxemia. Depending upon the degree of hypoxemia and resultant acidosis, the person may develop myocardial dysfunction and electrical instability, cardiac arrest, and central nervous system (CNS) ischemia. Asphyxia leads to relaxation of the airway, which permits the lungs to take in water in many individuals (previously referred to as *wet drowning*), although most patients aspirate <4 mL per kg of fluid. Approximately 10% to 20% of individuals maintain tight laryngospasm until cardiac arrest occurs and inspiratory efforts have ceased. These victims do not aspirate any appreciable fluid (previously referred to as *dry drowning*). Most individuals are found after having been submerged in liquid for an unobserved period of time.

In young children suddenly immersed in cold water (<20°C), the mammalian diving reflex may occur and produce apnea, bradycardia, and vasoconstriction of nonessential vascular beds with shunting of blood to the coronary and cerebral circulation.

The target organ of submersion injury is the lung. Aspiration of 1 to 3 mL per kg of fluid leads to significantly impaired gas exchange. Injury to other systems is largely secondary to hypoxia and ischemic acidosis. Additional CNS insult may result from concomitant head or spinal cord injury. Fluid aspirated into the lungs produces vagally mediated pulmonary vasoconstriction and hypertension. Fresh water moves rapidly across the alveolar–capillary membrane into the microcirculation. Surfactant is destroyed, producing alveolar instability, atelectasis, and decreased compliance with marked ventilation/perfusion (V/Q) mismatching. As much as 75% of blood flow may circulate through hypoventilated lungs.

In salt water near drowning, surfactant washout occurs, and protein-rich fluid exudates rapidly into the alveoli and pulmonary interstitium. Compliance is reduced, the alveolar–capillary basement membrane is damaged directly, and shunting occurs. This results in rapid induction of serious hypoxia. Fluid-induced bronchospasm also may contribute to hypoxia.

Pulmonary hypertension may occur secondary to inflammatory mediator release. In a minor percentage of patients, aspiration of vomitus, sand, silt, stagnant water, and sewage may result in occlusion of bronchi, bronchospasm, pneumonia, abscess formation, and inflammatory damage to alveolar capillary membranes. Postobstructive pulmonary edema following laryngeal spasm and hypoxic neuronal injury with resultant neurogenic pulmonary edema may also play roles. Uncommon pathogens, such as *Aeromonas*, *Pseudallescheria*, and *Burkholderia*, cause a significant portion of pneumonia in these patients. As such, pneumonia may present late and atypically.

CNS injury has proven to be a major determinant of subsequent outcome. If the period of ischemia is limited or the individual rapidly develops core hypothermia, injury may be limited and the individual may recover with minor neurologic sequelae.

Resultant autonomic instability may lead to hypertension, tachycardia, diaphoresis, agitation, and muscle rigidity. Rhabdomyolysis and acute tubular necrosis are also well-recognized sequelae of drowning.

72.2 CAUSES

- Water sports hazards, especially with personal watercraft
- Poor judgment and substance abuse (alcohol or other recreational drugs) in conjunction with boat operation

- Cervical spine injury and head trauma associated with surfing, water skiing, jet skiing, and scuba diving accidents
- In preschool-aged children, drownings occur most commonly in residential swimming pools.
- Many residential pools have no physical barrier between the pool and the home.
- Open gates are involved in up to 70% of drownings in cases involving fenced-in pools. Pools may also be accessed through unlocked windows when the pool area abuts the house.
- Young adults typically drown in ponds, lakes, rivers, and oceans. Approximately 90% of drownings occur within 10 yards of safety.
- Cervical spine injuries and head trauma, which result from diving into water that may be shallow or contain rocks and other hazards, have been implicated.
- Alcohol and, to a lesser extent, other recreational drugs are implicated in many cases. Australian, Scottish, and Canadian data showed that 30% to 50% of older adolescents and adults who drowned in boating incidents were inebriated, as determined by blood alcohol concentrations.
- Consider underlying disease/illness in all age groups.
  - Seizure disorder
  - Myocardial infarction (MI) or syncopal episode
  - Poor neuromuscular control, such as that seen with significant arthritis, Parkinson disease, or other neurologic disorders
  - Major depression/suicide
  - Anxiety/panic disorder
  - Diabetes, hypoglycemia
  - Other injuries (e.g., bites, stings, lacerations)

72.3 FREQUENCY

United States: Drowning deaths number more than 8,000 per year, with 1,500 of these deaths occurring in children. In 1995, the US Consumer Product Safety Commission found an overall submersion injury/death rate of 1.93 cases per 100,000 population in all age groups, with a peak of 3.22 cases per 100,000 children younger than 4 years. In 2002, the Centers for Disease Control and Prevention reported that 3,447 individuals had died secondary to unintentional drowning, with 1,158 (34%) of these individuals younger than 19 years. In fact, a bimodal distribution of deaths is observed, with an initial peak in the toddler age group and a second peak in adolescent to young adult males. In the toddler group, most incidents occur in bathtubs and swimming pools. In the adolescent and young adult groups (aged 15 to 24 years), most incidents occur in natural bodies of water. For every death from drowning, an estimated four individuals are hospitalized and 14 individuals visit the ED.

Despite preventive measures, the 1997 National Center for Health Statistics found drowning second only to motor vehicle collisions (MVCs) as the most common cause of injury and death in children aged 1 month to 14 years.

An additional 1,200 reported immersion deaths are boating related (90% of boating deaths), 500 are motor vehicle associated, and 1,000 reported drownings are of undetermined etiology. Scuba diving accounts for an estimated 700 to 800 deaths per year (etiologies include inadequate experience/training, exhaustion, panic, carelessness, and barotrauma).

Submersion-related injuries are the fifth leading cause of accidental death in the United States in all age groups; incidence is approximately 2.5 to 3.5 per 100,000 population. California reports approximately 25,000 ocean rescues on its beaches each year. However, true incidence of near drowning has yet to be defined accurately, since many cases are not reported.

International: Annually, approximately 150,000 deaths are reported worldwide from drowning, with an annual incidence probably closer to 500,000. Several of the most densely populated nations in the world fail to report near-drowning incidents. This, along with the fact that many cases are never brought to medical attention, renders accurate worldwide incidence approximation virtually impossible.

The incidence of near drowning has an estimated range of 20 to 500 times the rate of drowning.

72.4 MORTALITY/MORBIDITY

Morbidity and death in immersion injuries are due primarily to laryngospasm and pulmonary injury, resulting hypoxemia and acidosis, and their effects on the brain and other organ systems.

Prevention is as important as any measures that can be taken after the fact.

A high risk of death exists secondary to the development of adult respiratory distress syndrome (ARDS), which has been termed *postimmersion syndrome* or *secondary drowning*. Morbidity is due to neurologic insult as well as to multiple organ system failure.

The adult mortality rate is difficult to quantify because of poor reporting and inconsistent record keeping.

Thirty-five percent of immersion episodes in children are fatal; 33% result in some degree of neurologic impairment and 11% in severe neurologic sequelae.

In 2002, per CDC data, approximately 2,822 individuals were treated for drowning in US emergency departments.

72.5 HISTORY

The age of the victim, submersion time, water temperature, water tonicity, degree of water contamination, symptoms, associated injuries (especially cervical spine and head), presence of coingestants, underlying medical conditions, type and timing of rescue and resuscitation efforts, and response to initial resuscitation are all relevant factors.

Thermal conduction of water is 25 to 30 times that of air. The temperature of thermally neutral water, in which a nude individual's heat production balances heat loss, is 33°C.

Physical exertion increases heat loss secondary to convection/conduction up to 35% to 50% faster.

A significant risk of hypothermia usually develops in water temperatures <25°C, which is the temperature found in most US natural waters during the majority of the year.

Other important historical factors include the following:

- Shortness of breath, difficulty breathing, apnea

- Persistent cough, wheezing

- In stream, lake, or salt water immersion, possible aspiration of foreign material

- Level of consciousness at presentation, history of loss of consciousness, anxiety

- Vomiting, diarrhea

- Coincident alcohol or drug use

- Pertinent past medical history, particularly seizure disorder, diabetes mellitus, psychiatric history, severe arthritis, or neuromuscular disorder
- Bradycardia or tachycardia, dysrhythmia

72.6 PHYSICAL

A victim of a submersion incident may be classified initially into one of the following four groups:

- Asymptomatic
- Symptomatic (three groups)
  - Altered vital signs (e.g., hypothermia, tachycardia, bradycardia)
    - Anxious appearance
    - Tachypnea, dyspnea, or hypoxia: If dyspnea occurs, no matter how slight, the patient is considered symptomatic.
    - Metabolic acidosis (may exist in asymptomatic patients as well)
    - Altered level of consciousness, neurologic deficit
  - Cardiopulmonary arrest
    - Apnea
    - Asystole (55%), ventricular tachycardia/fibrillation (29%), bradycardia (16%)
    - Immersion syndrome
  - Obviously dead
    - Normothermic with asystole
    - Apnea
    - Rigor mortis
    - Dependent lividity
    - No apparent CNS function

72.7 TREATMENT

Bystanders should call 911 or equivalent immediately. They should never assume the individual is unsalvageable unless it is patently obvious that the individual has been dead for quite a while. If they suspect injury, they should move the individual the least amount possible and begin CPR.

Prehospital care is focused on the following important points:

- Optimal prehospital care is a significant determinant of outcome in the management of immersion victims. The victim should be removed from the water at the earliest opportunity. Rescue breathing should be performed while the individual is still in water, but chest compressions are inadequate because of buoyancy issues.

The patient should be removed from the water with attention to cervical spine precautions. If possible, the individual should be lifted out in a prone position. Theoretically, hypotension may follow lifting the individual out in an upright manner because of the relative change in pressure surrounding the body from water to air. Management of the ABCs is the priority, with particular attention to securing the earliest possible airway and providing adequate oxygenation and ventilation.

- In the patient with an altered mental status, the airway should be checked for foreign material and vomitus.
- Intrinsic compressions to remove water from the lungs is not recommended, as they have proven not to remove fluid, delay the start of resuscitation, and risk causing the patient to vomit and aspirate, and ventilation is achieved even if fluid is present in the lung. If the rescuer is unable to ventilate the patient, then an airway clearing method should be attempted.
- Immediately place the patient on 100% oxygen by mask. If available, continuous noninvasive pulse oximetry is optimal. If the patient remains dyspneic on 100% oxygen, or manifests a low oxygen saturation, use CPAP, if available. If it is not available, consider early intubation, with appropriate use of PEEP.

- Immobilize the neck if the patient has facial or head injury, is unable to give an adequate history, or may have been involved in a diving accident or MVA.

- Begin rewarming. Wet clothing is ideally removed before the victim is wrapped in warming blankets.

Emergency Department Care

Initial management of near drowning should place emphasis on immediate resuscitation and treatment of respiratory failure. Evaluate associated injuries early, as a cervical spine injury may complicate airway management. Provide all victims of a submersion injury with supplemental oxygen during their evaluations.

- ET intubation: Intubation may be required in order to provide adequate oxygenation in a patient unable to maintain a pO_2 of >60 to 70 mm Hg (>80 mm Hg in children) on 100% oxygen by face mask.

- In the alert, cooperative patient, use a trial of bilevel positive airway pressure (BiPAP)/CPAP, if available, to provide adequate oxygenation before intubation is performed.
- Other criteria for ET intubation include the following:
  - Altered level of consciousness and inability to protect airway or handle secretions
  - High alveolar–arterial (A-a) gradient: PaO_2 of 60 to 80 mm Hg or less on 15 L oxygen nonrebreathing mask
  - Respiratory failure: $PaCO_2 > 45$ mm Hg
  - Worsening ABG results
- Intubated victims of submersion injury may require PEEP with mechanical ventilation to maintain adequate oxygenation. PEEP has been shown to improve ventilation patterns in the noncompliant lung in several ways, including (1) shifting interstitial pulmonary water into the capillaries, (2) increasing lung volume via prevention of expiratory airway collapse, (3) providing better alveolar ventilation and decreasing capillary blood flow, and (4) increasing the diameter of both small and large airways to improve distribution of ventilation.
- Extra corporal membrane oxygenation (ECMO) has been shown to be helpful in individuals who remain hypoxic despite aggressive mechanical ventilation.
- Bronchoscopy may be needed to remove foreign material, such as aspirated debris or vomitus plugs, from the airway.

■ Rewarming: Hypothermic patients with core temperatures <30°C who have undergone sudden, rapid immersion may display slowing of metabolism and preferential shunting of blood to the heart, brain, and lungs, which may exert a protective effect during submersion. This is not, however, the case with most immersion victims, who have become hypothermic gradually and are at risk for ventricular fibrillation and neurologic injury. As such, vigorously rewarm hypothermic patients to normothermia.

- Many authors have postulated that a primitive mammalian diving reflex may be responsible for survival after extended immersion in cold water. The mechanism for this reflex has been postulated to be reflex inhibition of the respiratory center (apnea), bradycardia, and vasoconstriction of nonessential capillary beds triggered by the sensory stimulus of cold water touching the face; these responses preserve the circulation to the heart and brain and conserve oxygen, thereby prolonging survival. The sudden temperature drop may depress cellular metabolism significantly, limiting the harmful effects of hypoxia and metabolic acidosis.
- Place a nasogastric tube to assist in rewarming efforts and urinary catheter to assess urine output.
- Core rewarming with warmed oxygen, continuous bladder lavage with fluid at 40°C, and IV infusion of isotonic fluids at 40°C should be initiated during resuscitation.
- Warm peritoneal lavage may be required for core rewarming in patients with severe hypothermia.
- A cascade unit on the ventilator provides warm inspired air.
- Thoracotomy with open heart massage and warm mediastinal lavage may be effective. The hypothermic heart is typically unresponsive to pharmacotherapy and countershock.
- Extracorporeal blood rewarming may be used in patients with severe hypothermia who do not respond to lavage/thoracotomy or who are in arrest.
- Attempt central venous access cautiously in these patients in order to avoid stimulation of the hypothermic atrium and resultant dysrhythmias.
- Do not abandon resuscitation of a submersion victim until the patient has been warmed to a minimum of 30°C.

■ Initiate appropriate treatment of hypoglycemia and other electrolyte imbalances; seizures; bronchospasm; and cold-induced bronchorrhea, dysrhythmias, and hypotension, as necessary.

■ Patient disposition depends on the history, presence of associated injuries, and degree of immersion injury.

- Patients able to relay a good history of minor immersion injury, without evidence of significant injury and without evidence of bronchospasm, tachypnea/dyspnea, or inadequate oxygenation (by ABC analysis and pulse oximetry), can be safely discharged from the ED after 6 to 8 hours of observation. However, be aware that these studies did not include older individuals or those with underlying medical conditions that might place them at increased risk of hypoxic injury and acidosis.
- Victims of mild to moderately severe submersion, who only have mild symptoms that improve during observation and have

no abnormalities on ABC analysis or pulse oximetry and chest radiograph, should be observed for a more prolonged period of time in the ED or observation unit.

- Certain patients may display mild to moderately severe hypoxemia that is corrected easily with oxygen. Admit these patients to the hospital for observation. They can be discharged after resolution of hypoxemia if they have no further complications.
- Admit patients who require intubation and mechanical ventilation to the ICU. Varying degrees of neurologic as well as pulmonary insults typically complicate their courses.

CHAPTER

73

Return-to-Play

73.1 RETURN TO PLAY: LOWER LIMB MUSCLE INJURIES

Contributed by Prof. Emin Ergen, University of Ankara, Turkey; Chairman FITA Medical Committee.

- *Return to Play?* The most important determinant in making the decision regarding return to physical activity is the absence of pain; however, other parameters such as flexibility, range of motion, and strength should be considered carefully.

- *Flexibility testing*: In testing for flexibility, it should be considered that whether the restriction is due to muscular tightness or other sources of restriction such as lack of joint range of motion or pain.

- *Heel cord flexibility*: Patient sits with knee extended and is asked to actively dorsiflex the ankle. A goniometer is used for measurement. A value of at least 10 degrees beyond plantigrade value is considered normal. This may also be done with the knee flexed to assess thickness within the soleus (normal value should be at least 20 degrees beyond plantigrade).

- *Hamstring flexibility*: The athlete lies supine with hip at 90-degree flexion position and is asked to extend the knee actively without changing the hip position. A goniometer is used for the measurement. Less than 10 degrees short of full flexion is considered to be normal.

- *Quadriceps flexibility*: The athlete lies prone and the knee is flexed passively by the physician. A full knee flexion without tilting of the pelvis is considered to be normal.

- *Iliotibial band flexibility (modified Ober test)*: Patient lies on the opposite side, near the edge of the examination table, facing away from the physician. The hip is slightly extended and passively adducted by gravity. The iliotibial band should not slip anteriorly or posteriorly to the greater trochanter or allow lateral tilting of the pelvis. If the knee drops level to or below the level of the table, it is considered normal.

- *Strength testing.* Although there are many ways of assessing strength, it is best evaluated using dynamometers (static or isokinetic) providing objective results. For an event physician, manual testing can also be used due to the unavailability of dynamometric evaluation. Each sport has its own normative data. Return to full training and competition presupposes that strength has been regained to within 10% of normal. The agonist/antagonist ratios must be restored for the entire limb, not only the involved muscles.

These tests may also be used to evaluate how prone a muscle is to injury.

73.2 RETURN TO PLAY: JOINT INJURIES

Contributed by Prof. Emin Ergen, University of Ankara, Turkey; Chairman FITA Medical Committee.

In order to make a "return-to-play" decision, it is necessary to ensure the following:

- A careful clinical and field assessment is required to permit an athlete to return to sport.

- That functional and rehabilitative exercises can be performed without pain during or after activity.

Joint protection with taping or bracing may be required for a certain period of time depending on the instability and pain. Long-term use of external support is not recommended due to probable disuse of proprioceptive receptors and in turn leading to more severe functional instability. There are a number of methods to protect against reinjuries. Braces have the advantage of being easy to fit and adjust, lack of skin irritation, and reduced cost compared to taping over a lengthy period. Many athletes get skin reactions to prolonged taping.

73.3 RETURN TO PLAY: KNEE INJURIES

Contributed by Prof. Lars Engebretsen, University of Oslo, Scientific Director, IOC.

Medial or Lateral Collateral Ligament Rupture

Prognosis: Grades I and II collateral ligament injuries often normalize after 6 to 12 weeks. Grade III injuries depend on accompanying injuries and therefore usually take significantly longer time to heal. With the exception of major lateral injuries, the athlete can usually return to sport activity after rehabilitation without major problems.

Anterior Cruciate Ligament Rupture

Prognosis: Most athletes in pivoting sports will need a reconstruction if returning to sport. Approximately 60% to 70% are able to return within 6 to 12 months after surgery. The long-term prognosis is dependent upon meniscal and cartilage injuries.

In an isolated ACL tear, 20% of the patients will have radiographic osteoarthritis signs 10 years after injury, whereas as many as 50% to 70% of patients will have radiographic signs if they have meniscal injuries in addition to the ACL injury.

Athletes in nonpivoting sports will usually cope with extensive rehabilitation emphasizing strength and proprioception. They may return to their sport within 3 to 4 months.

Meniscal Injuries

Prognosis: Prognosis is generally good. A sutured meniscal injury requires rest for a period of at least 4 to 6 months before the athlete returns to sport activity in which the knee is subjected to torsional loading. The athlete may return to sport activity within 4 weeks of a minor resection. The long-term prognosis is not known. A total resection of the medial meniscus puts the patient at high risk for radiographic arthrosis 10 years later on, whereas a partial resection appears to cause only a moderately increased risk of arthrosis.

Dislocated Patella

Prognosis: The prognosis is very good. The athlete almost always returns to sporting activity after 3 or 4 months.

Femoral Condyle/Tibial Plateau Fracture

Prognosis: Prognosis depends entirely on the nature of the fracture, which may vary from major plateau compression in ski jumpers to minimal depression fractures in recreational slalom skiers. The normal healing period for minor injuries is 6 to 12 weeks but the athlete must reckon with 3 months away from sporting activity.

Posterior Cruciate Ligament Ruptures

Prognosis: Isolated PCL injuries seldom cause symptoms during sports activity. However, the knee may gradually become less stable, due to stretching of the secondary stabilizers. Some of these patients will eventually require surgery.

Knee Dislocation

Prognosis: This is such a severe injury that only a few patients return to sporting activity.

Quadriceps/Patellar Tendon Rupture

Prognosis: The prognosis is good, but the athlete often loses some flexion ability during the first year after injury.

Chondral and Osteochondral Injuries

Prognosis: Short-term prognosis is good. In the long term, lesions of more than 2 cm^2 increase the frequency of osteoarthritis and may significantly reduce knee function after 10 years.

Patellar Fracture

Prognosis: Prognosis is good in the short term, in the sense that a patellar fracture almost always heals within 6 to 8 weeks. The problem is often a long-term reduction in flexion, particularly from cartilage injuries where symptoms usually do not appear until about 3 to 12 months later, when the patient begins full loading.

Special Injuries in Children

Prognosis: Follow-up studies of children who undergo surgery for cruciate ligament avulsion show very good results with respect to stability and function. Epiphyseal injuries increase the risk of growth disturbances, but this rarely occurs if the patient has the most common grade I injury. The prognosis is also very good for cartilage and meniscus injuries in children and they seldom cause symptoms in later life.

73.4 RETURN TO PLAY: ABDOMINAL INJURY

Contributed by David McDonagh, FIMS, FIBT, and AIBA.

For the event physician, this can be a difficult decision. There are two main scenarios: (1) An athlete has received a potential spleen injury during an event and the EP must decide if the athlete can continue the event or not and (2) an athlete consults the EP before an event regarding a recent injury and requests an evaluation to allow participation in the upcoming event.

In answer to this second scenario, I would ascertain the date of injury and the presence or absence of splenic illness, examine the patient for splenic tenderness and splenomegaly, and consider the need for blood tests and radiologic investigation.

In the first case, where an athlete has to be evaluated immediately after an injury to the upper left abdomen, one must take a careful history and examination. It is difficult to evaluate the extent of a splenic injury immediately after the injury has taken place. If findings are normal, if the athlete shows no signs of paleness, sweating, or shock, and if the tenderness is over the costal margin rather than the spleen, then it is probably acceptable to allow the athlete to return to play. It can be advisable to observe the patient first for 10 to 15 minutes in case of deterioration. Athletes with occult problems, who have returned to play, often tend to leave the event for a second time as they experience increased discomfort. These athletes should be stabilized and sent to hospital for further evaluation. If the athlete completes the event without discomfort and is asymptomatic, then they should be warned of delayed onset complications and of the necessary appropriate action to be taken. Postevent alcohol should be avoided. After abdominal surgery, a break of 6 months is often recommended before commencing contact sports.

73.5 RETURN TO PLAY: EPILEPSY

Contributed by Geraint Fuller, Consultant Neurologist, Consultant Neurologist, Gloucester Royal Hospital, United Kingdom; Advisory consultant to the British Olympic Association.

First Seizure

A decision on immediate return to play is not relevant as a sports participant will be taken directly to hospital after a first seizure.

After a single seizure, about 50% of patients will go onto have a second seizure. The risk falls as time passes but takes about 12 months to fall close to the background population rate.

Subsequent return to sports participation will depend on a number of factors.

- The results of the investigations into the seizure. Most young adults who have had a first seizure will have no specific cause found. In some, there will be features that either lead to a diagnosis of epilepsy (such as a history of myoclonic jerks) or findings on EEG or MRI that indicate a higher risk of recurrence.

- The nature of the sport

Regulated Sports

Motor sports have specific regulations based on the driving regulations. In the United Kingdom, a patient will not be able to drive until 12 months free of seizures. This would be the minimum for those involved in motor sports. Some other sports have specific regulations, though these vary in different jurisdictions—for example, boxing excludes those with epilepsy. Professional Jockeys in the United Kingdom need to be free of seizures and off treatment for 10 years—the same standard as heavy goods vehicle drivers.

Most sports do not have specific regulations and the risks need to be considered on an individual basis. Issues that need to be considered relate to the pattern of epilepsy (the seizure type, the frequency of seizures, the warning of impending seizure, and its duration), the inherent risk involved in the sport, to both the patient with epilepsy and his or her teammates or other players, and what opportunities there are to reduce the risk. For example, most patients with epilepsy can swim in swimming pools with little risk, but open water swimming would require greater safety provision and would entail higher risk. In some sports, for example white water kayaking, it would be difficult to organize safe recovery in the event of a seizure, while this would be much more straightforward in flat water kayaking.

After a single seizure, the main issues to consider relate to the sport alone.

Risks associated with combat sports are difficult to determine. If a player had a seizure in a full contact martial art fight, he or she could suffer the consequences of an undefended attack—and potentially a significant injury. Where specific regulations do not exist the type and frequency of seizures and the type and duration of combat and attendant risks need to be considered.

As can be appreciated from the foregoing, the return-to-play decision will need to be considered on an individual basis, in discussion with the patient, the coaches, the neurologist, and the sports physician.

Return-to-Play Decisions in Patients with Epilepsy

Return-to-play decisions in patients with active epilepsy depend on the type of seizure, their speed of their recovery, their usual seizure pattern, as well as the sport played. The safety aspects of the sport will already have been considered.

Tonic–clonic seizures: The physical fatigue and confusion after a tonic–clonic seizure are such as to prevent immediate return to play. Return to training can then build up in the same way as following

a concussion. Patients are likely to have a good idea how quickly they have been able to build up following previous seizures.

Complex partial seizures, simple partial seizures, and absences: patients with active epilepsy will have these types of seizures more frequently than tonic–clonic seizures. The severity of these seizures varies enormously. Some patients will be able to continue their activities almost immediately after an absence (sometimes being unaware of having had one) while other patients will be muddled and need to sleep. Thus a patient with active epilepsy who has frequent brief simple partial seizures may be able to return to play on recovery—sometimes within minutes. Alternatively, someone with less frequent more severe complex partial seizures may take a few days to return to training.

The best approach for each patient will need to be arrived at individually.

Concussive Syncope

This is a manifestation of head injury and the guidelines developed for head injury should be followed. This has no implications for driving in the United Kingdom.

73.6 RETURN TO PLAY: EXERTIONAL HEAT STROKE

Contributed by Prof. Andreas Niess, University of Tübingen, Germany.

Recovery times from EHS show a large individual variability. Involvement of several organ systems in the pathophysiology of EHS underline the necessity of searching for persistent damage post-EHS, particularly in liver, heart, muscle, as well as the renal and neurologic system. However, scientific evidence in this area is lacking and recommendations for return to activity are based on common sense and caution. An ACSM position stand addressed this issue as followed:

- A minimum of one week of rest post-EHS is recommended.

- A physical examination of the organs/systems affected by EHS should precede the start of activity.

- Activity and training should be started under normal conditions, and if well tolerated, gradually increased by intensity and duration.

- If additional heat exposure and resulting acclimation reflect existing heat tolerance, an additional 2 to 4 weeks of training allow return to full activity including competitive sports.

- If return to activity proves to be difficult, additional heat tolerance testing should be considered.

73.7 RETURN TO PLAY: HYPOTHERMIA

Contributed by Peter Jenoure, IOC Medical Committee, Switzerland.

The return to competition after an episode of hypothermia will obviously very much depend on the severity of the disease and the type of event.

When a clinically relevant form of hypothermia occurs during a sporting event, the athlete will in practically all cases have to stop his ongoing activity. Therefore, he will be taken out of the race.

In a competition lasting many days, for instance a cycling tour with multiple stages, this will mean withdrawal from the event.

A particular situation could arise when an athlete finishes a race, but in a hypothermic situation. If this occurs, the hypothermia will presumably be of a mild level and the treatment simple. Depending on the type of the race, and if the athlete does not have his own medical support, the event physician may be asked to give recommendations regarding the athlete's further participation in the competition. This decision will obviously be taken on a medical basis, depending on the recovery status of the athlete, how demanding the next day's competition will be, the weather forecast, etc. This will not be an easy decision, but as already said, a difficult decision based on many important criteria.

73.8 RETURN TO PLAY: CONCUSSION

Contributed by Jon Patricios, Sports Concussion South Africa, Johannesburg, South Africa.

Any head injury is a potentially serious injury. Concussion is a common incidence in sports; however, the crucial point is to recognize that a concussion has happened.

"Sports concussion is defined as a complex pathophysiological process affecting the brain, induced by traumatic biomechanical forces."

Several common features that incorporate clinical, pathologic, and biomechanical injury constructs that may be utilized in defining the nature of a concussive head injury include the following:

- Concussion may be caused by a direct blow to the head, face, neck, or elsewhere on the body with an "impulsive" force transmitted to the head.

- Concussion typically results in the rapid onset of short-lived impairment of neurologic function that resolves spontaneously.

- Concussion may result in neuropathologic changes, but the acute clinical symptoms largely reflect a functional disturbance rather than structural injury.

- Concussion results in a graded set of clinical syndromes that may or may not involve loss of consciousness. Resolution of the clinical and cognitive symptoms typically follows a sequential course.

- Concussion is typically associated with grossly normal structural neuroimaging studies.

Grading scales have been abandoned in concussion. Instead, characteristics and observations in the recovery of the athlete should lead the individual return-to-play process.

Return to Play

One of the critical issues in concussion management is return to play. A *simple concussion* recovers spontaneously over several days. In these situations, it is expected that an athlete will proceed rapidly through the stepwise return-to-play strategy. In the first few days following an injury, physical AND cognitive rest is required. Activities requiring concentration and attention may aggravate the symptoms and delay recovery.

The return to play following a concussion needs to follow a stepwise process:

- No activity and complete rest. Once the athlete is asymptomatic, they proceed to level two. The athlete spends, at the minimum, one day at each stage.

- Light aerobic exercise such as walking or stationary cycling, no resistance training. Performing step two without symptoms allows the athlete to proceed to level three. If symptoms return, the athlete moves back one stage then continues.

- Sport-specific training (e.g., skating in hockey, running in football), progressive addition of resistance training at steps three or four. Performing step three without symptoms allows the athlete to proceed to level four.

- Noncontact training drills. Performing step four without symptoms allows the athlete to proceed to level five.

- Full contact training after medical clearance. Performing step five without symptoms allows the athlete to proceed to level six.

- Game play

In the case of complex concussion, rehabilitation will be more prolonged and return-to-play decisions will be more cautious. Such complex cases should be managed by physicians with a specific expertise in the management of concussion injury. An additional return-to-play consideration is that the concussed athlete should not only be symptom free but also should not be taking any medications that may effect or modify the symptoms of concussion.

73.9 RETURN TO PLAY: ANKLE SPRAIN

Contributed by Jack Taunton, Prof. University of BC, CMO, Vancouver 2010 Winter Olympic Games, Canada.

Fraser (2007) also presented the following functional return-to-sport criteria. This was developed from his work with university, national, and professional athletes with acute ankle sprains:

- Dorsiflexion of at least 7 cm on the knee to wall test

- Inversion of 70% and not painful on lateral cutting

- 30-second eyes closed balance test (<2 touch difference)

- Pain-free hop then to lateral hop

- 3 hop for distance test and must be 25 cm difference side to side

- Once these criteria are met, Fraser allows the athlete to progress through.

- Technical skill part of practice with minimal to no discomfort

- One-on-one offensive drills

- One-on-one defensive drills

- Scrimmage the progression to game play

CHAPTER 74

Emergency Equipment

Contributed by David McDonagh, FIBT and FIMS

74.1 EMERGENCY ROOM MEDICAL EQUIPMENT AT A SPORTS VENUE

The following lists were developed by David McDonagh and Prof. Inggard Lereim. They are now used as an equipment guideline for the International Skiing Federation (FIS). We are not saying that the following equipment should be obligatory, merely giving a proposal to allow one to upscale or downscale based on one's own needs. Thanks also to Drs. Costas Parisis and Demetri Pyrros, Athens 2004 Olympic Summer Games, for their contribution.

Arena Emergency Rooms

Each larger arena should have two emergency rooms: one emergency room for athletes and team members and one for spectators.

Emergency rooms should have easy-to-clean floors and walls, ample lighting, electric outlets, and running water. They should also have their own WC or at least a WC very close by.

The following services should be provided:

1. Emergency first aid, including the ability to treat acute, life-threatening situations
2. Treatment of diseases and injuries
3. Simple prescriptions
4. Storage function

Which types of equipment should be available?

1. Standard office furniture
2. Emergency medical equipment
3. Infusion liquids for patient treatment/storage
4. Pharmaceuticals for patient treatment
5. Disposables
6. Patient treatment modules
7. Wheelchair/stretcher

Standard Office Equipment

Stretcher unit: 1, mimimum

Surgical lamp with wheels: 1

Office table: 1

Stool: 1

Chairs: 2

Washing basin with elbow control: 1

Liquid soap bottle: 1

Paper towel box: 1

Waste paper bucket: 1

Toxic waste container: 1

Mirror: 1

Wheeled defibrillator table for emergency equipment: 1

Wheeled table for surgical instruments: 1

Wall cabinet for instruments and disposables: 1

Wall (lockable) cabinet for pharmaceuticals: 1

Shelves: 2

Refrigerator: 1

Telephone: 1

PC with electronic journal system: 1

Lamp, surgical, capacity 500 lux: 1

Boxes, trays for storage: 10

Curtain rail: 1

Curtain: 1

Emergency Medical Equipment

Defibrillator: 1

ECG: 1

Manual suction unit: 1

Ventilator, portable, with tubes/mask and quick-release attachment: 1

Oxygen tanks, 10 L, with wall attachment: 2

Oxygen tank trolley: 2

Portable oxygen units, 2.5 L with regulator: 1

Pressure-reducing valve with adjustable and volume-reducing controls: 2

Portable oximeter/pulsemeter: 1

Nebulizer, automatic: 1

Immobilization kit: 1

Infusion liquid warmer, capacity 10 L: 1

Otoscope/ophthalmoscope: 1 set

Thermometer (auricular) with strips: 1 set

Suture kit: 5 sets

Sphygmomanometer: 1

Stethoscope: 1

Patella hammer with pin and brush: 1

Infusion Liquid

Glucose, 1,000 mL: 2

Ringer's lactate, 1,000 mL: 6

Plasma expanders, 500 mL: 2

Calcium bicarbonate, 500 mL: 2

Manitol 150 mg/mL, l,500 mL: 2

Wall Cabinet for Pharmaceuticals/Urine Sticks/Urine Catheters

NB. Doping substances regulations

Solu-Cortef, 5×100 mg bottle: 1 set

Atropine sulfate (Atropin) inj., 0.6 mg/mL: 1 mL $\times 10$

Adrenaline inj., 1 mg/mL: 1 mL $\times 10$

Morphine chloride, 10 mg/mL ampules: 1 mL $\times 10$

Nitroglycerine sublingual tablets, 0.5 mg: 100 tablets

Furosemide inj., 10 mg/mL: 2 mL $\times 10$

Terbutaline sulfate inj., 0.5 mg/mL: 1 mL $\times 10$

Terbutaline sulfate turbuhaler: 3 boxes

Ventolin inhalation aerosol, 200 dosages: 3 boxes

Ventolin inhalation liquid, 1 mg/mL: 2.5 mL $\times 60$

Ipratropium bromide inhalation liquid, 0.25 mg/mL, 20 mL bottle: 1 bottle

Theophylline inj., 30 mg/mL: 10 mL $\times 5$

Noscapine mixture, 100 mL bottle: 5 bottles

Noscapine tablets, 50 mg: 100 tablets

Buscopan inj., 20 mg/mL: 1 m: $\times 10$

Diazepam inj., 5 mg/mL, 2 mL $\times 5$

Diazepam supp., 5 mg $\times 5$

Buprenorphine, 0.2 mg tablets: 10 tablets

Metoclopramide inj., 5 mg/mL: 2 mL $\times 20$

Xylocaine inj., 5 mg/mL: 20 mL $\times 3$

Xylocaine spray, 80 g: 1 bottle

Xylocaine gel, tube, 10 g: 10 tubes

Chlorhexidine 0.1%, 250 mL bottle: 4 bottles

Paracetamol tablets, 500 mg: 100 tablets

Paracetemol suppository, 1 g: 10 units

Ampicillin, 250 mg bottle: 2 bottles

Phenoxymethylpenicillin tablets, 660 mg: 100 tablets

Trimethoprim Sulfa tablets: 100 tablets

Azitromycin tablets, 500 mg: 50 tablets

Chloramphenicol eye salve 1%, 200 mg tube: 20 tubes

Chloramphenicol eye drops, 10 mL: 2 bottles

Canesten salve, 30 g: 1 tube

Fucidin salve: 1 tube

Fucidin bandages, 10 × 10 cm: 1 set

Flamazine, 50 mg tube: 6 tubes

Hydrocortisone salve, 30 g: 2 tubes

Flumethasone/clioquinol ear drops, 7.5 mL: 2 bottles

Xylometazoline nasal spray, 1 mg/mL, 10 mL: 4 bottles

Magnesium hydroxide/magnesium carbonate tablets: 20 tablets

Antidiarrhea mixture: 4 bottles

Lactulose mixture, 200 mL bottle: 1 bottle

Loperamide capsules, 2 mg, 16 tablets per pack: 2 packs

Glucose, 500 mg/mL, 50 mL: 3 bottles

Glucose, 50 mg/mL, 100 mL: 3 bottles

Ibuprofen tablets, 600 mg: 50 tablets

Sterile water, 50 mL: 5 bottles

Saline, 9 mg/mL, 50 mL: 5 units

Paracetamol codeine tablets: 100

Tetanus vaccine capsules: 5 units

Enteric-coated NSAID tablets: 100 tablets

Nitrazepam, 5 mg: 100 tablets

Histoacryl (skin adhesive): 5 tubes

Amiodarone, 50 mg/mL: 10 ampules

Calcium gluconate: 5 ampules

Hypertonic glucose solution 35%: 5 ampules

Heparin 5,000 IU/mL: 2 units

Verapamil, 2.5 mg/mL: 5 ampules

Isoproterenol, 0.2 mg/mL: 5 ampules

KCl 10%: 5 ampules

Normal saline 0.9%, 10 mL: 5 ampules

Procainamide, 100 mg/mL: 2 units

Urinary catheter, size 14: 5 units

Urinary catheter set, disposable: 5 units

Urine sticks, leucocytes, protein, sugar, ketones: 1 box

Blood sticks, sugar, ketones: 1 box

Lancets, disposable: 1 box

Eye bath, glass, plastic, disposable: 5 units

Eye bath liquid, bottle, 1 L: 2 bottles

74.2 PORTABLE EMERGENCY MEDICAL EQUIPMENT

Sled Unit

The sled unit should contain

Mounted oxygen tank, 2.5 L, with regulator: 1

Immobilization unit: 1

Survival sheet: 1

Body warmer (e.g., STK): 1

Infusion warmer, capacity 3 L: 1

Scoop stretcher: 1

Aluminum blanket: 1

Stretcher mattress: 1

Stretcher Unit

The stretcher unit should contain

Stretcher: 1

Immobilization unit: 1

Survival sheet: 1

Woolen blanket: 1

Aluminum blanket: 2

Stretcher mattress: 1

Mounted oxygen holder, 2.5 L, with clip: 1

Bandage Unit

Large bandage scissors, curved, 180 mm: 1

Thermal blanket: 1

Triangular sling: 5

Compresses, 100 × 100 mm, sterile: 10

Compresses, 200 × 300 mm, sterile: 2

Single gauze kit, 170 × 170 mm: 4

Single gauze kit, 200 × 260 mm: 2

Tourniquet, 20 × 40 cm: 1

DuoDERM sheets: 2

Water-Jel, 5 × 5 cm: 5

Water-Jel, 5 × 15 cm: 5

Water-Jel, 10 × 10 cm: 2

Elastoplast, 6 × 1,000 mm, roll: 1

Skin/bandage plaster, 25 × 1,000 cm, roll: 1

Gauze, 100 mm: 5

Tube gauze, head/leg: 4

Safety pins: 6

Forceps, disposable, sterile: 3

Protective gloves, nonsterile, pair: 5

Nasal tampon: 2

Pencil:1

Pencil, skin, red/blue: 1

Injury card with plastic coat: 10

Infusion Unit

Infusion liquid must be stored in a plastic encasement. Glass is not allowed. Infusion liquid must be stored in a specially designed, insulated heating unit. Infusion liquids should have a temperature of around 37°C, and as near physiological temperature as possible. Infusion liquids should not be warmer than physiological temperature.

Hyperbaric pressure cuff: 1

Tourniquet with Velcro: 2 (must also have a device for children)

Infusion set, with drop chamber, 1.8 m: 2

Infusion set, without drop chamber, 800 mm: 2

Clamp, infusion set: 20

Cannula, injection, paper pack, 0.8×40 mm: 15

Venous catheter, 1.0 mm: 2

Venous catheter, 1.4 mm: 4

Venous catheter, 1.7 mm: 4

Butterfly, 0.6 mm: 3

Syringe, 10 mL: 5

Syringe, 2 mL: 5

Elastoplast, 25 mm: 1

Thermal heat packs, small: 1

Splint, 15×25 cm: 1

Sterile swabs: 10

Ventilation Unit

Respiration bag, with valve: 1

Silicone facial mask, child: 1

Silicone facial mask, adult: 1, with neck fastener: 1

Mouth-to-mouth mask: 3

Simple suction unit, manual: 1

Nasogastric tube, ch 25, sterile: 2

Oropharyngeal airway, size 3, size 2, and size 1: 2

Airway Unit

Magill's forceps adult: 1

Magill's forceps child: 1

Manual suction unit: 1

Suction catheter, ch 10: 2

Suction catheter, ch 16: 2

Nasogastric tube, ch 25, sterile: 1

Laryngoscope: 1

blade, adult, with halogen bulb: 1

blade, child, with halogen bulb: 1

Laryngoscope batteries, reserve: 2

Laryngoscope bulbs, halogen, reserve: 2

Endotracheal tube with cuff, #9, #7, #5, #4, #3: 1 of each

End-tidal CO_2 monitor, handheld: 1

Arterial forceps: 1

Mandrin, for tubes 1–4: 1

Mandrin, for tubes 4–7: 1

Oropharyngeal airway, size 3, size 2, and size 1: 1 of each

Cuff syringe, 10 mL, disposable, sterile: 2

Gauze swabs, pack of 5: 1

Sticking plaster, 25 mm, silk: 1

Safety pins: 6

Cricothyroidotomy set: 1

Xylocaine gel 2%, 20 mL: 1 tube

Continuous Positive Airway Pressure (CPAP) Unit

CPAP Venturi unit, adjustable: 1

CPAP tube/mask/fastener/filter: 1 of each

PEEP valve, 7.5 mm: 1

Oxygen catheter: 1

Oxygen Unit, Portable

Oxygen tank, 2.5 L, with regulator: 1

Silicone respiration bag with valve: 1

Silicone facial mask, adult: 1

Neck fastener: 1

Tongue depressor, #2: 3

Manual suction unit: 1

Pharmaceutical Unit

NB. Doping substances

Atropine sulfate, 1.0 mg/mL: 1 m: × 2

Adrenaline, 1 mg/mL: 1 mL × 20

Morphine chloride, 10 mg/mL ampules: 1 mL × 10

Nitroglycerine sublingual tablets, 0.5 mg: 10 tablets

Terbutaline sulfate, 0.5 mg/mL: 1 mL × 5

Theophylline, 30 mg/mL: 10 m: × 5

Buscopan, 20 mg/mL: 1 mL × 5

Diazepam, 5 mg/mL, rectal: 2 mL: × 10

Metoclopramide, 5 mg/mL: 2 mL × 20

Phenoxymethylpenicillin tablets, 660 mg: 20 tablets

Flamazine, 50 mg tube: 1 tube

Flumethasone/clioquinol ear drops, 7.5 mL: 1 bottle

Glucose, 120 mg/mL, 50 mL bottle: 5

Blood sticks, sugar, ketones: 1 box

Lancets, disposable, paper-packed: 3

Sterile water, 50 mL, bottle: 1

Medical Equipment Unit

Large bandage scissors, curved Ig 180 mm: 1

Compresses, 100 × 100mm, sterile: 5

Gauze swabs, sterile, pack of 5: 2

Pencil, skin, red/blue: 1

Patient trauma cards: 10

Cannula, injection, paper pack, 0.8 × 40 mm: 10

Cannula, injection, paper pack, 0.6 × 25 mm: 5

Intracardiac needle: 1

Intraosseous needle: 1

Syringe, 10 mL: 2

Syringe, 2 mL: 3

Scalpel, #10, sterile, disposable: 1

Blade, scalpel, #10, sterile, disposable: 6

Needle holder, 160 mm: 1

Nonresorbable sutures, 4.0: 3

Arterial clamp, curved, 130 to 160 mm: 2

Arterial clamp, straight 130 to 160 mm: 2

Stethoscope with membrane: 1

Sphygmomanometer: 1

Sports Unit

Sports ice, small: 3

Warm packs, large: 2

Sports tape, 5 cm: 3 rolls

Tensoplast, 5 cm: 1 roll

Tensoplast, 10 cm: 1 roll

Elastic tape, 80 mm: 2 rolls

Elastic tape, 100 mm: 2 rolls

Immobilization Unit

Rigid cervical collars, set of 6 sizes (or adjustable) with mandibular/occipital support and tracheotomy entry port: 1 set

Vacuum mattress with pump: 1

Vacuum splints with pump: 1 set

Traction splint, lower extremity: 1 set (optional)

Emergency Belt Pack ("Fanny Pack"), Large

Small bandage scissors, curved Ig: 1

Pocket knife, small: 1

Thermal blanket: 1

Forceps, disposable, sterile: 1

Nasal tampons: 1

Triangular sling: 1

Compresses, 100 × 100 mm, sterile: 5

Compresses, 200 × 200 mm, sterile: 2

Large bandage, 200 × 400 mm: 1

Single gauze kit, 170 × 170 mm: 1

Combination bandage: 1

Band-Aid, 60 × 1,000 m, roll: 1

Elastoplast, 25 × 1,000 mm, roll: 1

Elastic bandage, 80 mm, roll: 1

Elastic bandage, 100 mm, roll: 1

Tube gauze, head/leg: 1

Safety pins: 6

Protective gloves, nonsterile, pair, large: 5

Pencil: 1

Notebook: 1

Patient trauma cards with plastic wallets: 5

Mouth-to-mouth mask: 1

Pencil flashlight with halogen bulbs: 1

For doctors and nurses:

Stethoscope: 1

Tongue depressor #3: 1

Tongue depressor #1: 1

Emergency Belt Pack ("Fanny Pack"), Small

Small bandage scissors, curved Ig: 1

Pocket knife, small: 1

Thermal blanket: 1

Forceps, disposable, sterile: 1

Nasal tampons: 1

Triangular sling: 1

Compresses, 100 × 100 mm, sterile: 5

Elastoplast, 25 × 1,000 mm, roll: 1

Elastic bandage, 100 mm, roll: 1

Tube gauze, head/leg: 1

Safety pins: 6

Protective gloves, nonsterile, pair, large: 5

Pencil: 1

Notebook: 1

Patient trauma cards with plastic wallets: 5

Mouth-to-mouth mask: 1

Pencil flashlight with halogen bulbs: 1

74.3 PULSE OXIMETERS

Pulse oximeters emit and receive red and infra-red light rays that have passed through or been reflected from peripheral blood vessels, thus allow-ing a microcomputer to calculate the relative oxy-genation of hemoglobin and then the SpO_2 value. In adults, normal arterial saturation is between 95% and 99%. Values between 90% and 94% indicate a mild hypoxemia, 85% to 89% saturation implies a moderate hypoxemia and the need for supplemen-tal oxygen, while 84% or less implies a severe hypox-emia and the need for supplemental oxygen and assisted ventilation. Though not as reliable as arte-rial blood gases, these simple noninvasive devices can give valuable information in the prehospital set-ting. False readings can occur if the tested finger is in motion, if the finger sensors are wet or moist, and if the sensor does not fit properly around the finger.

74.4 DEFIBRILLATORS (AEDs)

AEDs are now usually found in most ambulances, and the event physician will probably have access to one at larger sporting events. If the cause of the sud-den cardiac arrest is ventricular fibrillation (VF) or pulseless ventricular tachycardia, then victims have a greater chance of survival if electrical defibrillation is performed. Once the patient has gone over to an asys-tole, the chances of survival decrease. The chances of successful defibrillation reportedly decline by 7% to 10% with each minute that passes after the arrest, so earliest possible defibrillation is recommended.

AEDs have voice and visual prompts, most are semiautomatic, and some newer machines are fully automatic. The machines analyze the victim's car-diac rhythm and determine the need for a shock. Semiautomated AEDs inform the user that the patient needs to be shocked and the user has to press a button; automatic AEDs will deliver the shock automatically.

Defibrillation Procedure

Continue CPR while the pads are being applied: one pad to the right of the sternum, below the clavicle, and the other pad in the midaxillary line just at the lowest point of pectoralis major. Female breast tissue should be moved if necessary. Note lateral and vertical placement of pad. Do not worry if you use a right pad in the left position or vice versa. Do not remove pads as they may not adhere as well the second time. Remove chest hair if neces-sary. Pediatric pads are available.

1. Follow the voice/visual prompts.
2. Ensure that nobody touches the athlete during the rhythm analysis.

3. If a shock is indicated
   - Keep everybody away from the patient—do not touch the patient.
   - Press the shock button as directed by the prompt.
   - Follow other voice prompts.
4. If no shock is indicated, resume CPR immediately (30 compressions per two breaths) and continue to follow the voice prompts.

74.5 VACUUM MATTRESSES AND SPLINTS

A vacuum mattress is useful for the gentle immobilization of patients, especially in case of a spinal, pelvic, or femoral trauma. It is more comfortable to lie on than a backboard and is particularly useful when you want to avoid the compression of damaged tissue—for example, with spinal injuries and fracture dislocations. Vacuum splints are more flexible than rigid backboards, which can be both an advantage and a disadvantage.

It consists of a sealed bag containing small polystyrene balls, with a valve, straps, and handles. The bag can be molded around a patient. Using a pump, one can withdraw air from the bag and it molds itself around the whole patient (mattress) or a patient extremity (splint). Further straps are then applied to secure the patient and enhance immobilization.

Often, a combination of equipment is used. A patient is scooped onto a vacuum mattress, the air is evacuated, the mattress molds around a patient, and then the vacuum mattress is put on a stretcher. A sheet can be put on the vacuum mattress to protect the mattress from glass and also to limit patient sweating.

The vacuum mattress provides comparable spinal immobilization to the long spinal board with increased comfort.

74.6 TRACTION SPLINTS

As a rule, traction splints are used to treat major bone fractures, mostly femur but sometimes tibia fractures. They work by holding the broken bone immobile and by applying pressure along the bone length. The idea is that, by using a traction splint, you can prevent or correct the bone shortening that can occur due to muscular contraction or direct trauma.

There are four basic types: the Thomas splint (half-ring), the Hare traction splint, the Sager splint, and the Kendrick traction device. The basic principle is that one end of the traction splint is strapped to the upper thigh while another strap is applied around the foot and ankle: The different devices have different types of mechanisms that actively counteract the muscle tension and thus produce traction. Additional straps are then added to aid immobilization of the limb.

Obviously, traction splints should not be used if the splint can cause further damage, so they should be avoided if there is a risk of pelvic fracture, if there is sign of injury in the area where the straps are to be applied, or with an intra-articular knee injury.

74.7 LIFTING DEVICES AND BACKBOARDS

Lifting devices were developed so that patients could be lifted from the ground with a minimum of movement. They are particularly useful in lifting the unconscious, "floppy" patient who has not been otherwise immobilized. One such device, the scoop stretcher, is particularly effective in that it can be opened at one end and the board can be effectively placed under the patient with a minimum of patient movement.

Backboards are not primarily lifting devices and are usually rigid, straight, 2-m-long plastic boards used as spinal immobilizers when spinal injury is present or feared. Often, the patient is turned using a four-man log-roll technique, deviations from the spinal neutral position are corrected, a cervical collar and neck supports are applied, and the patient is turned and supported back onto the backboard.

Combi-boards that combine both these functions are also available.

When using a backboard, it is important to correctly position the athlete onto the board, usually after having log-rolled the athlete. When log rolling, it is important to roll the athlete in a controlled and coordinated manner, without compromising the integrity of the spine.

The athlete should be secured to the backboard by an adequate number of belts or straps. The head should have extra neck supports as cervical collars alone do not give total support with upper cervical or lower cervical lesions. Remember, the backboard is flat, but the spine is not, so correct padding of the back to support the hollows is recommended.

74.8 CERVICAL COLLARS

There are two types of cervical collars: soft collars and rigid collars. Rigid collars are used when a potential cervical fracture and/or spinal cord injury is suspected. I always have a set of rigid collars available at a sporting event; I never have soft collars. Soft cervical collars are made of foam and are often used in the treatment of minor strain injuries or in a transition period from a rigid cervical collar to no collar at all. They offer minimal movement restriction and in my opinion, should not be used with acute neck injuries; they give a false sense of security as far as immobilization is concerned and they may compress neck veins and hinder respiratory function.

Rigid collars, on the other hand, are necessary and effective splints. When applying a collar, it is best to be two care providers; this gives greater stability. These collars *limit* but do not prevent cervical movement and thus help protect a cervical fracture and/or a spinal cord injury. In order to prevent secondary spinal injury, the EP should choose a rigid cervical collar that can be applied with minimal movement and that will sufficiently restrict cervical motion during transport. The collar must also "fit" the athlete and must neither be too short (thus giving poor occipital–mandibular axis control) or too long (thus forcing the neck into hyperextension). The ideal cervical collar should support the occipital region and the mandible (thus limiting anteroposterior head movement) and prevent lateral flexion of the neck. Women have often long, thin necks while bigger men have shorter and thicker necks.

On the subject of women, some wear long, droopy metal earrings—the aluminum Christmas Tree variety. These must be removed if they are sharp as they may cut the athlete inside the collar. Finally, make sure that hair does not get caught in between the Velcro attachments as this may cause the collar to loosen.

Collars should be easy to apply and should be radiolucent and MRI and CT scan compatible. Collars should have an anterior opening to allow access for checking carotid pulses, assessing neck veins, and allowing for advanced airway procedures. Cervical collars should not compress neck veins and must not hinder respiration.

Finally, it must be remembered that rigid cervical collars *should not* be used if there is a traumatic fixed-neck deformity—in other words, if the neck is locked into a flexed, extended, or laterally flexed position due to vertebral dislocation or destruction. In these circumstances, the use of a rigid collar will probably worsen the situation by forcing the neck back into an anatomical position and possibly lacerating the spinal cord. In these situations, I have used a vacuum splint to mold around the neck and shoulders. It is an extremely difficult situation to manage as the neck requires constant manual support to the hospital, with preferably no movement, several assistants, and help from an anesthetist.

74.9 ORTHOPEDIC BRACES AND ORTHOTICS

Ankle Braces

The purpose of an ankle brace is to support the joint during ambulation. There are many products on the market, but one of the most used is the Aircast Air-Stirrup, which is a combination of semi-rigid outer plastic shells with preinflated air cells within the inner padding that provide support and produce graduated compression during ambulation. The compression promotes efficient edema reduction in addition to helping accelerate rehabilitation. These are efficient braces and are streamlined to fit in shoes for early protected weight bearing. They can be used for both acute injuries and chronic instability. Elbow braces are based on the same principle; they concentrate compression directly on the extensor muscle, not around the arm, for more support and less constriction. These are useful for a tennis elbow/golfer's elbow.

Knee Braces

Although rigid knee braces are used for extra protection against injury in some sports like motorsports, there are many contact sports in which they are not allowed to be used. There are two reasons for this conclusion: the first being that if you need to have a rigid brace, then the joint is probably too unstable to participate in sport, and secondly, rigid braces can cause injury to other athletes in contact sports. Rigid braces may of course be used in training, and they do play an important role in athlete rehabilitation. Otherwise, soft braces or orthotics, usually made from neoprene, are commonly used to provide support and sometimes compression during sporting competition.

Cryotherapy

While good, old-fashioned ice is hard to beat, it can at times be impractical. A very handy product is the cold compression cuff, which offers focused compression with cold therapy and helps minimize posttraumatic swelling and pain.

CHAPTER 75

Rapid Diagnostic Tests

Contributed by David McDonagh, FIBT and FIMS

Reviewers: Kristian Bjerva, Professor, Clinical Chemistry Department, and Svein A. Nordbø, Professor, Microbiology, St. Olavs University Hospital, NTNU, Trondheim, Norway

75.1 C-REACTIVE PROTEIN

The C-reactive protein (CRP) was first discovered by Tillett and Francis at the Rockefeller Institute in 1930. It is one of several substances that can be found after an acute inflammatory reaction—the so-called acute-phase response—be that an infection, immune, or allergic reaction, tissue trauma, surgery or even malignancy. For the EP, the presence of elevated C-reactive protein can be an invaluable tool for gauging the severity of infections in the athlete.

Other acute-phase protein markers such as the complement components C3, C4, C5, etc.; haptoglobin; ceruloplasmin; GA-1 trypsin inhibitor; fibrinogen; prothrombin; etc. can also be used to identify the presence of inflammation; however, CRP testing has become one of our most important parameters of infection recognition, and in particular in sports medicine, where the advent of rapid diagnostic tests is a great aid to the traveling sports physician. The erythrocyte sedimentation rate (ESR) is still an excellent test, but it takes several hours to complete. White blood cell counts can also give valuable information about the extent of infection, but test machines are expensive and not likely to be available at a sports event. At major world championships, it is not unusual to have a CRP machine in the athletes medical room and most EPs would recommend such a purchase. Prices and quality vary—it is important to purchase the tests with best sensitivity. Studies have shown that these rapid tests are not 100% reliable. Some studies show an excellent correlation between capillary whole blood CRP values and venous blood samples analyzed by hospital laboratories. Other studies show high "false normal" and "false elevated" rates. Study conclusions vary as do results from different products. It would appear that hospital venous blood sampling is more reliable, but rapid tests are much easier to use and give quicker results (Table 75.1).

Usually, the CRP plasma level in a healthy individual is under 10 mg per L. With rapid tests, capillary blood is used and normal values are usually defined as being <5 mg per L or <7 mg per L depending on the machine used. Mild to moderate viral infections may give values between 40 and 60 mg per L, whereas serious bacterial infections will often show values over 100, even >200 mg per L. Both capillary and plasma levels begin increasing within 4 to 6 hours after acute response and continue to increase for 24 to 48 hours. CRP remains elevated as long as the acute-phase response is active.

75.2 HUMAN CHORIONIC GONADOTROPIN—PREGNANCY TESTS

Pregnancy tests are now widely used both by athletes and physicians and they detect the presence of HCG in the urine. HCG can be found in small amounts in the blood and urine of nonpregnant subjects. HCG levels in blood start to rise 6 to 8 days after fertilization, reaching a peak after 7 to 10 weeks. Most modern pregnancy test kits reveal

TABLE 75.1	NycoCard vs. Afinion CRP Tests Properties		
	Time	**Testing Volume**	**CV**
NycoCard	Within 3 min	5μL blood, serum or plasma	Under 7%
Afinion	3:45 min	1.5μL blood, serum, plasma	<10% for CRP under 20 mg/L
			> 6% for CRP over 20 mg/L

positive results after 7 days, some as early as 3 or 4 days. False positive results are extremely unlikely. The levels of sensitivity and specificity of these tests are considered excellent. For example, the QuickVue One-Step HCG Urine test can detect low HCG levels as early as 2 to 3 days before expected menses, has an accuracy > 99%, needs only three drops of blood, gives results in 3 minutes, and can be stored at room temperature.

75.3 D-DIMER

D-dimer tests are useful diagnostic adjuncts when a hypercoagulability is suspected—most commonly DVT but also DIC. In sporting environments, they can be useful tests to have if you have a small clinic or office available. It can be difficult to differentiate between partial calf muscle ruptures, strains, and a DVT, and the D-dimer test can be a useful aid. A positive D-dimer indicates the presence of an elevated level of fibrin degradation products and can indicate the presence of a thrombus, but levels can also be elevated after recent surgery, trauma, infection, liver disease, pregnancy, eclampsia, heart disease, and some malignancies.

A negative test result can usually be relied upon—if the correct sample taking and testing procedures have been carried out. False positives may be seen if there is hemolysis or with elevated levels of rheumatoid factor, triglycerides, lipemia, and bilirubin. Some tests give a qualitative result within 3 minutes but have a CV of up to 15%.

75.4 STREP A

Throat infection with streptococcus bacteria should be treated with an antibiotic. Throat cultures have traditionally been used to detect streptococcal throat infections; however, one must wait several days before receiving an answer, due to transport, culture growth, and reporting procedures. Strep tests have been developed to identify the presence of *Streptococcus pyogenes* (group A streptococcus), which is one of the commoner (but by no means only) cause of bacterial pharyngitis. A sample is taken from the back of the throat and tonsils and effort must be made to take an appropriate sample. Several different types of rapid strep tests are available and results are available within minutes. Please note: These tests can only detect the presence of group A strep; they do not detect other groups of streptococci or other bacteria. A positive rapid strep test indicates the presence of group A streptococci, and antibiotics should be prescribed if there are positive clinical findings. A negative rapid strep test indicates the probable absence of group A *Streptococcus* as the causative bacteria; it does not exclude the bacterial pharyngitis diagnosis.

The QuickVue Dipstick Strep A test allows for rapid qualitative detection of group A streptococcal antigen directly from the throat. Time to result: Read at 5 minutes. It has a sensitivity of 92% and a specificity of 98%. Tests can be stored for 18 months at room temperature.

75.5 MONO TEST

These are heterophile antibody tests and are used to detect the presence of infectious mononucleosis due to Epstein-Barr virus (EBV). Commercially available test kits have varying sensitivity and specificity. As a rule, mono tests are usually not positive in the incubation period, the 4 to 6 weeks before symptom debut, so if a test is taken too early (i.e., before specific heterophile antibodies have developed), the test may be negative. If the mono test is initially negative and the EP still suspects an infectious mononucleosis, a blood test may be taken and sent to the lab for Epstein-Barr virus analysis.

Alternatively, the EP may repeat the mono test after a week, but by then the athlete has usually returned home. Tests are usually negative after the infection has subsided, usually after the fourth week of illness. The test is most reliable when the patient has symptoms of fever, malaise, pharyngitis, tender cervical lymphadenitis, and splenomegaly. Up to 10% of infected adolescents do not produce a heterophile antibody and will thus not have a positive monospot test. A white blood cell count is also useful in making the diagnosis—elevated levels may indicate a bacterial infection—as is a strep test to exclude strep throat (again remembering that strep tests only measure strep group A activity). Patients with negative mono tests and few or no reactive lymphocytes may be infected by another microorganism such as cytomegalovirus (CMV) or toxoplasmosis. As the test is specific for heterophile antibodies and not EBV, it can also be positive in patients with lymphoma, systemic lupus erythematosus (lupus), and some gastrointestinal cancers.

One kit is the Clearview IM mono test, which is a rapid immunoassay for qualitative detection of infectious mononucleosis IGM heterophile antibodies using whole blood, serum, or plasma. It has a sensitivity of whole blood: 95, 5%, and serum/plasma: 98, 5%; and a specificity of whole blood: 100%, and serum/plasma: 100%.

75.6 HIV/AIDS

Clinical studies show that these rapid HIV tests are as sensitive and as specific as enzyme immunoassay screening tests, so much so these tests are now used by the WHO. Clients with negative rapid HIV test results are told that they are not infected, the only proviso being that it is 3 months since the time of exposure. HIV antibodies take time to develop, so early tests may prove negative even if there is an infection present. Patients should be retested 3 months after the initial potential exposure. False-positive results do occur, so patients should be referred to supplemental laboratory tests such as a western blot or immunofluorescence assay. Never tell the patient that the rapid test was positive. Only on receipt of a positive supplemental test should this issue be addressed, preferably by experienced staff.

CHAPTER 76

Sport-Specific Injury Profiles: Winter Olympic Federations

Contributed by David McDonagh, Chair FIBT Medical Committee; and all the Chairpersons of the Winter Olympic International Federations whose names you will find below

76.1 BIATHLON (IBU)

The sport of biathlon combines two separate skills, cross-country skiing and rifle shooting.

What makes this sport so difficult is that the athletes have to be top-class skiers as well as top marksmen; they ski at full speed between the obligatory shooting posts (standing and lying).

Time penalties (extra laps) are given for missed shots. The winner is the athlete with the fastest time. There are sprint, individual, pursuit, and relay events for both men and women (Table 76.1).

76.2 BOBSLEIGH AND SKELETON (FIBT)

A bobsleigh, or bobsled, is an aerodynamic machine made of fiberglass and steel, mounted on four highly polished steel runners. The sled is driven down a man-made track. The two front runners have approximately three inches of lateral movement and are attached to ropes held by the driver, who steers the sled by pulling on these ropes. The brake handles are located on either side of the brakeman in the four-man sled and in front of the brakeman in the two-man sled. All sleds are standardized according to specifications set by the FIBT. Maximum weight of a four-man sled (including crew) is 630 kg. Maximum weight of a two-man sled (including crew) is 390 kg. There are two-person races for men and women. Men also have a four-man event. A skeleton, or toboggan, is a low profile but heavy sled, with a fiberglass "pod," which provides the aerodynamics to the lower part, mounted onto a steel chassis/frame. The sled runs on two highly polished steel runners. The runners are mounted such that the "bow" can be controlled, which assists in the steering of the sled. There are

no brakes on a skeleton sled, so the athlete and sled will stop by decelerating in the braking stretch. There are races for men and women. Bobsleigh and skeleton events are decided on time, and the athlete/athletes with the lowest combined time in all heats is the winner. The sports originated in St. Moritz, Switzerland (Table 76.2).

76.3 CURLING (WCF)

Developed in Scotland, curling is a competition between two teams with four players each. The game is played on ice, and the two teams take turns pushing a 19-kg stone down a track toward a series of concentric circles. The object is to get the stone as close to the center of the circles as possible. One athlete pushes the stone out on the track, while the other members may speed up the stone by brushing the ice ahead of the stone. The score is determined when all stones have been delivered. This is called an end. There are usually 10 ends and the team with the most points at the conclusion of ten ends is the winner (Table 76.3).

76.4 ICE HOCKEY (IIHF)

The origins of ice hockey are unclear, but it is believed that the first competitions and rules were developed at McGill University in Montreal, Canada. At the Olympic Winter Games, both men and women compete. A team has six players on the ice while play is in progress. A game consists of three 20-minute periods, with a 15-minute intermission between periods. Goals are scored by hitting the puck in goal. The winner is the team that scores most goals (Table 76.4).

TABLE 76.1 **IBU—International Biathlon Union**

Federation physician	Jim Carrabre, Cologne, MW, USA
E-mail	Athlondoc@aol.com
Accident type	Extremity injuries
	Overuse musculoskeletal disorders
	Eating disorders
Essential skills required by an event physician	Reanimation techniques
	Experience with general sports medical background
Essential equipment	Neck, spine, limb immobilization units
	Snow scooter/sled stretcher unit
Specific qualification requirements	Recommend certified sports medicine physicians

TABLE 76.2 **FIBT—International Bobsleigh and Skeleton Federation**

Federation physician	David McDonagh, Trondheim, Norway
E-mail	mcdonagh@ntnu.no
Accident type	
(1) Sled Crashes	(1) High-velocity injuries: head, neck, spinal injuries; friction burns on the back
(2) Start area accidents	(2) Muscle/hamstring ruptures at the push start phase; ocular foreign bodies, when sharpening blades
Essential skills required by an event physician	Safe helmet removal
	Ability to extricate an athlete from a bobsleigh
	Competency with neck, spine, extremity immobilization; wound care; ABC
Essential equipment	Neck, spine, limb immobilization
	Reanimation equipment
	Oxygen tank, ventilation mask, infusion set
Specific qualification requirements	None, but there is a clause in the rules saying that the physician "should be competent in emergency medical procedures"

TABLE 76.3 **WCF—World Curling Federation**

Federation physician	Evan L. Lloyd, Edinburgh, Scotland
E-mail	evlloyd@waitrose.com
Accident type	Occasional fall on ice (rare), leading to upper extremity and head injuries
Essential skills required by an event physician	Physician not always present and seldom busy in this safe sport
Essential equipment	None
Specific qualification requirements	None

TABLE 76.4	IIHF—International Ice Hochey Federation
Federation physician	Mark Aubry, Ottawa, Canada
E-mail	markaubry@rogers.com
Accident type	Contact sport: contusions, sprains, strains, fractures, head and neck injuries
Essential skills required by an event physician	ATLS
	ACLS
	Emergency medicine
	Sports medicine
Essential equipment	Resuscitative care equipment, including IV solutions, defibrillator
	Backboard
	Suture equipment and wound care
	Splints
	Paramedic care
Specific qualification requirements	No specific qualifications but suggest experience in sports medicine and emergency care

76.5 LUGE (FIL)

Luge is the French word for "sled." Luge, bobsleigh, and skeleton all share the same tracks. In luge, the athlete slides with his or her back on the sled, feet first, down the track, whereas in skeleton, the athlete slides head first with his or her stomach on the sled. Though sleds have been in Norway for over a thousand years, the first international sled race occurred in Davos, Switzerland. There are single and double events for both men and women (Table 76.5).

TABLE 76.5	FIL—International Luge Federation
Federation physician	Jörg Ellermeyer, Königsee, Germany
E-mail	ellermeyer@t-online.de
Accident type	Sled crashes, start area incidents
Essential skills required by an event physician	High-velocity injuries: head, neck, spinal injuries
	Friction burns on the back, elbows
	Fractures of metatarsals
	Ankle injuries
	Neck pain due to chronic strain
	Muscle/hamstring ruptures at the push start phase
	Ocular foreign bodies when sharpening blades
Essential equipment	Reanimation equipment
	Neck, spine, limb immobilization
	Bandage unit
Specific qualification requirements	None, but the physician must be proficient in emergency medical procedures

TABLE 76.6	ISU—International Skating Union
Federation physician	Jane Moran, Victoria, BC, Canada
E-mail	jane-moran@shaw.ca
Accident type	Fall from height, crashes into boards, blade lacerations
	Major blood vessel lacerations, cervical spine and spinal injuries, concussions
	Asthma exacerbations
	Epistaxis
Essential skills required by an event physician	Good emergency skills: be able to maintain airways, set up an intravenous drip, control hemorrhages, perform cervical and spinal immobilization, perform neurological assessment, manage a concussed patient, remove helmets in short track, stop epistaxis, and suture
Essential equipment	Bandage unit
	Suture unit
	Airway unit
	Cervical collars, spinal boards
Specific qualification requirements	Skilled in prehospital trauma care
	Proficient in ABC and spinal treatment

76.6 SKATING (ISU)

Skating is an age-old form of transportation from northern Europe, but the modern sport of skating was formalized in the late 1800s. There are several different skating disciplines.

Figure skating includes women's singles, men's singles, pairs, and ice dancing.

Short track speed skating races are now almost exclusively indoor events where the winner is the first athlete over the finish line. As these tracks are short, falls are not uncommon and races can be dramatic. As the athletes have sharp blades on their boots, this can be a dangerous sport. There are individual and team events for both men and women.

Speed skating is believed to have been developed in the Netherlands and consists of sprint events (500 m) up to long distance events (10,000 m) (Table 76.6).

Synchronized skating (groups of 8–20 skaters moving together) is not an Olympic Sport.

76.7 SKIING (FIS)

Skiing is another ancient form of transportation, probably originating in Norway. Alpine skiing evolved from cross-country skiing. The first alpine skiing competition was held in the 1850s in Oslo.

The first slalom was organized in 1922 in Mürren, Switzerland.

The FIS has several disciplines: alpine skiing, cross-country skiing, ski jumping, Nordic combined, snowboard, and freestyle skiing.

The *alpine events* are

- Downhill: Longest course, fewest turns, fastest speed. It is a single run event.

- Super-G (super giant slalom): The speed of downhill with the turns of giant slalom, shorter course than downhill but longer than a giant slalom. It is a single run event.

- Giant slalom: Similar to slalom, with fewer but wider turns. Each skier makes two runs down two different courses on the same slope on the same day.

- Slalom: The shortest course with the quickest turns. Each skier makes two runs down two different courses on the same slope on the same day.

- Combined: Consists of one downhill followed by two slalom runs.

Cross-country skiing has also several variations from sprints to marathon events, team and individual events, pursuits, interval starts, and mass starts.
Ski jumping has three basic forms: the normal hill, the large hill, and ski flying, all depending on the

TABLE 76.7	FIS—International Ski Federation
Federation physician	Chair, Herbert Hoerterer, Germany
	Vice Chair, Inggard Lereim, Trondheim, Norway
E-mail	mail@fisski.ch
Alpine skiing	
Accident type	
(1) Sled Crashes	(1) High-velocity injuries: head, neck, spinal, limb injuries
(2) Start area accidents	(2) Muscle/hamstring ruptures at the push start phase
Essential skills required by an event physician	Safe helmet removal
	Ability to extricate an athlete from a bobsleigh
	Competency with neck, spine, extremity immobilization; wound care; ABC
Essential equipment	Neck, spine, limb immobilization
	Reanimation equipment
	Oxygen tank, ventilation mask, infusion set
Specific qualification requirements?	None, but there is a clause in the rules saying that the physician "should be competent in emergency medical procedures"
Cross-Country skiing	
Accident type	Muscle/hamstring, joint strains
Falls	Hypothermia
	Respiratory problems
Essential skills required	General sports medical skills
Essential equipment	Neck, spine, limb immobilization
	Bandage unit.
	Reanimation equipment
	Oxygen tank ventilation mask infusion set
Ski jumping	
Accident type	(1) High-velocity injuries: head, neck, spinal injuries
Falls	
	(2) Muscle/ligament/joint injuries
Essential skills required by an event physician	Safe helmet removal
	Competency with neck, spine, extremity immobilization; wound care; ABC
	Should be competent in emergency medical procedures
Essential equipment	Neck, spine, limb immobilization
	Reanimation equipment,
	Oxygen tank, ventilation mask, infusion set
Nordic combined	
Accident type	As with ski jumping and cross-country skiing

(Continued)

TABLE 76.7	FIS—International Ski Federation (*Continued*)

Freestyle and Snowboard	
Accident type	(1) High-velocity injuries: head, neck, spinal injuries
Falls	(2) Muscle/ligament/joint injuries
Essential skills required by an event physician	Safe helmet removal
	Competency with neck, spine, extremity immobilization; wound care; ABC
	Should be competent in emergency medical procedures
Essential equipment	Neck, spine, limb immobilization
	Reanimation equipment,
	Oxygen tank, ventilation mask, infusion set

length of the take-off ramp. Normal hill competitions: Distances of up to and over 110 m can be reached. Large hill competitions: Distances of over 145 m can be obtained on the larger hills. Both individual and team competitions are run on these hills. Ski-flying competitions: The ski-flying World Record is currently 239 m (a soccer pitch and an American football field are approximately 110 m.)

Ski jumping is one of the two elements in the *Nordic combined* sport, the other being cross country skiing. Points are awarded first for the ski jump, then for the cross-country skiing.

Snowboarding was developed in the United States and became a FIS discipline in 1994. There are three main types of snowboarding events:

- Halfpipe: A half-cylinder–shaped course dug deep into the snow, where the athlete gains speed then slides up over the rim of the pipe and performs various aerial tricks. The more difficult the trick, the more points scored (like in gymnastics).

- Alpine: Parallel giant slalom—head-to-head races down a mountain.

- Snowboard cross: Head-to-head races involving jumps and obstacles.

Freestyle skiing, again, was developed in the United States and features moguls, aerials, and ballet.

- Moguls: The athlete skis down a steep hill full of small mounds (moguls).

- Aerials: The athlete skis down a steep hill then makes a ski jump containing acrobatic tricks (Table 76.7).

CHAPTER 77

Sport-Specific Injury Profiles: Summer Olympics Federations

Contributed by David McDonagh, AIBA and FIMS; and all the Chairpersons of the Summer Olympic International Federations whose names you will find below

In this chapter we will give a brief presentation of the Summer Olympic Sports and in particular the lesser known sports.

77.1 AQUATICS (FINA)

There are several aquatic disciplines: swimming, synchronized swimming, diving, water polo, and open-water swimming (Table 77.1). Whilst potentially dangerous sports, most swimming events are not associated with serious injuries, mostly due to the proper control placed on events by the international federation.

77.2 ARCHERY (FITA)

The first recorded archery contest of more recent times was staged in Finsbury, England, in 1583. Archery joined the Olympic Games as a men's sport in 1900 in Paris and then women archers in St. Louis. Individual events became a fixture in 1972. Team events were added in 1988.

There are several archery disciplines that basically involve shooting from different distances in different environments with various forms of equipment. The disciplines are outdoor, indoor, field, ski, 3-D, run, flight, and clout archery (Table 77.2).

77.3 ATHLETICS (IAAF)

Athletics can be divided into four main areas: track, field, combined, and road events.

- Track events include sprints, middle-distance running and long-distance running, hurdling, relays, and the steeplechase.
- Field events include jumping sports—long jump, high jump, triple jump, and pole vault—

and throwing sports—javelin, shot put, discus, and hammer throw.

- Combination events of the above sports include the heptathlon for women and the decathlon for men.
- Road events include the marathon and walking events.

As these sports include a multitude of disciplines, it is safe to say that most injuries can occur—just look at the decathlon—10 separate track-and-field events held on two consecutive days including the 100-m sprint, the long jump, the shot put, the high jump, and the 400-m run followed by the 110-m hurdle race, the discus throw, the pole vault, the javelin throw and the 1,500-m run. The heptathlon is seven track-and-field events held on two consecutive days including the 60-m sprint, the long jump, the shot put, and the high jump, followed by the 60-m hurdle race, the pole vault, and the 1,000-m run (Table 77.3).

77.4 BADMINTON (BWF)

Badminton has its history in a variety of sports: the ancient Chinese played a game called *Ti Zian Ji* in 500 BC, in which a shuttle was kicked with the feet. This may have spawned the development of battledore and shuttlecock, popular games in China, Japan, India, and Greece from the turn of the first millennium to the Middle Ages, when they became known as *jeu de volant* in mainland Europe. The closest modern variant of badminton was an Indian game called *poona*, which was brought to England by British army officers in the middle of the 1800s. A few years later, the Bath Badminton Club drew up the rules that form the basis of today's game. Badminton made its Olympic debut at the 1992 Summer Games in Barcelona, Spain, and has quickly become a popular part of

TABLE 77.1	FINA—International Acquatic Federation
Federation physician	Dr. Margo Mountjoy, Toronto, Canada
E-mail	mmsportdoc@aol.com
Accident type	*Swimming:* Overuse injuries, mainly shoulders, knees and lumbar spine
Aquatic sports are generally quite safe from a medical perspective.	*Synchronized swimming:* Overuse injuries + acute traumatic injuries from acrobatic lifts
	Water polo: Head/face trauma, finger trauma, contusions, lacerations, overuse injuries of shoulder and knees
	Diving: overuse injuries of the wrist, fingers and spine; traumatic injuries are rare.
	Open-water swimming: See Chapter 14.2
Essential skills required by an event physician	See FINA's medical rules and "Medical Guidelines for FINA Competitions," http://www.fina.org/H2O/index.php?option=com_content&view=category&id=89:medical-rules&Itemid=184&layout=default
Essential equipment	See "Medical Guidelines for FINA Competitions." Special medical equipment required for open-water swimming may be found in the *Open Water Swimming Manual.*
Specific qualification requirements	The event physician must be a "qualified medical officer."

TABLE 77.2	FITA—International Archery Federation
Federation physician	Emin Ergen, Ankara, Turkey
E-mail	ergen@medicine.ankara.edu.tr
Accident type	Soft-tissue problems (mainly overuse)
	Heat-related problems: sunburn, heat stroke
	Minor injuries or burns in hands when aiming arrows or carbon shafts are broken
Essential skills required	General medical skills
	Ability to treat musculoskeletal injuries
	Ability to remove ticks
Essential equipment	Bandage unit
	Thermometer
	Stethoscope
	IV infusion set
	Sphygmomanometer
	NaCl 0.9% isotonic solution
Specific qualification requirements	None

TABLE 77.3	IAAF—International Association of Athletics Federations
Federation physician	Juan Manuel Alonso, Madrid, Spain
	Gabriel Dollé, Monaco
E-mail	JM Alonso: dir.medico@rfea.as
	G Dollé: gabriel.dollé@hq.iaaf.org
Accident type	Muscle/tendon acute and chronic injuries
	Joint sprains/dislocations
	Bone fractures
	Concussion
	Heat-related illnesses
	Cardiac arrest
	Asthma crisis/metabolic disorders
Essential skills required by an event physician	Competence in management of musculoskeletal acute and chronic injuries
	Treatment of heat-related illnesses
	Cardiopulmonary resuscitation
	Spinal/extremity immobilization
	Skill at acute internal medical problems (asthma crisis, metabolic disorders, etc.)
Essential equipment	Reanimation equipment and defibrillator
	Emergency medicines
	Bandage unit
	Infusion sets
	Neck, spine, limb immobilization units
	Diagnostic equipment (ECG, glucose test, etc.)
Specific physician qualifications	Being prepared

the schedule. Athletes from China, Indonesia, Malaysia, and Korea have tended to dominate the medal tables (Table 77.4).

77.5 BASKETBALL (FIBA)

Basketball is played by two teams, made up of five players and seven substitutes. The aim of the game for each team is to get the ball into the elevated baskets at either end of the court more times than the opposition, while preventing the opposition from scoring at the same time. A game is made up of four periods, each lasting 10 minutes of actual playing time. If the scores are tied at the end of the game, extra 5-minute overtime periods are played until a winner is declared. There are strict limitations on how the ball can be moved by and between players, including strict time limits that make the games fast, furious, and physical. Basketball is an unusual sport in that one man created it—Canadian physical education teacher Dr James Naismith. He wanted an indoor sport to keep the students at the YMCA training school at Springfield College in Massachusetts fit during the harsh New England winters, and put together the 13 rules that form the basis of modern basketball in December 1891. As the years went by, its popularity spread around the world, leading to the creation of the International Basketball Federation in Switzerland in 1932. Basketball's appeal is truly global, however, with school children and adults playing the game from Europe to Asia. Basketball made its official Olympic debut in the 1936 Summer

TABLE 77.4 WBF—World Badminton Federation	
Federation physician	Gurchuran Singh, Malaysia
E-mail	gbr@pc.jaring.my
Accident type	Eye injuries (shuttlecock), lacerations (racquet)muscle: hamstring and calf injuries
	Achilles ruptures,
	Knee and ankle sprains including ACL injuries
	Low back strains
	Rotator cuff tears
	Abrasions
	Foot blisters (plantar) in hot climates
Essential skills required by an event physician	Accident and emergency medicine
	Reanimation equipment
Essential Equipment	Emergency medicines
	Infusion sets
	Limb immobilization units
	Stretcher
	Wheel chair.
Specific qualification requirements	Registered MD with diploma in sports medicine/emergency medicine

Games in Berlin, Germany. Women's basketball was introduced in the 1992 Summer Games in Barcelona, Spain (Table 77.5).

77.6 BOXING (AIBA)

Modern Olympic boxing is determined by regulations adapted from the famous "Queensberry Rules." Boxers fight in an elevated ring with a canvas and rubber floor, measuring 6.1 × 6.1 m. The sides are marked by four rows of ropes. There are two corners—blue and red—for each opponent to sit in between rounds. The boxers wear clothing to match the color of their corner. As with most combat sports, competitors are divided into weight divisions so that they face-off against opponents of equal size. In Beijing, there were 12 weight classes. Because of this, boxers are weighed on the opening day of competition and every day of the tournament to make sure that they are not heavier than their division's permitted maximum. Contests are scored by five judges, who award points when they feel contact has been made from a targeted punch. Events take place over four rounds of two minutes

each. At the end of the match, the boxer with the greatest number of points is the winner. Boxers can also win a match by knocking out their rivals (Table 77.6).

TABLE 77.5 FIBA—International Basketball Federation	
Federation physician	Heinz Günter, Vienna, Austria
E-mail	doc.heinz@inode.at
Accident type	Muscle injuries
	Ankle and knee joint injuries
Essential skills required by an event physician	None
Essential equipment	None
Specific qualification requirements	Orthopedic surgeons preferred

TABLE 77.6	**AIBA—International Boxing Association**
Federation physician	Charles Butler
Email	cbutlermd@gmail.com
Accident type	Cuts, abrasions, nasal injuries, head injuries
Essential skills required of an event physician	Boxing experience
	Ability to determine if athlete is fit to box
	Safe removal of head-guard and mouthpiece
	Ability to detect and take initiative to prevent serious head, thorax, abdominal injuries
	First aid skills
Essential equipment	Emergency ABC equipment
	Bandage unit (swabs, alcohol, gloves)
	Stethoscope
	Flashlight
	RR meter
	Cervical collar
	Injury severity card
Specific qualification requirements	Boxing experience.
	Must be approved as a ringside physician

77.7 CANOEING (ICF)

In flat-water racing events, paddlers race on a straight course, each boat in a separate lane, over three different distances: 200, 500, and 1,000 m. There are kayak events for men and women in single (K1), double (K2), and four (K4) boats, and canoe events, only for men, in single (C1), double (C2), and four (C4) boats. This form of racing became an Olympic discipline in 1936 and its program includes events over 500 m and 1,000 m. In a kayak, the paddler is seated and uses a two-blade paddle, while in a canoe, the paddler is kneeling on one knee, and uses a single-blade paddle.

In slalom racing, paddlers have to navigate the kayak or canoe through pairs of poles, called "gates," set up over the challenging rapids, waves, eddies, and currents on a 300-m stretch of rough water. If the paddler touches one of the poles, or misses a gate altogether, penalty times are added to the time achieved by the competitor on that run. There are single kayak (K) events for men and women, and canoe events, also for men and women, in single (C1) and double (C2) boats. There are also team events.

This discipline made its appearance in the Olympic Games in Munich in 1972 and then had to wait until 1992 to be reinstated to the Olympic program (Table 77.7).

77.8 CYCLING (UCI)

Cycling events include road, track, mountain bike, cyclo-cross, BMX, trials, indoor cycling, and para-cycling.

In April 1981, the International BMX Federation was founded, and the first World Championships were held in 1982. Since January 1993, BMX has been fully integrated into the International Cycling Union (UCI). BMX was included in the 2008 Olympic Summer Games in Beijing, China. The sport is based on motocross, and riders race around a track, leaping and banking corners and other obstacles. Eight riders compete in each heat (qualifying rounds, quarterfinals, semifinals, and finals), with the top four qualifying for the next round.

Track cycling is a very specialized indoor event. Races take place on an indoor velodrome—a 250- to 300-m wooden oval, with straights banked at 12 degrees and corners banked at 42 degrees. Events include short-distance sprints, time trials, and long-distance endurance races for both teams and individuals. Depending on the discipline, the

TABLE 77.7 **ICF—International Canoeing Federation**

Federation physician	Don McKenzie, Vancouver, Canada
E-mail	don.mckenzie@shaw.ca
Accident type	Primarily overuse in flat-water, some trauma in slalom (lacerations, shoulder dislocations, etc.)
	There are many disciplines in canoeing and the accident types are quite diverse. Any trauma/LOC could result in potential drowning.
Essential skills required by an event physician	Flat-water: First aid, understanding and appreciation of overuse injuries
	Slalom: General emergency medicine skills
Essential Equipment	First aid equipment
	Equipment for resuscitation
Specific qualification requirements	None

result is judged by time, by victory over an opponent, or by completion of a distance.

Mountain biking covers three different disciplines: downhill, four cross, and cross-country/marathon, of which only cross-country is included in the Olympics. Riders all start together and race over a course with laps of 3 or 6 km. A race lasts between 2 and 2½ hours.

Road racing has been part of the Olympics since the 1896 Summer Games in Athens, Greece. That year, competitors rode for two laps of the marathon route from Athens to Marathon and back—a distance of 87 km. Now, road races take place over 239 km for men and 120 km for women, with shorter time trials taking place over 46.8 km for men and 31.2 km for women (Table 77.8).

TABLE 77.8 **UCI—International Cycling Union**

Federation physician	Mario Zorzoli, 1860 Aigle, Switzerland
E-mail	mario.zorzoli@uci.ch
Accident type	High velocity injuries: head, neck, spinal injuries, collarbone and limb (especially elbow and wrist) fractures, thoracic trauma
	Burns and skin injuries
	Splinters on the track
Essential skills required by an event physician	Safe helmet removal
	Competency with neck, spine, extremity immobilization; wound care; ABC
Essential equipment	Neck, spine, limb immobilization
	Reanimation equipment
	Oxygen tank, ventilation mask, infusion set
	Adapted wound dressings
Specific qualification requirements	Experience in sports medicine and/or emergency medicine or traumatology
	In MTB events (downhill), experience in mountain rescue

77.9 EQUESTRIAN SPORTS (FEI)

The Fédération Équestre Internationale is the international governing body of equestrian sports. Recognized competition disciplines include dressage, combined driving, endurance riding, eventing, para-equestrianism, reining, show jumping, and vaulting. It does not govern or provide rules for horse racing or polo. The FEI headquarters are in Lausanne, Switzerland (Table 77.9).

77.10 FENCING (FIE)

In Olympic fencing, there are individual and team competitions for men and women in three disciplines: foil (a very light sword), épée (the sporting version of a rapier), and sabre. Athletes wear protective head and body equipment (Table 77.10).

77.11 FIELD HOCKEY (FIH)

A game consists of two 35-minute periods, with a 10-minute interval for half-time. For the men's competition, there are 12 teams of 16 players that are placed into two pools of six for the preliminary rounds. Each team plays every other team in that pool. The top two teams in each pool progress to the semifinals. The remaining teams play for classifications 5 through 12. Winners of the semifinals play for the gold medal, and losers of the semifinal play for the bronze. For women, there are 12 teams that are placed into two pools of six teams. Like the men's competition, each team plays every other team in that pool. The best two teams of each group progress to the semifinals, and the remaining teams play for classifications 5 through 12. Winners of the semifinals play for the gold medal, and losers of the semifinal play for the bronze (Table 77.11).

77.12 FOOTBALL (FIFA)

Football (Soccer) needs no introduction, it being the world's most played game. FIFA was founded in 1904 and had its Olympic debut in 1908. At the London 2012 Olympics women of all ages and men under 23 are allowed to compete (Table 77.12).

TABLE 77.9	FEI—International Equestrian Federation
Federation physician	Craig Ferrell
E-mail	Craig.ferrell@gmail.com
Accident type	Multitrauma
	Head injuries
	Spinal injuries
	Pelvis and extremity fractures
Essential skills required by an event physician	Emergency management
	Airway management including intubation
	Fluid resuscitation
	Fracture management
	Head injury evaluation
Essential equipment	Ambulance (ideally)
	Spine board
	IV fluids with appropriate catheters
	Airway and intubation tools and medications
	Oxygen
Specific qualification requirements	None at present

TABLE 77.10	FIE—International Fencing Federation
Federation physician	George Ruijsch van Dugteren, Cape Town, South Africa.
E-mail	vandug@iafrica.com
Accident type (1) Life-threatening injuries (2) Sports injuries	(1) Accidents are infrequent, but there is always the (rare) possibility of a very serious injury (e.g., penetration of head, neck, thorax, with trauma to vital structures with broken blade). Contingency plans must therefore be made for this possibility by taking the appropriate measures. (2) A wide range of acute injuries, mostly minor, may occur during competition or training, especially the limbs (ankle sprains, foot, knee, injuries, muscle strains, bruising, superficial lacerations, etc.).
Essential skills required by an event physician	(1) Medical doctor or paramedic, competent at and equipped for ALS. This is obligatory for all official FIE competitions. (2) Sports medicine–trained doctor, paramedic, or physiotherapist, competent at and experienced in dealing with acute and chronic sports injuries. Also obligatory. Roles (1) and (2) are often combined.
Essential equipment	(1) Resuscitation equipment (cardiac, respiratory); ambulance present or max 10 min away; efficient means of communication (2) Appropriate first aid equipment, not forgetting ice, bandages, dressings, stretcher, wheelchair, crutches, etc.

TABLE 77.11	FIH—International Hockey Federation
Federation physician	Fook Wong, San Jose, CA, USA
E-mail	fookywong@hotmail.com
Accident type	Athlete hit by ball or stick
	Fractures
	Sprains
	Lacerations
	Collisions
	Turf burns/skin abrasions
	Dental injuries
Essential skills required of an event physician	Cervical collar application
	Use of spinal board
	Limb splint application
	Safe removal from field of play
Essential equipment	Cervical collar
	Spinal transfer board
	Extremity splints
	Crutches
	Wheelchair
Specific qualification requirements	None. Usually orthopedists, physical rehabilitation specialists, or primary care physicians (general practitioners)

TABLE 77.12	FIFA—International Federation of Football Associations
Federation physician	Terence Babwah, Trinidad, West Indies
E-mail	terbab@hotmail.com
Accident type	50–70% contact injuries; 30–50% noncontact injuries
Contact: during tackles, contact with other players	90% injuries are soft-tissue injuries (e.g., muscle strains, tendon injuries, muscle contusions)
Noncontact: injuries not involving contact	10% are severe injuries: muscle tears, head and neck injuries, limb fractures
	70% of injuries involve the lower limb (most common are foot and ankle injuries; second are groin and thigh injuries) and 30% upper limb and back
Essential skills required by an event physician	Management of head and neck injuries on field with correct removal of unconscious or head-injured player from field of play
	CPR and use of defibrillator on field
	Immobilization of limbs after injuries
	Initial management of soft-tissue injuries
Essential equipment	Spine board
	Rigid collar
	Oxygen and face mask
	Airways
	Limb splints
	Current debate: external defibrillator
Specific qualification requirements	FIFA competitions require fully equipped emergency teams including trained physicians at all games. All FIFA requirements regarding staff and infrastructure are laid out in detail in the "Medical Services at FIFA Tournaments" document provided to the respective local organizing committee in preparation of the competition.
	At national level, large disparity at present depending on the role and standard of sports medicine in the respective member association and the level of the competition.
	At present, FIFA is aiming to establish requirements for team physicians trained in football medicine with all relevant related medical injuries, complaints, and illnesses to be covered.

77.13 GOLF (IGF)

Golf has reentered the Olympic program, last been Hosted at the 1904 St. Louis Games. At the 2016 Rio de Janeiro Olympic Games, a 72-hole individual stroke play competition featuring both 60 ranked men and women is planned (Table 77.13).

77.14 GYMNASTICS (FIG)

There are many various gymnastic events. In the Beijing Olympics, both the floor exercise and the horse vault events were for both men and women. Men also competed in the horizontal bar, parallel bars, pommel horse, rings, and in individual all-around and team artistic gymnastics. Women also competed

TABLE 77.13	IGF—International Golf Federation
Federation physician	
E-mail	
Accident type	Tendinitis and tendinosis of the shoulder, elbow, and wrist, often due to repetitive movements. Back pain—including disc problems, spondylolysis, spondylolisthesis, and myalgia. Hip problems, often myalgias, due to swing posture. Costal lesions. Head injuries due to being struck by a club or ball.
Essential skills required by an event physician	Should be experienced with treating stress and overuse injuries, head injuries, be able to treat asthma, allergies, and various bite wounds.
Essential equipment	Standard doctors bag with medication—in particular for asthma and allergy, and antibiotics, NSAIDs, nebulizer.
Specific qualification requirements	General practitioner with sports medical experience; sports medical doctor.

in asymmetric bars, balance beam, individual all-around, and team artistic gymnastics (Table 77.14).

77.15 HANDBALL (IHF)

Handball is considered one of the oldest games in the history of sport. References in Homer's *Odyssey* provide evidence of a game similar to handball, which was played on the island of the Faiakes (Corfu). Another sign is a third century BC bronze statuette found in Dodoni, showing a boy carrying a ball in his hand. Depictions of humans playing a "primitive" form of handball are also found on a marble plaque found at the Athens Acropolis, dating to about 600 BC. The sport reappeared in the indoor form, for men, at the Munich 1972 Olympic Games and, for women, in 1976 in Montreal (Table 77.15).

TABLE 77.14	FIG—International Gymnastics Federation
Federation physician	Michel Leglise, Paris, France
E-mail	info@fig-gymnastics.org
Accident type	Spinal injury
	Limb fracture/dislocation
	Hand and toe injuries
Essential skills required by an event physician	Neck and spinal immobilization
	Ability to reduce dislocations and fractures
	Ability to use limb splints
	Treatment of cuts and abrasions
	Ability to administer CPR
Essential equipment	Cervical collar
	Spinal board
	Limb splints
	Bandage unit for cuts and abrasions
	Suture material
Specific qualification requirements	None

TABLE 77.15	IHF—International Handball Federation
Federation physician	Francois Gnamian, Abidjan, Ivory Coast
E-mail	Fr.gnamian6002@yahoo.fr
Accident type	Joint dislocation/sprains (shoulder, elbow, knee, ankle)
	Finger sprains or fractures
	Concussion
	Facial injuries, nasal injuries
Essential skills required by an event physician	Competency with neck, spine, extremity immobilization
	Laceration, abrasion wound care
	Reanimation
Essential equipment	For international events, one ambulance for athletes
	Immobilization equipment
	Resuscitation equipment
	Wound care equipment
Specific qualification requirements	None. However, traumatologist, orthopedic surgeon, or sports medicine specialists are preferred

77.16 JUDO (IJF)

Judo has its origins in the Japanese martial arts. Judo was derived from jujitsu, the art of attacking others or defending oneself. In 1882, Dr. Kano Jigoro (the Father of Judo) made a comprehensive study of the ancient self-defense forms and integrated the best of these forms into a sport that is known as Kodokan judo. The term *judo* breaks down into *ju* (gentle) and *do* (way or path), or "the gentle way." Judo became an official event in the Olympic Games of Tokyo in 1964 (Table 77.16).

TABLE 77.16	IJF—International Judo Federation
Federation physician	Lauri Malinen, Finland
E-mail	lauri.malinen@pkssk.fi
Accident type	Joint dislocation (shoulder, elbow)
	Knee, finger, toe sprains or fractures
	Rib fractures
	Facial injuries, cuts around the eyes
Essential skills required by an event physician	Competency with neck, spine, extremity immobilization
	Laceration, abrasion wound care
	Reanimation
Essential equipment	Ambulance for spectators, ambulance for athletes
	Immobilization equipment
	Resuscitation equipment
Specific qualification requirements	Experience in judo

77.17 MODERN PENTATHLON (UIPM)

The modern pentathlon is the original military sport: It contains shooting, fencing, swimming (200-m freestyle), show jumping, and finally, a 3,000-m run. The final run is staggered, so the first person across the line is the winner. This is a demanding sport for the athlete as competitions are often carried out on one day. Both women and men compete in this sport (Table 77.17).

77.18 ROWING (FISA)

Founded in1892 in Turin, FISA was the first international sports federation to join the Olympic movement. It has been on the Olympic program since the 1896 Summer Olympics in Athens (even though the rowing events were cancelled due to high winds).

In Olympic rowing, there are many variations: There are events for men and women, lightweights and heavyweights, with one or two oars. There are single events and team events with 8, 4, or 2 athletes, without or without a coxswain (Table 77.18).

77.19 RUGBY (IRB)

Founded in England at Rugby School by William Webb Ellis, the game is now spread all over the world. Rugby union was played at the Olympic Games in 1900, 1908, 1920, and 1924. The executive board of the International Olympic Committee has reinstated rugby as an Olympic sport, in the sevens format, from 2016. Rugby sevens is the reduced version of the game, with seven rather than 15 players. The game is fast and furious and has fewer injuries than the full 15-man game and will make its debut in the 2016 Rio Olympics (Table 77.19).

77.20 SAILING (ISAF)

In Olympic sailing, there are many events. Common for men and women are the Laser one-person dinghy, windsurfers, 470 two-person dinghy, and keelboats, as well as men's skiff, Finn, and tornado classes. Sailing, which has had both kings and princesses participating in the Olympics, does not have a medical committee.

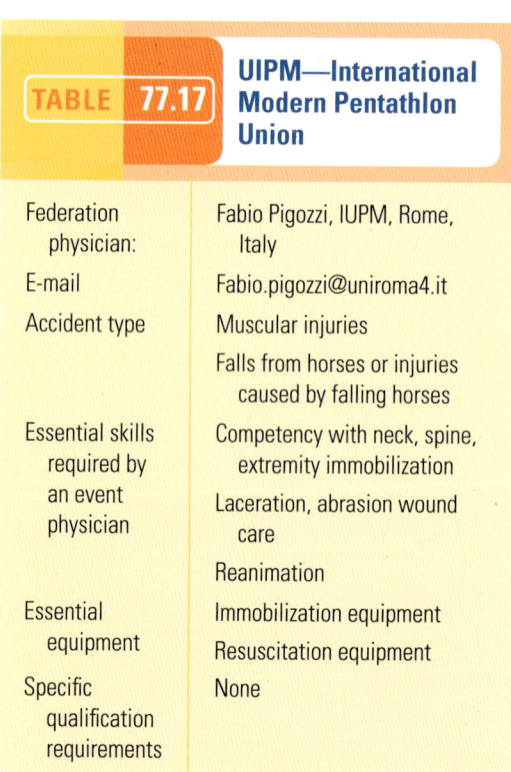

TABLE 77.17	UIPM—International Modern Pentathlon Union
Federation physician:	Fabio Pigozzi, IUPM, Rome, Italy
E-mail	Fabio.pigozzi@uniroma4.it
Accident type	Muscular injuries
	Falls from horses or injuries caused by falling horses
Essential skills required by an event physician	Competency with neck, spine, extremity immobilization
	Laceration, abrasion wound care
	Reanimation
Essential equipment	Immobilization equipment
	Resuscitation equipment
Specific qualification requirements	None

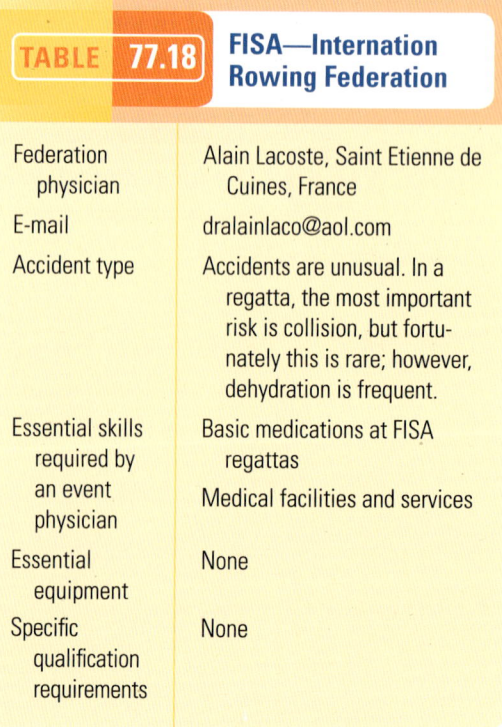

TABLE 77.18	FISA—Internation Rowing Federation
Federation physician	Alain Lacoste, Saint Etienne de Cuines, France
E-mail	dralainlaco@aol.com
Accident type	Accidents are unusual. In a regatta, the most important risk is collision, but fortunately this is rare; however, dehydration is frequent.
Essential skills required by an event physician	Basic medications at FISA regattas
	Medical facilities and services
Essential equipment	None
Specific qualification requirements	None

TABLE 77.19	IRB—International Rugby Board
Federation physician	Martin Raftery, Australia
E-mail	irb@irb.com
Accident type	Tackling, fall injuries
	Accidental blows, strains, and sprains
Essential skills required by an event physician	Neck, spine, extremity immobilization
	Soft-tissue injuries
	Knee, ankle, shoulder injuries
Essential equipment	Immobilization and resuscitation equipment
Specific qualification requirements	Experience in treating rugby injuries

77.21 SHOOTING SPORTS (ISSF)

Shooting has been on the Olympic Program since 1896. There are several different disciplines for men (9) and women (6) basically using pistols, rifles or shotguns to shoot various targets (Table 77.20).

77.22 TABLE TENNIS (ITTF)

Table tennis evolved, along with badminton and lawn tennis, in England from the ancient game of tennis (also known as *jeu de paume*, real tennis, court tennis, or royal tennis). The game had many

TABLE 77.20	ISSF—International Shooting Sports Federation
Federation physician	James M. Lally, California, USA
E-mail	drlally@primehealthcare.com
Accident type	Repetitive stress–type injuries, mostly musculoskeletal from holding a firing position
	Rarely, an eye injury from powder, particle, fragment blowback, especially since introduction of shooting safety glasses
Essential skills required by an event physician	Manipulative /manual medicine since most shooters are reluctant to take oral medications
	General medical knowledge/practices for those rare, unforeseen situations like new-onset seizure, cardiac arrest, heat injury, limb injury from fall
	Common sense, good humor, and lots of patience
Essential equipment	Stethoscope
	Blood pressure cuff
	Eye irrigation
	Liniment (Bengay)
	ACE wrap
	Minor first aid kit
	Water
Specific qualification requirements	None

TABLE **77.21**	ITTF—International Table Tennis Federation
Federation physician	Jean Francois Kahn, Paris, France
E-mail	kahn@ccr.jussieu.fr
Accident type	Sprains
	Muscular, tendon, joint strains
Essential skills required of an event physician	General medical skills
Essential equipment	General medical equipment
	Physiotherapy, massage
Specific qualification requirements	None

only kicks are permitted to the head/face, excluding the back of the head. One point is scored for a blow to the trunk, two points for a head/face kick, and three points for a knockout.

Most injuries are minor and do not lead to time loss. The range of time-loss (TL) injuries in adults was from 2 to 34 per 1,000 athlete-exposures (A-E). In children, the rates ranged from 7 to 30 per 1,000 A-E.

In adults, fractures ranged from 8% to 23% of total injuries. In children, the range was 3% to 11%. The foot is especially susceptible to fractures. Cerebral concussion rates ranged from 1 to 55 per 1,000 A-E (adults) and from 4 to 51 per 1,000 A-E (children).

The roundhouse kick is involved in the greatest number of injuries in adults and children, followed by the spinning back kick. For TL injuries in adults, the roundhouse kick was the most dominant injury mechanism.

In adults and children, the roundhouse kick was involved in most cases of cerebral concussion. The axe kick was the next commonest kick involved in concussion.

Without having the WTF's recommendations, it is difficult to say with certainty which skills are required, but it would appear that an ability to evaluate and treat head and neck injuries is essential.

77.24 TENNIS (ITF)

Tennis was one of the original nine Olympic sports in Athens in 1896, with Ireland's John Boland defeating Dionysios Kasdaglis of Greece to become the first Olympic tennis champion. Tennis withdrew from the Olympics after the 1924 Games but returned in Seoul in 1988 (Table 77.22).

77.25 TRIATHLON (ITU)

The triathlon is a relatively new event at the Olympics, having made its debut at the Sydney 2000 Summer Games. The medals were some of the first handed out in Sydney and the golds were awarded to Brigitte McMahon of Switzerland in the women's race and Canada's Simon Whitfield in the men's. There are always three events: open-water swimming, cycling, and finally running. In the Beijing Olympics, athletes swam for 1.5 km, cycled 40 km, and finally ran 10 km. The sport is reported to have been started in Hawaii, where athletes competed against each other to prove who was the fittest—runners or cyclists (Table 77.23).

different popular names initially, including ping pong, which also had its own governing body. The sport is now run by the ITTF, which was founded in 1928 (Table 77.21).

77.23 TAEKWONDO (WTF)

Contributed by Dr. Willy Pieter, Department of Physical Education, University of Asia and the Pacific, Pasig City, Metro Manila, Philippines.

The name is composed of three parts: "tae" means "foot" and refers to all leg techniques; "kwon" means "fist" and refers to all arm techniques; and "do" means "the way," which originally referred to the road to enlightenment. The match lasts three rounds of 2 minutes each with a 1-minute break in between rounds. In case of a tie at the end of the third round and after a 1-minute break, a sudden-death fourth round is contested. The athletes wear a helmet, chest protector, and gloves. They compete in eight weight divisions (four divisions at the Olympic Games) each for men and women. Junior taekwondo athletes compete in 10 weight divisions. Points may be scored on the trunk covered by the chest protector, excluding the spine. Kicks and punches are allowed to the trunk, while

TABLE 77.22	ITF—International Tennis Federation
Federation physician	Do not have a dedicated physician
Head of Science Commission	Stuart Miller, Roehampton, UK
E-mail	Stuart.Miller@itftennis.com
Accident type	See Chapter 14
Essential skills required by an event physician	Cardiac resuscitation
	Defibrillation
	Intravenous infusion
	Competent with limb immobilization
	Musculoskeletal examination
	Familiarity with doping list
Essential equipment	Resuscitation equipment
	AED
	Ventilation mask
	Infusion set
	Limb immobilization
	General medications
Specific qualification requirements	None

TABLE 77.23	ITU—International Triathlon Union
Federations name/Sport	ITU, Triathlon, Duathlon, Winter Triathlon
Federation physician	Sergio Migliorini,Cameri, Italy
E-mail	sermigliorini@aliceposta.it
Accident type	Oculofacial trauma and barotraumas
	Head, shoulder, hip, wrist injuries
	Low back pain
	Acute and overuse injuries
	Heat stroke
Essential skills required by an event physician	Competent in acute and overuse injuries, heat incidents, wound care, ABC
Essential equipment	Reanimation equipment and medication for acute respiratory and cardiac emergencies
	ECG, defibrillator
	Infusion sets
	Neck, spine, limb immobilization
	Bandage unit
	Blankets, towels, water
Specific qualification requirements	None, but two physicians must be present (also one physician per 200 athletes)

TABLE 77.24	**FIVB—International Volleyball Federation**
Federations name/Sport	FIVB, Volleyball and Beach volleyball
Federation physician	Roald Bahr, Oslo, Norway
E-mail	Roald.bahr@nih.no
Accident type	Acute ankle sprains, acute knee sprains
	Finger sprains, dislocations, fractures
	Beach volleyball: dehydration and hyperthermia
Essential skills required by an event physician	Competent in resuscitation with oxygen and defibrillator
	Beach volleyball: rehydration and cooling
Essential equipment	Reanimation equipment and defibrillator
	Infusion sets
Specific qualification requirements	Must have sports medical training and certification as provided by national authorities

TABLE 77.25	**IWF—International Weightlifting Federation**
Federation physician	Michael Irani, London, England
E-mail	mehernooshuk@hotmail.com
Accident type	Extremity and spinal injuries
	Overuse musculoskeletal disorders
	Acute patellar tendon rupture
	Shoulder and elbow dislocation
	Syncope
	Palm and shin abrasions
Essential skills required by an event physician	Knowledge of competition rules and spinal immobilization
	Ability to reduce dislocations and fractures, use limb splints, treat cuts and abrasions, administer CPR
Essential equipment	Guedel airways
	Ambu Bag and mask(s)
	Cervical collar
	Spinal board
	Limb splints
	Bandages and tape
	Antiseptic lotion
	Ice packs
	Surgical gloves
	Ambulance and accompanying personnel
	(A local doctor should be present to assist in logistics for injured athletes or spectators.)
Specific qualification requirements	Doctors must be proposed by their National Federation and selected at the Electoral Congress

77.26 VOLLEYBALL (FIVB)

The game of volleyball was invented in Springfield, Massachusetts, in 1895. Inventor William G. Morgan was a former student of the Canadian teacher James Naismith, the inventor of basketball. The game was spread by the American armed forces and grew in popularity outside of the United States more than it did within its country of origin. It became an official Olympic sport in 1964 (Table 77.24).

77.27 WEIGHTLIFTING (IWF)

Weightlifting was popular in ancient Greece and Egypt but did not feature in the ancient Olympics. The sport was included in the first modern Games in Athens in 1896. Women's events were introduced in Sydney in 2000. There are eight weight classes for men and seven for women.

Competitors must lift in two categories—first snatch, then clean and jerk—and the two lifts are put together to determine the final placement. Each competitor can have three attempts at each category. In the snatch, the competitor lifts the bar overhead in a single movement. In the clean and jerk, the weight is raised to shoulder level in one movement and then lifted overhead in a second movement (Table 77.25).

77.28 WRESTLING (FILA)

In wrestling, there are two main disciplines: freestyle and Greco-Roman. Female wrestling became an Olympic discipline at the Athens Games in 2004. In Greco-Roman wrestling, competitors are only allowed to use their arms and upper bodies to subdue and control their opponent, and to touch their opponent in the arms and upper bodies (Table 77.26).

TABLE 77.26	FILA—International Federation of Associated Wrestling Styles
Federation physician	Marc Demars
E-mail	marc.demars@wanadoo.fr
Accident type	Contusions
	Epistaxis
	Distortions of knee, ankle, elbow, wrist
	Luxations of shoulder and elbow
	Neck and spinal injuries (especially cervical injuries)
Essential skills required by an event physician	Competence in sports trauma management
	Neck and spinal immobilization
	Ability to reduce luxations
	Knowledge of osteopathy and rheumatology
Essential equipment	First aid kit/bandage unit
	Immobilization unit, including vacuum mattress
	Infusion unit
	Ventilation unit with oxygen
	Defibrillator
	Stretcher
Specific qualification requirements	Sports medicine specialist with emergency medical skills

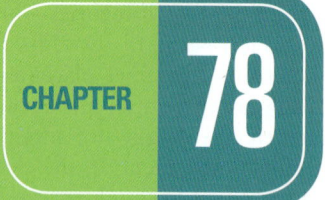
Sport-Specific Injury Profiles: International Paralympic Committee (IPC)

Contributed by Dr. Peter van de Vliet, Medical and Scientific Director, International Paralympic Committee, Bonn, Germany

The IPC acts as the International Federation for the following IPC sports:

- Alpine skiing
- Athletics
- Biathlon
- Cross-country skiing
- Ice sledge hockey
- Powerlifting
- Shooting
- Swimming
- Wheelchair dance sport

The IPC acts as the major event organizer for the Paralympic Summer and Winter Games with the following sports on the program:

Summer Games:

- Archery
- Athletics
- Boccia
- Cycling
- Equestrian
- Football: 5-a-side and 7-a-side
- Goalball
- Judo
- Powerlifting
- Rowing
- Sailing
- Shooting
- Swimming
- Table tennis
- Volleyball (sitting)
- Wheelchair basketball
- Wheelchair fencing
- Wheelchair rugby
- Wheelchair tennis

Winter Games:

- Alpine skiing
- Biathlon
- Cross-country skiing
- Ice sledge hockey
- Wheelchair curling

Here are some of the specific injuries and illnesses seen at paralympic events and the minimum of physician skill-sets and equipment needed to treat them (Table 78.1).

TABLE 78.1 IPC—International Paralympic Committee

Federation Name	International Paralympic Committee (IPC)
Sports	See above
Federation physician	IPC does not have a mandate for a medical officer, except for major events. All medicine-related questions should be addressed to Dr. Peter Van de Vliet, IPC Medical and Scientific Director
Address	International Paralympic Committee, Adenauerallee 212–214, D 531113 Bonn, Germany
E-mail	peter.vandevliet@paralympic.org
Accident type	The conditions observed in Paralympic athletes include cerebral palsy, paralysis, amputations, visual impairments, and certain intellectual disabilities.
	Besides regular sports-related accident types, medical teams should be aware that athletes with high spinal cord lesions, as well as athletes with cerebral palsy or brain injury, might suffer from reduced temperature regulation and have a greater risk of dehydration, independent of the temperature.
	A specific concern arises regarding skin breakdown in athletes with spinal cord lesion, and the deliberate induction of autonomic dysreflexia ("boosting") in athletes with high spinal cord lesion.
Essential skills required by an event physician	The medical program for athlete care should be consistent with that provided for the Olympic athletes.
	It is important for the medical team to understand that treating *elite athletes* with these disabilities can be very different than providing treatment to patients in typical physical medicine and rehabilitation or physiatrist practices.
	The athletes are often experts with regard to their disabilities and how they manage their health so they should be active participants in determining treatment options.
Essential equipment	Besides regular sports-related equipment, the medical teams must be sure they have experience in extricating athletes from adaptive equipment when Paralympic athletes are competing with such adaptive equipment (e.g., monoski shells, ice sledges).
Specific qualification requirements	Event physicians preferably have experience in providing care to athletes with disabilities and have background in sports medicine or rehabilitation medicine/physiatry.

CHAPTER 79

Sport-Specific Injury Profiles: Non-Olympic Sports

79.1 AMERICAN FOOTBALL (IFAF)

Contributed by Dr. James Macdonald, Team Doctor for the University of California at Santa Cruz (UCSC) and covers high school football games in Santa Cruz, California

American football is a type of "gridiron" football, which, as its name would suggest, is primarily played in the United States. The sport is spreading, with teams forming in Europe, Australia, the Pacific Islands, and Mexico; the Canadian version of the sport is very similar to what is played in the United States. The rules of American football evolved from rugby football code in the late 19th century.

The sport is a collision sport marked by bouts of intermittent anaerobic activity and large amounts of contact. There is a substantial injury rate, despite the use of special protective equipment, ranging from helmets with face masks to shoulder pads. Soft-tissue injuries, skin infections, hyperthermic illnesses, fractures, and dislocations are commonly seen; so, too, are more catastrophic injuries, such as closed head and cervical spine injuries. According to the National Center for Catastrophic Sport Injury Research, 28 football players died from direct football injuries in the years 2000 to 2005, with an additional 68 dying from dehydration, asthma, or other noninjury causes.

The International Federation of American Football is the governing body for American football with 45 member associations throughout the world. The digest of rules for the sport can be found at http://www.nfl.com/rulebook/digestofrules (Table 79.1).

79.2 CRICKET (ICC)

Cricket is believed to have originated in England and was definitely being played at the time of Henry VIII. With the expansion of the British Empire, the sport spread around the world and is played in more than 100 countries. It is a major sport in England, India, Australia, South Africa, India, Pakistan, and the West Indies.

In cricket, one team bats (with two batsmen at a time) trying to score as many runs as possible until being dismissed. A batsman can be dismissed by either being bowled out, run out, or if the ball is caught in the air. The team with the most runs wins. There are many variations of the game including test cricket, one-day events and limited overs cricket (e.g., 20/20). Bowlers can bowl at great speed (up to 160 km an hour) and aim for the batsmen (Table 79.2).

79.3 BASEBALL (IBAF)

Baseball is a simple game, with two teams who take turns batting and fielding, each trying to score more runs than the other. It has a range of complex rules and terminology and tactical subtleties and techniques, though, that make it a complex sport with a true depth of understanding. Baseball was spawned in the United States in the early 19th century, with its roots in the British games of rounders and cricket. In 1876, a national league was formed for teams across the country to compete against each other, and the tactics, terminology, history, and stars of the sport are now an ingrained part of

TABLE 79.1 IFAF—International Federation of American Football

Accident type	Injuries include concussions and other closed head injuries; cervical spine injuries; brachial plexus injuries ("stingers"); fractures and dislocations; lacerations, abrasions and contusions; severe ligamentous disruptions such ACL and MCL tears. The injury rate is high in American football.
Essential skills required by an event physician	Management of cervical spine trauma
	Evaluation of concussions
	Splinting of acute fractures and dislocations
	Laceration repair
	Injections (such as of the AC joint)
	Return-to-play decisions are made frequently in American football
Essential equipment	Especially important to have are tools to evaluate concussions and stabilize cervical spine injuries, including special equipment for removing face masks, and spine transport boards. Taping and bracing are frequently done both pregame and during the game to protect injured anatomy. Emergency medical transport should be at close hand for transfer from field to hospital.
Specific qualification requirements	Team rosters are typically large and the injury rate high, so coverage of games is usually done by physicians in concert with athletic trainers and standby emergency medicine personnel. No specific qualifications are required.

TABLE 79.2 ICC—International Cricket Council

Federation physician	Peter Harcourt
E-mail	peter.harcourt@vis.org.au
Accident type	Contusions
	Strains and sprains in the lower back, shoulder, elbow, knee, and foot
Essential skills required by an event physician	Competence in the diagnosis and care of musculoskeletal injuries and heat-related illnesses
Essential equipment	General medical and sports resuscitation equipment
Specific qualification requirements	Sports medicine experience essential, sports medicine specialist preferable

the language and culture in the United States. Over time, baseball's influence has spread worldwide. It is now hugely popular in Japan and Central and South America, with Cuba having won three gold medals from the four Olympic finals contested so far, and Japan being a regular medal finisher. Baseball became a full Olympic sport for the 1992 Summer Games in Barcelona, Spain, having been a demonstration sport a number of times in the past. Until the 2000 Summer Games in Sydney, the event was only open to amateur players, but that year the competition was opened up to professional players to let them represent their country. At the Olympic Games, each team plays the other seven teams once in a league, and the top four teams advance to the semifinals. The first-placed team then plays the fourth-placed team, and the second-placed plays the third. The winners of those semifinals meet to decide the gold and silver medals, with the two losing teams playing for the bronze. Baseball lost its Olympic position after the Beijing Games (Table 79.3).

TABLE 79.3	Baseball
Federation physician	Gianfranco Beltrami, Italy
E-mail	g.beltrami@alice.it
Accident type	Head and neck injuries. Blunt injuries to the trachea, larynx, heart (contusion, even rupture), abdomen (organs, viscera, or vessels), genitalia.
Essential skills required by an event physician	Competent in neck, spine and extremity immobilization; wound care; and ABC
Essential equipment	Immobilization unit
	Reanimation equipment
	Oxygen, ventilation mask
	Infusion unit
Specific qualification requirements	Experienced in emergency medical procedures

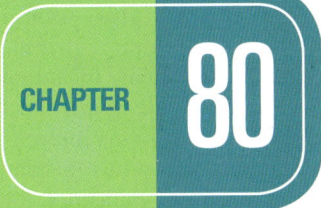

80

Coaches and Referees:
The BokSmart Project

Contributed by Wayne Viljoen, Justin Durandt, Pierre Viviers, and Clint Readhead, South African Rugby Medical Association Committee Members

While this next chapter may diverge somewhat from what may appear to be the direction of this manual (i.e., the training of Event Physicians), I include it as an example of how one may establish training courses to teach nonmedical staff in the absence of a trained physician. This may be an avenue that other federations or authors might want to explore—David McDonagh

BokSmart is a national rugby safety program developed in South Africa, and aims to make the game of rugby union safer for all participants involved in the game by teaching and implementing evidence-based injury prevention and injury management strategies to predominantly nonmedical personnel. It further aims to educate and teach safe and effective rugby techniques to assist in lowering the number of serious and/or catastrophic concussion, head, neck, and spine injuries associated with the game. The program is mainly focused on coaches and referees.

80.1 WHY WAS BOKSMART INTRODUCED?

A serious or catastrophic concussion, head, neck, or spine injury is a very real risk in a contact sport such as rugby union. However, very few of these injuries occur relative to the number of player exposure hours to the training and playing of rugby. Injuries can range from death to permanent damage such as quadriplegia, tetraplegia, paraplegia, or to what is commonly termed a "near-miss" injury; this refers to an acute brain or spinal cord injury with either complete recovery or partial recovery with some residual damage remaining after the injury. Due to the enormous following and immense amount of media exposure given to rugby union in South Africa, a huge amount of pressure has been placed on rugby's controlling body to make the game safer for all involved in the game and to reduce the risk of these injuries occurring.

In schoolboy rugby in South Africa, an average of seven injuries a year, and in rugby union as a whole, an average of 17 serious and/or catastrophic injuries a year have been reported to the Chris Burger/ Petro Jackson Players' Fund (www.playersfund. org.za/) between 2001 and 2008. This does not however account for those injured players missed or not picked up by the system (New Zealand has been averaging around 1 to 2 per year since 2001). However, there are between 400,000 and 500,000 rugby players in South Africa versus approximately 150,000 players in New Zealand, which represents around —two to three times more players exposed to rugby and the risk of serious and/or catastrophic injury. Regardless of this fact, the statistics are still too high, and one of these injuries is one too many. The common aim and ultimate goal of the various rugby injury prevention programs around the world (BokSmart [SA], Rugbysmart [NZ], Smart-rugby [AUS], Rugby Ready [IRB]) are to eliminate these injuries from the game.

80.2 WHAT ARE THE PROGRAM CONTENTS?

The strategic framework for BokSmart rests on five main pillars:

- Coaches and referees
- Medical protocols
- Research
- Legislation
- Marketing and communication

Coaches and Referees

The primary aim of BokSmart is to provide rugby coaches, referees, players, and administrators with the correct knowledge, skills, and leadership abilities to ensure that safety and best practice principles are incorporated into all aspects of contact rugby in South Africa.

At most matches played in SA, there are little or no medically qualified personnel, medical facilities, emergency medical equipment, or medical support available, and the same applies for practices. For this reason, coaches and referees are sometimes the only people available to intervene and ensure the safety of the players on the field, and are therefore viewed as the first line of defense in the prevention of serious and/or catastrophic injuries.

Medical Protocols

These protocols were developed to provide coaches, referees, and players with a better understanding of injuries—how to prevent them and how they should be managed appropriately both on and off the field. From a serious injury management perspective, a coach or referee will know, at the very least, what not to do, how to manage the situation, and how to engage appropriate medical support as quickly as possible.

Prevention is always better than cure, and the BokSmart program also addresses numerous topical issues around injury prevention, injury management, rugby safety, and performance.

Eating and Drinking Right for Rugby: This section focuses on providing relevant topical information and practical guidelines for rugby players on different components of nutrition.

Effective Play and Controlling the Game: Rugby is a contact sport with high-impact collisions, so there is always a risk of injury. It is essential to stress the point that players should be properly coached to play safe rugby, and this is especially important when teaching the correct execution in contact situations. Even more important is to highlight the fact that *safe rugby* is also *smart* and *winning rugby*. This section also brings in the referee's role in keeping players safe on the field during all aspects of play, and ensuring a fair and safe contest at all times.

Fair Play and the BokSmart Code of Conduct: This is to ensure that rugby is played in good spirit, in a disciplined and fair manner, and without any unnecessary rough play and malice.

Management of Rugby Injuries: This section encompasses various aspects of injury identification, prevention, and management, including on-field acute rugby injuries, acute spinal cord injuries, and concussion; specific injury prevention programs, rehabilitation, and return-to-play guidelines; and specific practical guidelines for a coach or referee on when an injury is serious enough to remove a player from the field of play or when to seek specialist medical opinion. BokSmart provides detailed clinical best practice guidelines in these areas via an educational DVD. Detailed injury prevention programs are provided on the BokSmart website; the most relevant being on preventative neck and shoulder conditioning. An instructional portion on neck conditioning is further provided on the DVD resource.

Physical Preparation and Recovery Techniques: Evidence-based and practical guidelines are provided regarding the various components and injury treatment and prevention, recovery, and performance.

Preparticipation Screening of Players: In the South African rugby environment, the medical screening of players during the preseason is not standard and very rarely practiced. For this reason BokSmart has devised a preparticipation screening tool for coaches. This is an easy-to-use questionnaire, which helps the coach to assess which players are at risk or require medical clearance or medical attention before participating in rugby training or in contact sessions—with particular emphasis on concussion, head, neck, and spine injuries. For every question answered with a "yes," there is a directive to assist the coach in suitably referring the player to a medical professional for clearance.

Preseason Testing and the Physical Profiling of Players: Testing of players prior to participating in rugby has become a very necessary and important part of injury prevention initiatives around the world and in all sports. It is important to ensure that players are adequately prepared physically for the game, and suitably conditioned, developed, and matched for their position and age-group–specific level. BokSmart has provided coaches with a basic rugby fitness testing battery to assess players' physical readiness for participating in rugby. This aims to prevent coaches from putting "at-risk" players onto the field where they are not suitably developed or conditioned for their positions and age-appropriate levels of play.

Protective Equipment in Rugby: Several commercial companies are involved in the design and production of a wide variety of protective equipment and clothing specific to rugby. Despite claims by these manufacturers, much controversy remains regarding the effectiveness of protective equipment. BokSmart provides practical guidelines regarding the most effective forms of protective equipment.

Safety in the Playing Environment: Because of the diversity and demographic vastness in South Africa, coaches and referees frequently have to make important safety decisions on whether a match should take place or not, or how to proceed if an emergency situation presents itself on the field. For this reason BokSmart has developed guidelines for minimum medical standards before a match can take place, and provides a basic medical resource and basic medical training for non-medical personnel in the DVD workshops.

Serious Injury Protocol: One of the medical protocol initiatives is a "serious injury" protocol, reporting form, and follow-up questionnaire, to study and understand from a practical perspective why the serious and/or catastrophic injuries are occurring, where they are occurring, and how one can prevent them. Every coach and referee will be educated in the DVD workshops on how to use this protocol effectively.

Strength and Conditioning for Effective Rugby: Resistance training and physical conditioning for rugby forms an extremely important part of injury prevention in rugby. A lack of strength and conditioning in a contact sport such as rugby union can lead to excessive fatigue on the field, which reduces concentration and control and thereby exposes one to an increased risk of severe injury.

BokSmart provides evidence-based resistance training guidelines and programs and rugby-specific fitness conditioning guidelines and programs for players at all levels of rugby (resistance exercises and fitness drills are detailed and explained in full on the BokSmart website, www.BokSmart.com).

Research

BokSmart aims to assist in establishing effective injury surveillance protocols on a national level, and monitor injury trends around the country. Research provides scientific credibility to the program by measuring the effects of the intervention. BokSmart has also utilized 34 experts to research

and provide all the evidence-based guidelines provided on the program.

Legislation

To ensure success, legislation forms a crucial cog in the wheel. BokSmart aims to legislate that no coach or referee may put a team on the field or blow a game, respectively, unless they have undergone the BokSmart training. They would have to renew their license every 2 years. BokSmart also aims to legislate and enforce specific medical protocols and minimum medical guidelines for rugby participation. BokSmart aims to motivate any other legislative changes in the game within South Africa on the basis of scientific evidence or current best clinical practice guidelines.

Marketing and Communication

BokSmart has developed a Web site that is accessible to the general public, coaches, referees, players, and anyone else who may be interested. When the program was launched, an extensive marketing campaign was put in place to message BokSmart to the entire rugby population and general public at large. Communication and education plays a massive role in keeping players safe on the field, and this forms the very basis of the BokSmart campaign.

80.3 HOW DOES BOKSMART TRAIN NONMEDICAL PERSONNEL?

BokSmart plans to educate and empower every coach and referee at all levels of play around the country to promote safe rugby techniques and basic medical and injury prevention practices. Every coach and referee at all levels of play will be trained on the BokSmart Rugby Safety Program at workshops provided around the country. At the BokSmart workshops, every attending coach and referee will receive an instructional booklet, an instructional DVD, and a pocket concussion guide, and will undergo a DVD-facilitated workshop.

The medical instructional section on the DVD uses expert EMS training personnel to explain and demonstrate the correct ways of identifying, grading, and managing a suspected serious head, neck, or spine injury. The section also details other concepts such as the primary injury survey, CPR, secondary injury survey, C-spine stabilization, the log roll, the vomit drill, basic emergency care, and treatment of acute soft-tissue injuries, to name but a few. Another key focus is on concussion, and coaches and referees are educated on this hot topic, and further provided with a compact instructional pocket "concussion guide," for identifying and managing a suspected concussed athlete properly. Frequently, referees and coaches do not understand or consider the potential effects of incorrectly managing a potentially serious concussion, head, neck, or spine injury on-field. Many times, peer pressure from a partisan crowd or spectators, a winning-at-all-cost approach, or a lack of understanding forces a coach or referee to make a decision that could permanently affect a player's life. These situations are life changing for both parties if something goes wrong.

Every coach and referee having attended the entire course will be licensed for a 2-year period. At the end of the 2-year period, they will have to attend another BokSmart workshop presented in a similar format and receive the most recent evidence-based rugby safety information at the time.

In addition to these courses, BokSmart has also developed a rugby-specific first aid training program, called the BokSmart Rugby Medic program. The Rugby Medic program provides coaches, referees, players, or any involved person within the rugby community, at the very least, with the primary skills necessary to be able to identify and manage a potentially serious or catastrophic concussion, head, neck, or spine injury.

The focus of the Rugby Medic program is mainly on the disadvantaged and underresourced areas, which do not have any appropriate equipment, training, or medical support. These clubs or schools are often identified by the unions or can directly request training, and BokSmart provides the Rugby Medic training at no cost to the school or club. The course is a 1-day practical course, and basic competency on the different components is assessed at the end of the course. If the trained rugby club or school does not possess the minimum emergency medical equipment required to appropriately stabilize and support a seriously injured player, and they comply with specific minimum criteria, BokSmart provides them with a complete set consisting of a spinal board, cervical collar, spider harness, and head blocks at no cost.

On top of this, BokSmart provides a toll-free national emergency telephone helpline called the BokSmart Spineline to expedite and fast-track the emergency treatment and management of a potentially seriously injured rugby player. The BokSmart Spineline is a dedicated emergency rugby helpline for serious concussion, head, neck, and spine injuries. The number (0800 678 678) is linked to a national emergency service provider, ER24, who provides the necessary advice, provides an initial telephone screen, and dispatches or arranges suitable transportation of the injured player to the nearest or most suitable medical facility as required. Part of the BokSmart training and Rugby Medic training is to educate everyone on the BokSmart Spineline's availability and how to utilize this service properly.

Additionally, the serious injury protocol that every coach and every referee receives provides step-by-step instructions and details the club, school, team, provincial union, and South African Rugby Union's responsibilities. The protocol also dictates that, in the case of such an injury, the home team's responsible person, coach, or referee needs to telephone the BokSmart Spineline helpline. The local emergency medical service provider will immediately notify the BokSmart Serious Injury Case Manager (SICM) to the injury. The SICM then ensures that all relevant parties are informed with regard to any serious and/or catastrophic injury associated with the game, and makes key decisions regarding the injured player's management en route to a suitable medical facility.

Following the incident, both the referee and coach have to independently submit a completed Serious Injury Report Form to the BokSmart SICM within 48 hours. The SICM will in the interim ensure that appropriate care and management of the player has been provided. The SICM then performs a standardized follow-up assessment with the injured player, coach/referee, and/or witnesses to better understand how the incident could have been prevented.

80.4 WHAT ARE THE DIFFICULTIES IN CONDUCTING SUCH A PROGRAM?

Given the diversity of the South African population, the demographic vastness of the country, and the great economical disparity between communities, it is a challenge to implement a program of this nature.

Another impediment for this type of program is that there are 14 provincial rugby unions in SA, and each union has its own unique educational format, demographic challenges, and structures in place. One of the provincial unions has six subunions within its structures, is extremely vast and covers almost a third of the country's surface area. To access one of the subunions within this union's borders requires a 1,000-km trip; another subunion is a 720-km trip. Many of the remaining unions have similar challenges in urban areas, towns, rural settlements, and villages that may be huge distances apart, thus posing challenges in gathering coaches and referees. BokSmart has therefore endeavored to ensure the respective unions present the rugby safety workshops within a structure suitable to their respective demographics.

South Africa also has 11 official languages. Given the extent and outreach of the program, it is not financially viable to produce such program in all 11 languages. BokSmart has used English as the language of choice. To make this work practically, the different regional trainers who are selected to present the workshops within their provincial union structures are required to have a specific skill set to be effective.

This presents another challenge. The selected facilitators have to be well-respected coaches or referees within their union and community. They need to have a good understanding of English and be able to communicate effectively and facilitate a workshop. Given the linguistic challenges in SA, it is also important that the facilitator be able to efficiently facilitate the discussions in the respective language applicable to the zone or region he or she is allocated within the union.

One of the biggest obstacles for participation in programs like these within the South African context is the fear of failure. The only criteria for licensing would be a compulsory attendance at the workshop. This same strategy has been used very effectively in New Zealand's Rugbysmart program.

80.5 RESULTS

It is presently too early to show any results, as the program is in its early stages, and the DVD workshops have not commenced as yet. Some of the aspects of the program have been active for a while such as the Rugby Medic program. BokSmart has not officially launched yet and has already reached over 300 clubs and school teams, and provided close to 100 sets of equipment in the last year. It has empowered certain clubs and teams that previously did not have any medical support at matches to have a basic level of medical care present in the event of a serious injury happening.

Having seen the effectiveness of a similar DVD-facilitated rugby safety program in New Zealand, BokSmart is confident that, through these initiatives, the number of serious and/or catastrophic injuries will be reduced via appropriate education.

80.6 ADVICE TO OTHERS WISHING TO INTRODUCE A SIMILAR PROGRAM

Important advice is to share knowledge and interact with other role players around the world. One cannot grow and develop an effective program of this nature without tapping into the resources of existing programs and learning from them. Do not however merely copy a successful program and expect it to work. Learn from other programs' mistakes, take the best of what has worked, and modify this to suit your own unique environment and circumstances. In the same light, be willing to share your information with others. Be cognizant of barriers to participation, and remove them where possible. Attendance on its own has shown to be effective in reducing serious injuries. Standardize the message of the program to ensure consistency. If you are providing training to between 30,000 and 55,000 coaches and referees around the country in a year, the message can change via different interpretation of the presenters. By using a DVD-facilitated workshop, the message that is provided is the same at every workshop, and the same message is always reinforced. This has also been shown to be a very effective strategy. To get coaches and referees to buy into a biennial certification system, you have to provide extras such as additional practical coaching or refereeing tips that can act as a drawcard to entice them to attend and participate. Be subtle in how you push safety and injuries. If you keep focusing just on safety and injury prevention, they will quickly lose interest. Finally, legislation is the key to the success of this type of program. If you do not have to attend, nine times out of ten, you will not.

CHAPTER 81

Major Championship Medical Plan: An Example

Contributed by Dr. Charles Butler, Chair, Amateur International Boxing Federation Medical Committee, Michigan, United States; Medical Plan from the AIBA World Championships, Chicago, United States, 2007

TABLE OF CONTENTS

MESSAGE FROM THE CHIEF MEDICAL OFFICER

Welcome to Chicago!

The Chicago Organizing Committee has spared no effort or expense to make this the best and safest Elite World Championship in history. In my six World Championships, I have never seen an organizing committee work as hard or achieve as much in strategic preparation for your safety.

We welcome you, the almost 700 athletes from 120 countries; you, the AIBA staff, technical delegates, judges, and referees; you, coaches, trainers, volunteers, and support personnel including my fellow physicians who will give their time to work for your safety.

We, as a team, have created this hard-copy medical plan so that everyone will be aware of the preparations made and resources available to take care of our athletes and guests. We have included names and telephone numbers of emergency personnel and facilities and the standardized schema for treatment of the stricken boxer. The more people who understand the plan, the more smoothly this plan is likely to run in time of need. While we have tried to plan for every eventuality, we want all to know that boxing is the safest of all contact sports. The concussion rate at World Championships is less than 0.75%. Amateur boxing has the fewest concussions and a rate of neurologic injury that approximates the general population.

Your medical officers, the AIBA medical jury, and team and volunteer physicians are here to serve you. We wish every athlete success. We anticipate a fiercely fought and fairly judged competition. We are available to serve in need. We sincerely wish you a safe, successful event.

Yours in Boxing,

Charles F. Butler

Charles F. Butler MD, PhD

81.1 INTRODUCTION

81.1.1 Purpose of Document

The goal of this medical plan is to cover all aspects of the sport, the facility, the equipment, and the athlete.

81.2 FACILITY EVALUATION (MEDICAL)

81.2.1 Inspect Practice Facility (UIC PEB)

On October 17, members of the AIBA medical commission shall inspect the practice facilities to ensure the following:

- All rings and equipment have been installed properly and safely (see "Ring Inspection," below)

- Emergency medical treatment plan is in place and understood by training center manager, George Hernandez. In case of accident or injury, call 911.

81.2.2 Inspect Competition Arena (UIC Pavilion)

On October 20, members of the AIBA medical commission and the CMO shall inspect the competition facilities to ensure the following:

- All rings and equipment have been installed properly and safely (see "Ring Inspection," below).

- Relationship, position, and distance of the rings from the fans are acceptable. Ringside personnel must be safe from fan activity.

- Dressing rooms (locker rooms) are an acceptable distance from the rings, and the route is convenient for athlete entrance and exit.

- An area for postbout exams has been established within the arena.

- A medical observation area has been established that is
  - Appropriate to privately examine, suture, or splint boxer
  - Well lighted in order to examine or suture athlete
  - Accommodating for examination of athletes either supine or standing
  - Stocked with suture equipment, local anesthetic, and simple examination tools (otoscope, ophthalmoscope, etc.)

- Tables have been installed adjacent to the ring in the neutral corner accommodate —three to four physicians at ringside. These tables should be stocked with plenty of gauze, gloves, and penlights.

- Stairs have been installed adjacent to the physician tables so that the physicians can mount ring apron quickly.

81.2.3 Ring Inspection

The following are standard criteria used to determine that both the training and competition rings have been installed properly and safely:

TABLE 81.1.2	Summary of Medical
Chief medical officer (CMO)	Dr. Charles Butler (269) 598-6000
Assistant CMO	Dr. Robin Goodfellow (269) 598-5533
AIBA Medical Commission chairman	Dr. Edward van Wijk
AIBA Medical Commission member	Dr. Vagner Mortensen
Training center manager	George Hernandez (773) 415-7620
Tournament hospital	Rush University Medical Center 1653 W. Congress Parkway, Chicago, IL 60612 (312) 942-5000
Hospital emergency contact	Hospital triage nurse (312) 942-3422
Ambulances	Two at UIC Pavilion during competition Zero stationed at UIC PEB (training center) Advance Ambulance 5567 N. Elston Ave., Chicago, IL 60630 (773) 774-8999
Medical insurance	1) USA Boxing Insurance for athlete accident/injury ($350,000 limit) 2) Optional MEDEX TravMed Abroad ($3/day/person for $100,000 limit)

- Rings of appropriate size (6.1 m)
- No dangerous seams or surface defects
- Floor at least 1-in wooden base
- Covering foam or Ensolite, 2.5 cm thick (not thicker)
- Tight-fitting canvas mat cover
- Ring posts padded
- Buckles covered
- No sharp edges
- Four ropes, proper tension, two spacers on each side

81.3 MEDICAL PROCEDURE

81.3.1 Medical Staff During Competition

The following are basic procedures for the medical jury during competition.

- Medical staff shall introduce themselves to the local metro officers and/or crowd control staff so that they know who is in charge case of a medical emergency.
- Referees shall face the medical table during the rest period.
- Referees shall make eye contact with medical staff to know who to signal into the ring.
- Ringside staff shall be the last ones to leave the arena after the fight.
- EMTs shall remain until all dressing rooms and medical rooms have been cleared.

81.3.2 Unconscious Victim

The protocol to manage an unconscious boxer shall be discussed in the first CMO/AIBA Medical Commission briefing before the competition.

- Check airway
- Remove mouthpiece
- Ensure cervical precautions (log roll, etc.)
- Place athlete on stretcher
- Provide oxygen

- Remove headgear at ringside
- Install cervical collar
- Check for movement (spinal cord intact)
- Load into ambulance; light and siren transport to hospital
- Notify Rush Hospital triage nurse @ 312-942-3422

81.3.3 Evacuation from UIC Pavilion

An evacuation route has been established for possible injured boxers to Rush Hospital. This route must be communicated to the AIBA medical commission, CMO, assistant CMO, on-site physicians, and EMTs.

EMTs and two ambulances should be established on-site at all times during competition.

EMTs shall be prepared to mount the ring if intubation and evacuation are necessary.

Volunteer Illinois licensed physicians shall be setup near the AIBA medical jury.

81.3.4 Medical Assistance for Tournament Personnel or Spectators

Basic medical assistance to spectators will be provided by the venue. Any emergencies shall be handled by a call to 911. A physician not serving at ringside could also assist.

Although basic first aid supplies are expected of UIC, the event shall additionally consider having the following on-site:

- Insulin/glucose for diabetics
- Nitroglycerine for cardiac patients

- Medications for acute allergic reactions
- Antihistamines
- Sedatives

81.3.5 Medical Assistance in Hotels

Basic medical assistance to hotel guests will be provided by the hotel. Any emergencies shall be handled by a call to 911.

In international tournaments, the federation team physicians will be responsible for medical treatment of their athletes.

81.3.6 Medical Assistance at Practice Facility

Basic first aid will be available to athletes by UIC at the training facility. All emergencies shall be handled by a call to 911.

In international tournaments, the federation team physicians will be responsible for medical treatment of their athletes.

81.4 STAFF

81.4.1 Medical Staff Officials

There will be eight physicians from AIBA's medical commission attending the competition in addition to the chief medical officer (CMO) and assistant CMO.

These medical officials shall be provided the following:

- VIP credentials allowing them to go anywhere
- Medical jury positioned at ringside in front of technical jury

TABLE 81.4.1	Medical Commission Members
Medical Official	**Title**
Dr. Charles Butler	Chief medical officer (CMO)
Dr. Robin Goodfellow	Assistant CMO
Dr. Edwin van Wijk	AIBA Medical Commission chairman
Dr. Vagner Mortensen	AIBA Medical Commission member
Dr. Odd Syverstad	AIBA Medical Commission member
Dr. Gideon Kendino	AIBA Medical Commission member
Dr. Erno Kiss	AIBA Medical Commission member
Dr. Jean Louis Llouquet	AIBA Medical Commission member
Dr. Hirofumi Nagatomi	AIBA Medical Commission member
Dr. Nirmolak Singh	AIBA Medical Commission member

- Three to four seats at physicians' table for medical jury (three jury, one extra physician)

- Steps to access ring by physician table (neutral corner)

- Car for AIBA physicians to get back and forth from hotel

- Transportation for doping doctor who must stay after others leave to get to hotel

- At least six seats for the AIBA medical commission

81.4.2 Federation (Team) Doctors

It is expected that nearly half of the federations will bring a doctor. These doctors will be used throughout the tournament to facilitate medical examinations. Specifically, all federation doctors (~42) will be required to assist with the initial weigh-ins and medical evaluations scheduled for 7:00 AM on October 23.

81.4.3 Volunteer Doctors

The local organizing committee plans to supplement the medical officials and team doctors with local doctor volunteers. The plan includes recruitment of five to ten local doctors to be present for the initial weigh-in and medical evaluations scheduled for 7:00 AM on October 23.

81.4.4 Medical Symposium

A medical symposium shall take place October 29 at 8:00 AM. The following are requirements for this seminar:

- Meeting shall last approximately 2 to 3 hours

- Physicians, coaches, trainers, and Referees and Judges (R/Js) are welcome to attend

- A suitable presentation room (50 to 75 chairs) is required (including capability to present in PowerPoint)

- Adequate communication of the seminar (date, location, etc.) in the official and boxer hotels

81.5 EQUIPMENT

81.6 MEDICAL INSURANCE

81.6.2 Athlete Injury/Accident Insurance (via USA Boxing)

Coverage is only applicable to *athlete* injuries/accidents incurred during the "usual activities" of our competition. This *excludes*

TABLE 81.5.1	Emergency Equipment at Ringside
Equipment	**Location**
Oxygen	FOP
Stretcher	FOP
Cervical collar	FOP
Oral airways, 2 sizes	FOP
Screw to pry teeth to secure airway	FOP
AmbuBag, valve, mask	FOP
Equipment for CPR	FOP
Laryngoscope	FOP
Adrenalin, etc.	FOP

FOP, Field of play.

- Coverage for foreign coaches, officials, referees, delegation members, guests, fans, etc. (USA delegation is covered)

- Sickness, disease, previous injury, assault and battery/fighting

- Air travel

Coverage includes the usual activities and travel to and from such activities, including the competition, shows, preshows, practices, and warm-ups.

Excess accident medical is $25,000 per person with an additional catastrophic injury policy with an aggregate limit of $350,000. Deductible is $100. Benefit period is 52 weeks.

81.6.3 Optional MEDEX TravMed Abroad Insurance

As healthcare is expensive in the United States, all event participants are encouraged to carry medical

TABLE 81.5.2	Miscellaneous Supplies
Equipment	**Location**
Diagnostic instruments	UIC Pav
Surgical instruments/supplies	UIC Pav
Orthopedic supplies	UIC Pav

TABLE 81.5.3 Forms

Form	Location
TUE	AIBA
Restriction forms	UIC Pav
USA Boxing Medical Claim Form	UIC Pav and UIC PEB
Printed cards for weigh-in	Palmer
Printed cards for doping checks	UIC Pav
Injury sheet with physician advice	UIC Pav

insurance during their stay in Chicago. The local organizing committee, working with USA Boxing, has negotiated a discounted rate for you. All accredited members of the World Boxing Championship can receive MEDEX TravMed Abroad insurance for *only $3 per day per person*. For participants purchasing the coverage for October 18 to November 4, the total cost will be $54.00 per person.

TravMed Abroad includes a $100,000 emergency medical and evacuation benefit and 24/7/365 multilingual MEDEX Assistance. The deductible is $25.00. This insurance provides not only medical services but also a variety of travel services (such as translation support). For more information on the benefits, services, and exclusions, please call MEDEX at 1-800-732-5309 or visit their Web site at http://www.medexassist.com/Individuals/Products/TravMedAbroad.aspx.

Note: This insurance product has been tailored to accommodate sport-related accidents and injuries, as well as foreign participants. The base product on the Web site does not reflect this.

81.6.3.1 Enrollment

Travelers *must* purchase coverage within 24 hours of checking into the World Boxing Championships or by the next business day. Visit the tournament services office (third floor of Palmer House) for assistance. The three available options for enrollment are

Phone registration

- Call this number to enroll: 1-800-732-5309
- Hours: 8:00 AM to 5:00 PM Monday through Friday

TABLE 81.6.1 Summary

Coverage Type	Carrier	Coverages
Accident medical coverage for boxers (US and foreign)	USA Boxing (through sanction of event)	Accident medical: $25,000/person Accidental death and dismemberment: $10,000 Deductible: $100 Covers usual competition activities (competitions, shows, preshow activities, practices, and warm-ups)
Catastrophic medical coverage for boxers (US and foreign)	USA Boxing (through sanction of event)	Catastrophic coverage: $350,000 Deductible: $25,000 Covers usual competition activities (competitions, shows, preshow activities, practices, and warm-ups)
Optional emergency accident and sickness medical insurance	MEDEX TravMed Abroad (Purchased by Federation $3/day/person)	Accident and sickness: $100,000/person Emergency dental: $200 Emergency medical evacuation and repatriation deductible: $25

- *Please be sure to mention USA Boxing to receive the special rate ($3/day/person).*

Fax registration

- Visit the tournament services office and complete the available form

- Fax to 1-410-308-7905

- *Please be sure to mention USA Boxing to receive the special rate ($3/day/person).*

E-mail registration
E-mail the following details to AMiller@medex-assist.com

1. Subject: World Boxing Championship TravMed Registration (Federation)

2. Federation: example, Ireland

3. Participant information for EACH person: first name, last name, date of birth, arrival date, departure date

4. Payment information:
   - Credit card type: American Express, VISA, or Mastercard
   - Credit card number
   - Expiration date
   - Cardholder name
   - Amount approved to charge ($3/day/person)

81.6.3.2 Corporate Contact
Our contact at MEDEX is Andrew Miller.
E-mail: amiller@medexassist.com
Direct Phone: (410) 308-7933

81.7 ANTIDOPING

81.7.1 Doping Control Overview

USADA (United States Anti-Doping Agency) will administer doping tests. USADA will provide training to all doping chaperones and staff to ensure that all rules are followed and no specimens are corrupted.

Athletes will be selected for doping tests per the following schedule:

October 23 to October 28 and October 30 to November 1: one athlete selected randomly. It has been suggested to randomly select athletes for doping from the first session.

November 2: six losing athletes randomly selected
November 3: all 11 gold-winning athletes

81.7.2 Doping Control Area Requirements

The doping control area shall be established per defined requirements, including the following:

- Three rooms shall be available—they must be connected. First, the waiting room, then the processing room, and then finally the sample collection room (requiring private area with adequate toilet rooms).

- The doping room shall have the ability to be locked.

- The doping room shall have a table at the entrance where the officials sign in boxers (give special badge and take the accreditation).

- There shall be one table per four to six athletes to be tested.

- There shall be a sufficient number of chairs (two per athlete, one per test personnel, two extra); finals shall test 11 athletes, so approximately 20 to 30 chairs will be required.

- There shall be a refrigerator or cooler stocked with at least eight 12–ounce, individually sealed (tamper evident) containers of soft drinks, water, and juice (no alcohol).

- USADA contact information shall be made available to medical officials.

- The doping room shall be located within a 1½-minute walking distance from the ring.

- There shall be a TV for the boxers who are tested (they want to follow other matches). Chaperones shall be available and responsible to bring the boxers from the ring to the doping room.

- The doping waiting room shall have a trash can.

- All doping rooms shall have adequate lighting.

- USDA shall make doping control chaperones and staff aware of special needs handling/process.

- Transportation shall be made available for both the doping doctor and the boxers to bring them back to the hotel (samples sometimes take hours to collect).

- Contact USAB for the lab to process doping tests and US procedures.

81.8 MEDICAL EVALUATION AND WEIGH-IN

81.8.1 Overview

The medical evaluation and weigh-in processes are determined by AIBA's technical delegates. This plan will substitute that listed below when made available to the local organizing committee.

On October 23 starting at 7:00 AM on the fourth floor of the Palmer House Hotel, all athletes shall be evaluated by a medical professional and weighed.

81.8.2 Installation and Setup Requirements

The following are requirements and instructions provided to the local organizing committee by the chief medical officer. These requirements were used in consideration of preparing for the design, setup, and installation of the medical evaluation and weigh-in process scheduled for October 23. These requirements include

- The medical evaluation and weigh-in location shall consist of three connecting rooms preceded by a practice scale. These rooms are
  - First room with two tables for technical delegates and AMC member to check passports and AIBA passbooks
  - Second room with EMTs and doctors to perform medical evaluations
  - Third room with scales for weigh-in
- The weigh-in location shall be flexible to adapt to the changing daily requirements per the following:
  - First day (October 23): 10 to 20 paramedics to test the blood pressure and temperature of the boxers and 15 to 29 tables for the doctors in charge to do the medicals
  - Daily (after October 23): 8 to 12 paramedics to test the blood pressure and temperature of the boxers and eight to 10 tables for the doctors in charge to do the medicals

  - Semifinals (November 2): six paramedics to test the blood pressure and temperature of the boxers and four to six tables for the doctors in charge to do the medicals
  - Finals (November 3): six paramedics to test the blood pressure and temperature of the boxers and four to six tables for the doctors in charge to do the medicals

- Staffing physical exams (excluding registering and weigh-ins) shall be supplemented with federation doctors and local volunteer physicians.

- Transportation shall be provided for doctors for the morning medicals.

- Establish a registration area consisting of two tables at the entrance for technical delegates and AMC members to check AIBA passbooks and passports.

- There shall be adequate space for boxers.

- There shall be adequate desks/tables and chairs for physicians.

- There shall be adequate light.

- There shall be proper temperature control and ventilation.

81.9 ATHLETE SERVICES

81.9.1 Beverage Requirements

Bottled water shall be available in adequate supply for all athletes.

Cold bottled water, pop, or coffee shall be available in adequate supply for officials, referees/judges, and physicians.

81.9.2 Food Requirements

Nutritional food appropriate for all ethnicities shall be available for athletes throughout the day.

Appendix

TRIATHLON EQUIPMENT

ACLS equipment and drugs: These are best supplied by trained paramedics but should be available with experienced personnel.

Lab available for serum electrolytes	Ice for injuries and over heating as required: up to 1 kg/4 athletes
Oral fluid: 1 L/4 competitors, depending upon the environment	Blankets and towels for up 10% to 15% of athletes
One set of blood pressure cuff/stethoscope per nurse and or physician	Bandage/dressings for 5% of athletes
IV setups for 5% or more of competitors, depending upon the environment	IV fluids: Should not be hypotonic unless serum electrolytes have been taken, and should not be given except to athletes who are clinically quite dehydrated and cannot take p.o. fluids.

A partial checklist (thanks to T.K. Miller, MD.), which should be evaluated, updated, and adjusted on a race-by-race basis:

Ace wraps, acetaminophen, alcohol wipes, ant- acid tablets, antiemetic/antinausea medications	Back/spine board, basins
Cervical collars + one clip board per cot	Epinephrine, eye pads, eye wash
Flash lights or penlights	Gauze pads 2 × 2 and 4 × 4, gloves, exam, gloves, sterile + glucose monitor, for example, finger stick
Goose neck lamp	Hibiclens + hydrogen peroxide
IV dressings + IV hangers + IV dressings	Lidocaine, injectable + lidocaine, viscous
Medical reporting forms	Needles, IV start and for injection
Oto-ophthalmoscope	Pads, abdominal + pens, writing one for each clipboard + polysporin/antibiotic ointment
Q tips	Saline irrigation + scissors + scrub brushes, sterile + slings, for upper extremity injury
Sheets + soap + Steristrips + suture kits + syringes	Tape, adhesive for bandages + Telfa pads (i.e., nonstick bandages) + thermometers
Tongue blades, tourniquets for blood draw and IV starts	Valium ampoules for injection, Vasoline + Ventolin or similar inhaler
Wipes, sterile	

TERRAIN SPORT EQUIPMENT

See Table A1.

ACSM—CONSENSUS STATEMENTS

See pages 16–24 and 528–529.

TABLE A1 Equipment and Medical Supplies in Medical Tents in OTW 2007

Items from Warehouse and Central Sterilizing Supplies Department

Wound Management	Unit	Total	Wound Management	Unit	Total
Elastic dressing pad	box	110	Bowl 6"	pc	25
Strapping micropore ½"	roll	29	Kidney dish 10"	pc	37
Strapping micropore 1"	roll	94	Gallipot (2 oz)	pc	85
Adhesive zinc oxide	roll	175	Plastic dissecting forceps	pc	70
Elastoplast	roll	175	Dx. applicator w/cw tip	pc	19700
Crepe bandage 3"	roll	1710	Nonsterile gauze	100/pk	42
Crepe bandage 4"	roll	1710			
Tubigrip "E"	box	20			
Tubigrip "F"	box	28			
Duoderm	pc	18			
Wooden tongue Depressor	box	18			
Triangular bandage	pc	70			
Sufratulle dressing pack	pc	60			

Monitor and Tools	Unit	Total	Monitor and Tools	Unit	Total
Lancet	pc	190	Pen	pc	41
Torch	pc	10	Book (shorthand)	pc	11
Small torch	pc	35	Small note book	pc	30
Battery (size D)	pc	52	Thermometer	pc	44
Battery (size AA)	pc	120	Oral disposable thermometer sheath	pc	200
Latex small gloves (Vinyl)	pc	1600	Razor	pc	11
Latex medium gloves (Vinyl)	pc	3100	Sphygmomanometer	pc	11

(continued)

TABLE A1 Equipment and Medical Supplies in Medical Tents in OTW 2007 (continued)

Monitor and Tools	Unit	Total
Latex large gloves (Vinyl)	pc	1900
Scissors	pc	83
Surgical masks	box (50 pc each)	18

IV Line	Unit	Total
BGS with pump	set	11
Syringes 2.5 mL	box	1300
JMS infusion set	set	38
Needle 21 G	pc	1000
Angiocath 16 G	pc	24
Angiocath 18 G	pc	24
Angiocath 20 G	pc	24
Angiocath 22 G	pc	24
Tegaderm	pc	24
Tourniquet	metre	11
Sharp box	pc	12

Monitor and Tools	Unit	Total
Stethoscope	pc	11
Pocket mask	pc	11
Hemostix machine	pc	11

Others	Unit	Total
Machintosh plastic sheet	sheet	11
Tape Adhesive Packaging Clear 430 mm × 40 m	roll	11
Bed sheet	sheet	11

Items from Pharmacy

Antiseptics	Unit	Total
0.015% chlorhexidine gluconate with 0.15% cetrimide (Salvon)	1 L/bottle	20
0.015% chlorhexidine gluconate with 0.15% cetrimide (Salvon)	25 mL/pack	90
NS for irrigation	1 L/bottle	32

Local Application	Unit	Total
Vaseline 100 g/bottle	100/bottle	80
Anthisan/Eurax Cream	tube	12
Analgesic Balm	tube	1662

Monitor and Tools	Unit	Total
Haemo-Glukotest	pc	165

IV Line	Unit	Total
Dextrose 10%, 500 mL	bottle	22
Dextrose 50%, 500 mL	bottle	12
Normal saline, 500 mL	bottle	22

Oral Drugs	Unit	Total
Paracetamol	tab	750
Dologesic	tab	750
Triact	tab	750
Glucose powder	500 g/pack	?????
GES	sac	455
Aspirin 300 mg	tab	190
Buscopan 1 mg	tab	275
Maxalon	tab	225
Imodium (Loperamide) 2 mg	tab	225
Loratadine 10 mg	tab	130
Ventolin inhaler	tube	11
Stemetil	tab	225
Naprosyn	tab	285
Antiseptic handrub	bottle	25
Alcohol swab	box	28

Team Physician Consensus Statement

SUMMARY

The objective of the Team Physician Consensus Statement is to provide physicians, school administrators, team owners, the general public, and individuals who are responsible for making decisions regarding the medical care of athletes and teams with guidelines for choosing a qualified team physician and an outline of the duties expected of a team physician. Ultimately, by educating decision makers about the need for a qualified team physician, the goal is to ensure that athletes and teams are provided the very best medical care.

The Consensus Statement was developed by the collaboration of six major professional associations concerned about clinical sports medicine issues: American Academy of Family Physicians, American Academy of Orthopaedic Surgeons, American College of Sports Medicine, American Medical Society for Sports Medicine, American Orthopaedic Society for Sports Medicine, and the American Osteopathic Academy of Sports Medicine. These organizations have committed to forming an ongoing project-based alliance to "bring together sports medicine organizations to best serve active people and athletes."

EXPERT PANEL

Stanley A. Herring, M.D., Chair, Seattle, Washington
John A. Bergfeld, M.D., Cleveland, Ohio
Joel Boyd, M.D., Edina, Minnesota
William G. Clancy, Jr., M.D., Birmingham, Alabama
H. Royer Collins, M.D., Phoenix, Arizona
Brian C. Halpern, M.D., Marlboro, New Jersey
Rebecca Jaffe, M.D., Chadds Ford, Pennsylvania
W. Ben Kibler, M.D., Lexington, Kentucky
E. Lee Rice, D.O., San Diego, California
David C. Thorson, M.D., White Bear Lake, Minnesota

TEAM PHYSICIAN DEFINITION

The team physician must have an unrestricted medical license and be an M.D. or D.O. who is responsible for treating and coordinating the medical care of athletic team members. The principal responsibility of the team physician is to provide for the well-being of individual athletes—enabling each to realize his/her full potential. The team physician should possess special proficiency in the care of musculoskeletal injuries and medical conditions encountered in sports. The team physician also must actively integrate medical expertise with other healthcare providers, including medical specialists, athletic trainers, and allied health professionals. The team physician must ultimately assume responsibility within the team structure for making medical decisions that affect the athlete's safe participation.

QUALIFICATIONS OF A TEAM PHYSICIAN

The primary concern of the team physician is to provide the best medical care for athletes at all levels of participation. To this end, the following qualifications are necessary for all team physicians:

- Have an M.D. or D.O. in good standing, with an unrestricted license to practice medicine
- Possess a fundamental knowledge of emergency care regarding sporting events
- Be trained in CPR
- Have a working knowledge of trauma, musculoskeletal injuries, and medical conditions affecting the athlete

In addition, it is desirable for team physicians to have clinical training/experience and administrative skills in some or all of the following:

- Specialty Board certification
- Continuing medical education in sports medicine
- Formal training in sports medicine (fellowship training, board recognized subspecialty in sports medicine [formerly known as a certificate of added qualification in sports medicine])
- Additional training in sports medicine
- Fifty percent or more of practice involving sports medicine
- Membership and participation in a sports medicine society
- Involvement in teaching, research and publications relating to sports medicine
- Training in advanced cardiac life support
- Knowledge of medical/legal, disability, and workers' compensation issues
- Media skills training

DUTIES OF A TEAM PHYSICIAN

The team physician must be willing to commit the necessary time and effort to provide care to the athlete and team. In addition, the team physician must develop and maintain a current, appropriate knowledge base of the sport(s) for which he/she is accepting responsibility. The duties for which the team physician has ultimate responsibility include the following:

Medical management of the athlete

- Coordinate pre-participation screening, examination, and evaluation

- Manage injuries on the field
- Provide for medical management of injury and illness
- Coordinate rehabilitation and return to participation
- Provide for proper preparation for safe return to participation after an illness or injury
- Integrate medical expertise with other health care providers, including medical specialists, athletic trainers and allied health professionals
- Provide for appropriate education and counseling regarding nutrition, strength and conditioning, ergogenic aids, substance abuse, and other medical problems that could affect the athlete
- Provide for proper documentation and medical record keeping

Administrative and logistical duties

- Establish and define the relationships of all involved parties
- Educate athletes, parents, administrators, coaches, and other necessary parties of concerns regarding the athletes
- Develop a chain of command
- Plan and train for emergencies during competition and practice
- Address equipment and supply issues
- Provide for proper event coverage
- Assess environmental concerns and playing conditions

EDUCATION OF A TEAM PHYSICIAN

Ongoing education pertinent to the team physician is essential. Currently, there are several state, regional and national stand-alone courses for team physician education. There are also many other resources available. Information regarding team physician specific educational opportunities can be obtained from the organizations listed to the right.

Team physician education is also available from other sources such as: sport-specific (e.g., National Football League Team Physician's Society) or level-specific (e.g., United States Olympic Committee) meetings; National Governing Bodies' (NGB) meetings; state and/or county medical societies meetings; professional journals; and other relevant electronic media (Web sites, CD-ROMs).

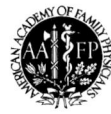

- American Academy of Family Physicians (AAFP)
  11400 Tomahawk Creek Pkwy.
  Leawood, KS 66211-2672
  1-800-274-2237

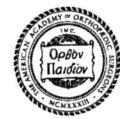

- American Academy of Orthopaedic Surgeons (AAOS)
  6300 N. River Rd.
  Rosemont IL 60018
  1-800-346-AAOS

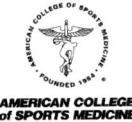

- American College of Sports Medicine (ACSM)
  401 W. Michigan St.
  Indianapolis, IN 46202-3233
  (317) 637-9200

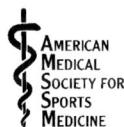

- American Medical Society for Sports Medicine (AMSSM)
  11639 Earnshaw
  Overland Park KS 66210
  (913) 327-1415

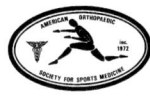

- American Orthopaedic Society for Sports Medicine (AOSSM)
  6300 N. River Rd. Suite 200
  Rosemont IL 60018
  (847) 292-4900

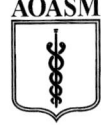

- American Osteopathic Academy of Sports Medicine (AOASM)
  7611 Elmwood Ave., Suite 201
  Middleton, WI 53562
  (608) 831-4400

CONCLUSION

This Consensus Statement establishes a definition of the team physician, and outlines a team physician's qualifications, duties and responsibilities. It also contains strategies for the continuing education of team physicians. Ultimately, this statement provides guidelines that best serve the health care needs of athletes and teams.

Reprinted with permission of the project-based alliance for the advancement of clinical sports medicine, comprised of the American Academy of Family Physicians, the American Academy of Orthopaedic Surgeons, the American College of Sports Medicine, the American Medical Society for Sports Medicine, the American Orthopaedic Society for Sports Medicine, and the American Osteopathic Academy of Sports Medicine © 2000.

Pocket SCAT2

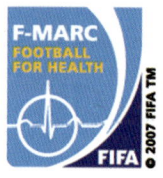  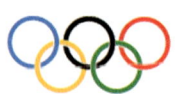 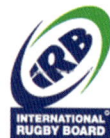

Concussion should be suspected in the presence of **any one or more** of the following: symptoms (such as headache), or physical signs (such as unsteadiness), or impaired brain function (e.g. confusion) or abnormal behaviour.

1. Symptoms

Presence of any of the following signs & symptoms may suggest a concussion.

- Loss of consciousness
- Seizure or convulsion
- Amnesia
- Headache
- "Pressure in head"
- Neck Pain
- Nausea or vomiting
- Dizziness
- Blurred vision
- Balance problems
- Sensitivity to light
- Sensitivity to noise
- Feeling slowed down
- Feeling like "in a fog"
- "Don't feel right"
- Difficulty concentrating
- Difficulty remembering
- Fatigue or low energy
- Confusion
- Drowsiness
- More emotional
- Irritability
- Sadness
- Nervous or anxious

2. Memory function

Failure to answer all questions correctly may suggest a concussion.

"At what venue are we at today?"
"Which half is it now?"
"Who scored last in this game?"
"What team did you play last week/game?"
"Did your team win the last game?"

3. Balance testing

Instructions for tandem stance
*"Now stand heel-to-toe with your **non-dominant** foot in back. Your weight should be evenly distributed across both feet. You should try to maintain stability for 20 seconds with your hands on your hips and your eyes closed. I will be counting the number of times you move out of this position. If you stumble out of this position, open your eyes and return to the start position and continue balancing. I will start timing when you are set and have closed your eyes."*

Observe the athlete for 20 seconds. If they make more than 5 errors (such as lift their hands off their hips; open their eyes; lift their forefoot or heel; step, stumble, or fall; or remain out of the start position for more that 5 seconds) then this may suggest a concussion.

Any athlete with a suspected concussion should be IMMEDIATELY REMOVED FROM PLAY, urgently assessed medically, should not be left alone and should not drive a motor vehicle.

SCAT2

 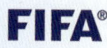 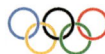

Sport Concussion Assessment Tool 2

Name _____

Sport/team _____

Date/time of injury _____

Date/time of assessment _____

Age _____ Gender ☐ M ☐ F

Years of education completed _____

Examiner _____

What is the SCAT2?[1]

This tool represents a standardized method of evaluating injured athletes for concussion and can be used in athletes aged from 10 years and older. It supersedes the original SCAT published in 2005[2]. This tool also enables the calculation of the Standardized Assessment of Concussion (SAC)[3,4] score and the Maddocks questions[5] for sideline concussion assessment.

Instructions for using the SCAT2

The SCAT2 is designed for the use of medical and health professionals. Preseason baseline testing with the SCAT2 can be helpful for interpreting post-injury test scores. Words in Italics throughout the SCAT2 are the instructions given to the athlete by the tester.

This tool may be freely copied for distribtion to individuals, teams, groups and organizations.

What is a concussion?

A concussion is a disturbance in brain function caused by a direct or indirect force to the head. It results in a variety of non-specific symptoms (like those listed below) and often does not involve loss of consciousness. Concussion should be suspected in the presence of **any one or more** of the following:

- Symptoms (such as headache), or
- Physical signs (such as unsteadiness), or
- Impaired brain function (e.g. confusion) or
- Abnormal behaviour.

Any athlete with a suspected concussion should be REMOVED FROM PLAY, medically assessed, monitored for deterioration (i.e., should not be left alone) and should not drive a motor vehicle.

Symptom Evaluation

How do you feel?

You should score yourself on the following symptoms, based on how you feel now.

	none	mild		moderate		severe	
Headache	0	1	2	3	4	5	6
"Pressure in head"	0	1	2	3	4	5	6
Neck Pain	0	1	2	3	4	5	6
Nausea or vomiting	0	1	2	3	4	5	6
Dizziness	0	1	2	3	4	5	6
Blurred vision	0	1	2	3	4	5	6
Balance problems	0	1	2	3	4	5	6
Sensitivity to light	0	1	2	3	4	5	6
Sensitivity to noise	0	1	2	3	4	5	6
Feeling slowed down	0	1	2	3	4	5	6
Feeling like "in a fog"	0	1	2	3	4	5	6
"Don't feel right"	0	1	2	3	4	5	6
Difficulty concentrating	0	1	2	3	4	5	6
Difficulty remembering	0	1	2	3	4	5	6
Fatigue or low energy	0	1	2	3	4	5	6
Confusion	0	1	2	3	4	5	6
Drowsiness	0	1	2	3	4	5	6
Trouble falling asleep (if applicable)	0	1	2	3	4	5	6
More emotional	0	1	2	3	4	5	6
Irritability	0	1	2	3	4	5	6
Sadness	0	1	2	3	4	5	6
Nervous or Anxious	0	1	2	3	4	5	6

Total number of symptoms (Maximum possible 22) ▭

Symptom severity score
(Add all scores in table, maximum possible: 22 x 6 = 132) ▭

Do the symptoms get worse with physical activity? ☐ Y ☐ N
Do the symptoms get worse with mental activity? ☐ Y ☐ N

Overall rating

If you know the athlete well prior to the injury, how different is the athlete acting compared to his / her usual self? Please circle one response.

no different	very different	unsure

Cognitive & Physical Evaluation

1 ## Symptom score (from page 1)
22 **minus** number of symptoms | of 22

2 ## Physical signs score
Was there loss of consciousness or unresponsiveness? | Y | N
If yes, how long? _____ minutes
Was there a balance problem/unsteadiness? | Y | N

Physical signs score (1 point for each negative response) | of 2

3 ## Glasgow coma scale (GCS)

Best eye response (E)

No eye opening	1
Eye opening in response to pain	2
Eye opening to speech	3
Eyes opening spontaneously	4

Best verbal response (V)

No verbal response	1
Incomprehensible sounds	2
Inappropriate words	3
Confused	4
Oriented	5

Best motor response (M)

No motor response	1
Extension to pain	2
Abnormal flexion to pain	3
Flexion/Withdrawal to pain	4
Localizes to pain	5
Obeys commands	6

Glasgow Coma score (E + V + M) | of 15

GCS should be recorded for all athletes in case of subsequent deterioration.

4 ## Sideline Assessment – Maddocks Score

"I am going to ask you a few questions, please listen carefully and give your best effort."

Modified Maddocks questions (1 point for each correct answer)

	0	1
At what venue are we at today?	0	1
Which half is it now?	0	1
Who scored last in this match?	0	1
What team did you play last week/game?	0	1
Did your team win the last game?	0	1

Maddocks score | of 5

Maddocks score is validated for sideline diagnosis of concussion only and is not included in SCAT 2 summary score for serial testing.

5 ## Cognitive assessment
Standardized Assessment of Concussion (SAC)

Orientation (1 point for each correct answer)

	0	1
What month is it?	0	1
What is the date today?	0	1
What is the day of the week?	0	1
What year is it?	0	1
What time is it right now? (within 1 hour)	0	1

Orientation score | of 5

Immediate memory

"I am going to test your memory. I will read you a list of words and when I am done, repeat back as many words as you can remember, in any order."

Trials 2 & 3:

"I am going to repeat the same list again. Repeat back as many words as you can remember in any order, even if you said the word before."

Complete all 3 trials regardless of score on trial 1 & 2. Read the words at a rate of one per second. Score 1 pt. for each correct response. Total score equals sum across all 3 trials. Do not inform the athlete that delayed recall will be tested.

List	Trial 1	Trial 2	Trial 3	Alternative word list		
elbow	0 1	0 1	0 1	candle	baby	finger
apple	0 1	0 1	0 1	paper	monkey	penny
carpet	0 1	0 1	0 1	sugar	perfume	blanket
saddle	0 1	0 1	0 1	sandwich	sunset	lemon
bubble	0 1	0 1	0 1	wagon	iron	insect
Total						

Immediate memory score | of 15

Concentration

Digits Backward:

"I am going to read you a string of numbers and when I am done, you repeat them back to me backwards, in reverse order of how I read them to you. For example, if I say 7-1-9, you would say 9-1-7."

If correct, go to next string length. If incorrect, read trial 2. One point possible for each string length. Stop after incorrect on both trials. The digits should be read at the rate of one per second.

Alternative digit lists

	0	1			
4-9-3	0	1	6-2-9	5-2-6	4-1-5
3-8-1-4	0	1	3-2-7-9	1-7-9-5	4-9-6-8
6-2-9-7-1	0	1	1-5-2-8-6	3-8-5-2-7	6-1-8-4-3
7-1-8-4-6-2	0	1	5-3-9-1-4-8	8-3-1-9-6-4	7-2-4-8-5-6

Months in Reverse Order:

"Now tell me the months of the year in reverse order. Start with the last month and go backward. So you'll say December, November ... Go ahead"

1 pt. for entire sequence correct

Dec-Nov-Oct-Sept-Aug-Jul-Jun-May-Apr-Mar-Feb-Jan | 0 | 1

Concentration score | of 5

[1] This tool has been developed by a group of international experts at the 3rd International Consensus meeting on Concussion in Sport held in Zurich, Switzerland in November 2008. The full details of the conference outcomes and the authors of the tool are published in British Journal of Sports Medicine, 2009, volume 43, supplement 1.
The outcome paper will also be simultaneously co-published in the May 2009 issues of Clinical Journal of Sports Medicine, Physical Medicine & Rehabilitation, Journal of Athletic Training, Journal of Clinical Neuroscience, Journal of Science & Medicine in Sport, Neurosurgery, Scandinavian Journal of Science & Medicine in Sport and the Journal of Clinical Sports Medicine.

[2] McCrory P et al. Summary and agreement statement of the 2nd International Conference on Concussion in Sport, Prague 2004. British Journal of Sports Medicine. 2005; 39: 196-204

[3] McCrea M. Standardized mental status testing of acute concussion. Clinical Journal of Sports Medicine. 2001; 11: 176-181

[4] McCrea M, Randolph C, Kelly J. Standardized Assessment of Concussion: Manual for administration, scoring and interpretation. Waukesha, Wisconsin, USA.

[5] Maddocks, DL; Dicker, GD; Saling, MM. The assessment of orientation following concussion in athletes. Clin J Sport Med. 1995;5(1):32–3

[6] Guskiewicz KM. Assessment of postural stability following sport-related concussion. Current Sports Medicine Reports. 2003; 2: 24-30

6 Balance examination

This balance testing is based on a modified version of the Balance Error Scoring System (BESS)[6]. A stopwatch or watch with a second hand is required for this testing.

Balance testing

"I am now going to test your balance. Please take your shoes off, roll up your pant legs above ankle (if applicable), and remove any ankle taping (if applicable). This test will consist of three twenty second tests with different stances."

(a) Double leg stance:
"The first stance is standing with your feet together with your hands on your hips and with your eyes closed. You should try to maintain stability in that position for 20 seconds. I will be counting the number of times you move out of this position. I will start timing when you are set and have closed your eyes."

(b) Single leg stance:
"If you were to kick a ball, which foot would you use? [This will be the dominant foot] Now stand on your non-dominant foot. The dominant leg should be held in approximately 30 degrees of hip flexion and 45 degrees of knee flexion. Again, you should try to maintain stability for 20 seconds with your hands on your hips and your eyes closed. I will be counting the number of times you move out of this position. If you stumble out of this position, open your eyes and return to the start position and continue balancing. I will start timing when you are set and have closed your eyes."

(c) Tandem stance:
*"Now stand heel-to-toe with your **non-dominant foot** in back. Your weight should be evenly distributed across both feet. Again, you should try to maintain stability for 20 seconds with your hands on your hips and your eyes closed. I will be counting the number of times you move out of this position. If you stumble out of this position, open your eyes and return to the start position and continue balancing. I will start timing when you are set and have closed your eyes."*

Balance testing – types of errors
1. Hands lifted off iliac crest
2. Opening eyes
3. Step, stumble, or fall
4. Moving hip into > 30 degrees abduction
5. Lifting forefoot or heel
6. Remaining out of test position > 5 sec

Each of the 20-second trials is scored by counting the errors, or deviations from the proper stance, accumulated by the athlete. The examiner will begin counting errors only after the individual has assumed the proper start position. **The modified BESS is calculated by adding one error point for each error during the three 20-second tests. The maximum total number of errors for any single condition is 10.** If a athlete commits multiple errors simultaneously, only one error is recorded but the athlete should quickly return to the testing position, and counting should resume once subject is set. Subjects that are unable to maintain the testing procedure for a minimum of **five seconds** at the start are assigned the highest possible score, ten, for that testing condition.

Which foot was tested: ☐ Left ☐ Right
(i.e. which is the **non-dominant** foot)

Condition	Total errors
Double Leg Stance (feet together)	of 10
Single leg stance (non-dominant foot)	of 10
Tandem stance (non-dominant foot at back)	of 10
Balance examination score (30 **minus** total errors)	of 30

7 Coordination examination

Upper limb coordination
Finger-to-nose (FTN) task: *"I am going to test your coordination now. Please sit comfortably on the chair with your eyes open and your arm (either right or left) outstretched (shoulder flexed to 90 degrees and elbow and fingers extended). When I give a start signal, I would like you to perform five successive finger to nose repetitions using your index finger to touch the tip of the nose as quickly and as accurately as possible."*

Which arm was tested: ☐ Left ☐ Right

Scoring: 5 correct repetitions in < 4 seconds = 1

Note for testers: Athletes fail the test if they do not touch their nose, do not fully extend their elbow or do not perform five repetitions. Failure should be scored as 0.

Coordination score	of 1

8 Cognitive assessment

Standardized Assessment of Concussion (SAC)

Delayed recall
"Do you remember that list of words I read a few times earlier? Tell me as many words from the list as you can remember in any order."

Circle each word correctly recalled. Total score equals number of words recalled.

List	Alternative word list		
elbow	candle	baby	finger
apple	paper	monkey	penny
carpet	sugar	perfume	blanket
saddle	sandwich	sunset	lemon
bubble	wagon	iron	insect

Delayed recall score	of 5

Overall score

Test domain	Score
Symptom score	of 22
Physical signs score	of 2
Glasgow Coma score (E + V + M)	of 15
Balance examination score	of 30
Coordination score	of 1
Subtotal	**of 70**
Orientation score	of 5
Immediate memory score	of 5
Concentration score	of 15
Delayed recall score	of 5
SAC subtotal	**of 30**
SCAT2 total	**of 100**
Maddocks Score	**of 5**

Definitive normative data for a SCAT2 "cut-off" score is not available at this time and will be developed in prospective studies. Embedded within the SCAT2 is the SAC score that can be utilized separately in concussion management. The scoring system also takes on particular clinical significance during serial assessment where it can be used to document either a decline or an improvement in neurological functioning.

Scoring data from the SCAT2 or SAC should not be used as a stand alone method to diagnose concussion, measure recovery or make decisions about an athlete's readiness to return to competition after concussion.

Athlete Information

Any athlete suspected of having a concussion should be removed from play, and then seek medical evaluation.

Signs to watch for

Problems could arise over the first 24-48 hours. You should not be left alone and must go to a hospital at once if you:

- Have a headache that gets worse
- Are very drowsy or can't be awakened (woken up)
- Can't recognize people or places
- Have repeated vomiting
- Behave unusually or seem confused; are very irritable
- Have seizures (arms and legs jerk uncontrollably)
- Have weak or numb arms or legs
- Are unsteady on your feet; have slurred speech

Remember, it is better to be safe.
Consult your doctor after a suspected concussion.

Return to play

Athletes should not be returned to play the same day of injury. When returning athletes to play, they should follow a stepwise symptom-limited program, with stages of progression. For example:

1. rest until asymptomatic (physical and mental rest)
2. light aerobic exercise (e.g. stationary cycle)
3. sport-specific exercise
4. non-contact training drills (start light resistance training)
5. full contact training after medical clearance
6. return to competition (game play)

There should be approximately 24 hours (or longer) for each stage and the athlete should return to stage 1 if symptoms recur. Resistance training should only be added in the later stages.
Medical clearance should be given before return to play.

Tool	Test domain	Time	Score			
		Date tested				
		Days post injury				
SCAT2	Symptom score					
	Physical signs score					
	Glasgow Coma score (E + V + M)					
	Balance examination score					
	Coordination score					
SAC	Orientation score					
	Immediate memory score					
	Concentration score					
	Delayed recall score					
	SAC Score					
Total	SCAT2					
Symptom severity score (max possible 132)						
Return to play			Y N	Y N	Y N	Y N

Additional comments

Concussion injury advice (To be given to concussed athlete)

This patient has received an injury to the head. A careful medical examination has been carried out and no sign of any serious complications has been found. It is expected that recovery will be rapid, but the patient will need monitoring for a further period by a responsible adult. Your treating physician will provide guidance as to this timeframe.

If you notice any change in behaviour, vomiting, dizziness, worsening headache, double vision or excessive drowsiness, please telephone the clinic or the nearest hospital emergency department immediately.

Other important points:
- **Rest and avoid strenuous activity for at least 24 hours**
- **No alcohol**
- **No sleeping tablets**
- **Use paracetamol or codeine for headache. Do not use aspirin or anti-inflammatory medication**
- **Do not drive until medically cleared**
- **Do not train or play sport until medically cleared**

Clinic phone number

Patient's name

Date/time of injury

Date/time of medical review

Treating physician

Contact details or stamp

Index

Note: Page numbers in Italics indicate Figure and page number followed by t indicate tables.